Pulmonary Hypertension

Bradley A. Maron • Roham T. Zamanian
Aaron B. Waxman

Editors

Pulmonary Hypertension

Basic Science to Clinical Medicine

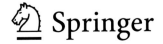 Springer

Editors
Bradley A. Maron
Cardiovascular Medicine Department
Harvard Medical School Brigham
and Women's Hospital
Boston, MA
USA

Roham T. Zamanian
Pulmonary and Critical Care Medicine
Stanford University Medical Center
Stanford, CA
USA

Aaron B. Waxman
Pulmonary Critical Care Medicine Department
Cardiovascular Medicine Department
Brigham and Women's Hospital
Harvard Medical School
Boston, MA
USA

ISBN 978-3-319-23593-6   ISBN 978-3-319-23594-3   (eBook)
DOI 10.1007/978-3-319-23594-3

Library of Congress Control Number: 2015955472

Springer Cham Heidelberg New York Dordrecht London

Printed on acid-free paper

Springer International Publishing AG Switzerland is part of Springer Science+Business Media (www.springer.com)

Bradley Maron:
"I dedicate this book to my parents, Dr. Barry and Donna Maron, my beautiful wife Dr. Jill Maron, and, with tremendous love our children Alexis and Jack for their beautiful spirit and inspiration."

Aaron Waxman:
"For my wife, Dr. Sue J. Goldie, who has been a driving force in everything I do. In fact, without her encouragement I would not ever have been in a position to work on this book. And to my boys Jacob and Matthew, always making me proud, forever onward."

Roham Zamanian:
"To all of my mentors, especially C Kees Mahutte, an inspiring and superb teacher, and to my loving and supportive wife Julie and sons Andreas, Kamran, and Oliver."

Foreword

Since its initial description in 1891 by von Romberg (Über Sklerose der Lungenarterie. Dtsch Arch Klin Med 1891;48:197–206), pulmonary hypertension has evolved from a single disease to a complex pathophenotype of many different etiologies, ranging from intrinsic lung disease to pulmonary arterial pathobiology. The last 25 years, in particular, have led to remarkable progress in understanding subtleties in pathophysiology, the complex causative and adaptive molecular events, and therapies for many forms of pulmonary hypertension. This broad expansion of our knowledge of the classification, causation, and treatment of pulmonary hypertension has led to the establishment of a rich discipline that defines the contemporary field.

With these rapid advances in epidemiology, pathobiology, and therapeutics, the field of pulmonary hypertension clearly warrants a definitive textbook. In *Pulmonary Hypertension: Basic Science to Clinical Medicine*, Maron, Zamanian, and Waxman have provided just what the field needs at this stage in its development. Beginning with a review of historical perspective, the chapters that follow offer unique, comprehensive, and highly useful insights into the current state of the disease. How best to define the phenotype(s), disease epidemiology, and the role of inflammation, neurohumoral factors, and metabolic adaptation are summarized in clearly written, up-to-date chapters by authors who have led their respective fields in these burgeoning areas of investigation. Novel approaches to disease, including modern genomics and genetics, the role of noncoding RNAs, and network biology are also presented in well-written, clearly presented chapters on these complex topics.

These basic chapters are followed by timely, rigorous, and practical presentations on cardiopulmonary hemodynamic assessment in the evaluation of patients with dyspnea and suspected pulmonary hypertension, the challenge of relevant clinical endpoints in clinical trials of patients with pulmonary hypertension, advanced imaging strategies, and the growing field of biomarkers of disease activity and response to therapy. These initial clinical chapters are followed by up-to-date reviews of current pharmacotherapies and surgical therapies, including devices and lung or heart-lung transplantation. Chapters on newer molecular targets, special clinical considerations in subsets of patients with pulmonary hypertension of which any physician caring for these complicated patients should be aware, and what the future holds for the syndrome round out this thorough textbook.

The complexity of the pathobiology, clinical presentation, and clinical course of patients with pulmonary hypertension is what makes the syndrome interesting to study and challenging to treat. Maron, Zamanian, and Waxman have done a superb job in compiling an excellent roster of chapter contributors who provide a contemporary, comprehensive overview of the field in all of its complexity, and do so with clarity and great care. For these reasons, I believe this textbook is essential for the any physician or scientist with an interest in pulmonary hypertension that will establish itself in short order as a definitive reference for the discipline.

Boston, MA, USA   Joseph Loscalzo, MD, PhD

Acknowledgment

The editors wish to acknowledge the assistance and support of Ms. Stephanie Tribuna in the completion of this project.

Contents

Contributors

Manyoo Agarwal, MBBS Pulmonary Critical Care Medicine,
Center for Pulmonary Heart Disease, Brigham and Women's Hospital,
Heart and Vascular Center, Boston, MA, USA

Nadine Al-Naamani, MD Pulmonary, Critical Care and Sleep Division,
Pulmonary Hypertension Center, Tufts Medical Center, Boston, MA, USA

Mary Bartlett, MSN, FNP Division of Pulmonary and Critical Care,
Department of Medicine, Winthrop University Hospital, Mineola, NY, USA

Department of Pulmonary Medicine, Winthrop University Hospital, Mineola, NY, USA

Christian Bermudez, MD Division of Cardiovascular Surgery, Hospital of the University
of Pennsylvania, Philadelphia, PA, USA

David Boulate, MD, MSc Thoracic, Vascular and Heart-Lung Transplantation,
Marie Lannelongue Hospital, Le Plessis-Robinson, France

Yonatan Buber, MD Department of Cardiology, Boston Children's Hospital and Brigham
and Women's Hospital, Harvard Medical School, Boston, MA, USA

Heart Institute, Sheba Medical Center, Tel Aviv University Faculty of Medicine, Ramat Gan, Israel

Sackler Faculty of Medicine, Tel Aviv University, Tel Aviv, Israel

Murali M. Chakinala, MD Internal Medicine, Washington University, St. Louis, MO, USA

Pulmonary and Critical Care Division, Washington University School of Medicine,
St. Louis, MO, USA

Gaurav Choudhary, MD Division of Cardiology, Department of Medicine,
Providence VA Medical Center, Alpert Medical School of Brown University, Providence,
RI, USA

Wendy K. Chung, MD, PhD Molecular Genetics in Departments of Pediatrics and
Medicine, Columbia University Medical Center, New York, NY, USA

Vinicio De Jesus Perez, MD Department of Medicine, Stanford University Medical Center,
Stanford, CA, USA

Division of Pulmonary and Critical Care, Stanford University Medical Center,
Stanford, CA, USA

Karim C. El Kasmi, MD, PhD Department of Pediatrics, Children's Hospital Colorado,
Aurora, CO, USA

Elie Fadel, MD, PhD Thoracic and Vascular Surgery and Heart-Lung Transplantation,
Marie Lannelongue Hospital, Le Plessis-Robinson, France

Harrison W. Farber, MD Division of Pulmonary, Allergy, Sleep and Critical Care Medicine, Pulmonary Hypertension Center, Boston University School of Medicine, Boston Medical Center, Boston, MA, USA

Wassim H. Fares, MD, MSc Pulmonary, Critical Care and Sleep Medicine, Yale University, School of Medicine, New Haven, CT, USA

Joshua P. Fessel, MD, PhD Division of Allergy, Pulmonary and Critical Care Medicine, Department of Medicine, Vanderbilt University School of Medicine, Nashville, TN, USA

Robert P. Frantz, MD Division of Cardiovascular Diseases and Internal Medicine, Mayo Pulmonary Hypertension Clinic, Mayo Clinic College of Medicine, Rochester, MN, USA

Maria G. Frid, PhD Department of Pediatrics, University of Colorado Denver, Aurora, CO, USA

Nicholas M. Furiasse, MD, MS Division of Cardiology, Department of Medicine, Northwestern University Feinberg School of Medicine, Chicago, IL, USA

Evgenia Gerasimovskaya, PhD Department of Pediatrics, University of Colorado Denver, Aurora, CO, USA

Jose Gomez-Arroyo, MD, PhD Department of Anesthesiology and Critical Care Medicine, Johns Hopkins University, Baltimore, MD, USA

Brian B. Graham, MD Program in Translational Lung Research, Department of Medicine, University of Colorado Denver, Aurora, CO, USA

Julien Guihaire, MD, PhD Adult Cardiac Surgery, Centre Hospitalier Universitaire de Rennes, Rennes, France

Fravncois Haddad, MD Biomarker and Phenotype Core Laboratory, Stanford Cardiovascular Institute, Palo Alto, CA, USA

Nathan D. Hatton, MS, MD Division of Pulmonary Medicine, Department of Medicine, University of Utah, Salt Lake City, UT, USA

Traci Housten, RN, MS Pulmonary and Critical Care Medicine, Johns Hopkins University, Baltimore, MD, USA

Jessica Huston, MD Division of Cardiovascular Medicine, Department of Medicine, University of Utah, Salt Lake City, UT, USA

Geeshath Jayasekera, MBChB, MRCP Scottish Pulmonary Vascular Unit, Golden Jubilee National Hospital, Glasgow, UK

Naftali Kaminski, MD Section of Pulmonary, Critical Care and Sleep Medicine, Department of Medicine, Yale University, School of Medicine, New Haven, CT, USA

Martha Kingman, BSN, MS, DNP Heart and Lung Center, University of Texas Southwestern Medical Center at Dallas, Dallas, TX, USA

Kristina T. Kudelko, MD Department of Medicine, Stanford University, Stanford, CA, USA

Division of Pulmonary and Critical Care, Stanford University Medical Center, Stanford, CA, USA

Rahul Kumar, PhD Division of Pulmonary Sciences and Critical Care Medicine, Department of Medicine, University of Colorado, Denver, Aurora, CO, USA

Jane A. Leopold, MD Division of Cardiovascular Medicine, Department of Cardiovascular Medicine, Brigham and Women's Hospital and Harvard Medical School, Boston, MA, USA

Lijiang Ma, MD, PhD Molecular Genetics in Department of Pediatrics, Columbia University Medical Center, New York, NY, USA

Departments of Pediatrics and Medicine, Columbia University Medical Center, New York, NY, USA

Balakrishnan Mahesh, MD, FRCS, PhD Division of Cardiothoracic Transplantation, Department of Cardiothoracic Surgery, University of Pittsburgh Presbyterian Medical Center, Pittsburgh, PA, USA

Bradley A. Maron, MD Division of Cardiovascular Medicine, Department of Medicine, Brigham and Women's Hospital and Harvard Medical School, Boston, MA, USA

Department of Cardiology, Veterans Affairs Boston Healthcare System, Boston, MA, USA

Colleen A. McEvoy, MD Pulmonary and Critical Care Division, Washington University School of Medicine, St. Louis, MO, USA

Olaf Mercier, MR, PhD Surgical Research Laboratory, Marie Lannelongue Hospital, Le Plessis-Robinson, France

Matthew Moll, MD Internal Medicine, Boston Medical Center, Boston, MA, USA

Robert Naeije, MD, PhD Hypertension artérielle pulmonaire, médecine du sport, Erasme Hospital, Brussel, Belgium

Ivana Nikolic, MD Division of Cardiology, Department of Medicine, Harvard Medical School, Brigham and Women's Hospital, Boston, MA, USA

Eva Nozik-Grayck, MD Department of Pediatrics, University of Colorado Denver, Aurora, CO, USA

William M. Oldham, MD, PhD Division of Pulmonary and Critical Care Medicine, Department of Medicine, Brigham and Women's Hospital and Harvard Medical School, Boston, MA, USA

Alexander R. Opotowsky, MD, MPH, MMSc Department of Cardiology, Boston Children's Hospital, Brigham and Women's Hospital and Harvard Medical School, Boston, MA, USA

Kusum V. Pandit, MBBS, PhD Department of Medicine, University of Pittsburgh Medical Center, Pittsburgh, PA, USA

Division of Pulmonary, Allergy and Critical Care Medicine, Dorothy P. and Richard P. Simmons Center for Interstitial Lung Disease, University of Pittsburgh School of Medicine, Pittsburgh, PA, USA

Myung H. Park, MD Division of Cardiovascular Medicine, Department of Cardiology, University of Maryland School of Medicine, Baltimore, MD, USA

Division of Heart Failure, Department of Cardiology, Houston Methodist DeBakey Heart & Vascular Center, Houston Methodist Hospital, Houston, TX, USA

Andrew J. Peacock, MPhil, MD Scottish Pulmonary Vascular Unit, Regional Heart and Lung Centre, Golden Jubilee National Hospital, Glasgow, UK

Abby Poms, BS, RRT, CCRP Department of Pulmonary and Critical Care Medicine, Duke University Pulmonary Vascular Disease Center, Durham, NC, USA

Jens Poth, MD, PhD Department of Pediatrics, University of Colorado Denver, Aurora, CO, USA

Ioana R. Preston, MD Pulmonary, Critical Care and Sleep Medicine Division, Pulmonary Hypertension Center, Tufts Medical Center, Boston, MA, USA

Steven C. Pugliese, MD Division of Pulmonary Sciences and Critical Care Medicine, Department of Medicine, University of Colorado Denver, Aurora, CO, USA

Jonathan D. Rich, MD Division of Cardiology, Department of Medicine, Northwestern University Feinberg School of Medicine, Chicago, IL, USA

Franz Rischard, MD Pulmonary, Allergy, Critical Care & Sleep Medicine, Arizona Health Sciences Center, Tucson, AZ, USA

Jeffrey C. Robinson, MD Division of Pulmonary Sciences and Critical Care Medicine, Department of Medicine, University of Colorado, Denver, Aurora, CO, USA

John J. Ryan, MD, FAHA, FACC Division of Cardiovascular Medicine, Department of Medicine, University of Utah, Salt Lake City, UT, USA

Division of Cardiovascular Medicine, Department of Medicine, University of Utah Health Science Center, Salt Lake City, UT, USA

Mayank Sardana, MBBS Department of Medicine, Boston Medical Center, Boston, MA, USA

Kurt R. Stenmark, MD Department of Pediatrics, University of Colorado Denver, Aurora, CO, USA

Thomas E. Stephens, BA Department of Medicine, Brigham and Women's Hospital, Boston, MA, USA

Victor F. Tapson, MD, FCCP, FRCP Cedars-Sinai Medical Center, Beverly Hills, CA, USA

Pulmonary and Critical Care Division, Clinical Research for the Women's Guild Lung Institute, Cedars-Sinai Medical Center, Los Angeles, CA, USA

Glenna L. Traiger, RN, MSN, CNS-BC Division of Pulmonary and Critical Medicine, David Geffen School of Medicine at UCLA, Los Angeles, CA, USA

Rubin M. Tuder, MD Division of Pulmonary Sciences & Critical Care Medicine, Department of Medicine, University of Colorado Hospital, Aurora, CO, USA

Corey E. Ventetuolo, MD, MS Division of Pulmonary, Critical Care and Sleep Medicine, Departments of Medicine and Health Services Policy and Practice, Rhode Island Hospital, Alpert Medical School of Brown University, Providence, RI, USA

Aaron B. Waxman, MD, PhD, FACP, FCCP, FPVRI Pulmonary and Critical Care Medicine, Cardiovascular Medicine, Brigham and Women's Hospital Heart and Vascular Center, Harvard Medical School, Boston, MA, USA

Paul B. Yu, MD, PhD Division of Cardiovascular Medicine, Department of Medicine, Harvard Medical School, Brigham and Women's Hospital, Boston, MA, USA

Roham T. Zamanian, MD Division of Pulmonary and Critical Care, Stanford University Medical Center, Stanford, CA, USA

Historical Perspective on the Classification and Nomenclature of Pulmonary Hypertension

Myung H. Park

Introduction

The history of how nomenclature and classification of pulmonary hypertension (PH) has evolved is a tribute to the dedication, scientific curiosity, and courageous risks undertaken by notable scientists and clinicians spanning over three centuries. The challenges in understanding the complex pathophysiology of cardiopulmonary systems are illustrated by series of misconceptions that took place through the years that are beginning to be understood. Indeed, the dilemma the medical community faced in their quests to name the conditions currently known as pulmonary hypertension and pulmonary arterial hypertension (PAH), and in deriving at a working classification, underscores the complexity of cardiopulmonary medicine. A sensible nomenclature and a well-organized classification scheme are important in order to provide structure and framework for any disease process, especially one as complex as pulmonary hypertension. They serve as a foundation for the medical community by providing a common language and framework for patient care, furthering research, and collaborating in clinical trials. This chapter will discuss the notable individuals, their discoveries and contributions, which have shaped the field and helped to achieve the advances in pulmonary hypertension (Table 1.1).

M.H. Park, MD
Division of Cardiovascular Medicine, Department of Cardiology, University of Maryland School of Medicine, Baltimore, MD, USA

Division of Heart Failure, Department of Cardiology, Houston Methodist DeBakey Heart & Vascular Center, Houston Methodist Hospital, 6550 Fannin St, Suite 1901, Houston, TX, 77030, USA
e-mail: mpark@medicine.umaryland.edu;
Mhpark@houstonmethodist.org; parkm9093@gmail.com

Key Contributors with Keen Observations: The Evolution in Understanding Pulmonary Circulation

The study of circulatory system dates back to the Ancient Greeks with most significant contribution accredited to studies by Galen [1, 2]. Born in 129 AD in Pergamum, Asia Minor (currently Bergama, western Turkey) during the rule of the Roman Empire, he acquired training when he was appointed as the surgeon to the gladiators. His reputation as the leading medical authority quickly rose where he was ultimately appointed as Physician to the Emperor. Through his experiments with animals and experiences in the field treating soldiers, he formulated a series of observations of the circulation and physiology. He claimed that the cardiovascular function was an open-ended system being comprised of two distinct networks of arteries and veins, where blood and air dissipated at the ends of arteries and veins according to the needs of the local tissues [1, 3].

This belief was held firm for 15 centuries until challenged by the scientific findings of William Harvey with his historic publication of *Exercitatio Anatomica de Motu Cordis et sanguinis in Animabilus* in 1628 [3–5]. In this monumental work written from his observations and experiments, Harvey correctly portrayed the circulatory system as a closed system where the blood circulates from the heart to the tissues via arteries and back to the heart through the veins and the lungs. Furthermore, he also surmised that there were pores in the lungs that allowed the blood to return to the heart. Indeed, these pores were later shown to be vascular capillaries once microscopy was available by Malpighi in 1661 [6]. He also had the incredible insight to differentiate the functions of the two ventricles as he stated: "So it appears that whereas one ventricle, the left, suffices for distributing the blood to the body and drawing it from the vena cava, as is the case in all animals lacking lungs, nature was compelled when she wished to filter blood through the lungs to add the right ventricle...Thus the right ventricle may be said to be made for the sake of transmitting blood through

Table 1.1 Major milestones in development of nomenclature and classifications in pulmonary hypertension

Date/time range	Key figure/event	Contribution
1628	William Harvey	Publication of his book *Exercitatio Anatomica de Motu Cordis et sanguinis in Animabilus*
1891	Ernst von Romberg	Description of abnormal findings in autopsy as "pulmonary vascular sclerosis", first name given for PH
1901	Abel Ayerza	Key lecture integrating cyanosis and right heart failure, named the condition as "cardiac negro" (black cardiac)
1913	F. C. Arrillaga	Syphilitic arteriosclerosis assigned as etiology of PH; changed the name of disease to "Ayerza's Disease"
1929	Werner Forssman	Demonstrated that it was possible to perform right sided catheterization in humans by performing catheterization on himself
1951	David Dresdale	Coined the term "primary pulmonary hypertension", PPH
1956	Forssman, Cournand, Richards	Awarded Nobel Prize for their contributions to the discovery of circulatory and cardiopulmonary systems
1958	Paul Wood	Published *Pulmonary Hypertension with Special Reference to the Vasoconstrictive Factor*
1965–1970s	First PPH Epidemic	Related to approval of Aminorex
1973	1st WHO Meeting in PH	Landmark meeting in PPH; provided recommendations for future directions
1981	PPH Registry	Landmark multicenter U.S. study characterizing natural history and clinical features of PPH
1996–1970s	Second PPH Epidemic	Due to approval of "fen-phen"
1998	2nd World Symposium on PH	Formation of Evian Classification of PH; introduction of term "pulmonary arterial hypertension", PAH
2003	3rd World Symposium on PH	Venice Classification; idiopathic PAH introduced to replace term PPH
2008	4th World Symposium on PH	Dana Point Classification; modification of genetic category, among others in Group 1
2013	5th World Symposium on PH	Nice Classification; further modifications of genetic category, among others in Group 1
2014	International Right Heart Failure Foundation Working Group	Development of a comprehensive nomenclature of right heart failure: defining distinction between right heart failure and right ventricular failure, components of right heart system, and definition of right heart failure

the lungs, not for nourishing them." Harvey's astute observations on human circulatory system started the beginnings of modern cardiology [5].

For the next few centuries, medical community was intrigued by reports from autopsy findings of abnormalities in pulmonary arteries and it was being accepted that pulmonary arteriosclerosis was morphological evidence of chronic pulmonary hypertension. However, the etiological basis for these findings remained a mystery. In 1891, a German physician and pathologist named Ernst von Romberg proceeded to categorize the abnormal findings in pulmonary arteries during autopsy simply as "pulmonary vascular sclerosis", providing the first name of many to follow for this elusive disease [7–9].

The first few decades of 1900s witnessed emergence of several different explanations as the cause for pulmonary hypertension. One notable contributor in furthering the field was Dr. Abel Ayerza, professor of medicine at the University of Buenos Aires, Argentina, when he delivered his key clinical descriptions in a landmark lecture to his students on August 20, 1901 [10]. He described 38-year-old male who had suffered from pneumonia at 20 and 32 years of age and

subsequently developed chronic respiratory symptoms. He presented with constellation of findings comprising of chronic cough and sputum production, dyspnea at rest, central cyanosis, clubbed fingers and tachypnea. The examination was significant for blood pressure of 150 mmHg (diastolic blood pressure was not able to be determined at that time), heart rate of 112 beats per minute, wet crackles and wheezing in the lungs with cardiovascular examination showing features of right heart failure (jugular venous distention, hepatomegaly, hepatojugular reflux, ascites and lower extremity edema). The laboratory findings revealed polycythemia of 6,560,000 red blood cells per mm^3 and white blood cells were 5,250 cells per mm^3. The patient died 24 days after admission to the hospital. His autopsy findings showed enlarged heart with thickened right ventricular wall, dilated right atrium, and normal left atrium and ventricle. Histological examinations of the pulmonary arteries revealed hyperplasia of the middle layer and intima, along with thrombus obstructing flow. Dr. Ayerza called this condition "cardiac negro" (black cardiac) to differentiate from other diseases due to the extreme degree of cyanosis seen in these patients.

This clinical and pathologic correlative description created marked interest among physicians worldwide and speculations started to emerge regarding the etiology [9, 10]. In 1905, Pedro Escudero proposed that "black cardiac" was secondary to a chronic pulmonary process and subsequently attributed the disease to complications of syphilis causing obliterating sclerosis of the pulmonary artery [9–11]. This misconception resulted in a considerable amount of debate of the role of the spirochete that lasted for two decades. In the midst of the controversy, Dr. F.C. Arrillaga, a student of Dr. Ayerza, focused on collecting information on patients with similar presentations who were described as "black cardiac". In 1913, he published his findings that consisted of a review of a selected group of 11 patients, including the first patient described by Dr. Ayerza, covering the varied causes, pathology and clinical manifestations [10, 12]. As a result, the disease became known worldwide as "Ayerza's disease." Dr. A.S. Warthin of University of Michigan described the first case in USA at the 34th Annual Meeting of the American Society for Medicine in 1919 as "A case of Ayerza's disease: chronic cyanosis, dyspnea, and erythema associated with syphilitic arteriosclerosis of the pulmonary artery" [13].

Despite his role in propagating the misconception of syphilis as the etiology, Dr. Arrillaga formulated a critical concept that shaped the nomenclature and classification of pulmonary hypertension by stating "sclerosis of the pulmonary artery was always primary and that it could be isolated or secondary to chronic pulmonary process" [10, 14]. Thus the theory of sclerosis of the pulmonary artery being the primary cause of Ayerza's disease, independent of a chronic lung process, initiated the practice of classifying the condition as "primary" pulmonary hypertension, now known as "idiopathic".

The notion of syphilitis being the cause of pulmonary hypertension was ultimately dispelled by a British physician named Dr. Oscar Brenner in 1935. As the Rockefeller Traveling Fellow at Massachusetts General Hospital (MGH), he reviewed 100 case reports of PH in the MGH autopsy files, of which 25 were categorized as "Ayerza's disease." He correctly arrived at the conclusion that that syphilis was not the cause but that clinical manifestations of the disease were due to heart failure secondary to pulmonary disease [15]. He made a significant contribution to the field by noting the presence of small muscular arteries and arterioles as the source of pulmonary hypertension. However, being mainly a histopathologist, he failed to recognize the role of vasoconstriction in the pathogenesis of pulmonary hypertension and its effect in the pathophysiology between pulmonary vascular lesions and right ventricular hypertrophy, viewing each as a separate entity due to an "unknown cause" [9, 15, 16].

Accessing the Inaccessible: Introduction of Right Heart Catheterization

The start of the twentieth century marked the birth of modern cardiopulmonary medicine with advances in understanding of physiology of pulmonary hemodynamics through innovations in technology to directly measure pulmonary circulation, which until then had been inaccessible. The initial studies were performed by measuring pulmonary arterial pressures in anesthesthetized, open-chest animals under artificial respiratory support [5, 17]. These experiments allowed development of accurate readings pulmonary pressures and methods to calculate pulmonary vascular resistance and the measurement of left arterial pressures. Among the key contributors in the study of pulmonary hemodynamics and physiology include Otto Frank (1865–1944) and Ernest Henry Starling (1866–1927) whose heart-lung preparations resulted in series of experiments under controlled setting to measure cardiac mechanical and physiologic causes and effect which led to the discovery of Frank-Starling law of the heart [15].

The other major discovery involved figuring out ways to measure pulmonary blood flow. August Krogh and Johannes Lindhard were the first to obtain indirect pulmonary blood flow measurement by using nitrous oxide gas uptake method in humans in 1912 [18]. To overcome limitations present in using the gas exchange technique, a direct approach to measure cardiac output was proposed by Adolph Fick in 1870 [5, 19]. It would take several decades for Fick's principles to be applied to measure cardiac output in humans due to many complexities inherent in its application, one of which included obtaining mixed venous blood. Werner Forssman made this possible by being the first to demonstrate the feasibility of obtaining direct cardiac measurements in humans by catheterizing himself via the antecubital vein and obtaining a radiographic picture of his heart in 1929 [20]. By showing that the right side of the heart could be safely catheterized by peripheral vein, Forssman disapproved the widely held belief that was prevalent in the medical community that placement of catheter in cardiac chambers would result in morbid or fatal complication. Although his courageous self-experiment propelled the field of invasive cardiology, his actions resulted in criticism and condemnation by his colleagues and administrators [5, 15, 21]. His contribution made it feasible to obtain cardiac output and pulmonary vascular resistance measurements which are critical components to define pulmonary arterial hypertension.

The potential applications of assessing right-sided hemodynamics were quickly realized throughout Europe, South American and United States. Dickinson W. Richards and Andre F. Cournand of the Bellevue Service of Columbia University College of Physicians and Surgeons began experiments placing catheters in the right atrium first in large animals and finally in humans by 1940 [22, 23]. Many discoveries were made by the team led by Cournand and Richards during the next couple of decades that included establishing the wide range of variations in pressure and flow seen in health and disease states and hemodynamics associated with congenital heart defects and valvular disease [23–25]. Forssman, Cournand and Richards won the Nobel Prize in 1956 in physiology and/or medicine for their contributions to the discovery of circulatory and cardiopulmonary system [21, 24, 25]. Advances in science and technology, including development of a flow-directed catheter with an inflatable balloon to measure left atrial pressure in animals followed by a modified technique of measuring pulmonary "capillary" pressure in humans, set the stage for wide use of right sided catheterizations in laboratories across the country [26, 27]. In 1970, William Ganz and Harold J C Swan introduced a multi-lumen, balloon tipped catheter that enabled the procedure to be performed from the fluoroscopy suite to the bedside [28].

Obtaining Insights into Cardiopulmonary Physiology: Measuring Hemodynamics in Health and Disease

The rapid advances in technology in the field of invasive hemodynamics in the twentieth century created a marked interest that propelled research in the field of cardiopulmonary medicine that resulted in the start of formal nomenclature and classification for pulmonary hypertension. David Dresdale, a trainee of Cournand and Richards, was the first to report in 1951 hemodynamic profiles of patients with pulmonary hypertension without evident etiology and coined the name "primary pulmonary hypertension (PPH)" [29]. This was a significant event since prior to this, PPH did not have an accepted terminology which impeded effective communication and research relating to the condition. Furthermore, Dresdale also contributed to the key concept on the role of vasoconstriction in the pathophysiology of pulmonary hypertension and the effects of vasodilators. He performed functional studies in animals that demonstrated acute hypoxia elicited pulmonary vasoconstriction and that administration of a pulmonary vasodilator tolazoline relieved pulmonary hypertension in patients with PPH [30, 31]. However, this resulted in some controversy because tolazoline also produces systemic vasodilatory effects, which raised the question if the effect on the pulmonary circulation was due to systemic vasodilation [9].

Another key contributor furthering the field of cardiopulmonary physiology was Paul Wood by performing a wide range of hemodynamic studies in his patients with valvular heart disease, congenital heart disease and pulmonary hypertension. In his seminal publication of "Pulmonary Hypertension with Special Reference to the Vasoconstrictive Factor", he outlined many seminal, critically important physiologic principles. First, he defined normal pulmonary hemodynamics from his laboratory at the Institute of Cardiology and at the Brompton Hospital: "The normal pulmonary pressure in a series of 60 normal controls….was 16/7 mm Hg…with mean being 11 mm. and the range 8/2-28/14 mm. The mean cardiac output was 8 liters a minute, and the common range 5.5 to 10.5 liters a minute." He also gave a definition of pulmonary hypertension stating: "Pulmonary hypertension literally implies a pulmonary blood pressure above 30/15 mm. which is the upper limit of the normal range. In practice serious pulmonary hypertension usually means a pressure at or around systemic level, but rarely in excess of 150 mm" [32]. Furthermore, he proposed a "working classification of pulmonary hypertension" based on physiologic distinctions differentiating into five types: Passive, Hyerkinetic, Obstructive, Obliterative, Vasoconstrictive, Polygenic, with a claimer stating that "…it may help to add a sixth (polygenic), to describe cases of mixed etiology" [32]. He also described the significance and meanings behind "reactive" versus "passive", with discussions centered around what he had learned from his experiments with intravenous injection of acetylcholine. This substance, being eliminated during a single passage through the pulmonary circulation, demonstrated the effect of a selective pulmonary vasodilator in that it decreased pulmonary pressures in his patients with pulmonary hypertension secondary to mitral stenosis [32, 33]. He confirmed the importance of the role of vasoconstriction in pulmonary hypertension, as well as the potent pulmonary vasodilatory effect of acetylcholine in patients who were subjected to pretreatment with hypoxic-inspired air [34, 35]. Furthermore, Paul Wood included 26 patients whom he labeled as "primary pulmonary hypertension", 21 of them being female between the ages 9 and 48, similar to the cohort that would be described 20 years later in the NIH Registry [35, 36].

It is noteworthy that with introduction of the name "primary pulmonary hypertension" enabled the medical community to focus and publish their findings by having a common language. Paul Wood also led the studies on hemodynamics of pulmonary hypertension of different etiologies with his descriptions of Eisenmenger's and mitral stenosis, which were corroborated by similar findings by other physicians in similar cohorts. Some of the critical works that emerged during this time include pathologic descriptions by Heath and Edwards in 1958 on Eisenmenger's patients, and Wagenvoort and Wagenvoort in 1970, that provided a first detailed post mortem descriptions [37, 38]. The publication by the Wagenvoorts was a landmark work titled "Primary Pulmonary Hypertension. A Pathologic Study of the Lung Vessels in 156 Clinically Diagnosed Cases" of confirmed PPH cases from 51 medical centers and pathologic laboratories in 14 different countries [38].

Primary Pulmonary Hypertension Takes Front Stage: The Aminorex Epidemic

Against the backdrop of a century of significant progress in the field of pulmonary hypertension, the epidemic of aminorex-induced PPH broke out in the late 1960s propelling this rare condition to the center stage [39]. Aminorex fumarate (Menocil®) shares similar chemical structures with epinephrine and amphetamines and its toxic effects have been reported to be predominately due to the release of catecholamines and norepinephrine [40, 41]. Aminorex became available as over-the-counter drug appetite suppressant to promote weight loss in 1965 in Switzerland, Austria, and Germany which was followed by a tenfold increase in the incidence of PPH reported in the three countries over the next 7 years [41].

The drug was withdrawn from the market in 1968 due to the alarming rate of PPH cases [9, 40]. However, important scientific advances resulted from this unfortunate event in that several key questions were raised followed by important observations regarding PPH which pushed the field forward. For one, it was observed that only 2 % of those who took aminorex developed PPH suggesting genetic predisposition playing an important role. Follow up experiments in animals to reproduce PPH were largely unsuccessful, which further supported the concept of genetic basis playing an important factor. The time frame of disease progression was also uncovered with appreciation of the latent period between the start of aminorex ingestion and onset of clinical manifestations, which appeared to peak at 6 months. In addition, it was observed that the changes related to PPH often progressed after the drug had been stopped and that in 12 of 20 patients who were followed for >17 years, the disease regressed demonstrating that in some patients PPH seemed reversible [9, 39, 41].

The First World Health Organization Meeting on Primary Pulmonary Hypertension: Geneva Meeting (1973)

Culminating from the urgent need to that rose by the epidemic and the many imminent questions that surfaced, the World Health Organization (WHO) convened its first meeting on PPH that took place on October 15–17, 1973 in Geneva, Switzerland. There were 19 attendees representing 10 countries (5 from USA and Switzerland, each, with largest number of participants). The "Primary Pulmonary Hypertension: Report on a WHO meeting" contains an account of the meeting based on the papers submitted by the participants, as well as their discussions. Of note, the introduction of the report starts with mention of the first WHO meeting on pulmonary circulation on cor pulmonale that was held on 1960 (Table 1.2). In the Classification of Chronic

Table 1.2 Classification of chronic cor pulmonale according to causative diseases

The diseases that may cause chronic pulmonary heart disease are listed below, classified into broad etiological groups.

1. Diseases primarily affecting air passages of the lung and the alveoli
    1.1 Chronic bronchitis with generalized airways obstruction with or without emphysema
    1.2 Bronchial asthma
    1.3 Emphysema without bronchitis or asthma
    1.4 Pulmonary fibrosis, with or without emphysema, due to:
        (a) Tuberculosis
        (b) Pneumoconiosis
        (c) Bronchiectasis
        (d) Other pulmonary infections
        (e) Radiation
        (f) Mucoviscidosis
    1.5 Pulmonary granulomata and infiltrations
        (a) Sarcoidosis
        (b) Chronic diffuse interstitial fibrosis
        (c) Berylliosis
        (d) Eosinophilic granuloma or histiocytosis
        (e) Malignant infiltration
        (f) Scleroderma
        (g) Disseminated lupus erythematosus
        (h) Dermatomyositis
        (i) Alveolar microlithiasis
    1.6 Pulmonary resection
    1.7 Congenital cystic disease of the lungs
    1.8 High-altitude hypoxia
2. Diseases primarily affecting the movements of the thoracic cage
    2.1 Kyphoscoliosis and other thoracic deformities
    2.2 Thoracoplasty
    2.3 Pleural fibrosis
    2.4 Chronic neuromuscular weakness—e.g., poliomyelitis
    2.5 Obesity with alveolar hypoventilation
    2.6 Idiopathic alveolar hypoventilation
3. Diseases primarily affecting the pulmonary vasculature
    3.1 Primary affections of the arterial wall
        (a) Primary pulmonary hypertension
        (b) Polyarteritis nodosa
        (c) Other arteritis
    3.2 Thrombotic disorders
        (a) Primary pulmonary thrombosis
        (b) Sickle cell anaemia
    3.3 Embolism
        (a) Embolism from thrombosis outside the lungs
        (b) Schistosomiasis (bilharziasis)
        (c) Malignant embolism
        (d) Other embolism
    3.4 Pressure on main pulmonary arteries and veins by mediastinal tumours, aneurysm, granuloma, or fibrosis

Reprinted from WHO Technical Report Series, No. 213, 1961 [42], Table 1, pp 7–8, with permission from World Health Organization (WHO)

Cor Pulmonale According to Causative Disease, PPH is listed in the 3rd group among the "Diseases primarily affecting the pulmonary vasculature", which is most likely the first formal proposed classification [42].

Among the many important discussions that took place during that seminal meeting, one lengthy deliberation was centered on the dilemma surrounding the nomenclature of the term "primary pulmonary hypertension" being used in two distinct ways. Clinically, PPH referred to "indicate the presence of elevated pulmonary arterial pressures in the absence of discernable cause". Its meaning also designated morphological changes found in pulmonary vascular pattern of PPH, namely concentric intimal fibrosis, necrotizing arteritis, and plexiform lesions. The group came to a consensus that it was not practical to abolish the term "primary pulmonary hypertension" due to its wide acceptance and use. Instead, they agreed to the term "primary pulmonary hypertension" to be used only to mean "pulmonary hypertension of unknown cause" and that the term "plexogenic pulmonary arteriopathy" be used to designate the constellation of morphologic changes associated with PPH [43]. It is interesting to note that this same debate will be held 25 and 30 years later at the next two subsequent WHO meetings.

The participants also discussed the definition of the disease that was initially reported during the WHO Expert Committee on Chronic Cor Pulmonale, stating "The mean pressure in the pulmonary artery does not normally exceed 15 mm Hg when the subject is at rest in a lying position. This value is little affected by age and never exceeds 20 mm Hg. Hypertension is definitely present if the pressure exceeds 25 mm Hg" [42, 43]. The group confirmed the findings initially stated by Paul Wood and set a formal cutoff value to define pulmonary hypertension which is used to present day. Discussion on left sided filling pressure was also held, with the group agreeing that the normal range is 6–9 mmHg and "may even reach 12 mm Hg" based on the measurements in normal individuals [43, 44]. It is noteworthy that the current upper limit range of 15 mmHg. used to define pulmonary arterial hypertension (PAH) was not set at the first WHO meeting. Other topics that were discussed include the value of end diastolic pressure of the pulmonary artery as an indicator of the left ventricular end diastolic pressure, with the group concluding that end diastolic pressures were not reliable in reflecting the left sided filling pressure in those with pulmonary vascular disease [43, 45]. The controversy surrounding relevance and accuracy of diastolic pulmonary gradient in patients with pulmonary hypertension due to left heart disease is ongoing to present day and studies are being conducted to help answer the question [46]. The effect of exercise on pulmonary pressures were also a major item of discussion: "Some forms of pulmonary hypertension are latent and become apparent only when there is an increase in blood flow. It is therefore important to know the response of the normal pulmonary circulation to effort" [43]. The participants pointed out that for "…an output of 20 liters or more, the mean

pulmonary artery pressure does not normally exceed 30 mm Hg" based on prior study on hemodynamics during exercise, the value used as a cut off to define "exercise-induced pulmonary hypertension" formally stated during the 2003 Evian meeting was later retracted at the 2008 Dana Point meeting due to insufficient data to justify the definition [47–49]. Indeed, similar questions relating to effects of age and state of physical conditioning affecting pulmonary pressures with exercise were raised during the Geneva meeting as would be raised in others to follow. The recommendation that "…more information needs to be obtained on the various pressures and the resistance in the lesser circulation under clearly defined exercise conditions" set forth by the members would be restated during the Dana Point meeting [49].

The most significant outcome that resulted from the 1st WHO meeting was based on the series of proposed recommendations, one of which called for the "establishment of a central register of patients with primary pulmonary hypertension seen in centers throughout the world" [43]. In place of an international registry, the National Heart, Lung and Blood Institute (NHLBI) of the National Institute of Health (NIH) created a National Registry of Patients with PPH in 1981 [50]. The Registry had three core groups, namely one focusing on statistics and epidemiology, a core dedicated to pathology, and 32 clinical centers collaborating to collect patient information. The Registry completed its 194 patient enrollment in 1987, a historic accomplishment resulting in contributing critical information on the natural history, epidemiology, and clinical features of the disease that led the participants in future collaborations in clinical trials [9, 50, 51].

The Second PPH Epidemic: As Unprecedented Advances in PH Unfolds

The outbreak of the second PPH epidemic related to the agent "fen-phen" in U.S. in the early 1990s is a sober tale of historical lessons not learned. Despite numerous reports that were emerging which demonstrated definite link between fenfluramine and dexfenfluramine and PPH in both animal experiments (induction of PPH in rats with high consumption of fenfluramine) and epidemiological studies throughout Europe (7 % in control versus 32 % among aminorex users among affected patients), it was believed that a safer form of the drug could be formulated by using smaller doses of fenfluramine in combination with phentermine (an amphetamine-like agent) [52–54]. Though several prominent members of the pulmonary hypertension community vocally opposed the release of another appetite suppressant agent, in April 1996 the Food and Drug Administration approved dexfenfluramine (Redux®) and fenfluramine (Pondimin®) for the treatment of obesity. The drug sales skyrocketed, as did the reports of PPH (23-fold increase among patients ingesting the drug for more than 3 months) and valvular heart disease [55]. Reports of fatality linked to "fen-phen" ingestion led the FDA to remove the drug from the market in September 1997. Though the etiology of this form of pulmonary hypertension has not been clearly identified, it is thought to be caused by effects of high levels of serotonin in blood due to failure of adequate clearance from the lungs along with genetic predisposition [41, 56].

The 2nd World Symposium on Pulmonary Hypertension: Evian Meeting (1998)

The Second World Symposium on Pulmonary Hypertension, held 25 years after the first meeting in Evian, France in 1998, occurred during a period of unprecedented amount of heightened interest in pulmonary hypertension from many segments of society: medical community, including clinicians and basic scientists in quest to learn more about this elusive "orphan" disease; lay public and the media related to the "fen-phen" epidemic; pharmaceutical industry with focused interest in developing PAH-targeted treatments; and regulatory agencies recognizing the need to provide effective, yet safe, therapies for this deadly condition. Marking the 25th anniversary of the first meeting, clinical scientists convened from around the world to review the body of work that had been accomplished during the last 25 years since the first WHO meeting followed by discussions regarding relevant merits and synopsis on the current state of knowledge and concluding with recommendations for future studies. Focused areas of discussions included a pathology section with significant information that had emerged relating to endothelial dysfunction in pulmonary hypertension, as well as in depth descriptions of the abnormalities found in pulmonary vessels [57]. Other sections were dedicated to assessing risk factors for developing pulmonary hypertension, with drugs such as aminorex and fenfluramine/dexfenfluramine, HIV, scleroderma spectrum of diseases, liver disease/portal hypertension, and families with documented PPH, and indications for screening for those with risk factors; genetics of pulmonary hypertension with studies that illustrated the prevalence and patterns of transmission among family members with history of PPH; and methods of evaluation and work up. The committee on therapeutics focused on epoprostenol which had been approved in 1996, first PAH-targeted treatment and demonstrated survival benefit, as well as the use of calcium channel blockers for minority of patients who demonstrated acute vasoreactivity [57, 58].

The most significant proposal that emerged from the meeting was the formation of clinical classification of the different etiologies of pulmonary hypertension, which was one of six recommendations that was stated during the first meeting in Geneva in 1973: "A classification is recommended, taking into account both clinical (etiological) and morphological characteristics. A separate clinical and morphological nomenclature is suggested" [43]. The committee worked to achieve this goal which was felt to be "helpful in communicating about individual patients and in standardizing diagnosis and treatment" [57]. It was further mentioned that "several previous classification have proven to be problematic…. This classification reflects recent advances in the understanding of pulmonary hypertensive disease, and recognizes the similarity between primary pulmonary hypertension and pulmonary hypertension of certain known etiologies" [57].

The Evian Classification proposed five categories that grouped different forms of pulmonary hypertension sharing similarities in pathophysiological mechanisms, clinical presentations, and therapeutic options. Group 1 was named "Pulmonary arterial hypertension", which was the first time this terminology was formally used and included a subgroup under the heading of PPH that designated those without identifiable cause for the disease, both sporadic and familial forms. The second subgroup included PAH occurring related to a variety of underlying diseases, including collagen vascular disease (referred to now as connective tissue disease), congenital systemic to pulmonary shunts, portal hypertension, human immunodeficiency virus (HIV), drugs and toxins (including anorexigens and others), persistent PH of the newborn, and other. Though diverse in etiologies, these conditions have in common the localization of lesions to the small pulmonary muscular arterioles and share similar clinical presentations and responsiveness to PAH-specific treatment, such as epoprostenol [58, 59].

A methodology for categorizing risk factors and associated conditions for pulmonary hypertension was also proposed. A risk factor was defined as any factor or condition that was thought to play a role in the development of the disease such as drugs, other diseases, or a clinical state. Risk factors were defined as those factors that were present prior to the onset of the disease and were categorized based on the strength of the association with PPH regarding their probable causal role: "Definite" indicated an association based on several concordant observations, including a major controlled study or a clear epidemic role; "Very likely" was based on several concordant observations or a general expert-based consensus; "Possible" designated an association based on case series, registries, or expert opinion; "Unlikely" indicated risk factors that have been proposed but without evidence of any associations from controlled studies [57].

Groups 2 through 5 included pulmonary hypertension that occurs secondary to systemic processes. Group 2, "Pulmonary Venous Hypertension", included those with predominantly left-sided valvular or myocardial diseases. This category also included extrinsic compression of the pulmonary vein and pulmonary veno-occlusive disease (PVOD), which share similar clinical features as PPH. Group 3 referred to "Pulmonary Hypertension Associated with Disorders of the Respiratory System or Hypoxemia" where the predominant cause is inadequate oxygenation of arterial blood occurring as a result of parenchymal and/or airway lung disease, impaired control of breathing, or high altitude effect. Group 4, "Pulmonary Hypertension Due to Chronic Thrombotic and/or Embolic

Disease", was categorized as thromboembolic obstruction of proximal pulmonary arteries and distal pulmonary arteries, which included sickle cell disease. Group 5 included "Pulmonary Hypertension due to Disorders Directly Affecting the Pulmonary Vasculature" such as PH stemming from inflammatory processes or mechanical obstruction (i.e. schistosomiasis, sarcoidosis) [57, 60]. As recommended during the first meeting in Geneva, the group also set forth a new pathologic classification that outlined recommendations for the pathologic characterization based on histologic findings as well as a functional classification based on the severity of symptoms [57].

The 3rd World Symposium on Pulmonary Hypertension: Venice Meeting (2003)

The 3rd World Symposium on Pulmonary Hypertension held in Venice, Italy in 2003 provided an opportunity to assess the usefulness of the Evian classification and determine areas that needed modifications. The impact of Evian classification was evaluated through a questionnaire that was sent to those who attended the Venice meeting with questions focusing on clinical acceptance and use in practice as well as its usefulness for drug evaluation and basic science. The responses received were overwhelmingly favorable to all queries. Another evidence that demonstrated the significant impact the Evian classification was that both the U.S. Food and Drug Administration and European Agency for Drug Evaluation also started to use the classification system for the labeling of new PAH-targeted therapies. Therefore, the task force agreed to maintain the overall organization of the clinical classification system [60].

The task force members proposed several important changes to the Evian classification. The most significant one involved the decision to replace the term "primary pulmonary hypertension" which has been used for more than 50 years since coined by Dresdale to designate unexplained or idiopathic PAH [29]. The major reason for this change in terminology centered around the recognition that several conditions, such as ingestion of appetite suppressants, connective tissue disease, and HIV infection, can produce pulmonary vascular disease which share similar clinical and pathologic presentations as PPH. All of these conditions were grouped under the heading of "secondary pulmonary hypertension," along with all the other conditions listed under Groups 2 through 5 in the Evian classification. Thus the term "secondary pulmonary hypertension" was dropped in the Evian classification for it had lost its usefulness for diagnosis and treatment. In contrast, the term PPH was kept because it was well accepted and recognized. However, it was agreed that in order to use the term "primary", there had to be a "secondary" to differentiate the two conditions. The decision therefore was to replace PPH with "idiopathic pulmonary arterial hypertension" (IPAH) [60].

The other change in the classification included reclassifying PVOD and pulmonary capillary hemangiomatosis (PCH)

as part of Group 1 PAH from Group 2 Pulmonary Venous Hypertension as initially proposed in the Evian Classification supported by findings that the two diseases manifest histological changes (intimal fibrosis, medial hypertrophy, plexiform lesions) that is similar to PAH [60–63]. A new category named "Miscellaneous" was added as Group 5 to include sarcoidosis, histiocytosis X, lymphangiomatosis, and compression of pulmonary vessels. The revised classification also contained a guideline for the classification of congenital systemic-to-pulmonary shunts.

The 4th World Symposium on Pulmonary Hypertension: Dana Point Evian Meeting (2008)

The international group of experts who convened at the 4th World Symposium on PH at Dana Point, California achieved the general consensus to maintain the overall structure of the prior Evian-Venice classifications with updates to reflect new information that had emerged in the past 5 years [64]. Majority of the changes were made to Group 1 (PAH) category, one of which involved replacing the term "familial PAH" with "heritable PAH" as a result of studies demonstrating that mutations in the gene encoding the bone morphogenetic protein receptor type II (BMPR2), localized to chromosome 2q33, have been detected in 11–40 % of apparently idiopathic cases with no family history [64–67]. Thus it was determined that the distinction between idiopathic and familial BMPR2 mutations is artificial. Furthermore, in 20 % or fewer families with PAH, no BMPR2 mutations could be identified. The other major modification included moving schistosomiasis from Group 4 (PH due to chronic thrombotic and/or embolic disease) to Group 1 (PAH) with recent publications that showed PH associated with schistosomiasis with similar histologic lesions as IPAH, including development of plexiform lesions [67–69]. In addition, chronic hemolytic anemias was added as a new subcategory of PAH which had been listed under Group 1 "Other" conditions in Venice classification. This change was based on published studies showing that PAH appeared to be a complication of chronic hereditary and acquired hemolytic anemias, especially sickle cell disease (SCD) [70, 71]. The initial studies reported a high prevalence of PH among SCD patients of 32 %, but these studies were based on echo based findings with only 9 % of the cohort meeting the criteria for PH when confirmed by right heart catheterization [71, 72]. Furthermore, a large proportion of the patients with SCD were reported to have pulmonary venous hypertension and differing pathologic findings. This group would be re-categorized under Group 5 Miscellaneous at the next WHO meeting.

An update on the PAH risk factors was provided with addition of St. John's Wort, phenylpropanolamine (an agent found in over-the-counter weight loss drugs), selective serotonin reuptake inhibitors (SSRIs) in association with pregnancy in the "Possible" category, and addition of amphetamine use as "Likely" risk factor. Congenital heart disease category was updated providing a more detailed description of each condition to emphasize the four distinct phenotypes [73–75]. Furthermore, PVOD and PCH were categorized as 1' to designate the fact that they share similar characteristics as IPAH but with a number of distinct clinical differences [76, 77].

Updates in Groups 2 through 5 PH reflected growing knowledge in the cause and effect in the development of PH stemming from systemic conditions. Changes in Group 2 PH included recognition of heart failure with preserved ejection fraction (HFpEF), or diastolic dysfunction, as a common cause of pulmonary venous hypertension resulting in three categories: left heart systolic dysfunction, left heart diastolic dysfunction, and left heart valvular disease [78]. For Group 3 PH, the primary modification included adding a category of lung disease characterized by a mixed obstructive and restrictive pattern. Group 4 PH was changed to include only chronic thromboembolic pulmonary hypertension (CTEPH), deleting the prior designation of two subgroups of proximal and distal CTEPH due to recognition that this distinction was not clinically uniform across centers. Group 5 was named "Pulmonary Hypertension with Unclear Multifactorial Mechanisms" with four subcategories: hematologic disorders, systemic disorders, metabolic disorders and others [64].

The 5th World Symposium on Pulmonary Hypertension: Nice Meeting (2013)

During the most recent 5th World Symposium in Pulmonary Hypertension in 2013 held in Nice, France, the consensus among the committee members was to maintain the general scheme of previous classifications with a few modifications, mostly for Group 1 PAH [79] (Table 1.3a). To reflect the recent discoveries in the field of genetics, new gene mutations were added to the list for the heritable PAH group. These are rare mutations in other genes belonging to the TGF-β super family: activin-like receptor kinase-1 (ALK₁), endoglin (ENG) and mothers against decapentaplegic 9 (Smad 9). Furthermore, 2 new gene mutations have been identified: namely a mutation in caveolin-1 (CAV1) which encodes a membrane protein of caveolae which is present in endothelial cells of the lung, and KCNK3, a gene encoding potassium channel super family K member-3 [79–82]. These mutations are not closely related to TGF-β family, providing new insights into the pathogenesis of PAH. Several drugs were added to the list of toxin induced PAH: benfluorex (a derivative of fenfluramine) and SSRIs for definite association; interferon alpha and beta and amphetamine-like drugs for possible; and dasatinib, a tyrosine-kinease inhibitor used in treatment of chronic myeloproliferative (CML) disorders with likely association [74, 79, 83–86].

The CHD was updated with categories that cover the four different phenotypes of the disease. This classification offers a simple and a clinically useful way to approach CHD. Furthermore, with the recognition that CHD is a lifelong disease, it has been integrated with the Nice Pediatric classification to provide a comprehensive classification for

Table 1.3a Updated classification of pulmonary hypertension (Nice 2013)

1. Pulmonary arterial hypertension
1.1 Idiopathic PAH
1.2 Heritable PAH
1.2.1 BMPR2
1.2.2 ALK-1, ENG, **SMAD9, CAV1, KCNK3**
1.2.3 Unknown
1.3 Drug and toxin induced
1.4 Associated with:
1.4.1 Connective tissue disease
1.4.2 HIV infection
1.4.3 Portal hypertension
1.4.4 Congenital heart diseases
1.4.5 Schistosomiasis
1'. Pulmonary veno-occlusive disease and/or pulmonary capillary hemangiomatosis
1″. Persistent pulmonary hypertension of the newborn (PPHN)
2. Pulmonary hypertension due to left heart disease
2.1 Left ventricular systolic dysfunction
2.2 Left ventricular diastolic dysfunction
2.3 Valvular disease
2.4 **Congenital/acquired left heart inflow/outflow tract obstruction and congenital cardiomyopathies**
3. Pulmonary hypertension due to lung diseases and/or hypoxia
3.1 Chronic obstructive pulmonary disease
3.2 Interstitial lung disease
3.3 Other pulmonary diseases with mixed restrictive and obstructive pattern
3.4 Sleep-disordered breathing
3.5 Alveolar hypoventilation disorders
3.6 Chronic exposure to high altitude
3.7 Developmental lung diseases
4. Chronic thromboembolic pulmonary hypertension (CTEPH)
5. Pulmonary hypertension with unclear multifactorial mechanisms
5.1 Hematologic disorders: **chronic hemolytic anemia,** myeloproliferative disorders, splenectomy
5.2 Systemic disorders: sarcoidosis, pulmonary histiocytosis, lymphangioleiomyomatosis
5.3 Metabolic disorders: glycogen storage disease, Gaucher disease, thyroid disorders
5.4 Others: tumoral obstruction, fibrosing mediastinitis, chronic renal failure, **segmental PH**

Reprinted from Simonneau et al. [79], Table 1, with permission from Elsevier

5th WSPH Nice 2013. Main modifications to the previous Dana Point classification are in **bold**

BMPR bone morphogenic protein receptor type II, *CAV1* caveolin-1, *ENG* endoglin, *HIV* human immunodeficiency virus, *PAH* pulmonary arterial hypertension

Table 1.3b Updated clinical classification of pulmonary arterial hypertension associated with congenital heart disease

1. Eisenmenger syndrome
Includes all large intra- and extra-cardiac defects which begin as systemic-to-pulmonary shunts and progress with time to severe elevation of pulmonary vascular resistance (PVR) and to reversal (pulmonary-to-systemic) or bidirectional shunting; cyanosis, secondary erythrocytosis and multiple organ involvement are usually present
2. Left-to-right shunts
Correctable†
Noncorrectable
Include moderate to large defects; PVR is mildly to moderately increased systemic-to-pulmonary shunting is still prevalent, whereas cyanosis is not a feature
3. Pulmonary arterial hypertension (PAH) with coincidental congenital heart disease
Marked elevation in PVR in the presence of small cardiac defects, which themselves do not account for the development of elevated PVR; the clinical picture is very similar to idiopathic PAH. To close the defects in contraindicated
4. Post-operative PAH
Congenital heart disease is repaired but PAH either persists immediately after surgery or recurs/develops months or years after surgery in the absence of significant postoperative hemodynamic lesions. The clinical phenotype is often aggressive

Reprinted from Simonneau et al. [79], p. D39, Table 3, with permission from Elsevier

† Correctable with surgery or intravascular nonsurgical procedure

wider applicability [79, 87, 88] (Table 1.3b). Some types of PH in association with CHD that do not share similarities with Group 1 were moved to Group 2 and Group 5. Chronic hemolytic anemia, originally categorized in Group 4 (chronic thromboembolism) in Evian classification, was moved to Group 1 (PAH) in the Venice and Dana Point classifications. New studies have emerged demonstrating that pre-capillary PH associated with SCD has markedly different characteristics than other forms of PAH in pathologic findings from autopsies, hemodynamic profiles, and response to PAH-specific treatments. Thus in the Nice classification, SCD was moved from Group 1 (PAH) to Group 5 (unclear multifactorial mechanisms) [79, 89–91]. The other main change was designating persistent pulmonary hypertension of the newborn (PPHN) as number 1" to designate that it carries more differences than similarities with other types of PAH [92].

Nomenclature and Classification on Right Heart Failure: Right Heart Failure Summit (2013)

Though William Harvey had the incredible insight to make a case for the role of the right ventricle when he stated, "The right ventricle may be said to be made for the sake of transmitting blood through the lungs, not for nourishing them…" in 1628 in *Exercitation Anatomica de Motu Cordis et*

Sanguinis in Animalibus, the appreciation of the importance of right ventricular function and its contribution in determining functional and end organ outcome is now being recognized [4]. Indeed, the fact that the "knowledge about the role of the right ventricle in health and disease has lagged behind that of the left ventricle" and the consequence of this void in fully comprehending the mechanics of cardiopulmonary system has resulted in the medical community to strive to attain a better understanding of the physiology and mechanisms of right heart function and its responses to different forms of cardiac pathology [93]. Significant strides have been achieved in response to this call to learn about the right ventricle, from its unique embryonic origins and anatomic composition, its separate yet integrated function that is as important as the left ventricle, and the plasticity of its unique adaptive responses to hemodynamic perturbations [93, 94]. A large segment of the growing appreciation of the critical role of the right ventricle comes from studying patients with pulmonary arterial hypertension that clearly have shown that it is the state of the right ventricle which determines the outcome [51, 58, 95, 96]. Indeed, numerous studies have been reported with irrefutable evidence clearly delineating that the presence of pulmonary hypertension and right ventricular dysfunction has significant influence in the outcome in all forms of heart disease – systolic, diastolic, valvular – and lung disease [97–100].

Many unanswered questions remain, however, in our understanding of the unique make-up of the right ventricle from its distinct cellular components and anatomic composition to the intricate patho-biological pathways that govern its responses to abnormal hemodynamics and lead to the vicious cycle of right heart failure. The growing interest from the medical community in learning more about the unique and critical role of the right heart system has galvanized in the formation of the International Right Heart Failure Foundation (IRHFF) Working Group in developing a nomenclature in order to form an integrative and a common language that effectively describes right heart disease that is relevant to scientists and clinicians [101]. In this effort, the IRHFF Working Group provides definitions that distinguish between the right heart failure and right ventricular failure by outlining the components of right heart system. Thus the importance in recognizing that right heart failure represents a disturbance in any of the components that constitute the right heart circulatory system, which is defined as from the systemic veins up to the pulmonary capillaries at which point the deoxygenated blood transitions to oxygenated blood, is clearly outlined. How to best define right heart failure is also proposed "as a clinical syndrome due to an alteration of structure and/or function of the right heart circulatory system that leads to sub-optimal delivery of blood flow (how or low) to the pulmonary circulation and/or elevated venous pressure – at rest or with exercise". The four critical components of the nomenclature system are outlined which include: etiology (what is the primary cause); anatomy (what is the primary defect); physiology (what is the primary aberration); and clinical function (what is the clinical expression in the patient) [101] (Table 1.4). The goals of the scientific and clinical community are aligned in attaining the level of understanding of right heart system to develop effective therapies that target right heart failure.

Table 1.4 Development of a comprehensive nomenclature of right heart failure: framework, components and issues (International Right Heart Failure Foundation Scientific Working Group)

1. **Etiology: What is the primary cause?**

(a) Draw upon existing classification systems for congenital heart disease.

(b) Advance current descriptions of acquired etiologies.

(The novel aspect lies in the expanded definition of right heart failure to include pre-cardiac and post-pulmonary valvular compartments.)

2. **Anatomy: Where is the primary defect?**

(a) Describe the anatomic constituents of the right heart circulatory system.

(b) Describe the anatomic defects within the right heart circulatory system (systemic circuit and pulmonary circuit) and left heart circulatory system.

3. **Physiology: What is the primary aberration?**

(a) Define the appropriate hemodynamic and non-hemodynamic definitions and assessments of three distinct physiologic disturbances in the domains of *Preload stress*, *Contractile* insufficiency and *After-load* stress.

4. **Clinical function: What is the clinical expression in the patient?**

(a) Functional class components:

A. Subjective component

(a) Patient's reported symptom (Modified NYFIA functional class).

(b) Assessment of patient's activity profile (sedentary, active, etc.).

(c) Quality of life (Most appropriate assessment to be determined).

B. Objective component

(a) 6MWT (include Borg score, percent predicted value).

(b) Pending results and/or clinical situation, proceed with cardiopulmonary stress test (CPEX) (availability, safety and consistency in interpretation of data presenting as barriers to be further discussed).

(i) Assess hemodynamic and/or ventilator response/ insufficiency.

C. Modifiers to functional assessment (non-cardiovascular contributors to symptoms).

(a) Body mass index (BMI).

(b) Orthopedic limitations.

(c) Systemic processes.

(b) How should secondary modifiers (secondary organ function) be incorporated?

(i) Renal dysfunction—as measured by GFR?

(ii) Hepatic dysfunction—as measured by MELD.

(Should these elements be treated under physiologic aberrations or functional aspects?).

Reprinted from Mehra et al. [101], with permission from Elsevier

Conclusion

The past five decades have witnessed tremendous advances in gaining understanding in key areas of pulmonary hypertension: pathophysiology, epidemiology and genetics, diagnostics, therapeutics and prognosis. These achievements have been facilitated through the evolution of nomenclature and classifications over the years, which instituted changes to reflect the current concepts by providing a foundation of organization and structure for clinicians and scientists to engage in productive dialogue. One of key the demonstration of the success is the development and approval of 12 PAH-specific treatments in the past two decades, which have significantly improved the quality of life and survival in patients with pulmonary hypertension. However, further work is needed in to attain better understanding in several of key areas of pulmonary hypertension, in particular in the areas of PH associated with left heart disease and lung disease that impact a large number of patients in the aging population. The progress will be reflected in the changes seen in future nomenclature and classification systems that will document the ongoing progresses made in the field of pulmonary hypertension and right heart failure.

References

1. Aird WC. Discovery of the cardiovascular system: from Galen to William Harvey. J Thromb Haemost. 2011;9 Suppl 1:118–29.
2. Nutton V. Ancient medicine. London/New York: Routledge; 2004.
3. Silva JM. Da descoberta da circulacao sanguinea aos primeiros factos hemorreologicos. Rev Port Cardiol. 2009;28(11):1245–68.
4. Harvey W. Exercitatio de motu cordis et sanguiis in animalibus. Francoforti Guilelmi Fitzeri, 1628 (trans: CD Leake). Springfield: Charles C. Thomas; 1928.
5. Newman JH. Centennial review. Pulmonary hypertension. Am J Respir Crit Care Med. 2005;172:1072–7.
6. Malpighi M. De pulmonibus. 1661. Available from http://www.anatomist.co.uk/FamousAnatomists.
7. Romberg E. Ueber Sklerose der Lungen arterie. Dtsch Archiv Klin Med. 1981;48:197–206.
8. Larrabee WF, Parker RL, Edwards JE. Pathology of intrapulmonary arteries and arterioles in mitral stenosis. Proc Mayo Clin. 1949;24:316–26.
9. Fishman AP. Primary pulmonary arterial hypertension. A look back. J Am Coll Cardiol. 2004;43:2S–4.
10. Mazzei JA, Mazzei ME. A Tribute: Abel Ayerza and pulmonary hypertension. Eur Respir Rev. 2011;20:220–1.
11. Escudero P. The Black Cardiacs and the Ayerza's disease. Paris: Revue Critique; 1911.
12. Arrillaga FC. Sclerose de l'artere pulmonaire secondaire a certains etats pulmonaries chroniques (cardiaques noires) [Sclerosis of the pulmonary artery secondary to certain chronic pulmonary diseases (black cardiac)]. Arch Mal Coeur. 1913;6:518–29.
13. Warthin AS. A case of Ayerza's disease. JAMA. 1919;76:716.
14. Arrillaga FC, editor. La Arteritis Pulmonar: Cardiacos Negros [Pulmonary arteritis: Black Cardiacs]. Pedro Garcia: Buenos Aires; 1925.
15. Fishman AP. Historical perspective: a century of primary (idiopathic) pulmonary hypertension. In: Hill NS, Farber HW, editors. Pulmonary hypertension. Totowa: Humana Press; 2010. p. 1–14.

16. Brenner O. Pathology of the vessels of the pulmonary circulation. Arch Intern Med. 1935;56:211–37.
17. Wiggins CJ. The pressure pulses in the cardiovascular system. New York: Longmans; 1928.
18. Krogh A, Lindhard J. Measurement of the blood flow through the lungs of man. Skan Arch Physiol. 1912;27:100–25.
19. Fick A. Uber die Messung des Blutquantums in den Herzventrikeln. Sitx der Physik-Med ges Wurzburg. 1870;2:16.
20. Forssman W. Die Sonderung des rechten Herzens. Klin Wockschr 1929;45:2085.
21. Forssman W. Nobel Lecture: the role of heart catheterization and angiography in the development of modern medicine. In: Nobel lectures, physiology of medicine. Amsterdam: Elsevier Publishing; 1964.
22. Richards DW. The Burns Amberson Lecture: the right heart and the lung. Am Rev Respir Dis. 1966;94:691–702.
23. Cournand AW, Ranges HA. Catheterization of the right auricle in man. Proc Soc Exp Biol Med. 1941;46:62.
24. Richards DW. Nobel Lecture: the contributions of right heart catheterization to physiology and medicine with some observations of the physio-pathology of pulmonary heart disease. In: Nobel lectures: physiology or medicine. Amsterdam: Elsevier Publishing; 1964.
25. Cournand AF. Control of the pulmonary circulation in man with some remarks on methodology. Nobel lecture, December 11, 1956. In: Nobel lectures: physiology or medicine. Amsterdam: Elsevier Publishing; 1964.
26. Lategola M, Rahn H. A self-guiding catheter for cardiac and pulmonary arterial catheterization and occlusion. Proc Soc Exp Biol Med. 1953;84:667–8.
27. Hellems HK, Haynes FW, Dexter L. Pulmonary "capillary" pressure in man. J Appl Physiol. 1949–1950;2:24–9.
28. Swan HJ, Ganz W, Forrester J. Catheterization of the heart in man with use of a flow-directed balloon-tipped catheter. N Engl J Med. 1970;283:447–51.
29. Dresdale DT, Schulz M, Mitchtom RJ. Primary pulmonary hypertension: I. Clinical and hemodynamic study. Am J Med. 1951;11:686.
30. Von Euler US, Liljestrand G. Observations on the pulmonary arterial blood pressure in the cat. Acta Physiol Scan. 1946;12:301–20.
31. Motley HL, Cournand A, Werko L, Himmelstein A, Dresdale DT. The influence of short periods of induced anoxia upon pulmonary artery pressure in man. Am J Physiol. 1947;150:315–20.
32. Wood P. Pulmonary hypertension with special reference to the vasoconstrictive factor. Br Heart J. 1958;20:557–70.
33. Wood P, Besterman EM, Towers MK, McIlroy MB. The effect of acetylcholine on pulmonary vascular resistance and left atrial pressure in mitral stenosis. Br Heart J. 1957;19:279–86.
34. Harris P. Influence of acetylcholine on the pulmonary artery pressure. Br Heart J. 1957;19:272–86.
35. Fritts HW, Harris Jr P, Clauss RH, Odell JE, Cournand A. The effect of acetylcholine on the human pulmonary circulation under normal and hypoxic conditions. J Clin Invest. 1958;37:99–108.
36. Rich S, Dantzker DR, Ayres SM, Bergofsky EH, Brundage BH, Detre KM, Fishman AP, Goldring RM, Groves BM, Koerner SK, et al. Primary pulmonary hypertension: a national prospective study. Ann Intern Med. 1987;107:216–28.
37. Heath D, Edwards JE. The pathology of hypertensive pulmonary vascular disease: a description of six grades of structural changes in the pulmonary arteries. Circulation. 1958;18:533.
38. Wagenvoort CA, Wagenvoort N. Primary pulmonary hypertension: a pathologic study of the lung vessels in 156 clinically diagnosed cases. Circulation. 1970;42:1163–84.
39. Gurtner HP. Aminorex pulmonary hypertension. In: Fishman AP, editor. The pulmonary circulation: normal and abnormal. Mechanisms, management and the National Registry. Philadelphia: University of Pennsylvania Press; 1990. p. 397–411.
40. Mielke H, Seiler KU, Stumpf U, Wasserman O. Relation between serotonin metabolism and pulmonary hypertension in rats following administration of various anorectic drugs. Z Kardiol. 1973;62:1090–8.
41. Fishman AP. Aminorex to Fen/Phen. An epidemic foretold. Circulation. 1999;99:156–61.
42. Report of the WHO Expert Committee on chronic cor pulmonale. WHO Technical Report Series, No. 213; 1961.
43. Hatano S, Strasser R, editors. Primary pulmonary hypertension. Geneva: World Health Organization; 1975.
44. Walstor A, Kendall ME. Comparison of pulmonary wedge and left arterial pressure in man. Am Heart J. 1973;86:159–64.
45. Herbert WH. Limitations of pulmonary artery end-diastolic pressure as the reflection of the left ventricular end-diastolic pressure. N Y State J Med. 1972;72:229–32.
46. Vachiery JL, Adir Y, Barbera JA, et al. Pulmonary hypertension due to left heart disease. J Am Coll Cardiol. 2013;62:D100–8.
47. Ekelund LG, Holmgren A. Central haemodynamics during exercise. Circ Res. 1967;20 Suppl 1:33–43.
48. Barst RJ, McGoon M, Torbicki A, et al. J Am Coll Cardiol. 2004;43:40S–7.
49. Badesch DB, Champion HC, Gomez Sanchez MA. J Am Coll Cardiol. 2009;54:S55–66.
50. Fishman AP. Induction to the national registry on primary pulmonary hypertension. In: Fishman AP, editor. The pulmonary circulation: normal and abnormal. Mechanisms, management and the National Registry. Philadelphia: University of Pennsylvania Press; 1990. p. 437–9.
51. D'Alonzo GE, Barst RJ, Ayres SM, et al. Ann Intern Med. 1991;115:343–9.
52. Atanossoff PG, Weiss BM, Scjmid ER, Tornic M. Pulmonary hypertension and dexfenfluramine. Lancet. 1992;339:436.
53. Abenhaim L, Moride Y, Brenot F, et al. Appetite-suppressant drugs and the risk of primary pulmonary hypertension. International Primary Pulmonary Hypertension Study Group. N Engl J Med. 1996;335:609–16.
54. Weintraub M, Hasday JD, Mushlin AI, Lockwood DH. A double-blind clinical trial in weight control: use of fenfluramine and phenteramine along and in combination. Arch Intern Med. 1984;144:1143–8.
55. Connolly HM, Crary JL, McGoon MD, et al. Valvular heart disease associated with fenfluramine-phentermine. J Engl J Med. 1997;337:581–8.
56. Robiolio PA, Rigolin VH, Wilson JS, et al. Carcinoid heart disease. Correlation of high serotonin levels with valvular abnormalities detected by cardiac catheterization and echocardiography. Circulation. 1995;92:790–5.
57. Rich S, editor. World Health Organization executive summary from the world symposium on primary pulmonary hypertension. 1998. http://web.archive.org/web/20020408173726/http://www.who.int/ncd/cvd/ppph.html. Accessed 15 Jan 2015.
58. Barst RJ, Rubin LJ, Long WA, et al. A comparison of continuous intravenous epoprostenol (prostacyclin) with conventional therapy for primary pulmonary hypertension. The Primary Pulmonary Hypertension Study Group. N Engl J Med. 1996;334:296–302.
59. Badesch DB, Tapson VF, McGoon MD, et al. Continuous intravenous epoprostenol for pulmonary hypertension due to the scleroderma spectrum of disease. A randomized, controlled trial. Ann Intern Med. 2000;132:425–34.
60. Simonneau G, Galie N, Rubin LJ, et al. Clinical classification of pulmonary hypertension. J Am Coll Cardiol. 2004;43:5S–12.
61. Schraufnagel DE, Sekosan M, McGee T, et al. Human alveolar capillaries undergo angiogenesis in pulmonary veno-occlusive disease. Eur Respir J. 1996;9:346–50.
62. Daroca PJ, Mansfield RE, Ichinose H. Pulmonary veno-occlusive disease: report of a case with pseudoangiomatous features. Am J Surg Pathol. 1977;12:349–55.

63. Peitra GG. The pathology of primary pulmonary hypertension. In: Rubin LJ, Rich S, editors. Primary pulmonary hypertension: lung biology in health and disease. New York: Marcel Dekker; 1997. p. 19–61.

64. Simonneau G, Robbins IM, Beghetti M, et al. Updated clinical classification of pulmonary hypertension. J Am Coll Cardiol. 2009;54:S43–54.

65. Lane KB, Machado RD, Pauciulo MW, et al., for the International PPH Consortium. Heterozygous germ-line mutations in BMPR2, encoding a TGF-β receptor, cause familial primary pulmonary hypertension. Nat Genet. 2000;26:81–4.

66. Machado RD, Aldred MA, James V, et al. Mutations of the TGF-β type II receptor BMPR2 in pulmonary arterial hypertension. Hum Mutat. 2006;27:121–32.

67. Thomson JR, Machado RD, Pauciulo MW, et al. Sporadic primary pulmonary hypertension is associated with germline mutations of the gene encoding BMPR-II, a receptor of the TGF-β family. J Med Genet. 2000;37:741–5.

68. Chaves E. The pathology of the arterial pulmonary vasculature in Manson's schistosomiasis. Chest. 1966;50:72–7.

69. Lapa M, Dias B, Jardim C, et al. Cardio-pulmonary manifestations of hepatosplenic schistosomiasis. Circulation. 2009;119:1518–23.

70. Casto O, Hoque M, Brown BD. Pulmonary hypertension in sickle cell disease: cardiac catheterization results and survival. Blood. 2003;101:1257–61.

71. Gladwin MT, Sachdev V, Jison ML, et al. Pulmonary hypertension as a risk factor for death in patients with sickle cell disease. N Engl J Med. 2004;350:886–95.

72. Parent F, Egels S, Stzyrmf B, et al. Haemodynamic characteristics of patients wit sickle cell disease and suspected pulmonary hypertension on the basis of a tricuspid regurgitation jet velocity >2.5 m/s on Doppler echocardiography. Eur Respir J. 2006;28:544.

73. Walker AM, Langleben D, Korelitz JJ, et al. Temporal trends and drug exposures in pulmonary hypertension: an American experience. Am Heart J. 2006;152:521–6.

74. Chambers CD, Hernanez-Diaz S, Van Marter LJ, et al. Selective serotonin-reuptake inhibitors and risk of persistent pulmonary hypertension of the newborn. N Engl J Med. 2006;354:579–87.

75. Chin KM, Channick RN, Rubin LF. Is methamphetamine use associated with idiopathic pulmonary arterial hypertension? Chest. 2006;130:1657–63.

76. Runo JR, Vnencak-Jones CL, Prince M, et al. Pulmonary veno-occlusive disease caused by an inherited mutation in bone morphogenetic protein receptor II. Am J Respir Crit Care Med. 2003;167:889–94.

77. Lantuejoul S, Sheppard MN, Corrin B, et al. Pulmonary veno-occlusive disease and pulmonary capillary hemangiomatosis: a clinicopathologic study of 35 cases. Am J Surg Pathol. 2006;30:850–7.

78. Oudiz RJ. Pulmonary hypertension associated with left-sided heart disease. Eur Respir J. 2006;27:108–13.

79. Simonneau G, Gatzoulis MA, Adatia I, et al. Updated clinical classification of pulmonary hypertension. J Am Coll Cardiol. 2013;62(25):D34–41.

80. Harrison RE, Flanagan JA, Sankelo M, et al. Molecular and functional analysis identifies ALK-1 as the predominant cause of pulmonary hypertension related to hereditary haemorrhagic telangiectasia. J Med Genet. 2003;408:65–71.

81. Nasim MT, Ogo T, Ahmed M, et al. Molecular genetic characterization of SMAD signaling molecules in pulmonary arterial hypertension. Hum Mutat. 2011;32:1385–9.

82. Austin ED, Ma L, LeDuc C, et al. Whole exome sequencing to identify a novel gene (Caveolin-1) associated with human pulmonary arterial hypertension. Circ Cardiovasc Genet. 2012;5:336–43.

83. Boutet K, Frachon I, Jobic Y, et al. Fenfluramine-like cardiovascular side-effects of benfluorex. Eur Resp J. 2009;33:684–8.

84. Montani D, Bergot E, Gunther S, et al. Pulmonary hypertension in patients treated with dasatinib. Circulation. 2012;125:2128–37.

85. Dhillon S, Kaker A, Dosanjh A, et al. Irreversible pulmonary hypertension associated with the use of interferon alpha for chronic hepatitis C. Dig Dis Sci. 2010;55:1785–90.

86. Kieler H, Arama M, Engeland A, et al. Selective serotonin reuptake inhibitors during pregnancy and risk of persistent pulmonary hypertension in the newborn: population based cohort study from the five Nordic countries. BMJ. 2011;344:d8012.

87. Marelli AJ, Mackie AS, Ionescu-Ittu R, et al. Congenital heart disease in the general population: changing prevalence and age distribution. Circulation. 2007;115:163–72.

88. Lowe BS, Therrien J, Ionescu-Ittu R, Pilote L, et al. Diagnosis of pulmonary hypertension in the congenital heart disease adult population impact on outcomes. J Am Coll Cardiol. 2011;26:538–46.

89. Parent F, Bachir D, Inamo J, et al. A hemodynamic study of pulmonary hypertension in sickle cell disease. N Engl J Med. 2011;365:44–53.

90. Fonseca GH, Souza R, Salemi RM, et al. Pulmonary hypertension diagnosed by right heart catheterization in sickle cell disease. Eur Respir J. 2012;39:112–8.

91. Machado RF, Barst RJ, Yovetich NA, et al. Hospitalization for pain in patients with sickle cell disease treated with sildenafil for elevated TRV and low exercise capacity. Blood. 2011;118:855–64.

92. Ivy D, Abman SH, Barst RJ, et al. Pediatric pulmonary hypertension. J Am Coll Cardiol. 2013;62(Suppl):D118–27.

93. Voelkel NF, Quaife RA, Leinwand LA, et al. Right ventricular function and failure. Report of a National Heart, Lung, and Blood Institute Working Group on cellular and molecular mechanisms of right heart failure. Circulation. 2006;114:1883–91.

94. Chin KM, Kim NHS, Rubin LR. The right ventricle in pulmonary hypertension. Coron Artery Dis. 2005;16:13–8.

95. van de Veerdonk MC, Kind T, Marcys JT, et al. Progressive right ventricular dysfunction in patients with pulmonary arterial hypertension responding to therapy. J Am Coll Cardiol. 2011;58:2511–9.

96. Vonk-Noordegraaf A, Hadda F, Chin KM, et al. Right heart adaptation to pulmonary arterial hypertension. J Am Coll Cardiol. 2013;62:D22–33.

97. Ghio S, Gavazzi A, Campana C, et al. Independent and additive prognostic value of right ventricular systolic function and pulmonary artery pressure in patients with chronic heart failure. J Am Coll Cardiol. 2001;37:183–8.

98. Ding WH, Lam YY, Duncan A, et al. Predictors or survival after aortic valve replacement in patients with low-flow and high gradient aortic stenosis. Eur J Heart Fail. 2009;11:897–902.

99. Lam CS, Roger VL, Rodeheffer RJ, et al. Pulmonary hypertension in heart failure with preserved ejection fraction: a community based study. J Am Coll Cardiol. 2009;53:1119–26.

100. Seeger W, Adir Y, Barbera JA, et al. Pulmonary hypertension in chronic lung disease. J Am Coll Cardiol. 2013;62:D109–16.

101. Mehra MR, Park MH, Landzberg MJ, et al. Right heart failure: toward a common language. J Heart Lung Transplant. 2014;33(2):123–6.

The Defining Characteristics of Pulmonary Arterial Hypertension

2

Rahul Kumar, Jeffrey C. Robinson, and Rubin M. Tuder

Introduction

Over 50,000 research articles and 7000 reviews in the last two decades have witnessed the remarkable progress in the field of pulmonary hypertension (PH), however, a unifying pathobiologic definition of the disease remains to be validated. The current classification of PH remains largely based on the concepts instituted by the WHO-Conference in Nice (2013), in which the term pulmonary arterial hypertension (PAH) is distinguished from pulmonary hypertension (PH) due to left heart disease, pulmonary disease, chronic thromboembolic pulmonary hypertension (CTEPH) and PH of miscellaneous etiologies [1]. This classification is largely based on the perception, based on the available medical knowledge, that PH in these settings is pathobiologically distinct. However, the key criteria for the disease is finding of mean pulmonary arterial pressure (mPAP) exceeding 25 mmHg with normal capillary wedge pressure as measured by right-heart catheterization; this common definition obscures the potential for distinct pathobiological processes underlying the heterogeneity of PH. It is not therefore surprising that most of our current understanding of PH derives from investigation of the entities clustered under the PAH group, particularly idiopathic pulmonary arterial hypertension (IPAH).

PAH is a progressive cardiopulmonary disease in which extensive obliterative changes occur in small to midsized pulmonary arteries. Alterations in structure and function of the endothelium occur in conjunction with growth of neointimal, medial, and adventitial layers, culminating in an occlusive arteriopathy associated with high resistance to blood flow and ultimately right heart failure and death [2]. The persisting challenge in understanding the pathobiology of PH is to define how the structural, cellular and molecular characteristics of the normal pulmonary circulation change in the disease setting [2]. Complicating this is the fact that PH is a heterogeneous disease with a myriad of associated factors. Further, much of the mechanistic study has been concentrated in WHO group 1 and III (PAH and hypoxia-dependent PH, respectively), which limits our ability to globally define shared pathologic and molecular traits among classes of PH. Nevertheless, we seek to provide first a summary of the modern descriptive characterization of PAH, and then elaborate on several more evolved and interrelated paradigms in the field, including the role of inflammation, hypoxia signaling, and metabolic dysfunction that drive the characteristic vascular remodeling (Table 2.1). Finally, we examine the potential therapeutic opportunities within each of these realms.

Pathological Characteristics of Intima, Media and Adventitial Remodeling

Vascular remodeling in PAH is characterized by smooth muscle cell proliferation, hypertrophy of the medial layer, arteriolar muscularization and endothelial cell proliferation. However, we will review the overall pathological changes in rodent and human vasculature that characteristically defines PAH. The pathological diagnosis of pulmonary vascular remodeling has benefited from the progressive use of cell-specific immunohistochemistry to better define the structure and cellular composition of the pulmonary vascular lesions through pathological interpretation of PH. Remodeling in pulmonary artery (PA) e.g., intima, media and adventitia is probably the major contributor to reduced cardiac output (CO) and enhanced pulmonary vascular resistance (PVR).

Author contributed equally with all other contributors.

R. Kumar, PhD (✉) • J.C. Robinson, MD
Division of Pulmonary Sciences and Critical Care Medicine,
Department of Medicine, University of Colorado, Denver,
Research Complex 2, Room 9001, Mail stop C-272,
12700 East 18th Avenue, Aurora, CO, 80045, USA
e-mail: rahul.2.kumar@ucdenver.edu

R.M. Tuder, MD
Division of Pulmonary Sciences and Critical Care Medicine,
Department of Medicine, University of Colorado Hospital,
Aurora, CO, USA

Table 2.1 Predominant pathobiologic mechanisms in the development of pulmonary arterial hypertension

Hypoxic signaling	Mitochondrial dysfunction
HIF-1α/HIF-2α	Mitochondrial hyperpolarization
TGF-β	Suppressed mitophagy
ERK1/2	Increased mROS generation
Increased Ca++	HIF-1α and aerobic glycolysis
Quasi malignancy	**Inflammation**
Clonal endothelial cell proliferation	Perivascular T-cell and macrophages
Microsatellite instability	Activated TGF-β signaling
Somatic chromosomal abnormalities	Increased IL-6, IL4, IL-13
Dysregulated energetic metabolism	CCL5/RANTES

Therefore, reduction of PA luminal area is probably the critical factor in the increase in PVR in PAH and other forms of PH [3].

In recent years, the Pulmonary Hypertension Breakthrough Initiative (PHBI) allowed us the unique opportunity to determine the pattern of pulmonary vascular remodeling in a large set of lung tissues with PAH [2]. There are numerous potential predictions regarding how pulmonary artery remodeling might be present in patients with the disease. Previously, we already have provided data regarding the relationship between the numbers of profiles of pulmonary vascular lesions and parameters of hemodynamics in PAH [4]. However, based on physiological coupling between the heart and lung during rest and exercise, it has been predicted that overall surface area could be required to decrease by 80 % by the time PH develops [2]; the specific contribution of pulmonary vascular remodeling vis-a-vis vasoconstriction is unclear. However, the PHBI cohort provided us with several key findings and advanced our understanding of the spectrum of the pathology of the disease.

Intima remodeling involves proliferation of endothelial cells (forming the plexiform lesions), accumulation of myofibroblasts (intima obliteration or fibrosis) and accumulation of extracellular matrix including collagen and mucopolysaccharides [5]. The intima remodeling, irrespective of specific proportions of each of these individual components, leads to almost complete obliteration of the vascular lumen, forming intima lesions, the most characteristic morphological finding in severe PH. These lesions are associated with congenital heart malformations and located at branching points, often as isolated lesions [6, 7]. Although plexiform lesions are seen predominantly in idiopathic PAH (IPAH), their precursor and importance as a trigger of severe PAH remains unclear. We speculate that endothelial cell proliferation and fibrosis in luminal area could be due to environmental insult as a key process that might precede occlusive intima lesions. The later consisted of eccentric intima thickening, fibrotic, plexiform, concentric, and dilation/angiomatoid lesions and represent a process of misguided angiogenesis based on the findings of expression of vascular endothelial growth factor (VEGF), its receptors 1 (flt) and 2 (kdr), and hypoxia inducible factor (HIF)-1α and β [8]. Focal eccentric lesions and thickening can be detected in normal lungs, but these lesions are more widespread and impinge to a larger extent on the vascular lumen in PH. However, variable degrees of eccentric thickening have been reported in cigarette smokers lungs associated with pulmonary endothelial cell dysfunction, with or without evidence of PH [9].

The potential role for early endothelial cell apoptosis in the pathogenesis of uncontrolled proliferation of pulmonary endothelial cells was first documented in the rat model of severe pulmonary hypertension caused by the combination of VEGF receptor blockade with SU5416 and chronic hypoxia [10]. Moreover, the role of endothelial cell apoptosis in the pathogenesis of PH was also extended to the monocrotaline model [11]. Initial endothelial cell apoptosis might favor the emergence of apoptosis-resistant endothelial cells, with potential for uncontrolled proliferation [10, 12]. Further, dysfunctional ECs can either release factors that stimulate smooth cell (SMC) proliferation or fail to produce agents that usually suppress proliferation of SMCs in response to growth factors, such as apelin [13, 14].

A prominent feature of vascular remodeling is medial thickening where medial smooth muscle cells elaborate extracellular matrix proteins, alters lumen size by contraction and relaxation [15]. The medial smooth muscle cell layer represents approximately 10–15 % of the outside diameter of normal muscularized pulmonary arteries, while it approaches 30–60 % of the outside diameter in vessels of IPAH lungs [16–19]. More precisely, we mentioned that medial smooth muscle cell hypertrophy is a characteristic pathological feature of PH that involves muscularized arteries (ranging between 70 and 500 μm in diameter), and precapillary vessels (below 70 μm in diameter) [5]. Although careful morphometric assessments of medial remodeling are still lacking non-IPAH PH, it is apparent that medial thickening occurs in mild/moderate or severe PH and in cases of normal individuals exposed to cigarette smoke with no evidence of PH [9]. Although media remodeling was correlated with hemodynamic parameters, three of the four quartiles of media remodeling in PAH were equally shared with control lungs, however, only the fourth quartile with more extensive media thickness fell well above the thickness seen in control lungs. Of note, intima lesions appeared more severe than intima remodeling seen in control lungs, the combination of intima and media remodeling had the most significant correlation with pulmonary artery pressures. Nevertheless, medial thickening probably plays an important role in the pathogenesis of PH, hitherto it is difficult to relate the morphological identification of medial remodeling to specific levels of pulmonary artery pressures, degrees of severity of PAH, or potential for response to vasodilators [5].

The vascular adventitia compartment acts as a pathobiological "processing center" for the retrieval, integration, storage and release of key regulators of vascular wall function in health and disease and thus, considered as the principal "injury-sensing site" of the pulmonary vessel wall [20]. The adventitia is mostly composed of fibroblasts, it also contains local and circulating progenitor cells that differentiate into smooth muscle and endothelial cells and contributes to pathophysiological changes in vascular structure [21, 22]. The normal adventitia represents approximately 15 % of the external diameter of pulmonary arteries larger than 50 μm in diameter. In IPAH arteries, the adventitial thickness increases to 28 % of artery diameter, predominantly due to collagen deposition [16]. Whether the adventitia is thickened or presents with a heterogeneous stromal cell population in other forms of PH remains unclear. Adventitia remodeling failed to correlate significantly with hemodynamics in our cohort of PAH lungs despite an earlier extensive study of remodeling in IPAH [16]. This discrepancy can be explained by methodological differences and the difficulty in precisely defining adventitia boundaries. Our data do not detract from the growing importance of the adventitia niche in coordinating media remodeling and perivascular inflammation, a key process in PH.

Inflammatory Pathology and Pathobiology of PAH

The pathophysiological mechanisms of pulmonary hypertension are not fully understood. Although the exact pathophysiology remains unknown, there is increasing evidence to suggest an important role for inflammation to the development of pulmonary hypertension in particular in PAH. There is a high correlation and statistically significant association between perivascular inflammation and pulmonary artery pressures and pulmonary vascular remodeling [4]. While inflammation in PAH has been relatively well described [23], whether it is cause or consequence in the pathogenesis of this disease remains unexplored. Recent studies have pointed Inflammation as a cause of PH as it precedes to altered immune processes leading to vascular remodeling that underlie the development of pulmonary arterial hypertension [24, 25]. Inflammation has been defined as a complex series of interactions among immunological soluble factors and cells that can arise in response to environmental insult to cardiopulmonary system [26].

Several animal models like monocrotaline (MCT), chronic hypoxia, and increased pulmonary blood flow have been studied to investigate pathological contribution of inflammation in the pathophysiology of PH. These animal models along with the mouse model of BMPR II gene deletion [27], the vasoactive intestinal polypeptide deletion model [28], the simian immunodeficiency virus macaque model (a model of HIV-PAH) [29], the mouse model of schistosomiasis-induced PAH [30] and the vascular endothelial growth factor (VEGF) receptor-2 blockade model using SU5416 revealed perivascular inflammatory cell infiltrates around remodeled vessels [10]. The common inflammatory cells involved consist mainly of bone-marrow-derived macrophages [31] immature dendritic cells (DCs) [32] and a minority of lymphocytes. Elevated serum and pulmonary cytokine and chemokine levels precede the development of pulmonary vascular remodeling.

Histopathology and Inflammatory Chemokines and Cytokines in PAH

Evidence from clinical and experimental studies suggests that inflammation is a key in progression of vascular remodeling in PAH. Lung biopsies from patients with PAH including animal models of PH showed by varying degrees of perivascular inflammatory infiltrates, comprising T- and B-lymphocytes, macrophages, dendritic cells, and mast cells compared with control vessels [33, 34]. Recently, correlations of the degree of perivascular inflammation score with intima plus media and adventitia thickness, respectively, and with mean pulmonary arterial pressure supports a role for perivascular inflammation in the processes of pulmonary vascular remodeling [3]. The increased prevalence of PAH in patients with various inflammatory diseases further indicates an important role for the inflammatory and immunological process in the pathogenesis of the disease [35, 36].

Consistent with an exaggerated acquired immunologic response in IPAH, T regulatory cells were decreased around remodeled pulmonary arteries. Overall, these findings support the concept of impaired immunity in both IPAH and APAH associated with collagen vascular disease; there is compelling evidence of or frank autoimmunity in the latter, and possibly in IPAH as well. The concept of an autoimmune [37] and inflammatory component to PH is supported by the presence of autoantibodies in patients with IPAH [38], the immunologic basis of collagen vascular diseases [39], and the presence of markers of inflammation systemically in patients with IPAH [23, 40]. Recent pathological and pathobiological assessment on human and animal models provide evidence that both pulmonary vascular cells and inflammatory cells are important local sources of chemokines and cytokines that can lead to pulmonary vascular remodeling in PAH [41, 42]. These include interleukin (IL)-1β, IL-6, IL-4, IL-13, TGF-β, monocyte chemoattractant protein-1, fractalkine, CCL5/RANTES, and tumor necrosis factor (TNF)-α.

Chemokines are small proteins, with a molecular weight of around 8–10 kilodalton (kDa), which act in cell signaling and/or as cytokines. Chemokines, like CCL2/MCP-1, CCL5/

RANTES and CX3CL1/Fractalkine, play a significant role in the pathogenesis of PH. For instance, MCP-1 (CCL2) is produced by vascular cells that stimulate monocytes/macrophage activation and migration through chemokine (C-C motif) receptor mediated response; plasma and lung tissue of patients with IPAH showed elevated levels of MCP-1 [43]. Furthermore, pulmonary artery smooth muscle cells (PASMC) and endothelial cells (EC) from patients with IPAH overexpressed MCP-1 and exhibited exaggerated migratory and proliferative responses by increased levels of the chemokine (C-C motif) receptor. Further, MCP-1-blocking antibodies blocked the migratory and proliferative response [43]. Likewise, RANTES (or CCL5) mediated the trafficking and homing of T-lymphocytes, monocytes monocytes, basophils, eosinophils, and natural killer cells through different chemokine receptors [44]. Moreover, Fractalkine (CX3CL1) is expressed as soluble or membrane-bound forms, with its actions being mediated through chemokine (C-X3-Cmotif) receptor 1 (fractalkine receptor) (CX3CR1). Fractalkine was upregulated on both CD4 and CD8 T lymphocytes in PAH [45] and it is likely that the increased expression of CX3CR1 on diseased PASMC contributes to the perivascular inflammatory cell influx and induce PASMC proliferation in MCT-induced PH [46].

Cytokines represent a large group of signaling proteins that are produced and secreted by cells of the immune system and regulate numerous biological processes including inflammation, immunity and hematopoiesis [47]. Inflammatory cytokines and chemokines seem to play a crucial role in the development of pulmonary hypertension. Cytokines emerged as major contributing factors in the pathogenesis of pulmonary hypertension as they can be used as biomarkers both for diagnosis and clinical outcome of patients with PH [44, 45, 48]. Here, we will review a few important common cytokines that have been well defined in clinical settings and studied experimental and transgenic animal models of PH like monocrotaline (MCT), Sugen + hypoxia and schistosoma-induced PH models. While these models cannot recapitulate human PAH, they provide a mechanistic insight into the connection between the host immune response and the pulmonary vascular disease, thus underscoring their utility as promising physiological surrogate of the human disease [4, 47].

IL-6 is an important signaling molecule and is produced by inflammatory cells, i.e. monocytes and T-lymphocytes. Studies have shown an increase in IL-6 in patients with PAH, and in rodents over-expression of IL-6 is adequate to cause experimental PH. Pharmacological blockade of IL-6 suppresses hypoxia-induced PH [49–51]. The IL6 – STAT3 – miR-17/92 – BMPR2 pathway play plausible role and may contribute in the pathogenesis of the pulmonary arterial remodeling [47]. Mice exposed to *S. mansoni*, as well as in the lung tissue of patients who died of this condition, showed

a significant increase in IL-6/STAT3 signaling [52]. However, lack of IL-6 signaling by IL-6 genetic deficiency or with a pharmacologic STAT3 inhibitor resulted into more severe PH phenotype, including worse remodeling and RV hypertrophy [52]. This finding suggests that in mice exposed to *Schistosoma*, IL-6/STAT3 signaling is upregulated but in a compensatory manner, and that blockade of this pathway is detrimental.

Patients with PAH in association with connective tissue diseases showed higher IL-8 serum levels than patients without PAH and thereby play an important role in the development of PAH [53]. IL-8 is known to have proangiogenic and anti-apoptotic activities and acts as a growth factor for endothelial cells [54]. IL-8 might be involved in the hypoxic pressure response of pulmonary vessels as it was found elevated in early stages of high altitude pulmonary edema [55]. Similarly, IL-10 is also implicated in PAH as elevated levels were found in patients to counterregulate against inflammatory response in lung [47]. Further, injections of IL-10 reduced the mean pulmonary arterial pressure in MCT rats and significantly improved survival [56]. Overall, experimental data, however, suggest a protective role of the anti-apoptotic and anti-inflammatory cytokine IL-10.

The prototypic TH-2 cytokines IL-4 and IL-13 are critical in *Schistosoma* infection in the mouse [57]. One of the potential mechanisms underlying the pathogenesis of schistosomiasis-associated PAH is inflammation. IL-13 is a key inducer of several Type-2 cytokine-dependent pathologies. IL-13 regulates inflammation, mucus production, tissue remodeling, and fibrosis. IL-13Rα1 is the canonical IL-13 signaling receptor, whereas IL-13Rα2 is thought to be a competitive non-signaling decoy receptor. Other studies have shown that dysregulation of IL-13 signaling is present in human PAH; whether IL-13 is pro-proliferative or anti-proliferative remains unclear [30, 58, 59]. Favoring the pro-proliferative role(s) of IL-13, we found evidence of enhanced PH in *S. mansoni*-infected mice lacking IL-13Rα2, suggesting that IL-13 signaling is an important mediator of the granulomatous and vascular response to schistosomiasis infection [60]. Thus, IL-13 ligand and receptors may serve as novel biomarkers in PH and a potential target for receptor-directed biologic therapies.

Th1 and Th2 Immune Response Mediated Inflammatory Response in PAH

The effector responses of CD4+ T cells are generally divided into Th1, Th2, and Th17 responses; all there subsets appear to be involved in the pathogenesis of PH. In the Th1/Th17-skewed response, the arteriole may be invaded by mononuclear cells, including cytotoxic T cells, autoreactive B cells, autoantibodies, mast cells, and activated macrophages expressing granulocyte-macrophage colony-stimulating factor (GM-CSFR), inducible nitric oxide synthase (iNOS), and leukotriene B4 (LTB4). Th17 effector cells are induced in parallel to Th1 (producing interferon-γ, TNFs and IL-2), and, such as Th1, polarized Th17 cells have the capacity to cause inflammation and autoimmune disease. Both Th1 and Th17 colocalize regionally and may require each other for recruitment into the region [61]. Th17 cells not only produces IL-17 but it also produce cytokines like, IL-6, TNF-α, GM-CSF, IL-21, and IL-22. Th2 cells produce the cytokines IL-4, IL-5, and IL-13, which are involved in allergic responses and the clearance of extracellular worm driven antigens. When immune dysregulation favors TH1/TH17 immunity reactions, TNF-α and IL-6 seem harmful mediators promoting vascular remodeling [50, 62], whereas IL-6 may exert a protective effect in pulmonary vascular injury induced by Schistosomiasis [52]. In Th2-driven responses, there are unique inflammatory patterns. The inflammatory response is characterized by the recruitment of Th2 lymphocytes, mast cells, eosinophils and macrophages to the lung, and by elevated expression of allergen-specific immunoglobulin-E (IgE) in the serum [63]. It has been suggested that the chronicity of Th2 cytokine-mediated airway inflammation that is characteristic of allergic asthma is explained by the presence of a macrophage-like antigen-presenting cell population that persists in the airway lumen [64]. Further, transforming growth factor-β-mediated immunity response is closely linked with enhanced Th2 cytokines, e.g. IL-4 and IL-13 activity (Fig. 2.1), which then drives a destructive PH phenotype through pSTAT-6 signaling [65].

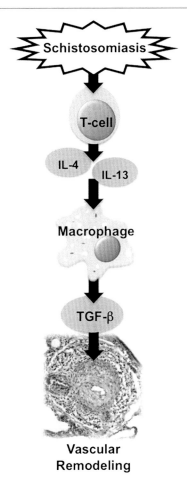

Fig. 2.1 Inflammatory pathways involved in the development of pulmonary arterial hypertension, highlighting the elucidated pathways triggered by *Schistosoma* infection

Macrophages and TGF-β Signaling in Pulmonary Vascular Remodeling

Among the inflammatory cells implicated in PAH, the monocyte/macrophage lineage has been consistently correlated with PH [31, 66–69]. However, macrophages efficiently respond to environmental signals with remarkable plasticity and undergo different forms of polarized activation that can be (simplistically) divided as classically activated (M1), alternatively activated (M2), and of an anti-inflammatory (regulatory) phenotype [70, 71]. Classically activated macrophages are effector phagocytes activated by interferon-γ and tumor necrosis factor (TNF-α). They produce inducible nitric oxide synthase and interleukin (IL)-12 and exhibit enhanced microbicidal or tumoricidal capacity [70]. On the other hand, M2-polarized macrophages are activated mostly by TH2 immune response mediated cytokines, IL-4 or IL-13 and express arginase-1 (Arg-1), found in inflammatory zone-1 (Fizz1), chitinase-3-like-3 (Ym1), and mannose receptor, C type lectin-1 [70–72]. M2 macrophages have been implicated in the pathogenesis of lung and other disorders via their ability to promote trophic, profibrotic, and angiogenic functions [73, 74]. The major characteristic of the third population, regulatory or anti-inflammatory macrophages, is the production of high IL-10 and low IL-12 levels and the promotion of immunosuppression [70, 72]. In the case of *Schistosoma* associated-PAH, once induced by Th2-CD4+ T-cells, macrophages stimulated by infection become alternatively activated (M2 phenotype) and, in the vascular adventitia, they can potentially represent the main cellular source of TGF-β (Fig. 2.1).

TGF-β signaling controls a plethora of cellular responses and is a member of a large family of multifunctional cytokines playing critical roles in embryogenesis, growth, wound repair, inflammation; TGF-β family has an important role in vascular homeostasis [75]. Abnormal TGF-β family signaling has been extensively linked to human PAH [76–78], and we and others have observed that blockade of TGF-β signaling suppresses PH due to monocrotaline or hypoxia in rodent models [65, 79, 80]. Recent studies have revealed significant insight into the mechanisms of the activation of TGF-β receptors through ligand binding, the activation of

Smad proteins through phosphorylation, the transcriptional regulation of target gene expression, and the control of Smad protein activity and degradation [81, 82]. Recently, we found the Th2 cytokines IL-4 and IL-13 to be necessary for TGF-β activation in mice exposed to *Schistosoma*; previously, we observed IL-13 gain-of-function to be sufficient for TGF-β activation [60, 65]. We also found up-regulation of the TGF-β signaling pathway manifest by increased Smad2/3 phosphorylation in areas of vascular remodeling in both the mouse model and human tissue from subjects who died from schistosomiasis-associated PH [60, 65]. *Schistosoma-induced* PH phenotype in mice was partially suppressed by blockade at the level of the TGF-β ligand, type 1 receptor function, or the intracellular signaling molecule Smad3. Coupled with the finding of IL-4 and IL-13 suppression by TGF-β signaling blockade, there may be a positive feedback loop of IL-4/IL-13 and TGF-β propagating the disease [65]. Thus, another potential target for patients with PAH is blockade of TGF-β signaling.

Recently, it has been shown that the accumulated macrophages expressed high levels of leukotriene A4 hydrolase (LTA4H), the biosynthetic enzyme for leukotriene B4 (LTB4) in both clinical tissue and the SU5416 (SU)/athymic rat model of severe PH [83].

In addition several growth factors, including PDGF, epidermal growth factor, VEGF, serotonin, and fibroblast growth factor 2, play an important role in the apoptosis-resistant phenotype and vascular remodeling in PAH [38, 84]. Some inflammatory cytokines, notably IL-6, trigger vascular smooth muscle cell proliferation through upregulated expression of VEGF and its receptor VEGFR2 [50]. Further, inflammatory end points can also be restrained by growth factors as serotonin reuptake inhibition attenuates matrix remodeling through reduced metalloproteinases as well as through reduced inflammatory cytokine expression in the MCT mouse model [85].

The Quasi Malignancy Paradigm of PAH

In their landmark 1962 paper describing altitude-related hypoxic PH, Vogel et al made the intriguing description of proliferative pulmonary vascular lesions:

> We have found what appear to be minute tumors of the lung… these tumors do not line the air spaces in any sense of the word. They are interstitial in position and are characteristically separated by a crown of capillaries from the airspace, thus establishing their interstitial location [86].

Since these early descriptions, it is now recognized that idiopathic PAH as well as other forms of PAH demonstrate lumen obliterating vascular lesions, often located at arterial bifurcations, termed 'plexiform lesions' [4]. Since this pathologic descriptive relationship was identified, further work

has delineated a molecular phenotype within these lesions that closely parallels neoplasia. For instance, vascular lesions in primary PAH have an abundance of clonal proliferative endothelial cells [87], microsatellite instability with disordered proliferation and apoptosis [88], somatic chromosomal abnormalities [89], and deregulated energetic metabolism [90]. Together, these properties share many of the hallmarks seen in cancer (albeit without the propensity for metastasis) as defined by Hanahan and Weinberg in their landmark review [91]. This work has led to a paradigm shift in the world of vascular biology away from a concept of increased vasomotor tone and elevated shear stress leading to PAH, to a more representative pathogenic concept of deregulated proliferative capacity of pulmonary vascular cells due to genetic susceptibility, surrounding inflammation, disordered angiogenesis, and aberrant growth/apoptotic signaling [92]. By parsing out the intricate pathobiology of these driving mechanisms in pulmonary vascular disease, there is hope for deriving therapies aimed at the primary defect of proliferative vascular lesions, in contrast to current therapies, which primarily target vasoconstriction. To illustrate, we will focus on two emerging – and interconnected – paradigms within pulmonary vascular disease, the role of hypoxic signaling as well as deregulated energetic metabolism, both features that parallel malignancy.

Hypoxia Signalling and PH

Many diseases associated with pulmonary hypertension, such as chronic obstructive pulmonary disease (COPD), interstitial lung disease, and obstructive sleep apnea result in either continuous or intermittent hypoxia. Many of these conditions have concomitant inflammation and parenchymal injury that may contribute to the vascular changes and resultant PH, but it remains clear that hypoxia and hypoxia signaling remain a driving force in not only WHO group III PH, but other forms – including PAH. The concept that PH and vascular remodeling can occur solely from hypoxia exposure is supported by observations of humans living at altitude. Persons living at high altitude are at risk for developing chronic elevations in PA pressure, only a fraction of which has a reversal with supplemental oxygen. Additionally, the lungs of high-altitude dwellers with PH have been shown to have vascular remodeling consisting of increased smooth muscularization of the small pulmonary arteries and thickened media and adventitia in the more proximal vessels [93]. Much of the work discussed is derived from animal models of PH, many incorporating hypoxia as the inducer of pulmonary vascular remodeling (Fig. 2.2). While there are inherent limitations in these models, they have illuminated aspects of pathobiology that are relevant to human disease and aid our understanding of how hypoxia contributes to the endothelial, smooth muscle, and adventitial phenotype of PH.

Fig. 2.2 Key mediators of hypoxia-induced pulmonary vascular disease, which result in increased vasomotor tone as well as pathologic vascular remodeling

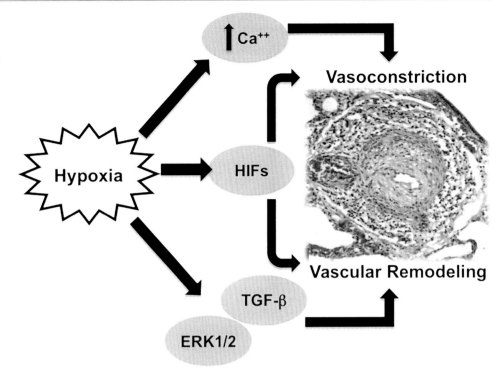

Murine modeling of hypoxic PH reveal that in the large PAs, there is an early adventitial expansion in response to hypoxia, with an increase in proliferating fibroblasts. Medial thickening follows thereafter, with a modest increase in proliferative and hypertrophied smooth muscle cells accompanied by increased matrix deposition [94]. It can be speculated that this initial vascular remodeling may be adaptive, as the adventitial and medial thickening decreases wall stress.

Mechanistically, there is a paucity of information regarding what pathways confer the proliferative phenotype to both the adventitial fibroblasts and medial smooth muscle cells. Studies of subpopulations of SMC that respond to hypoxia with a proliferation have been shown to have increased protein kinase C responses and activation of G-protein coupled receptor activation of ERK1/2 (Fig. 2.2), a signal transduction pathway demonstrated to be essential for hypoxia-triggers proliferation [95, 96]. Hypoxia inducible factor 1a (HIF-1α) activity in smooth muscle cells has also be critical for development of PH in a murine model of chronic hypoxic PH, the mechanism by which this transcriptional program confers vascular remodeling is yet to be delineated [97]. There is evidence to suggest that hypoxic conditions alter calcium homeostasis and ionic balance within PA SMCs (Fig. 2.2), leading to reduced potassium channel expression and increased [Ca2+], leading to enhanced pulmonary vasoconstriction and perhaps proliferation [98, 99]. Additionally, serotonin signaling appears to be necessary for PH related to chronic hypoxia [100].

The increase in matrix production – specifically elastin and collagen – is thought to be mediated through increased TGF-β signaling, a critical mediator of collagen synthesis. The importance in pulmonary vascular disease is revealed though use of a murine model containing a dominant negative mutation in the TGF-β receptor where chronic PH was attenuated [101]. Additionally, several groups have data that suggests that adventitial or interstitial lung fibroblasts can be activated by hypoxia with subsequent migration and differentiation into a perivascular smooth-muscle-like cell [102, 103].

As described above, PH is characterized by hypertrophy and proliferation of endothelial cells, along with subendothelial thickening – changes also observed with chronic hypoxic exposure. Hypoxia has been shown to lead to focal disruption and detachment between PA endothelial cells, along with damaged cell surface [104]. This hypoxia-induced endothelial damage increases expression of tissue factor, leading to a procoagulant state, along with increasing IL-1, IL-6, and a host of adhesion molecules that likely contribute to the inflammatory state of the pulmonary hypertensive response [105, 106]. It is also becoming increasingly clear that mitochondrial dysfunction within endothelial cells is a critical mediator of pulmonary vascular disease – a topic that will be explored below.

Disordered Mitochondria and Cellular Metabolism in PH

Mitochondrial function is of such critical importance, in the setting of hypoxia there is a highly conserved global program among all metazoan and mammalian cells to shift production of ATP from oxidative phosphorylation to lactic acid fermentation and glycolysis – a process known as the 'Pasteur effect'. However, this same phenomenon has been observed – first in tumor cells in the 1950s by Otto Warburg – in the setting of normal oxygen levels, termed the 'Warburg effect' [107]. In cancer cells, despite the considerably lower yield of ATP generated by glycolysis (2 molecules of ATP produced per glucose molecule from glycolysis versus 36 from oxidative metabolism), the Warburg effect is adaptive, allowing for increased ADP/ATP ratios, NADPH synthesis, and macromolecule generation (such as fatty acids, nucleotides, and carbohydrates) that is critical to support rapid and uncontrolled cellular proliferation [108]. A major paradigm shift has occurred in pulmonary vascular biology with the recognition that pulmonary artery smooth muscle and endothelial cells obtained from patients with IPAH have a dramatically increased glycolytic rate, further supported by [18F]fluoro-deoxy-D-glucose positron emission tomography scanning [109, 110]. This critical observation is opening new understanding into the pathobiology of PH, connecting inflammation and hypoxic signaling, and offers unique therapeutic targets to be explored.

Hypoxia Inducible Factors and Disordered Cellular Energenetics in PH

The glycolytic shift observed in normal physiologic adaptation to hypoxia, as well as in metabolically deranged tumor cells has been largely attributed to the up-regulation or increased stabilization of the hypoxia-inducible factors. HIF-α subunits, when combined with its β-subunit, transcriptionally activates more than 100 genes involved in energetic metabolism, apoptosis, cell cycle control, cellular migration, and angiogenesis [90]. In normoxic non-diseased states, hypoxia-inducible factors (consisting of HIF-1α or HIF-2α, each with different tissue expression patterns and collectively termed 'HIF') are subjected to rapid proteasomal degradation via prolyl hydroxylase and subsequent recognition and ubiquitination via the von Hippel-Lindau tumor suppressor protein [111]. The HIF transcriptional program is of critical importance in PH, as evidenced by increased expression of HIF-1α and HIF-1β in IPAH vascular lesions, in conjunction with increased HIF target vascular endothelial growth factor [8]. Additionally, in experimental models of PH, heterozygous knockout of either HIF-1α or HIF-2α is protective against development of PH [112, 113].

The contribution of HIF transcriptional regulation to the PH phenotype is varied. Increased HIF-1α expression has been shown to reduce voltage-gated K$^+$ channel currents in PASMCs, abrogating the hypoxic vasoconstriction response. Further, HIF-1α regulated expression of endothelin-1, a potent vasoconstrictor of the pulmonary vascular bed and

whose receptor is a common target of modern therapies [114]. HIF-1α has been shown to regulate the PASMC hypertrophic response in hypoxia via transient receptor potential Ca^{2+} channels [115]. However, HIF can also be directly linked to the disordered metabolic phenotype and disrupted mitochondrial function displayed by pulmonary vascular cells in PH.

HIF has potent effects on the metabolic status and mitochondrial function of pulmonary vascular cells. HIF transcriptional activity can be linked to a variety of extra- and intra-mitochondrial alterations. Pyruvate dehydrogenase kinase isozyme 1 (PDK1) is a ubiquitously expressed cytoplasmic inhibitor of pyruvate dehydrogenase (PDH) that is transcriptionally induced by HIF-1α [116, 117] (though PDK2 and 4 are the main forms expressed in pulmonary arteries-whether they are regulated by HIF-1α is unclear). PDH can be viewed as a mitochondrial 'gate keeper' enzyme as it is the critical regulator of pyruvate entry in the mitochondria. Glucose oxidation (resulting in conversion of pyruvate to acetyl-CoA) is mediated by PDH – inhibited by HIF-1α via PDK1 – and a fundamental step in the glycolytic switch observed in PH [118]. HIF acts at several other critical steps within the glycolysis pathway, for instance upregulation of GLUT1 and GLUT3, uniporter proteins that facilitate influx of glucose substrate. Additionally, HIF-1α induces lactate dehydrogenase A, leading to conversion of pyruvate into lactate, which in pulmonary microvascular endothelial cells has been shown to be critical for sustained rapid cell growth rates [119].

It is hypothesized that increased HIF in the vascular lesions may be the result of either direct hypoxia-like stabilization of HIF or deranged cell signaling that converges into enhanced normoxic HIF transcription. *In vitro* data, utilizing cultured endothelial cells from IPAH patients, suggests that HIF-1α may be stabilized via reduced NO mediated by decreased expression of manganese superoxide dismutase-2 (MnSOD2), which was previously observed in IPAH pulmonary tissue [120, 121]. Though the triggers of increased HIF in pulmonary vascular cells remains to be deciphered, there is a preponderance of data from human and animal studies pointing towards the importance of this transcriptional program in contributing to the vascular and metabolic remodeling in pulmonary vascular disease. Further, pulmonary vascular disease is associated with other aspects of mitochondrial dysfunction that lead to cellular apoptosis resistance, reduction in cellular mitochondrial content, and suppressed signaling results in the proproliferative vascular state of PH.

Mitochondrial Dysfunction in PH

Mitochondria play a key role in apoptosis as the source for proapoptotic molecules such as cytochrome C and apoptosis-inducing factor, which efflux to the cytoplasm through the mitochondrial transition pore. This voltage- and redox-sensitive channel is closed – conferring a resistance to apoptosis – by hyperpolarization of the mitochondrial membrane. Like many cancer cells, PASMCs have been demonstrated to have hyperpolarization of the mitochondrial membrane. Several mechanisms contribute to mitochondrial membrane polarization, but the foremost is carbohydrate metabolism (as detailed above). With PDH inhibition such as that seen in PH, there is resultant decrease in oxidative phosphorylation. This, in turn, leads to activation and translocation of glycogen synthase kinase 3β to the mitochondrial outer membrane, where it binds to the mitochondrial transition pore, trapping anions in the mitochondria and leading to increased membrane potential [122].

IPAH pulmonary artery endothelial cells have been shown to have a reduction in mitochondrial numbers per cell, as well as reduced mitochondrial DNA content [109]. Cellular mitochondrial content is continuously maintained by mitogenesis and selective degradation termed mitophagy. Mitophagy, when suppressed, is thought to result in accumulation of dysfunctional mitochondria. The intracellular mitochondrial network is critical for maintaining mitochondrial signaling and appropriate proliferative and apoptotic signaling. Fission is largely dependent on the HIF-1α regulated protein dynamin-related protein 1 (DRP-1), a GTPase that assembles into an oligomeric ring in the outer mitochondrial membrane and allowing for fair distribution of mitochondria when cell division occurs. It has been observed that PASMCs from PAH patients have increased activity of DRP-1, and when inhibited there is decreased proliferation that attenuated PAH in several animal models of the disease [123].

An essential byproduct of oxidative phosphorylation is mitochondrial-derived reactive oxygen species (mROS) in the form of superoxide – which is increasingly recognized as an important cellular signaling molecule rather than simple toxic byproduct. mROS is altered to stable H_2O_2 via MnSOD, subsequently diffusing to extra-mitochondrial targets such as membrane voltage-gated K^+ channels, leading to influx of Ca^{2+}, and an increased vasoconstriction and proliferative response [124]. Though disordered metabolism is an emerging component of the complex pathobiologic understanding of PAH, informed by decades of work in cancer biology, there is hope that it will provide new therapeutic angles for patients with PAH.

Conclusion

A detailed descriptive pathologic understanding of PAH has been informed by over a decade of work detailing the complex immunologic, hypoxic signaling, and disordered metabolic state that underlies the diseased pulmonary vasculature. While current therapies – including prostanoids, endothelin receptor antagonists, and phosphodi-esterase inhibitors – primarily target the vasoconstrictive component of PAH, there is hope that novel therapies targeted at the underlying pathobiologic mechanisms described herein will result in stabilization or even reversal of the pulmonary vasculopathy, resulting in improved outcomes for patients.

References

1. Simonneau G, Gatzoulis MA, Adatia I, et al. Updated clinical classification of pulmonary hypertension. J Am Coll Cardiol. 2013;62:D34–41.
2. Tuder RM. How do we measure pathology in PAH (lung and RV) and what does it tell us about the disease. Drug Discov Today. 2014;19:1257–63.
3. Stacher E, Graham BB, Hunt JM, et al. Modern age pathology of pulmonary arterial hypertension. Am J Respir Crit Care Med. 2012;186:261–72.
4. Tuder RM, Stacher E, Robinson J, Kumar R, Graham BB. Pathology of pulmonary hypertension. Clin Chest Med. 2013;34:639–50.
5. Tuder RM, Marecki JC, Richter A, Fijalkowska I, Flores S. Pathology of pulmonary hypertension. Clin Chest Med. 2007;28:23–42. vii.
6. Yaginuma G, Mohri H, Takahashi T. Distribution of arterial lesions and collateral pathways in the pulmonary hypertension of congenital heart disease: a computer aided reconstruction study. Thorax. 1990;45:586–90.
7. Cool CD, Stewart JS, Werahera P, et al. Three-dimensional reconstruction of pulmonary arteries in plexiform pulmonary hypertension using cell-specific markers. Evidence for a dynamic and heterogeneous process of pulmonary endothelial cell growth. Am J Pathol. 1999;155:411–9.
8. Tuder RM, Chacon M, Alger L, et al. Expression of angiogenesis-related molecules in plexiform lesions in severe pulmonary hypertension: evidence for a process of disordered angiogenesis. J Pathol. 2001;195:367–74.
9. Santos S, Peinado VI, Ramirez J, et al. Characterization of pulmonary vascular remodelling in smokers and patients with mild COPD. Eur Respir J. 2002;19:632–8.
10. Taraseviciene-Stewart L, Kasahara Y, Alger L, et al. Inhibition of the VEGF receptor 2 combined with chronic hypoxia causes cell death-dependent pulmonary endothelial cell proliferation and severe pulmonary hypertension. FASEB J. 2001;15:427–38.
11. Campbell AI, Zhao Y, Sandhu R, Stewart DJ. Cell-based gene transfer of vascular endothelial growth factor attenuates monocrotaline-induced pulmonary hypertension. Circulation. 2001;104:2242–8.
12. Sakao S, Taraseviciene-Stewart L, Lee JD, Wood K, Cool CD, Voelkel NF. Initial apoptosis is followed by increased proliferation of apoptosis-resistant endothelial cells. FASEB J. 2005;19:1178–80.
13. Thompson K, Rabinovitch M. Exogenous leukocyte and endogenous elastases can mediate mitogenic activity in pulmonary artery smooth muscle cells by release of extracellular-matrix bound basic fibroblast growth factor. J Cell Physiol. 1996;166:495–505.
14. Alastalo TP, Li M, Perez VJ, et al. Disruption of PPARgamma/beta-catenin-mediated regulation of apelin impairs BMP-induced mouse and human pulmonary arterial EC survival. J Clin Invest. 2011;121:3735–46.
15. Poiani GJ, Tozzi CA, Yohn SE, et al. Collagen and elastin metabolism in hypertensive pulmonary arteries of rats. Circ Res. 1990;66:968–78.

16. Chazova I, Loyd JE, Zhdanov VS, Newman JH, Belenkov Y, Meyrick B. Pulmonary artery adventitial changes and venous involvement in primary pulmonary hypertension. Am J Pathol. 1995;146:389–97.

17. Palevsky HI, Schloo BL, Pietra GG, et al. Primary pulmonary hypertension. Vascular structure, morphometry, and responsiveness to vasodilator agents. Circulation. 1989;80:1207–21.

18. Yi ES, Kim H, Ahn H, et al. Distribution of obstructive intimal lesions and their cellular phenotypes in chronic pulmonary hypertension. A morphometric and immunohistochemical study. Am J Respir Crit Care Med. 2000;162:1577–86.

19. Yamaki S, Wagenvoort CA. Comparison of primary plexogenic arteriopathy in adults and children. A morphometric study in 40 patients. Br Heart J. 1985;54:428–34.

20. Stenmark KR, Davie N, Frid M, Gerasimovskaya E, Das M. Role of the adventitia in pulmonary vascular remodeling. Physiology (Bethesda). 2006;21:134–45.

21. Hu Y, Zhang Z, Torsney E, et al. Abundant progenitor cells in the adventitia contribute to atherosclerosis of vein grafts in ApoE-deficient mice. J Clin Invest. 2004;113:1258–65.

22. Torsney E, Hu Y, Xu Q. Adventitial progenitor cells contribute to arteriosclerosis. Trends Cardiovasc Med. 2005;15:64–8.

23. Dorfmuller P, Perros F, Balabanian K, Humbert M. Inflammation in pulmonary arterial hypertension. Eur Respir J. 2003;22: 358–63.

24. Tamosiuniene R, Tian W, Dhillon G, et al. Regulatory T cells limit vascular endothelial injury and prevent pulmonary hypertension. Circ Res. 2011;109:867–79.

25. Rabinovitch M, Guignabert C, Humbert M, Nicolls MR. Inflammation and immunity in the pathogenesis of pulmonary arterial hypertension. Circ Res. 2014;115:165–75.

26. Nathan C. Points of control in inflammation. Nature. 2002;420: 846–52.

27. Hong KH, Lee YJ, Lee E, et al. Genetic ablation of the BMPR2 gene in pulmonary endothelium is sufficient to predispose to pulmonary arterial hypertension. Circulation. 2008;118:722–30.

28. Hamidi SA, Prabhakar S, Said SI. Enhancement of pulmonary vascular remodelling and inflammatory genes with VIP gene deletion. Eur Respir J. 2008;31:135–9.

29. Marecki JC, Cool CD, Parr JE, et al. HIV-1 Nef is associated with complex pulmonary vascular lesions in SHIV-nef-infected macaques. Am J Respir Crit Care Med. 2006;174:437–45.

30. Crosby A, Jones FM, Southwood M, et al. Pulmonary vascular remodeling correlates with lung eggs and cytokines in murine schistosomiasis. Am J Respir Crit Care Med. 2010;181:279–88.

31. Sahara M, Sata M, Morita T, Nakamura K, Hirata Y, Nagai R. Diverse contribution of bone marrow-derived cells to vascular remodeling associated with pulmonary arterial hypertension and arterial neointimal formation. Circulation. 2007;115:509–17.

32. Perros F, Dorfmuller P, Souza R, et al. Dendritic cell recruitment in lesions of human and experimental pulmonary hypertension. Eur Respir J. 2007;29:462–8.

33. Cool CD, Kennedy D, Voelkel NF, Tuder RM. Pathogenesis and evolution of plexiform lesions in pulmonary hypertension associated with scleroderma and human immunodeficiency virus infection. Hum Pathol. 1997;28:434–42.

34. Mauad T, Pozzan G, Lancas T, et al. Immunopathological aspects of schistosomiasis-associated pulmonary arterial hypertension. J Infect. 2014;68:90–8.

35. Thurnheer R, Jenni R, Russi EW, Greminger P, Speich R. Hyperthyroidism and pulmonary hypertension. J Intern Med. 1997;242:185–8.

36. Fagan KA, Badesch DB. Pulmonary hypertension associated with connective tissue disease. Prog Cardiovasc Dis. 2002;45:225–34.

37. Mouthon L, Guillevin L, Humbert M. Pulmonary arterial hypertension: an autoimmune disease? Eur Respir J. 2005;26:986–8.

38. Hassoun PM, Mouthon L, Barbera JA, et al. Inflammation, growth factors, and pulmonary vascular remodeling. J Am Coll Cardiol. 2009;54:S10–9.

39. Dib H, Tamby MC, Bussone G, et al. Targets of anti-endothelial cell antibodies in pulmonary hypertension and scleroderma. Eur Respir J. 2012;39:1405–14.

40. Soon E, Holmes AM, Treacy CM, et al. Elevated levels of inflammatory cytokines predict survival in idiopathic and familial pulmonary arterial hypertension. Circulation. 2010;122: 920–7.

41. Huertas A, Perros F, Tu L, et al. Immune dysregulation and endothelial dysfunction in pulmonary arterial hypertension: a complex interplay. Circulation. 2014;129:1332–40.

42. Ricard N, Tu L, Le HM, et al. Increased pericyte coverage mediated by endothelial-derived fibroblast growth factor-2 and interleukin-6 is a source of smooth muscle-like cells in pulmonary hypertension. Circulation. 2014;129:1586–97.

43. Sanchez O, Marcos E, Perros F, et al. Role of endothelium-derived CC chemokine ligand 2 in idiopathic pulmonary arterial hypertension. Am J Respir Crit Care Med. 2007;176:1041–7.

44. Dorfmuller P, Zarka V, Durand-Gasselin I, et al. Chemokine RANTES in severe pulmonary arterial hypertension. Am J Respir Crit Care Med. 2002;165:534–9.

45. Balabanian K, Foussat A, Dorfmuller P, et al. CX(3)C chemokine fractalkine in pulmonary arterial hypertension. Am J Respir Crit Care Med. 2002;165:1419–25.

46. Perros F, Dorfmuller P, Souza R, et al. Fractalkine-induced smooth muscle cell proliferation in pulmonary hypertension. Eur Respir J. 2007;29:937–43.

47. Groth A, Vrugt B, Brock M, Speich R, Ulrich S, Huber LC. Inflammatory cytokines in pulmonary hypertension. Respir Res. 2014;15:47.

48. Price LC, Wort SJ, Perros F, et al. Inflammation in pulmonary arterial hypertension. Chest. 2012;141:210–21.

49. Savale L, Tu L, Rideau D, et al. Impact of interleukin-6 on hypoxia-induced pulmonary hypertension and lung inflammation in mice. Respir Res. 2009;10:6.

50. Steiner MK, Syrkina OL, Kolliputi N, Mark EJ, Hales CA, Waxman AB. Interleukin-6 overexpression induces pulmonary hypertension. Circ Res. 2009;104:236–44. 28p.

51. Humbert M, Monti G, Brenot F, et al. Increased interleukin-1 and interleukin-6 serum concentrations in severe primary pulmonary hypertension. Am J Respir Crit Care Med. 1995;151:1628–31.

52. Graham BB, Chabon J, Kumar R, et al. Protective role of IL-6 in vascular remodeling in Schistosoma pulmonary hypertension. Am J Respir Cell Mol Biol. 2013;49:951–9.

53. Riccieri V, Stefanantoni K, Vasile M, et al. Abnormal plasma levels of different angiogenic molecules are associated with different clinical manifestations in patients with systemic sclerosis. Clin Exp Rheumatol. 2011;29:S46–52.

54. Li A, Varney ML, Valasek J, Godfrey M, Dave BJ, Singh RK. Autocrine role of interleukin-8 in induction of endothelial cell proliferation, survival, migration and MMP-2 production and angiogenesis. Angiogenesis. 2005;8:63–71.

55. Kubo K, Hanaoka M, Hayano T, et al. Inflammatory cytokines in BAL fluid and pulmonary hemodynamics in high-altitude pulmonary edema. Respir Physiol. 1998;111:301–10.

56. Ito T, Okada T, Miyashita H, et al. Interleukin-10 expression mediated by an adeno-associated virus vector prevents monocrotaline-induced pulmonary arterial hypertension in rats. Circ Res. 2007;101:734–41.

57. Chiaramonte MG, Schopf LR, Neben TY, Cheever AW, Donaldson DD, Wynn TA. IL-13 is a key regulatory cytokine for Th2 cell-mediated pulmonary granuloma formation and IgE responses induced by Schistosoma mansoni eggs. J Immunol. 1999;162: 920–30.

58. Cho WK, Lee CM, Kang MJ, et al. IL-13 receptor alpha2-arginase 2 pathway mediates IL-13-induced pulmonary hypertension. Am J Physiol Lung Cell Mol Physiol. 2013;304:L112–24.

59. Hecker M, Zaslona Z, Kwapiszewska G, et al. Dysregulation of the IL-13 receptor system: a novel pathomechanism in pulmonary arterial hypertension. Am J Respir Crit Care Med. 2010;182:805–18.

60. Graham BB, Mentink-Kane MM, El-Haddad H, et al. Schistosomiasis-induced experimental pulmonary hypertension: role of interleukin-13 signaling. Am J Pathol. 2010;177:1549–61.

61. Luger D, Silver PB, Tang J, et al. Either a Th17 or a Th1 effector response can drive autoimmunity: conditions of disease induction affect dominant effector category. J Exp Med. 2008;205:799–810.

62. Fujita M, Shannon JM, Irvin CG, et al. Overexpression of tumor necrosis factor-alpha produces an increase in lung volumes and pulmonary hypertension. Am J Physiol Lung Cell Mol Physiol. 2001;280:L39–49.

63. Wynn TA, Chawla A, Pollard JW. Macrophage biology in development, homeostasis and disease. Nature. 2013;496:445–55.

64. Julia V, Hessel EM, Malherbe L, Glaichenhaus N, O'Garra A, Coffman RL. A restricted subset of dendritic cells captures airborne antigens and remains able to activate specific T cells long after antigen exposure. Immunity. 2002;16:271–83.

65. Graham BB, Chabon J, Gebreab L, et al. Transforming growth factor-beta signaling promotes pulmonary hypertension caused by *Schistosoma mansoni*. Circulation. 2013;128:1354–64.

66. Tuder RM, Groves B, Badesch DB, Voelkel NF. Exuberant endothelial cell growth and elements of inflammation are present in plexiform lesions of pulmonary hypertension. Am J Pathol. 1994;144:275–85.

67. Pinto RF, Higuchi ML, Aiello VD. Decreased numbers of T-lymphocytes and predominance of recently recruited macrophages in the walls of peripheral pulmonary arteries from 26 patients with pulmonary hypertension secondary to congenital cardiac shunts. Cardiovasc Pathol. 2004;13:268–75.

68. Frid MG, Brunetti JA, Burke DL, et al. Hypoxia-induced pulmonary vascular remodeling requires recruitment of circulating mesenchymal precursors of a monocyte/macrophage lineage. Am J Pathol. 2006;168:659–69.

69. Vergadi E, Chang MS, Lee C, et al. Early macrophage recruitment and alternative activation are critical for the later development of hypoxia-induced pulmonary hypertension. Circulation. 2011;123:1986–95.

70. Mosser DM, Edwards JP. Exploring the full spectrum of macrophage activation. Nat Rev Immunol. 2008;8:958–69.

71. Edwards JP, Zhang X, Frauwirth KA, Mosser DM. Biochemical and functional characterization of three activated macrophage populations. J Leukoc Biol. 2006;80:1298–307.

72. Gordon S, Martinez FO. Alternative activation of macrophages: mechanism and functions. Immunity. 2010;32:593–604.

73. Mora AL, Torres-Gonzalez E, Rojas M, et al. Activation of alveolar macrophages via the alternative pathway in herpesvirus-induced lung fibrosis. Am J Respir Cell Mol Biol. 2006;35:466–73.

74. Shaykhiev R, Krause A, Salit J, et al. Smoking-dependent reprogramming of alveolar macrophage polarization: implication for pathogenesis of chronic obstructive pulmonary disease. J Immunol. 2009;183:2867–83.

75. Shi Y, Massague J. Mechanisms of TGF-beta signaling from cell membrane to the nucleus. Cell. 2003;113:685–700.

76. Deng Z, Morse JH, Slager SL, et al. Familial primary pulmonary hypertension [gene PPH1] is caused by mutations in the bone morphogenetic protein receptor-II gene. Am J Hum Genet. 2000;67:737–44.

77. Lane KB, Machado RD, Pauciulo MW, et al. Heterozygous germline mutations in BMPR2, encoding a TGF-beta receptor, cause familial primary pulmonary hypertension. Nat Genet. 2000;26:81–4.

78. Richter A, Yeager ME, Zaiman A, Cool CD, Voelkel NF, Tuder RM. Impaired transforming growth factor-beta signaling in idiopathic pulmonary arterial hypertension. Am J Respir Crit Care Med. 2004;170:1340–8.

79. Ma W, Han W, Greer PA, et al. Calpain mediates pulmonary vascular remodeling in rodent models of pulmonary hypertension, and its inhibition attenuates pathologic features of disease. J Clin Invest. 2011;121:4548–66.

80. Zaiman AL, Podowski M, Medicherla S, et al. Role of the TGF-beta/Alk5 signaling pathway in monocrotaline-induced pulmonary hypertension. Am J Respir Crit Care Med. 2008;177:896–905.

81. Kamato D, Burch ML, Piva TJ, et al. Transforming growth factor-beta signalling: role and consequences of Smad linker region phosphorylation. Cell Signal. 2013;25:2017–24.

82. You H, Gobert GN, Jones MK, Zhang W, McManus DP. Signalling pathways and the host-parasite relationship: putative targets for control interventions against schistosomiasis: signalling pathways and future anti-schistosome therapies. Bioessays. 2011;33:203–14.

83. Tian W, Jiang X, Tamosiuniene R, et al. Blocking macrophage leukotriene b4 prevents endothelial injury and reverses pulmonary hypertension. Sci Transl Med. 2013;5:200ra117.

84. Perros F, Montani D, Dorfmuller P, et al. Platelet-derived growth factor expression and function in idiopathic pulmonary arterial hypertension. Am J Respir Crit Care Med. 2008;178:81–8.

85. Li XQ, Wang HM, Yang CG, Zhang XH, Han DD, Wang HL. Fluoxetine inhibited extracellular matrix of pulmonary artery and inflammation of lungs in monocrotaline-treated rats. Acta Pharmacol Sin. 2011;32:217–22.

86. Vogel JH, Weaver WF, Rose RL, Blount Jr SG, Grover RF. Pulmonary hypertension on exertion in normal man living at 10,150 feet [Leadville, Colorado]. Med Thorac. 1962;19:461–77.

87. Lee SD, Shroyer KR, Markham NE, Cool CD, Voelkel NF, Tuder RM. Monoclonal endothelial cell proliferation is present in primary but not secondary pulmonary hypertension. J Clin Invest. 1998;101:927–34.

88. Yeager ME, Halley GR, Golpon HA, Voelkel NF, Tuder RM. Microsatellite instability of endothelial cell growth and apoptosis genes within plexiform lesions in primary pulmonary hypertension. Circ Res. 2001;88:E2–11.

89. Aldred MA, Comhair SA, Varella-Garcia M, et al. Somatic chromosome abnormalities in the lungs of patients with pulmonary arterial hypertension. Am J Respir Crit Care Med. 2010;182:1153–60.

90. Tuder RM, Davis LA, Graham BB. Targeting energetic metabolism: a new frontier in the pathogenesis and treatment of pulmonary hypertension. Am J Respir Crit Care Med. 2012;185:260–6.

91. Hanahan D, Weinberg RA. Hallmarks of cancer: the next generation. Cell. 2011;144:646–74.

92. Rai PR, Cool CD, King JA, et al. The cancer paradigm of severe pulmonary arterial hypertension. Am J Respir Crit Care Med. 2008;178:558–64.

93. Arias-Stella J, Saldana M. The terminal portion of the pulmonary arterial tree in people native to high altitudes. Circulation. 1963;28:915–25.

94. Kobs RW, Muvarak NE, Eickhoff JC, Chesler NC. Linked mechanical and biological aspects of remodeling in mouse pulmonary arteries with hypoxia-induced hypertension. Am J Physiol Heart Circ Physiol. 2005;288:H1209–17.

95. Dempsey EC, Das M, Frid MG, Stenmark KR. Unique growth properties of neonatal pulmonary vascular cells: importance of time- and site-specific responses, cell-cell interaction, and synergy. J Perinatol. 1996;16:S2–11.

96. Lanner MC, Raper M, Pratt WM, Rhoades RA. Heterotrimeric G proteins and the platelet-derived growth factor receptor-beta contribute to hypoxic proliferation of smooth muscle cells. Am J Respir Cell Mol Biol. 2005;33:412–9.

97. Ball MK, Waypa GB, Mungai PT, et al. Regulation of hypoxia-induced pulmonary hypertension by vascular smooth muscle

hypoxia-inducible factor-1alpha. Am J Respir Crit Care Med. 2014;189:314–24.

98. Weir EK, Olschewski A. Role of ion channels in acute and chronic responses of the pulmonary vasculature to hypoxia. Cardiovasc Res. 2006;71:630–41.

99. Remillard CV, Yuan JX. High altitude pulmonary hypertension: role of K+ and Ca2+ channels. High Alt Med Biol. 2005;6:133–46.

100. Launay JM, Herve P, Peoc'h K, et al. Function of the serotonin 5-hydroxytryptamine 2B receptor in pulmonary hypertension. Nat Med. 2002;8:1129–35.

101. Chen YF, Feng JA, Li P, et al. Dominant negative mutation of the TGF-beta receptor blocks hypoxia-induced pulmonary vascular remodeling. J Appl Physiol. 2006;100:564–71.

102. Jones R, Jacobson M, Steudel W. alpha-smooth-muscle actin and microvascular precursor smooth-muscle cells in pulmonary hypertension. Am J Respir Cell Mol Biol. 1999;20:582–94.

103. Sobin SS, Tremer HM, Hardy JD, Chiodi HP. Changes in arteriole in acute and chronic hypoxic pulmonary hypertension and recovery in rat. J Appl Physiol Respir Environ Exerc Physiol. 1983;55:1445–55.

104. Barbera JA. Mechanisms of development of chronic obstructive pulmonary disease-associated pulmonary hypertension. Pulm Circ. 2013;3:160–4.

105. Ten VS, Pinsky DJ. Endothelial response to hypoxia: physiologic adaptation and pathologic dysfunction. Curr Opin Crit Care. 2002;8:242–50.

106. Ali MH, Schildt SA, Chandel NS, Hynes KL, Schumacker PT, Gewertz BL. Endothelial permeability and IL-6 production during hypoxia: role of ROS in signal transduction. Am J Physiol. 1999;277:L1057–65.

107. Cottrill KA, Chan SY. Metabolic dysfunction in pulmonary hypertension: the expanding relevance of the Warburg effect. Eur J Clin Invest. 2013;43:855–65.

108. Kaelin Jr WG, Thompson CB. Q&A: Cancer: clues from cell metabolism. Nature. 2010;465:562–4.

109. Xu W, Koeck T, Lara AR, et al. Alterations of cellular bioenergetics in pulmonary artery endothelial cells. Proc Natl Acad Sci U S A. 2007;104:1342–7.

110. Marsboom G, Wietholt C, Haney CR, et al. Lung [1][8] F-fluorodeoxyglucose positron emission tomography for diagnosis and monitoring of pulmonary arterial hypertension. Am J Respir Crit Care Med. 2012;185:670–9.

111. Semenza GL. Oxygen sensing, hypoxia-inducible factors, and disease pathophysiology. Annu Rev Pathol. 2014;9:47–71.

112. Yu AY, Shimoda LA, Iyer NV, et al. Impaired physiological responses to chronic hypoxia in mice partially deficient for hypoxia-inducible factor 1alpha. J Clin Invest. 1999;103:691–6.

113. Brusselmans K, Compernolle V, Tjwa M, et al. Heterozygous deficiency of hypoxia-inducible factor-2alpha protects mice against pulmonary hypertension and right ventricular dysfunction during prolonged hypoxia. J Clin Invest. 2003;111:1519–27.

114. Whitman EM, Pisarcik S, Luke T, et al. Endothelin-1 mediates hypoxia-induced inhibition of voltage-gated K+ channel expression in pulmonary arterial myocytes. Am J Physiol Lung Cell Mol Physiol. 2008;294:L309–18.

115. Wang J, Weigand L, Lu W, Sylvester JT, Semenza GL, Shimoda LA. Hypoxia inducible factor 1 mediates hypoxia-induced TRPC expression and elevated intracellular Ca2+ in pulmonary arterial smooth muscle cells. Circ Res. 2006;98:1528–37.

116. Bowker-Kinley MM, Davis WI, Wu P, Harris RA, Popov KM. Evidence for existence of tissue-specific regulation of the mammalian pyruvate dehydrogenase complex. Biochem J. 1998;329(Pt 1): 191–6.

117. Hitosugi T, Fan J, Chung TW, et al. Tyrosine phosphorylation of mitochondrial pyruvate dehydrogenase kinase 1 is important for cancer metabolism. Mol Cell. 2011;44:864–77.

118. Kim JW, Dang CV. Multifaceted roles of glycolytic enzymes. Trends Biochem Sci. 2005;30:142–50.

119. Parra-Bonilla G, Alvarez DF, Al-Mehdi AB, Alexeyev M, Stevens T. Critical role for lactate dehydrogenase A in aerobic glycolysis that sustains pulmonary microvascular endothelial cell proliferation. Am J Physiol Lung Cell Mol Physiol. 2010;299:L513–22.

120. Fijalkowska I, Xu W, Comhair SA, et al. Hypoxia inducible-factor1alpha regulates the metabolic shift of pulmonary hypertensive endothelial cells. Am J Pathol. 2010;176:1130–8.

121. Bowers R, Cool C, Murphy RC, et al. Oxidative stress in severe pulmonary hypertension. Am J Respir Crit Care Med. 2004;169: 764–9.

122. Paulin R, Michelakis ED. The metabolic theory of pulmonary arterial hypertension. Circ Res. 2014;115:148–64.

123. Marsboom G, Toth PT, Ryan JJ, et al. Dynamin-related protein 1-mediated mitochondrial mitotic fission permits hyperproliferation of vascular smooth muscle cells and offers a novel therapeutic target in pulmonary hypertension. Circ Res. 2012;110:1484–97.

124. Platoshyn O, Golovina VA, Bailey CL, et al. Sustained membrane depolarization and pulmonary artery smooth muscle cell proliferation. Am J Physiol Cell Physiol. 2000;279:C1540–9.

Pulmonary Hypertension in Patients Without Pulmonary Arterial Hypertension

Jessica Huston, Nathan D. Hatton, and John J. Ryan

Introduction

Pulmonary Hypertension (PH) in clinical practice is more commonly secondary to chronic left sided heart disease and/ or chronic hypoxic lung disease, than due to idiopathic Pulmonary Arterial Hypertension (iPAH) (Fig. 3.1) [1, 2]. In the current World Health Organization (WHO) classification system of PH, PH secondary to left heart disease is categorized as Group 2 PH, with PH secondary to chronic lung disease being classified as Group 3 PH [3]. The causes of Group 2 PH include heart failure with reduced ejection fraction (HFrEF), heart failure with preserved ejection fraction (HFpEF), mitral and aortic valve disease [4], in addition to restrictive and constrictive physiology (Fig. 3.2). Group 3 PH is most commonly caused by chronic hypoxic lung disease, in particular chronic obstructive pulmonary disease (COPD) and interstitial lung disease (ILD) (Fig. 3.3) [5]. Many of the risk factors for cardiac and pulmonary etiologies of PH overlap, such as smoking, sleep apnea and obesity, and therefore characterizing patients as Group 2 or Group 3 PH can be challenging. Other syndromes such as sarcoidosis and connective tissue disease (especially scleroderma) can involve both the heart and lung tissue, thereby creating a clinical phenotype of PH that is difficult to define. In this chapter we will discuss the epidemiology, cellular mechanisms, clinical diagnosis and evaluation, management and outcomes of Group 2 and Group 3 PH (Table 3.1; Fig. 3.4). We will also discuss syndromes and scenarios where there is difficulty in ascertaining the etiology of PH. We will finally discuss future directions in therapeutics and diagnostics of Group 2 and Group 3 PH.

J. Huston, MD
Division of Cardiovascular Medicine, Department of Medicine, University of Utah, Salt Lake City, UT USA

N.D. Hatton, MS, MD
Division of Pulmonary Medicine, Department of Medicine, University of Utah, Salt Lake City, UT USA

J.J. Ryan, MD, FAHA, FACC (✉)
Division of Cardiovascular Medicine, Department of Medicine, University of Utah, Salt Lake City, UT USA

Division of Cardiovascular Medicine,
University of Utah Health Science Center,
30 North 1900 East, Room 4A100, Salt Lake City,
UT 84132, USA
e-mail: john.ryan@hsc.utah.edu

Pulmonary Hypertension Secondary to Left Sided Heart Disease

Epidemiology

Up to 250,000 patients in the United States have Group 2 PH, thereby making it much more prevalent than other causes of PH [7]. Approximately 60–70 % of patients with HFpEF and HFrEF develop PH [8] and up to half of patients referred to heart transplant clinics have pulmonary vascular resistance (PVR) greater than 2 Wood Units [9]. The development of PH in these patient populations is associated with a poor prognosis [10, 11]. In a study of HFrEF patients assessed for PH by echocardiogram, the 28 month mortality was almost 57 % in patients with PH compared to 17 % in HFrEF patients without PH [12]. Additionally, transplanted patients with PH have a greater risk of developing post-operative right ventricular failure and an increased risk of mortality [13]. In a community study of HFpEF patients, evidence of PH on echocardiography independently predicted survival [8]. However, treating patients with PH secondary to severe systolic heart failure with pulmonary vasodilators (prostaglandins) has caused pulmonary edema and death [13]. Thus, although PH predicts mortality, targeted PH treatments in PH-HFpEF may not improve outcomes, as will be subsequently discussed [4].

Pathophysiology

Elevated LV filling pressures lead to a passive increase in mPAP in order to maintain forward flow. Typically, this

© Springer International Publishing Switzerland 2016
B.A. Maron et al. (eds.), *Pulmonary Hypertension: Basic Science to Clinical Medicine*, DOI 10.1007/978-3-319-23594-3_3

Fig. 3.1 The prevalence "of pulmonary hypertension in Armadale, Australia and surrounding regions, December 2009 (Reproduced with permission from [1])

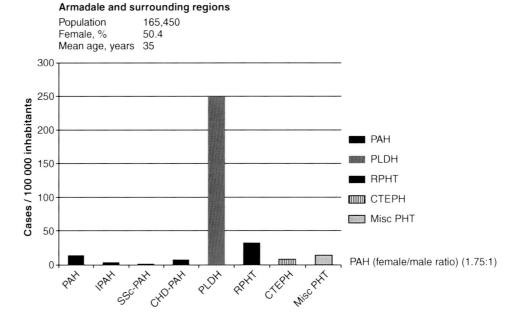

Fig. 3.2 Causes of Group 2 PH (Reproduced with permission from [4])

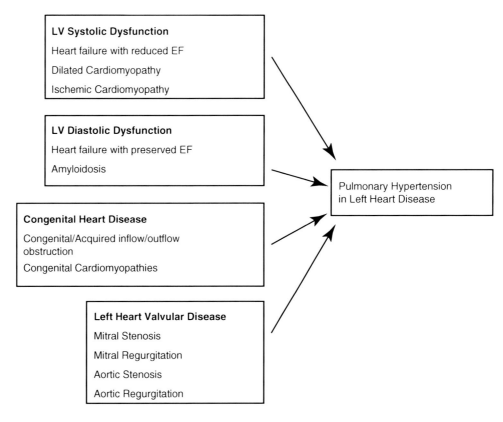

increase in mPAP is "proportionate" to the elevated LV filling pressure with a normal transpulmonary gradient and pulmonary vascular resistance ($\leq$12 mmHg and $\leq$2.5 WU, respectively). This is referred to as "proportionate" or "passive" PVH. However, in some patients with left heart disease, the mPAP increases quite markedly in response to the elevated left sided filling pressure due to vasoconstriction or remodeling of the pulmonary arteries similar to PAH. This results in an elevated transpulmonary gradient (TPG) and PVR (>12 mmHg and >2.5 WU, respectively), referred to as mixed or reactive pulmonary venous hypertension. Mixed PVH can be either reversible with vasodilators when vasoconstriction is dominant or is fixed due to remodeling of the pulmonary arteries [14].

Fig. 3.3 Causes of Group 3 PH

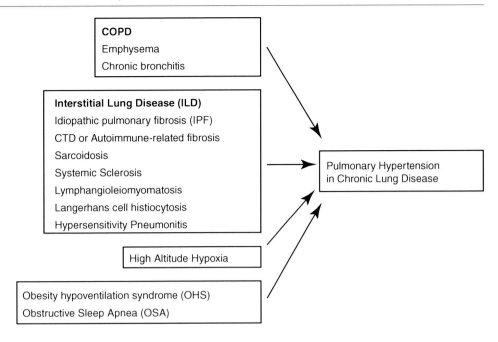

Table 3.1 Comparison of Group 2 and 3 diagnostic findings

	Group 2 PH	Group 3 PH
History	Dyspnea on exertion Lower extremity swelling	Dyspnea out of proportion to lung findings Nighttime awakenings, fatigue, morning headaches, snoring
Risk factors	Rheumatic fever Hypertension OSA CAD, history of MI	Smoking Asbestos, Silica, Talc, Coal dust Autoimmune disease
Examination	Elevated JVP Carotid bruits Irregular rhythm, murmur, S3 gallop, displaced PMI Crackles, dullness to percussion on lungs Hepatosplenomegally, ascites Lower extremity edema	Central obesity Barrel-chested Uveitis Pulmonary rales Clubbing of the extremities Erythema nodosum
CXR	Cardiomegally Pleural effusions Pulmonary edema	Bilateral infiltrates Hyperinflation with flattened diaphragms
Echocardiogram	Decreased EF Impaired relaxation Dilated, non-collapsible IVC	Mildly elevated RVSP Diastolic dysfunction
PFTs	Restrictive pattern	Obstructive or restrictive patterns Decreased DL_{CO}

Recently, the summary documents from the 5th World Symposium on Pulmonary Hypertension discussed the forms of pulmonary hypertension in left sided heart disease. In this document, it was suggested that the term "out-of-proportion" PH should no longer be used in patients with severe post-capillary PH with increased left atrial pressure (LAP). Instead, increasing recognition was offered to the importance of describing the presence of a pre-capillary component in some cases of PH from left heart disease. In this setting, the authors proposed 2 types of PH from left heart disease, on the basis of the level of the diastolic pressure difference (DPD). DPD is defined as pulmonary artery (PA) diastolic pressure minus pulmonary capillary wedge pressure (PCWP). In this setting, "isolated post-capillary PH" is defined as: PCWP > 15 mmHg and DPD < 7 mmHg, and "combined post-capillary PH and pre-capillary PH" is defined as PCWP > 15 mmHg and DPD > 7 mmHg (Table 3.2) [4].

In Group 2 PH, similar to Group 1, arteriolar remodeling is observed. Elevated left atrial pressure (LAP) is common to all forms of Group 2 PH. Backward transmission of this increase in LAP can mediate vascular changes. Acutely, an increase in LAP results in an increase in pulmonary venous pressure and, subsequently, pulmonary edema. Persistent increase in LAP produces fractures in the structure of the alveolar-capillary barrier by hydraulic forces [15], an event referred to as "capillary stress fracture" [16]. In this instance, the endothelial barrier is damaged and the extracellular matrix becomes weakened [17]. However, the pulmonary-capillary interface is typically able to restore its integrity with normalization of LAP [18]. With chronic elevation of LAP, the capillaries undergo vascular remodeling characterized by increased alveolar-capillary membrane thickness and increased deposition of collagen IV in the extracellular matrix (ECM) [19, 20]. This increase in membrane thickness can result in a decrease in diffusion capacity [15]. In HFpEF with PH there is pronounced medial hypertrophy in the small pulmonary

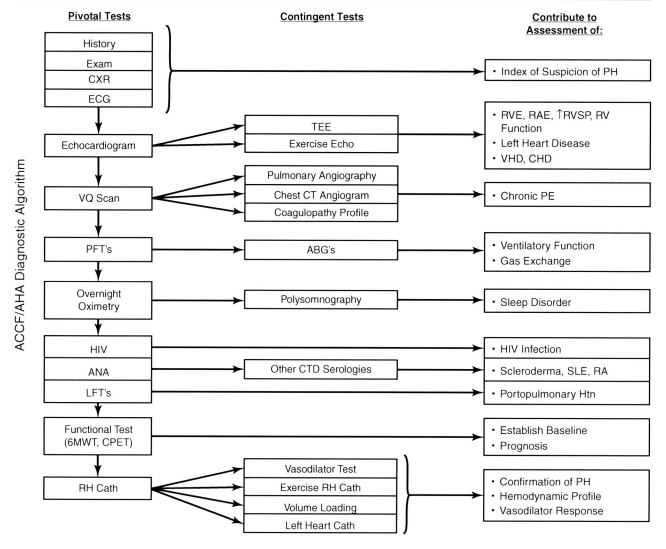

Fig. 3.4 ACCF/AHA PH diagnostic algorithm (Reproduced with permission from [6])

Table 3.2 Definition and classification of PH-LHD; LHD: Left heart disease

Terminology	PCWP (mmHg)	Diastolic PAP-PCWP (mmHg)
Isolated post-capillary PH	>15	<7
Combined post-capillary and pre-capillary PH	>15	≥7

Adapted from Vachiéry et al. Pulmonary hypertension due to Left Heart disease [4]

arteries (PAs) along with the formation of a neointimal layer similar to what is observed in Group I PAH [21].

The variability in PA pressures in patients with heart failure (systolic or diastolic) has not been fully explained. There does appear to be an element of genetic variability. Serotonin (5HT) transporter polymorphisms have been found to influence the degree of increased PA pressure in patients with systolic heart failure [22]. This is relevant in light of the known vasoconstrictor properties of 5HT. In a study of patients with congestive heart failure (CHF), those patients who were homozygous for the LL genotype of the 5HT promoter had significantly higher mean pulmonary artery pressures (mPAP) compared to those CHF patients who were heterozygous for the promoter [22]. Interestingly, in patients with Group 2 PH secondary to mitral valve disease, decreased bone-morphogenetic protein (BMPR) expression has been reported, suggesting a common pathway to PAH in the development of PH in PVH [23].

Role of Nitric Oxide in Group 2 PH

Nitric oxide (NO) derived from the pulmonary vascular endothelial cells plays an important role in maintaining resting pulmonary vascular tone and pulmonary vasodilatation response to endothelium-mediated triggers [24, 25]. The constitutive enzyme, endothelial nitric oxide synthase (eNOS), in the pulmonary vascular endothelial cells produces NO from arginine. NO then diffuses from the endothelial cells to the neighboring pulmonary artery smooth muscle cells where it stimulates soluble guanyl cyclase, leading to increased cyclic guanosine monophosphate (cGMP). cGMP relaxes pulmonary artery smooth muscle by inhibiting the release of calcium from sarcoplasmic reticulum. Consistent with this, infusion of NG-monomethyl-L-arginine (L-NMMA), a nonspecific inhibitor of eNOS, produces dose-dependent pulmonary vasoconstriction in normal adults and in children with congenital heart disease. In addition, cGMP reduces smooth muscle proliferation [26].

Experimental studies from animal models of chronic heart failure and chronic heart failure patients have shown reduced pulmonary endothelial cell derived NO in both populations [27]. Pulmonary arteries isolated from rats with chronic heart failure induced by ligation of the left coronary system showed reduced relaxation to acetylcholine, an eNOS agonist. Porter and colleagues studied the response of pulmonary arteries to acetylcholine infusion in heart failure patients with and without PH using intravascular ultrasound [28]. Patients with heart failure and PH had significantly reduced pulmonary vasodilatation in response to acetylcholine whereas those with normal pulmonary artery pressure had enhanced pulmonary vasodilatation. Similarly, Cooper and colleagues assessed pulmonary artery response to inhibition of NO with L-NMMA in CHF patients with and without elevated PVR by measuring segmental pulmonary arterial flow using Doppler wire [29, 30]. Taken together these studies demonstrate that PH due to left heart failure is associated with decreased pulmonary endothelium derived NO.

In addition to regulating vascular tone, endothelial-derived NO inhibits smooth muscle cell proliferation and thus decreased expression in heart failure begets more chronic changes in mPAP through vascular remodeling and platelet aggregation [31]. In light of this, strategies that increase pulmonary endothelial cell derived NO have attracted attention in the treatment of Group 2 PH.

Diagnosis

Diagnostic differentiation involves clinical features, echocardiogram assessment and invasive hemodynamics [21]. Risk factors for left ventricular dysfunction include increased age, hypertension, coronary artery disease (CAD), type 2 diabetes mellitus (DM2), obesity and atrial fibrillation [32, 33]. PH secondary to valvular disease or systolic heart failure can be determined through echocardiography relatively easily (Fig. 3.5). In contrast, it can be very difficult to distinguish between PAH and HFpEF. Assessing for clinical risk factors can accurately differentiate between PH secondary to

HFpEF and PAH with more than 90 % accuracy [32]. Echocardiographic findings that favor a diagnosis of Group 2 rather than Group 1 PH include left atrial enlargement, concentric remodeling, left ventricular hypertrophy and evidence of impaired relaxation by Doppler measurements [34]. Opotowsky and colleagues developed an echocardiographic scoring system to distinguish between PH from HFpEF and PAH [35]. In this model, the presence of an E:e' ratio of >10 (where E=mitral inflow velocities and e'=mitral annular Doppler velocity) and left atrial dimension of greater than 4.2 cm had marked sensitivity for PH from HFpEF (Fig. 3.6).

Thenappan and colleagues demonstrated a mean PVR of 1.6 (1.3–2.0) Wood Units in HFpEF without PH, and a mean PVR of 4.8 (3.0–8.4) Wood Units in HFpEF with PH [32]. This range in PVR demonstrates that the PVR observed in some PH-HFpEF patients can rival that seen in PAH, thus underscoring the distinct pulmonary vascular disease (PVD) that can develop in these patients [32]. Left atrial enlargement, which had been successfully used to differentiate PAH from PVH, did not differentiate HFpEF from PH-HFpEF. However, right atrial enlargement was more commonly seen in PH-HFpEF than HFpEF, likely due to the increase in RV afterload secondary to the PVD [35]. PH-HFpEF patients have poorer functional capacity than HFpEF patients, reflective of the RV dysfunction observed. This finding highlights the need to distinguish these cohorts in clinical trials. Although hypertension, obesity and DM2 are known to increase the risk of developing diastolic dysfunction [36], none of these risk factors preferentially favored the development of PH-HFpEF over HFpEF alone or *vice versa*.

Despite advances in imaging, invasive hemodynamics are often required to definitively measure left sided filling pressures, through left ventricular end-diastolic pressure (LVEDP) or pulmonary capillary wedge pressure measurements (PCWP) [37]. When measuring PCWP, recording mean end-expiratory PCWP values is critical, as opposed to mean PCWP recorded by automated catheterization laboratory equipment, which may underestimate the left sided filling pressures in up to a third of patients [38].

In the setting of elevated pulmonary pressures, vasoreactivity testing with systemic and/or pulmonary vasodilator agents is used to assess if the PH is "fixed" in nature [39]. Currently, there is no standard internationally accepted protocol defining "fixed" or "reversible" PH or a consensus on the procedure to use in evaluation of PH. However, patients whose PVR decreases to less than 2.5 Wood Units with vasodilation in the setting of CHF, have improved outcomes at time of heart transplantation [9] Protocols to assess vasoreactivity include the use of nitroglycerin, nitroprusside, milrinone, among others [3], and vary by institution.

Resting catheterization is often insufficient to definitively rule in or out left ventricular dysfunction as the cause of PH.

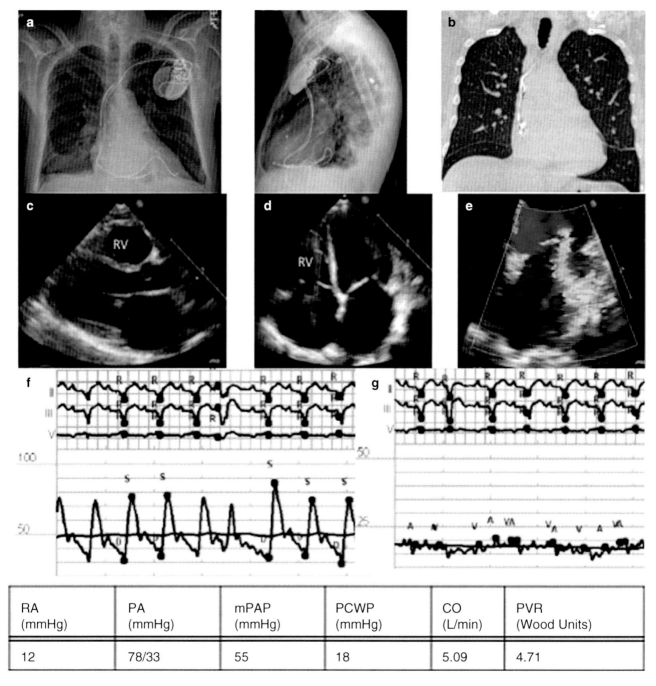

RA (mmHg)	PA (mmHg)	mPAP (mmHg)	PCWP (mmHg)	CO (L/min)	PVR (Wood Units)
12	78/33	55	18	5.09	4.71

Fig. 3.5 Group 2 PH from left sided valvular disease – Mitral regurgitation. (**a**) CXR showing ICD, small pleural effusions, (**b**) Chest CT with apical septal thickening, a sign of pulmonary veno-occlusive disease, (**c**) Parasternal long axis, large LA, (**d**) Apical 4 chamber with large atria, (**e**) Color Doppler showing MR jet, RHC pressure tracings, (**f**) pulmonary artery pressures, mPAP 55, (**g**) PCWP tracing, PCWP 18

For example, at the time of catheterization left sided filling pressures can normalize secondary to diuresis [40]. Additionally, in early stages of HFpEF, neurohormonal activation is not as advanced resulting in less pronounced fluid retention. In these circumstances, right heart catheterization performed at rest and with exercise can distinguish between PH secondary to HFpEF (with increased PCWP at exercise) and exercise-induced PAH (which retains a normal PCWP) [41, 42]. In HFpEF, with exercise the increase in PA pressures associates closely with the increase in PCWP [3]. However, what defines an abnormal PCWP with exercise is not well described with most investigators suggesting a threshold of 15–25 mmHg. There is also uncertainty as to whether assessments should be performed supine or upright, with arms or legs exercising [33].

Alternative techniques to differentiate between Group 1 and Group 2 PH in the catheterization laboratory include

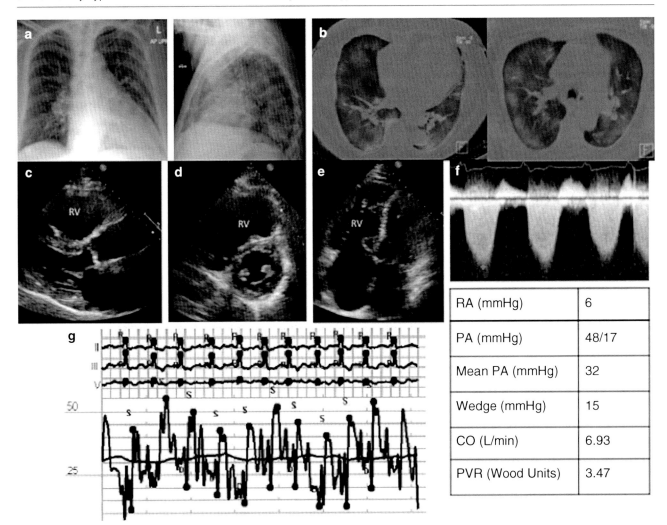

RA (mmHg)	6
PA (mmHg)	48/17
Mean PA (mmHg)	32
Wedge (mmHg)	15
CO (L/min)	6.93
PVR (Wood Units)	3.47

Fig. 3.6 Group 2 PH from heart failure with preserved ejection fraction. (**a**) PA/lateral CXR with cardiomegally and pulmonary edema, (**b**) Ventilation-Perfusion scan showing matched defects, (**c**) Parasternal long axis: large RV, (**d**) Parasternal short axis: large RV, (**e**) Apical 4 chamber: Large RV annexing the apex, (**f**) Tricuspid Doppler: TR velocity 359 cm/s, RVSP estimated at 52 mmHg, (**g**) RHC tracings of the pulmonary artery pressures, mPAP 32

rapid volume loading with saline infusion or leg lifting. A fluid challenge with 500 mL of normal saline over 5–10 min can identify patients with HFpEF and normal baseline PCWP, which may help reduce inappropriate diagnoses of PAH in patients with HFpEF [43, 44] However, even in healthy subjects a large volume fluid bolus can increased PCWP, thereby further confusing the role of this technique to distinguish between Group 1 PH and Group 2 PH secondary to HFpEF [45].

Management

The first step in managing Group 2 PH is treating the underlying disease process [4]. The priority is optimization of left sided filling pressures. Although pulmonary artery pressures can be expected to decrease significantly after appropriate treatment of the underlying etiology, targeted interventions may fail to remodel the pulmonary vasculature adequately to normalize pulmonary artery pressures.

In mitral stenosis, based on the American College of Cardiology (ACC)/American Heart Association (AHA) Valvular Heart Disease guidelines [46], percutaneous balloon mitral valvuloplasty (PBMV) is indicated for asymptomatic patients with moderate or severe MS and a pulmonary artery systolic pressure (PASP) > 50 mm Hg at rest or >60 mmHg with exercise. Exercise testing with hemodynamic assessment (Doppler or invasive) is recommended to evaluate the response of the mean mitral gradient and pulmonary artery pressure in patients with MS when there is a discrepancy between clinical symptoms or signs and resting echocardiographic findings [47]. An increase in RV systolic pressure to 60–70 mmHg should prompt consideration for valve surgery.

For patients with New York Heart Association class II-IV symptoms and mitral stenosis, surgical valve replacement should be pursued even if severe PH is present if the valve is not amenable to PBMV. Although PA pressures fall immediately after PBMV, in correlation with the reduction in mitral valve gradient [48], the maximal effect can be delayed up to 6 months after surgery [49].

In the setting of mitral regurgitation (MR), the 2014 ACC/AHA valve guidelines recommend earlier intervention for chronic MR [50] and in fact offer a Class IIa recommendation that mitral valve repair is reasonable for asymptomatic patients with chronic severe MR and resting pulmonary hypertension (PA systolic arterial pressure >50 mmHg). PH frequently complicates significant MR from flail leaflet being found in up to 25 % of patients [51]. When present, PH with MR is associated with major outcome implications, approximately doubling the risk of heart failure and death. Mitral valve surgery remains beneficial for these patients through either mitral valve repair or replacement.

Residual PH after mitral valve surgery is predictive of poor outcomes [52]. Although mitral valve repair or replacement is the optimum management of PH secondary to mitral valve disease, the rate and amount of regression of PH after mitral valve surgery varies considerably [53]. Patients with a decrease in left ventricular ejection fraction pre-operatively and fibroelastic deficiency as the underlying cause of mitral regurgitation are at increased risk of residual PH after mitral regurgitation surgery [54].

PH in aortic stenosis (AS) occurs secondary to diastolic dysfunction of the left ventricle and the accompanying left ventricular hypertrophy and elevated filling pressures [55]. In patients with severe symptomatic AS, about 50 % of patients have at least mild PH and 15–30 % of patients have severe PH with mean PAP > 50 mmHg [56–58]. PH is also more likely in AS if there is an accompanying decrease in LVEF and mitral regurgitation [59]. AS patients with severe PH have increased perioperative mortality in aortic valve replacement versus AS patients without PH. Furthermore, moderate to severe persistent pulmonary hypertension after aortic valve replacement for AS is associated with a decreased survival compared to normal pulmonary artery pressures or mild PH [60]. However, PA pressures do gradually decline post-operatively [61].

In the modern era of transcatheter aortic valve replacement (TAVR), the severity of PH before TAVR is associated with 2-year mortality rates of 14 %, 27 %, and 48 % for PA systolic pressures <30 mmHg, 30–60 mmHg, and >60 mmHg, respectively (p=0.001). Patients who have persistently severe PH after TAVR have a worse prognosis than those whose PA systolic pressures decrease below 60 mmHg (2-year mortality rate: 50.0 % vs. 18.6 %; p=0.001). PA systolic pressures can fall significantly within 90 days after TAVR [62], and by itself PH should not be a contraindication to valve replacement.

PH is found in 10–20 % of patients with aortic regurgitation (AR) [63] and occurs secondary to elevations in LVEDP. Unlike other valve lesions, historical reports suggest that there is no significant increase in operative mortality in patients undergoing aortic valve replacement (AVR) for AR with severe PH compared to those with mild PH or normal PA pressures [64]. Additionally, PA pressures decrease more predictably in patients after AVR for AR to near-normal levels as compared to AS [64].

Although treatment of advanced heart failure with decreased LVEF focuses on pharmacologic therapy, these patients are often considered for orthotopic heart transplantation. When PVR is greater than 2.5 Wood units and TPG is greater than 15 mmHg, mortality at 3 month and 1 year post-transplant is increased [65]. In those patients with a PVR <2.5 Wood Units, mortality at 1 year post-transplant is 5 % compared with 24 % in those with PVR >2.5 Wood Units [66]. Of note, in patients with a pre-transplant PVR > 2.5 Wood units in whom the PVR decreases to <2.5 Wood units with nitroprusside, mortality at 3 month post-transplant is considerably lower than those with "fixed" PH (3.8 % versus 40.6 %) [9]. Thus, fixed PH appears to portend a worse prognosis than reversible PH in heart transplant patients.

More recently, left ventricular assist device (LVAD) therapy has increased the options available for patients with systolic heart failure. In a retrospective study of 145 patients with systolic heart failure and severe PH treated by LVAD support, significant improvements were seen in mPAP, PVR and TPG after 6 months of LVAD support [67]. LVAD therapy for 6 months may be sufficient to adequately remodel the pulmonary vasculature and optimize patients for transplant. However, treatment beyond 6 months does not appear to have any additive effect on pulmonary vasculature [67]. There is perhaps an expanding role for the LVAD therapy a bridge to heart transplant in the management of patients with severe left ventricular systolic HF and PH [68].

Constriction and Restriction

Constrictive pericarditis is a pericardial compressive syndrome due to scarring, fibrosis, and pericardial calcification. The compressive phenomenon contributes to significant impairment of ventricular filling which is characterized by elevation of both left and right ventricular filling pressures and equalization of left and right ventricular diastolic pressures [69]. The causes of constrictive pericarditis include collagen vascular diseases (systemic lupus erythematosus), infection (tuberculosis) or as a consequence of trauma and traumatic hemorrhagic pericardial effusion. Treatment requires surgical removal of the pericardium, which should result in normalization of filling pressures and resolution of PH (Fig. 3.7) [70].

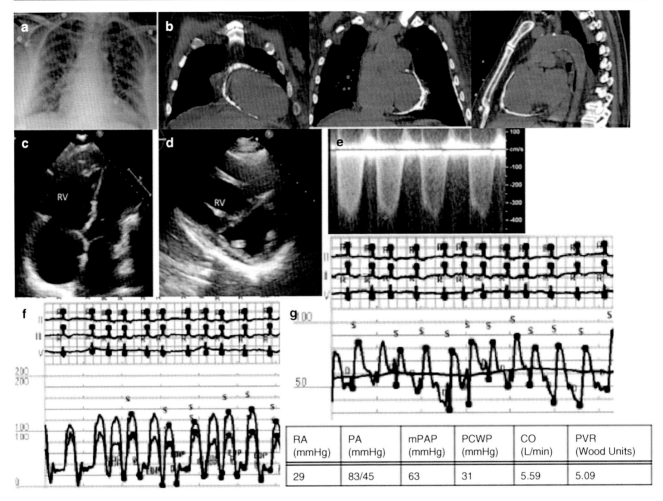

RA (mmHg)	PA (mmHg)	mPAP (mmHg)	PCWP (mmHg)	CO (L/min)	PVR (Wood Units)
29	83/45	63	31	5.59	5.09

Fig. 3.7 Group 2 PH from constrictive pericarditis. (**a**) CXR with pulmonary edema and cardiomegally, (**b**) CT scan showing pericardial calcification, (**c**) Apical 4 chamber with septal flattening and RV bowing into the LV, (**d**) Parasternal short axis with septal bowing into the LV creating A "D" shaped LV, (**e**) TR velocity, RVSP estimated at 46.8 mmHg, (**f**) RV/LV tracing showing discordance of the ventricular pressure with inspiration, (**g**) RHC tracing of the pulmonary artery pressures, mPAP 63 mmHg

Restrictive cardiomyopathy is a myocardial disease characterized by decreased myocardial relaxation and increased myocardial stiffness, resulting in elevation of left ventricular end-diastolic pressures. The resultant increase in LAP contributes to postcapillary PH. The postcapillary PH can, in turn, cause an increase in right ventricular end-diastolic pressure, which can cause equalization of the diastolic pressures in restrictive cardiomyopathy. Amyloidosis is the most common cause of restrictive cardiomyopathy. Other causes are endomyocardial fibrosis, and eosinophilic myocarditis. Treatment is targeted at the underlying condition and in certain circumstances requires heart transplantation.

These conditions are best diagnosed with invasive hemodynamics. Simultaneous right and left ventricular pressure tracings will show a "dip-and-plateau" pattern in both these conditions and equalization of the diastolic pressures. Constrictive pericarditis is characterized by discordant change in RV and LV pressures seen with respiration. In restrictive physiology, the changes in RV and LV pressures are concordant with respiration (Fig. 3.7).

The Role of Pulmonary Vasodilators

Many of the currently available agents for PAH, namely, endothelin receptor antagonists (ERA), prostacyclins, phosphodiesterase 5 inhibitors (PDE5i), and soluble guanylate cyclase stimulators (sGCs), have been studied in Group 2 PH and have failed to demonstrate clinical benefit (Table 3.3) [3]. In the Flolan International Randomized Survival Trial (FIRST), patients with systolic heart failure (LVEF < 25 % and New York Heart Association (NYHA) IIIB or IV) were randomized to intravenous epoprostenol or conventional therapy. Although epoprostenol decreased pulmonary artery pressure and PVR, there was no observed benefit in morbidity or 6-min walk distance (6MWD). In fact, the trial was

Table 3.3 Pulmonary vasodilators studied in left heart failure

Study and year published	Methods	Inclusion criteria	PH at entry	Average mPAP at entry (mmHg)	Results
Guazzi et al. [71] 2004	Sildenafil 50 mg once or placebo n=32 Randomized	>18 yrs NYHA II–III CHF LVEF<40 %	No	mPAP=33.6±3.3	Decreased mPAP Improved DLco Increased VO₂ Improved ventilator efficiency
Lewis et al. [72] 2007	Sildenafil 25–75 mg tid or placebo 12-week study n=34 Randomized	>18 yrs NYHA II-IV on conventional therapy LVEF<40 % mPAP >25 mmHg	Yes	mPAP=33±3	Decreased mPAP Improved peak VO₂ Increased 6MWD Decreased hospitalization
Guazzi et al. [73] 2007	Sildenafil 50 mg bid or placebo 6-month study n=46 Observational	<65 yrs NYHA II–III Cardiomyopathy LVEF <45 %	No	mPAP=33.7±3.1	Decreased mPAP Improved peak VO₂ Improved ventilator efficiency
Lewis et al. [74] 2008	Sildenafil 25–75 mg tid or placebo 12-week study n=30 Randomized	>18 yrs NYHA II–IV LVEF<40 % mPAP>25 mmHg	Yes	mPAP=30±7	Decreased mPAP Improved ventilator efficiency (decreased VE/VCO₂ slope) Increased RVEF
Behling et al. [75] 2008	Sildenafil 50 mg tid or placebo 4-week study n=19 Randomized	>20 yrs CHF on standard stable therapy LVEF<45 %	No	mPAP=59±18	Decreased mPAP Improved peak VO₂ Improved ventilator efficiency
Guazzi et al. [76] 2009	Sildenafil 25 mg tid or placebo 6-month study n=40 Observational	Age 65.3±7.3 yrs LVEF 37.2±7.4 %	No		Heart rate recovery improved
Guazzi et al. [77] 2011	Sildenafil 50 mg tid or placebo 12-month study n=44 Randomized	HFpEF LVEF>50 % Sinus rhythm No hospitalizations in prior 6 mo	Yes	mPAP=54.5±6.3	Decreased mPAP Improved RV function Decreased PVR Increased DLCO
Guazzi et al. [78] 2011	Sildenafil 50 mg tid or placebo 12-month study n=45 Randomized	NYHA II–III LVEF<40 % No hospitalizations in prior 6 mo Diabetic patients excluded	No	mPAP=38.4±3.0	Improved LVEF Decreased PASP Improved LV diastolic function Improved functional capacity
Guazzi et al. [79] 2012	Sildenafil 50 mg tid or placebo 12-month study n=32 Randomized	NYHA III–IV LVEF <45 %. mPAP 25–35 mmHg Females excluded	Yes	mPAP=34.8±4	Reversal of exercise oscillatory breathing Improved functional capacity Decreased PAP
Reichenbach et al. [80] 2012	Sildenafil 20–60 mg tid or nothing 3-month study n=47 Non-randomized	NYHA II–IV LVEF<40 %	Yes	mPAP=45±6	Decreased PVR Increased CO Increased TAPSE Decreased RV dimension
RELAX [81] Ongoing	Sildenafil 20 mg tid for 12 weeks followed by Sildenafil 60 mg tid × 12 weeks n=216 enrolled Randomized	>18 yrs NYHA II–III HFpEF, EF >50 % NT-proBNP>400 pg/ml	No		1° endpoint: Change in VO₂ 2° endpoint: 6MWD, composite clinical score
Givertz et al. [82] 2000	Sitaxsentan IV 1.5, 3, 6 mg/kg over 15 min n=48 Randomized	≥21 yrs NYHA III–VI ACEI+diuretics PCWP ≥15 CI ≤2.5	Yes	mPAP=60±2	Decreased PASP, PVR, mPAP Unchanged CI, SVR

Table 3.3 (continued)

Study and year published	Methods	Inclusion criteria	PH at entry	Average mPAP at entry (mmHg)	Results
HEAT Luscher et al. [83] 2002	Darusentan 30, 100, 300 mg/day 3 week study n = 157 Randomized	NYHA III EF ≤35 % PCWP ≥ 12 CI ≤2.6	No		Increased CI Unchanged PCWP, MPAP, PVR Unchanged BNP
Perez-Villa et al. [84] 2006	Bosentan 62.5 mg BID × 4 weeks , then 125 mg BID 6 week study n = 7 Non-randomized	Heart transplant candidates PVR > 2.5 Woods units	Yes	mPAP = 48 ± 9	Decreased PVR
Kaluski et al. [85] 2008	Bosentan 8–125 mg BID 5 month study n = 94 Randomized	NYHA IIIB–IV EF <35 % SPAP >40 mmHg	Yes	PASP = 51.8 ± 10.3	No change in sPAP Unchanged CI
Hefke et al. [86] 2012	Bosentan 62.5 mg BID up to 125 mg BID 12 month study n = 115 Observational, non-randomized	Heart transplant candidates mPAP >35 PVR >240 dyn TPG >15 mmHg	Yes	mPAP = 45.2 ± 8.7	Decreased PVR Decreased mPAP Decreased SVR Mortality much higher in placebo group
Padeletti et al. [87] 2013	Bosentan 62.5 mg BID for 1 month increased to 125 mg BID 4 month study n = 17 Non-randomized	>18 yrs NYHA III EF <35 % PASP >50, PVR >3 Woods units, or TPG >10 mmHg	Yes	mPAP = 41 ± 7	Decreased mPAP Decreased PVR Decreased TPR Unchanged CO
Montalescot et al. [88] 1998	Epoprostenol 4 ng/kg/ min increase by 2 every 5 min to reach 15 % decreased in SBP n = 19	>18 years Heart transplant candidates PASP >30	Yes	mPAP = 41 ± 2	Decreased mPAP Increased CO Increased PVC
Weston et al. [89] 2001	Inhaled Iloprost 580 μg single dose n = 6 Non-randomized, Observational	Heart transplant candidates mPAP >25 Resistant to Nitroprusside	Yes	mPAP = 40.6 ± 10.9	Decreased PASP Decreased MPAP Decreased TPG
Sablotzki et al. [90] 2002	Inhaled Iloprost 50 μg n = 29 (all male) Non-randomized, Observational	Heart transplant candidates Elevated PVR	Yes	PVR = 206 ± 94	Decreased mPAP, PVR Increased CI, SI
PROPHET [91] Scheidt et al. 2006	IV PGE₁ 50 ng/kg/min up until PVR decreased n = 92	Heart transplant candidates PVR >2.5 Woods Units TPG >12 mmHg	Yes	mPAP = 39 ± 9 PVR = 4.1 ± 2	Decreased MPAP, SVR, PVR Increased CO
Serra et al. [92] 2011	IV PEG1 2.5 ng/kg/min up to optimal dose, continuously for 72 h n = 22	NYHA III–IV EF <35 % ECHO-sPAP >3 m/s	Yes	PASP = 57.65 ± 3.4	Increased EF, NYHA class and PASP Improved 3 year mortality 27 % vs. 44 %
LEPHT [93] Bonderman et al. 2013	Riociguat 1 mg TID, 2 mg TID 16 week study n = 201 Randomized	>18 yrs mPAP ≥25 EF ≤40 % Optimal medical therapy × 30 days	Yes	mPAP = 40.4 ± 1.2	Unchanged mPAP Increased CI, SVI Decreased PVR Improved quality of life

Abbreviations: *PH* pulmonary hypertension, *PASP* pulmonary artery systolic pressure, *n* number, *yrs* years old, *NYHA* New York Heart Association, *CHF* congestive heart failure, *LVEF* left ventricle ejection fraction, *mPAP* mean pulmonary artery pressure, *DLco* diffusion capacity, *VO²* peak oxygen consumption, *tid* three times a day, *6MWD* 6 min walk distance, *bid* twice a day, *HFpEF* heart failure with preserved ejection fraction, *mo* months, *RV* right ventricle, *PVR* pulmonary vascular resistance, *PVC* pulmonary vascular compliance, *EF* ejection fraction, *LVEF* left ventricular ejection fraction, *PGE1* prostaglandin E1, *TPG* transpulmonary gradient, *ACEI* angiotensin converting enzyme inhibitor, *CI* cardiac index, *SVI* stroke volume index, *CO* cardiac output, *BNP* brain natriuretic peptide, *SVR* systemic vascular resistance

stopped early due to concerns for increased mortality in the epoprostenol arm [94]. The Endothelin Antagonist Bosentan for Lowering Cardiac Events in Heart Failure (ENABLE) study met with a similar fate [95]. In this study, 1,613 patients with LVEF<35 % and NYHA IIIB or IV were randomized to bosentan or conventional therapy. In this trial, the results of which have never fully been published, there was an increased risk of heart failure hospitalization in the bosentan arm, presumably due to fluid retention or decreased right ventricular function [96].

PDE5i have a less clear effect in Group 2 PH. Sildenafil had been shown to improve 6MWD and decrease hospitalization in a small trial of 34 patients with systolic heart failure and PH [72]. In this study, there was not a significant reduction in pulmonary artery pressures, despite the observed clinical benefit [72]. Larger trials of PDE5i have yet to be completed [97] and a trial of tadalafil in Group 2 PH has recently been terminated by the funding agency [98]. Therefore the role of PDE5i in systolic heart failure and Group 2 PH currently remains unanswered. sGCs also act through the nitric oxide pathway on the pulmonary vasculature in a similar mechanism to PDE5i. Riociguat, currently the only available sGCs for PAH in the United States, has been studied in a phase IIb trial in systolic heart failure [93]. In this study, after 16 weeks of therapy, there was no observed change in pulmonary artery pressures.

The role of pulmonary vasodilators in Group 2 PH from HFpEF is also understudied. In a placebo-controlled study of 44 patients with Group 2 PH secondary to HFpEF, sildenafil improved exercise capacity and decreased pulmonary artery pressures after 6 months of therapy [77]. However, in a larger, multicenter study of 216 patients with HFpEF (median PASP was 41 mmHg), after 24 weeks of sildenafil versus placebo, there was no change in peak VO$_2$, the study's primary endpoint [99]. Admittedly in this trial, patients were not stratified by PH status, therefore the effect of this therapy on the pulmonary vasculature is as such undefined [100].

Future Directions

There remains considerable interest in using pulmonary vasodilators in the treatment of Group 2 PH. Clinical trials are ongoing and hopefully will provide insight into the merit of targeting pulmonary artery pressures [101, 102]. However, the lack of clinical benefit despite rigorous attempts to lower pulmonary artery pressures in Group 2 PH challenges the relevance of targeting PH in HFrEF and HFpEF [100].

Technological advances now permit the measurement of ambulatory hemodynamics with implantable monitors. For example, the CardioMEMS™ device is implanted into the branch pulmonary arteries and allows transmission of pulmonary artery pressure measurements, through a radiofrequency-based wireless pressure sensor. In the randomized, single-blind CHAMPION trial of 550 patients with NYHA functional class III heart failure, clinicians were directed to use a medical algorithm to achieve protocol specific hemodynamic targets: PASP 15–35 mmHg, Pulmonary Artery Diastolic Pressure (PAD) 8–20 mmHg, and mean PAP 10–25 mmHg. The CardioMEMS arm was associated with a 28 % relative risk reduction in HF hospitalization over the 6-month study period. In patients with PH who were managed with the CardioMEMS™ device, clinicians made more changes to HF medications, primarily decongestive in nature (diuretics, nitrates, vasodilators etc.) [103]. The accuracy of pressure measurement obtained was comparable to that obtained invasively with right heart catheterization [104]. Wearable technology as well as indwelling, continuous monitoring such as that performed by the CardioMEMS™ device, present a unique opportunity to characterize hemodynamics in patients when engaged in activities of daily living and will hopefully provide insight on optimal treatment practices.

Pulmonary Hypertension Secondary to Chronic Hypoxic Lung Disease

Chronic hypoxic lung disease commonly causes pulmonary hypertension (PH) with a variety of phenotypes. Among hospitalized patients with chronic lung disease, up to 28 % have exhibited elevated mean pulmonary arterial pressures (mPAP) [105]. This patient cohort is ever expanding with an aging, overweight population that smoked tobacco and had significant pulmonary exposures. It is important to recognize the lesser-known complications of chronic lung disease for prognostication and focused treatment.

Epidemiology

Chronic Obstructive Pulmonary Disease (COPD)

COPD often leads to an elevation of pulmonary pressures, affecting 30–70 % of patients [106]. These patients typically have advanced stage COPD, with mild to moderate elevation of their mean pulmonary arterial pressures (mPAP). However, there is a small population (5 %) of COPD patients that have severe PH. This cohort typically has mPAP >40 mmHg, with less severe airflow obstruction and hypoxemia [21, 107].

In emphysematous type COPD, worsening PH correlates with worsening airflow obstruction. Minai and colleagues found that 38 % of patients with severe emphysema had PH, 69 % of those being pre-capillary PH. It is important to note that COPD patients may show evidence of Group 2 PH as well, given that smoking is a strong risk factor for CAD [108]. Chronic bronchitis pattern COPD has been less thoroughly studied, although there is some data showing reversal of PH in chronic bronchitis when treated with oxygen therapy [109].

Five year survival for COPD patients diagnosed with PH treated with oxygen therapy is 36 % compared to non-PH survival of 62 % [110]. Elevated pulmonary pressures in COPD correlate with increased hospitalizations and exacerbations [5, 111].

Interstitial Lung Disease (ILD)

The prevalence of PH ranges widely in patients with ILD and current prevalence is based on data primarily from patients referred for lung transplantation who had right heart catheterization (RHC). Idiopathic pulmonary fibrosis (IPF) is the most common form of ILD and as such has been studied most thoroughly. Rates of PH in IPF range from 31 to 84 %, depending upon the population studied [112, 113].

Prognostically, mPAP and FVC are the strongest predictors of survival in IPF [5]. A small subset of individuals with combined pulmonary fibrosis and emphysema are especially prone to PH and have high short term mortality with median survival ranging from 2.1 to 8.5 years [114]. In this cohort, the severity of PH and DLCO reduction do not correlate with the severity of obstructive lung disease [5]. Overall, in regards to lung disease, IPF carries a poor prognosis, with a median survival of 4.1 years and concomitant PH worsens that prognosis to a median survival of 0.7 years [115, 116].

ILD related PH also occurs in patients with pulmonary manifestations of connective tissue diseases, autoimmune disease and sarcoidosis. Similar to COPD, ILD related PH rarely exceeds the mild to moderate range with most mPAP<40 mmHg [117]. In sarcoidosis the prevalence of pulmonary hypertension is extremely wide (5–75 %) with the latter finding in lung transplant candidates [118, 119]. Sarcoidosis manifests in many ways resulting in PH through different mechanisms that will be discussed subsequently.

Other autoimmune diseases typically included in the Group 1 PH category can manifest as Group 3 PH as well. In scleroderma-associated ILD, for instance, the incidence of PH has been estimated to be up to 22 % and a low PaO_2 has been shown to correlate with development of PH more strongly than extent of lung fibrosis [120–123]. The prevalence of PH varies widely in all forms of ILD and there can be overlap of Group 1, 2 and 3 PH among the connective tissue disease and autoimmune patient populations.

High Altitude Pulmonary Hypertension (HAPH)

Increasing elevation portends a decrease in barometric pressure and concomitantly a decrease in the partial pressure of oxygen, most notably observed in patients at altitudes of 2,100 meters or greater above sea level. This atmospheric change manifests as worsened arterial oxygen saturation of hemoglobin with increasing altitude. The human body has multiple adaptation mechanisms to survive at altitude, which manifest as initial increases in cardiac output, followed by increase in hemoglobin production and decrease in plasma volume [124]. For the more than 140 million people living above 2,500 meters, this relative hypoxia can have significant health consequences, including PH. The primary geographic areas of the high altitude populations studied include the Himalayas, the Andes and the Rocky Mountains. Unfortunately, in a large number of these studies the mode of identifying patients with possible HAPH is EKG evidence of right heart strain and few of these patients undergo RHC. Studies of South American patients living at greater than 3,200 meters elevation have estimated prevalence of PH between 5 and 18 %; a few studies have shown higher pulmonary pressures in children than adults, especially those under the age of 5 [125, 126]. In a study of a Kyrgyz population, 14 % of adults were found to have EKG findings of right heart strain. A separate group of 136 Kyrgyz patients who underwent RHC showed that 20 % met criteria for PH [127].

There are many variables that influence the development of HAPH including elevation, sex, age and genetic susceptibility. HAPH is more common in men than women and in patients with OSA. The incidence also increases with higher elevation and older age as well. The prognosis of HAPH is favorable with removal of the stimulus, high altitude hypoxia, with a return of mPAP to normal values to be expected by 2 years at sea level [128].

Obesity-Hypoventilation Syndrome (OHS) and Obstructive Sleep Apnea (OSA)

Increasing rates of obesity have produced an increase in the number of patients with two, often overlapping, medical conditions that are associated with pulmonary hypertension: obesity-hypoventilation syndrome (OHS) and obstructive sleep apnea (OSA). Studies of patients with OHS on treatment with non-invasive positive pressure ventilation (NIPPV) have shown rates of PH up to 43 % by RHC, in which DL_{CO} was lower and body mass index (BMI) was higher in the patients with elevated pulmonary pressures [129]. Previous studies of OHS patients not treated with NIPPV had shown a prevalence of 59 %, although it is important to note that both studies used mPAP>20 mmHg diagnostic criteria for PH. PH is more common in OHS patients, as compared to purely OSA patients [130]. Minai and colleagues demonstrated that among patients with OSA, women have a higher rate of PH (86 % vs. 58 %) and those with Group 2 PH have higher frequency and length of nocturnal desaturations, as compared to those with Group 2 PH or normal mPAP [131]. The 8-year survival for patients with OSA and PH is significantly worse than those without PH (43 % vs. 76 %) [131]. PH in this setting will often improve with treatment of the underlying disease. Exercise capacity is also decreased when PH was present with OSA [131]. RV failure typically occurs in these patients when co-morbidities are present, such as left heart disease or hypoxic lung disease [132].

Pathophysiology

The mechanisms by which chronic lung disease causes PH are as diverse as the primary diseases themselves. Hypoxia results in distal changes in the pulmonary arterial system, initially vasoconstriction and, over time, muscularization of the vasculature [21, 133]. In large proximal arteries, medial and adventitial hypertrophy is predominantly seen [133].

The basis of much of the data on vascular remodeling in hypoxia is from examination of those individuals with high altitude pulmonary hypertension. In this population there is a production of α-smooth muscle actin (α-SM-actin) in the small pulmonary arteries that typically have very little smooth muscle, creating distal extension of the smooth muscle [133]. The protein α-SM-actin is a part of the contractile apparatus of smooth muscle cells and is a common marker of myofibroblast differentiation and increased fibroblast contractile activity [134, 135]. Medial and adventitial thickening appears to be due to this smooth muscle proliferation and extracellular matrix deposition. The adventitia also exhibits increased cellularity as a result of recruitment of fibroblasts. Initially, there seems to be an overall decrease in the size of the pulmonary vascular bed due to loss of small vessels in chronic hypoxia, however, animal model research has illustrated the presence of pulmonary angiogenesis in an attempt to decrease resistance across the vascular bed [136].

Hypoxia-Inducible Factor Alpha

One mediator of the adaptive response to hypoxia is hypoxia-inducible factor-alpha (HIF-α). There are two forms, HIF-1α and HIF-2α, the former activates glycolysis by upregulating Glucose transporter-1 (Glut-1) and the latter initiates erythropoietin (EPO) [137]. Glut-1 induces a shift to glycolytic metabolism in pulmonary vascular cells that correlates with a pseudo-hypoxic environment in the setting of inappropriate HIF-α activation [138, 139]. In the setting of normoxia, HIF-1α is bound to von Hippel Lindau (VHL) tumor suppressor protein (pVHL) and, when bound, ubiquinated HIF-1α cannot interact with DNA to alter transcription [140]. HIF-1α reacts to hypoxia by binding hypoxia response elements (HREs) in the DNA for molecules like vascular endothelial growth factor (VEGF) and erythropoietin (EPO) [141]. Interestingly patients affected by Chuvash syndrome, characterized by the developmental of polycythemia and PH, have a pVHL mutation that destabilizes the relationship of pVHL-HIF-1α in normoxia. In this disease, one mechanism of pulmonary vascular dysfunction is secondary to a perceived chronic hypoxic response in the absence of hypoxia. In mice, the development of PH appears to be independent of polycythemia [140, 142, 143].

Erythrocytosis does appear to play an important role in the development of PH, even outside of the Chuvash patient population. In COPD patients with polycythemia, phlebotomy correlated with a decrease in PVR and mPAP [143]. Increased blood viscosity is the mechanism by which erythrocytosis exacerbates PH, but does not appear to be the primary cause of elevated pulmonary pressures. Excess hemoglobin in erythrocytosis is thought to exacerbate hypoxic vasoconstriction by binding and removing large amounts of NO from the pulmonary circulation [142, 143, 145].

Microcirculation

In PH secondary to IPF, pulmonary vessel density is not uniform across parts of the lungs. The vessel distribution is thought to be secondary to an imbalance of angiogenic (VEGF and interleukin (IL)-8) and angiostatic (pigment epithelium-derived factor, PEDF) molecules [146–148]. This finding may be partially explained by the fact that VEGF transcription is induced by HIF-2α [149]. VEGF is involved in NO and prostacyclin synthesis in the lung, which leads to vasodilatation [150]. On a cellular level, VEGF does not appear to have significant mitogen effects on smooth muscle cells, but does stimulate transcription of matrix metalloproteinases-1,-3 and −9, that contribute to smooth muscle cell migration and digestion of the basement membrane as a first step in angiogenesis [151]. Inhibition of VEGF also correlates with endothelial cell apoptosis and elevated pulmonary pressures. Farkas and colleagues showed that vascular endothelial cell apoptosis, with microvascular rarefaction and pulmonary arterial medial thickening, correlated with decreased levels of VEGF in worsening IPF [149]. This reinforces the importance of anti-apoptotic properties of VEGF in maintaining lower pulmonary pressures, as represented by a negative correlation between mPAP and VEGF levels [149]. In the setting of ILD, it has been found that higher endogenous VEGF levels correlate with higher levels of fibrosis and poorer lung function [152]. IL-8 receptor (IL-8R) binding induces chemo-attractant molecule production and recruitment of neutrophils and other inflammatory cells. In animal models, overexpression of IL-8R has been shown to be protective by reducing the inflammatory response [153]. In rat models of PAH, transfusion of endothelial cells overexpressing IL-8R accelerates adherence to the injured lung and inhibits subsequent remodeling, likely by blocking inflammatory cell recruitment [154]. In IPF, higher levels of IL-8 are also predictive of increased mortality [155]. IL-8 is upregulated by hypoxia and is elevated in patients with COPD, correlating with disease severity [156]. PEDF is also instrumental in the remodeling of the lung endothelium and has a role in regulating angiogenesis as an angiostatic factor. PEDF is an inhibitor of VEGF angiogenesis and inhibits endothelial cell apoptosis and fibroblast growth. This activity may contribute to the development of PH in patients with IPF and emphysema, given that PEDF is elevated in these populations [147, 149, 157].

VEGF has been shown to play an important role, not only lung in vasculature, but also lung structure maintenance. This molecule likely participates in emphysematous changes and it has been hypothesized that decreased expression of VEGF and VEGF Receptor-2 in emphysema leads to alveolar septal endothelial apoptosis as a mechanism for wall destruction [158]. Additionally, chronic inhibition of VEGF in rats has been shown to lead to emphysema and that the addition of caspase inhibitors to halt apoptosis results in prevention of emphysema. Reduced levels of VEGF and the release of elastase by activated macrophages are two of the mechanisms known to produce alveolar septal destruction in emphysema [158].

Inflammation

In addition to VEGF, endothelial cell markers such as vascular cell adhesion molecule 1 (VCAM-1) and other vascular remodeling molecules are a topic of recent research. VCAM-1 is an adhesion molecule upregulated in hypoxia that facilitates inflammatory cell migration. A number of pro-inflammatory cytokines and growth factors are similarly upregulated in hypoxia, including monocyte chemoattractant protein-1 (MCP-1), IL-6, Transforming Growth Factor (TGF)-β1 and C5, with correlating increases in their respective receptors. Persistent hypoxia in animals models results in a predominantly monocytic perivascular infiltrate [159]. The recruitment of mesenchymal precursors of the monocyte line is profound and the corresponding influx of cells that produce type 1 collagen and α-SM-actin contributes to the expansion of the extracellular matrix (ECM) in vascular remodeling [160]. The increase in ECM thickens the vascular wall, thus increasing the distance of capillary from the alveoli thereby producing a paradoxical decrease in DLCO, worsening the hypoxic response [161].

In COPD, IL-6 is significantly elevated and correlates positively with pulmonary pressures, such that the high circulating IL-6 levels in homozygous GG genotype is associated with higher pulmonary pressures [162]. Elevated serum IL-6 levels have also been documented in PAH, PH related to scleroderma, systemic lupus erythematosus and other inflammatory diseases [163–165]. Mouse studies have shown the IL-6 deficiency results in a blunted hemodynamic response to hypoxia [166].

Vasoactive Molecules

COPD patients exhibit endothelial dysfunction and imbalance of the vasoactive mediators NO, prostacyclin, endothelin-1 (ET-1) and angiotensin. Some of these molecules are integrated into the VEGF and TGF-β1 molecular pathways and may have anti-proliferative and anti-inflammatory effects. eNOS has decreased expression in smokers and COPD patients with PH, thereby contributing to decreased NO [167–169]. NO is also scavenged by deoxygenated hemoglobin, a mechanism by which polycythemia can worsen PH. Angiotensin II, a vasoconstrictor, is active in pulmonary vascular cell growth in PH, with an increase in Angiotensin converting enzyme (ACE) seen in the pulmonary vasculature [170]. Multiple animal models have shown a decrease in hypoxic PH with angiotensin converting enzyme inhibitor (ACEi) treatment and ACE production is increased locally in small pulmonary arterioles during hypoxia [171–173].

Leptin

Leptin resistance is thought to play a role in OHS. Leptin, a protein released from adipose tissue, acts at the hypothalamic level to increase respiratory drive. Obese patients have significantly higher leptin levels than non-obese, as leptin acts as an appetite suppressant via hypothalamic receptor binding [174]. Campo and colleagues studied 225 obese patients and found an association between elevated leptin and reduced ventilatory drive and hypercapneic response [175]. In addition, regular NIPPV has been shown to reduce leptin levels in OHS patients [176]. Leptin likely plays an important role in ventilation as well as other physiological responses in obese patients, however these qualities have still yet to be characterized.

Diagnosis

The individual diagnoses in Group 3 PH depend on history, laboratory testing and imaging. There are many important elements of a patients history that can lead to further exploration of chronic lung disease, including smoking history, occupational exposures, previous rheumatologic diagnoses, morbid obesity and sleep disturbances. On EKG these patients may have signs of RVH, however, this is not a specific finding and is not often present in mild PH [106]. Echocardiogram is the screening test of choice and if suspicion is high, invasive hemodynamic monitoring may be indicated.

COPD

COPD diagnosis is made by the presence of obstructive lung disease seen on spirometry, indicated by an FEV$_1$/FVC ratio of

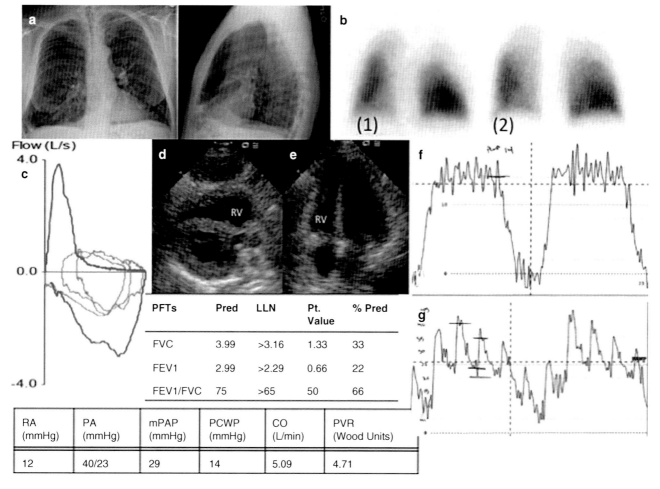

Fig. 3.8 Group 3 PH from chronic obstructive pulmonary disease. (a) CXR showing flatten diaphragms, hyperinflation, (b) (1) Ventilation (2) Perfusion scan with matched defects, (c) PFT's with severe obstruction, (d) Parasternal short axis, (e) Apical 4 chamber, RHC tracings, (f) PCWP 14 mmHg, (g) Pulmonary artery pressures, mPAP 34 mmHg

less than 70 % predicted (Fig. 3.8). Particularly important to the COPD diagnosis is smoking history, family history of early COPD and occupational exposures. In these patients which chest x-ray showing hyperinflation may also revealed large pulmonary artery shadows. Arterial blood gases may also aid in assessing the severity of hypoxia and thus increasing suspicion for secondary PH. Echocardiogram can be particularly difficult in these patients with large lung volumes [106].

ILD

Similar to COPD patients, it is important to take a careful history of exposures in suspected ILD patients. Many ILD patients will have a history of tobacco use or exposure to mining (radon, granite), sandblasting (silicosis) and asbestos for example. Laboratory testing includes anti-neutrophil antibodies (ANA), rheumatoid factor (RF) and erythrocyte sedimentation rate (ESR) to evaluate for autoimmune etiology such as scleroderma (Fig. 3.9). In addition kidney and liver function should be evaluated to explore associated syndromes. A chest x-ray may show important patterns of lobar predominance or

existence of obstruction as well as masses or calcified pleural plaques. Chest computer tomography (CT) can help to better characterize pulmonary parenchyma and patterns of disease. ILD patients should also undergo spirometric testing to determine severity of restriction and DL_{CO} reduction to help with assessing the severity of disease [177].

HAPH

High altitude pulmonary hypertension diagnosis is based on the exclusion of other causes of pulmonary hypertension and the history of living about 2,500 meters elevation. Screening with EKG to evaluate for RVH is often the first step followed by echocardiography. This is an additional population where exercise RHC may reveal pulmonary hypertension not seen on resting RHC.

OHS and OSA

The criteria for diagnosis of OHS include body mass index of greater than 30 kg/m², an awake arterial $PaCO_2$ greater than 45 mmHg and a polysomnogram with nocturnal

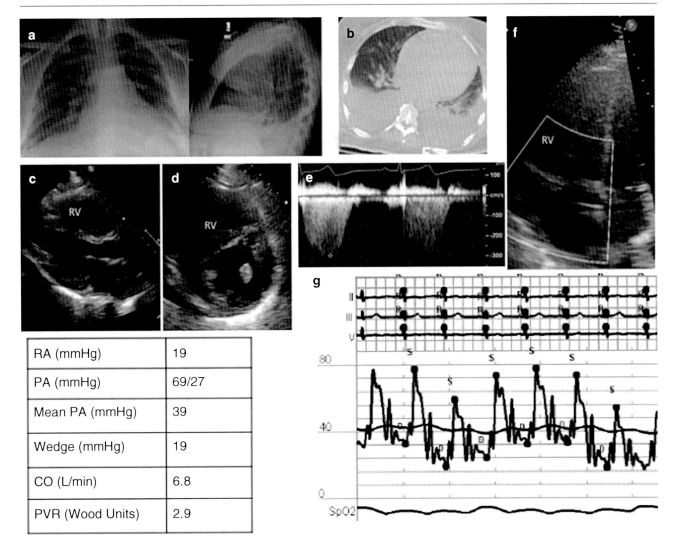

RA (mmHg)	19
PA (mmHg)	69/27
Mean PA (mmHg)	39
Wedge (mmHg)	19
CO (L/min)	6.8
PVR (Wood Units)	2.9

Fig. 3.9 PH from systemic sclerosis (Group 2/3 Overlap). (**a**) PA/Lat CXR with small lung volumes, no infiltrates, (**b**) Chest CT showing cardiomegally and bilateral pleural effusions, (**c**) Parasternal long axis showing a large RV, (**d**) Parasternal short axis showing a large RV and "D" shaped LV, (**e**) Tricuspid doppler with TR velocity 296 cm/s, RVSP estimated at 35 mmHg, (**f**) Apical 4 chamber showing a large RA and RV, (**g**) RHC tracing of pulmonary artery pressures, mPAP 39 mmHg

hypercapnea. Thus, polysomnogram and an arterial blood gas are required for diagnosis [174]. OSA diagnosis is based on a polysomnogram with episodes of apnea or hyponea quantified as an Apnea-Hyponea Index (AHI). An AHI of greater than or equal to 15 events per hour without symptoms or greater than or equal to 5 events per hour with symptoms is indicative of a positive test.

Management

Fundamentally, the management of PH in chronic hypoxic lung disease is to treat the underlying condition. If the patient has OSA, nocturnal positive pressure ventilation is recommended. In OHS, weight loss should be emphasized. In COPD patients, smoking cessation and oxygen therapy is stressed when appropriate. In autoimmune associated chronic hypoxic lung disease, oxygen therapy and immunosuppression are important considerations.

COPD

The treatments shown to improve survival in COPD include smoking cessation and oxygen therapy, however, there are multiple methods to reduce symptoms and morbidity. The mainstay of symptomatic control in COPD is bronchodilators, inhaled β-agonists and anticholinergics. Theophylline can produce a mild decrease in PVR, however drug levels must be closely monitored [178]. The Medical Research Council (MRC) and Nocturnal Oxygen Therapy Trial (NOTT) demonstrated that long-term oxygen therapy improves mortality independent of mild changes in pulmonary pressures [179, 180]. Normalization of the pulmonary pressures in a severe COPD population with long term oxygen therapy is rare [181]. Surgical intervention with lung volume reduction surgery (LVRS) has been used in patients with emphysema for symptom reduction, however, severe PH has traditionally been a contraindication to surgery. The effect of LVRS on PH has not been well defined. In some instances mPAP is increased post-operatively secondary to the decreased size of the vascular bed and, in other studies, improvements in right ventricular function were extrapolated to be secondary to improvements in right ventricular afterload [182, 183]. Transplantation is also an option for some patients and will be discussed independently.

Interstitial Lung Disease

No therapies currently exist that improve mortality in IPF, however, a few medications, such as nintedanib, an intracellular inhibitor that targets multiple tyrosine kinases, may be available soon [184]. It is very important to accurately diagnose the type of ILD, as some may respond to corticosteroids and immune modulators. Corticosteroids have been studied in controlled cohort studies if IPF patients without evidence of consistent benefit, however, sarcoidosis patients often improve with a course of prednisone [185]. Other immunosuppressants, such as methotrexate, azathioprine and cyclophosphamide have also been studied in IPF with disappointing results [186].

Other types of interstitial lung disease, including hypersensitivity pneumonitis (HP) and asbestosis, generally have accepted methods of treatment without controlled data. In treating HP and other exposure related lung disease, the first premise is to remove triggers including drugs, occupational exposures and smoking, as well as treating any gastroesophageal reflux symptoms. For connective tissue disease related ILD, the current method is to treat the underlying disease, primarily with immunomodulators [187].

N-acetylcysteine (NAC) has been studied as treatment in IPF with disappointing results. The IFIGENIA and PANTHER-IPF trials tested NAC as triple therapy with prednisone and azathioprine. The IFIGENIA trial illustrated a slower loss of FVC and DL_{CO} with the addition of NAC to prednisone and azathioprine but PANTHER-IPF was discontinued prior to completion, due to increase in deaths, hospitalizations and adverse events at which time the National Heart, Lung, and Blood Institute (NHLBI) issued a clinical alert against triple therapy [188, 189]. The Idiopathic Pulmonary Fibrosis Research Network published the results of the NAC versus placebo group, which showed no change in deterioration of FVC or DL_{CO}, as well as no improvement in quality of life measures, namely 6MWD or mortality [190].

High Altitude Pulmonary Hypertension

The primary treatment for HAPH is to relocate to a lower altitude, removing the hypoxic stimulus [128]. However,

pharmacological therapies should be used when PH is severe. Nifedipine has been shown to decrease mPAP in patients with HAPH [191]. Sildenafil decreased mPAP and increased 6MWD significantly at 3 months for HAPH patients [192]. Chronic mountain sickness is characterized by excessively elevated hemoglobin and hypoxemia often with moderate to severe PH. Acetazolamide has been used extensively for treating acute mountain sickness and studied in chronic mountain sickness to decreased erythropoesis, however the carbonic anhydrase inhibitors effects have yet to be studied in HAPH [193].

Obesity Hypoventilation Syndrome (OHS) and Obstructive Sleep Apnea (OSA)

In OHS and OSA the treatment strategies are very similar. The most common treatment for both of these entities, in addition to weight loss, is NIPPV during sleep. NIPPV helps mitigate concomitant reductions in FEV1 and FVC. OHS patients should also see a dietician and be started on a weight loss plan. Obesity alone causes decreased chest wall compliance and restrictive ventilation due to the weight of the chest wall. Weight loss has been shown to improve the respiratory mechanics and spirometry in these patients [194]. If necessary surgical weight loss procedures may be performed.

There are a few pharmacotherapies used in OHS with the therapeutic goal of increasing minute ventilation. Medroxyprogesterone has been shown to produce a decrease in $PaCO_2$ and an increase in PaO_2 [195]. These improvements do not come without risk, the most worrisome of which is the possibility of inducing a hypercoagulable state, thereby increasing risk of venous thromboembolism. Acetazolamide has also been studied in OHS, the goal to reduce serum bicarbonate and produce a mild metabolic acidosis to induce an increase in minute ventilation and decreased in $PaCO_2$ [196]. Medroxyprogesterone and acetazolamide may alter the acid base status to help increase minute ventilation, however, there are no strong recommendations for their use given the lack of data on long term safety or reductions in morbidity and mortality [174].

Lung Transplantation

In many of the diseases causing Group 3 PH, lung transplantation is the only therapy that can improve quality of life and prolong life. One of the most important steps is determining if a patient is a suitable transplant candidate. Relative contraindications include age ≥ 65 years, BMI ≥ 30 kg/m^2, severe osteoporosis, previous chest surgery, previous noncompliance and extracorporeal membrane oxygenation (ECMO) or mechanical ventilatory support [197]. The timing of transplantation is very important, in particular when considering the presence of right heart failure. IPF is the most common reason for lung transplantation worldwide, composing 23 % of those who have had the procedure, with a mean pulmonary arterial pressure >25 mmHg being one of the indications to consider transplantation [197, 198].

Lung transplant in itself has many complications and the median survival is around 5.7 years [199]. Of those transplanted, the median survival often correlates with disease process, with IPF and iPAH having the shortest median survival times at less than 5 years [199]. In patients with Group 3 PH, there has been shown to be an increased risk of reperfusion injury after transplant, but the survival is equivalent [200]. Better RV systolic function on exercise echocardiograms, were associated with better survival post lung transplant [201]. Overall, in lung transplant patients, exercise capacity and severity of exercise-induced hypoxemia have been shown to be good indicators of prognosis [202]. Of note, Huerd and colleagues showed that in patients with Group 3 PH who underwent single lung transplant, the survival outcomes were the same as those patients without pulmonary hypertension [203], however there is considerably variability in this practice.

Role of Pulmonary Vasodilators

As of today, there are no recommendations for the use of targeted PH therapy in Group 2 PH (Table 3.4).

COPD

Targeted PH therapy in COPD has been studied without observed benefit. The results of calcium channel blockers, for example, have been disappointing. In one study, the use of nifedipine improved mPAP, but inhibited hypoxia mediated vasoconstriction and, thus, worsened arterial oxygenation [223]. In a small study, the administration of inhaled iloprost worsened hypoxemia at rest and did not improve 6MWD [221]. Sildenafil has been shown to decrease brain natriuretic peptide (BNP) and pulmonary artery systolic pressure on echocardiogram, however, tadalafil did not change 6MWD or quality of life measures [212, 213]. Bosentan decreased PVR but did not change 6MWD or other echocardiographic parameters [215]. In emphysema there appears to be a downregulation of soluble guanylate cyclase (sGC) expression, and in a mouse model, riociguat, the sGC stimulator, protected against development of PH, vascular wall remodeling and right ventricular failure [224]. Thus far, targeted therapies have been inconsistent in their ability to improve 6MWD and hemodynamics, and, little data exists on the impact on morbidity and mortality in these populations.

ILD

In patients with lung fibrosis and hypoxia, vasodilators have been shown to worsen hypoxia, likely due to increased ventilation-perfusion mismatch from removal of hypoxia-mediated vasoconstriction. In IPF studies examining the effects of bosentan, ambrisentan and macitentan, these agents have all failed to show an effect on IPF progression and time to death. However, none of these studies focused on patients who had PH [216–218]. A recent pilot trial of riociguat for PH in ILD showed decrease in PVR with increase in CI and 6MWD [225]. One small study of subcutaneous treprostinil in IPF showed increase in 6MWD and improved hemodynamics [222]. Currently the B-PHIT trial is underway, evaluating bosentan in IPF patients with diagnosed PH [226] Tadalafil is also currently being studied in Group 3 PH by Maron and colleagues [227]. A few small studies have individually shown hemodynamic improvement or increased 6MWD for patients with IPF, however, the findings are not consistent across all studies [204–207, 211].

HAPH

Although, as previously mentioned, HAPH has been shown to correct after prolonged relocation to sea level, this may not be feasible for all sufferers [128]. In acute HAPH, short-term sildenafil has been shown to decrease mPAP elevations [125]. The use of fasudil, a Rho-kinase inhibitor and potent vasodilator, in HAPH showed significant decrease in mPAP [228]. Bosentan has also been studied in HAPH and produced an acute decrease in mPAP, while demonstrating that circulating ET-1 levels were significantly higher in HAPH compared with healthy high altitude inhabitants [229]. There is data showing changes in the Renin-Angiotensin-Aldosterone system in patients with HAPH, suggesting a possible therapeutic target in ACEi's [230]. Overall, small studies have shown benefit of targeted therapies, however, clinical use has not been widely accepted.

Future Directions

A few novel therapies are on the horizon, most notably pirfenidone for IPF. Pirfenidone is an oral anti-fibrotic and anti-inflammatory therapy that is thought to work by inhibiting fibroblast proliferation via DNA synthesis. It may also inhibit fibroblast proliferation, as well as TGF-β, thereby decreasing downstream fibronectin production [231]. Pirfenidone has been studied in randomized controlled trials of IPF patients; CAPACITY 1 and 2 found a reduced decline in FVC as well as progression-free survival [232]. King and colleagues demonstrated improvement in decline of FVC and death by 47.9 % with pirfenidone treatment [233]. Adverse events in both studies centered on gastrointestinal complaints including nausea, dyspepsia, elevated transaminases and anorexia. This medication recently finished Phase 3 trials and has been granted Breakthrough Therapy Designation by the FDA [233].

Nintedanib is another novel therapy that has shown recent promise in patients with IPF. Nintedanib is an inhibitor of tyrosine kinase targeting VEGF and fibroblast growth factor

Table 3.4 Pulmonary vasodilators studied in chronic hypoxic lung disease

Study and year published	Methods	Inclusion criteria	PH at entry	Average mPAP at entry (mmHg)	Results
Ghofrani et al. [204] 2002	Sildenafil 50 mg, Epoprostenol 8 ng/kg/min acute response during RHC n = 16 Randomized	Lung fibrosis patients mPAP > 35 mmHg PCWP < 15 mmHg	Yes	mPAP = 40 (25–60)	Decreased PVR in all groups
Madden et al. [205] 2006	Sildenafil 50 mg TID n = 7 8 week study Non-randomized	End stage COPD & IPF patients	Yes	mPAP = 39	Unchanged mPAP, CO Increase 6MWD
Collard et al. [206] 2007	Sildenafil 20–50 mg TID n = 14 12 week study	IPF patients mPAP ≥ 25 mmHg of catheterization or PASP ≥ 35 mmHg on Echo	Yes	mPAP = 30.7 ± 5.7	Improvement of 6MWD
Corte et al. [207] 2010	Sildenafil 10–25 mg TID 6 month study n = 15 Retrospective, non-randomized	ILD on Sildenafil compassionate use	Yes	mPAP = 41.3 ± 11 PASP = 73.8 ± 17.8	Decreased BNP Unchanged PASP Increased 6MWD
STEP-IPF [208] 2010	Sildenafil 20 mg TID n = 180 Randomized	Advanced IPF DLCO < 35 % predicted	No		Unchanged 6MWD Improved Shortness of Breath score, St George's QoL score Increased DLCO and PaO_2
Rao et al. [209] 2011	Sildenafil 20 mg TID 12 weeks n = 37 randomized	severe COPD 20 pack year TOB	Yes	mPAP = 52.7 ± 11.9	Increase 6MWD Decreased mPAP
Blanco et al. [210] 2010	Sildenafil 20 mg, 40 mg Once n = 20 randomized	COPD with PH	Yes	mPAP = 27 ± 10	Decreased mPAP Decreased PaO_2 at rest
Zimmermann et al. [211] 2014	Sildenafil 20 mg TID or Tadalafil 40 mg QD 12 month study n = 10 Non-randomized	ILD patients, stable within previous 3 months	Yes	mPAP = 42.9 ± 5.4	Increased CI Decreased mPAP (not significant) Decreased PVR
Sharif-kashani et al. [212] 2014	Sildenafil 25–50 mg BID vs. Amlodipine 2.5–7.5 mg QDay 2 week study n = 40 randomized	18–75 yrs RVSP > 45 mmHg COPD without hospitalization or exacerbation in 2 months NT-proBNP > 100	Yes (by Echo)	PASP = 60 ± 12.3	Decreased NT-proBNP levels Decreased PASP
Goudie et al. [213] 2014	Tadalafil 10 mg QD vs. placebo n = 113 Randomized	Moderate to Severe COPD (FEV1/FVC < 0.70) Age 35–85 years FEV1 < 80 % RVSP > 30 mmHg or Pulmonary Acceleration time < 120 ms	Yes		Unchanged in 6MWD Unchanged in quality of life measures
Seibold et al. [214] 2010	Bosentan 62.5 mg BID × 4 weeks then 125 mg BID 12 month study n = 163 Randomized	>18 yrs Interstitial pulmonary disease Systemic sclerosis DLCO < 80 % 6MWD 150–500 m or >500 mg with decreased O_2 sat	No		Unchanged 6MWD Unchanged DLCO and FVC

(continued)

Table 3.4 (continued)

Study and year published	Methods	Inclusion criteria	PH at entry	Average mPAP at entry (mmHg)	Results
Stolz et al. [215] 2008	Bosentan 62.5 mg BID 2 weeks the 125 mg BID 12 week study n=30 Randomized	COPD GOLD III-IV Optimal medical therapy No exacerbations within 1 month No heart failure	No	PASP=32±3	Unchanged 6MWD Decreased PVR, other Echo parameter unchanged
BUILD-3 King et al. [216] 2011	Bosentan 62.5 BID × 4 weeks, then 125 mg BID 20 months n=520 Randomized	≥18 yrs IPF (confirmed by lung biopsy)	No		Unchanged time to IPF worsening or death Unchanged QoL or dyspnea index
MUSIC Raghu et al. [217] 2013	Macitentan 10 mg Qday 1 year n=178 Randomized	>18 yrs IPF (confirmed by lung biopsy)			Unchanged worsening of FVC Unchanged time to first IPF worsening or death Improvement in dyspnea index
ARTEMIS-IPF [218] Raghu et al. 2013	Ambrisentan 5md/day × 2 weeks then 10 mg/day 34 weeks n=494 Randomized	40–80 yrs IPF diagnosed for at least 3 mos Excluded if >5 % honeycombing	No	mPAP=20.3±6.3	Stopped early No difference in DLco, FVC, 6MWD decline Increased disease progression Increased respiratory hospitalizations
Corte et al. [219] 2014	Bosentan 62.5 mg BID × 4 weeks then 125 mg BID 16 week study n=39 Randomized	ILD: IPF or NSIP	Yes	mPAP=36±8.9	Unchanged PVR Unchanged hemodynamic and Echo parameters
Olschewski et al. [220] 1999	IV Epoprostenol 2 ng/ kg/min up to max dose of 16 ng/kg/min, then Inhaled prostacyclin 54–68 µg total n=8	PASP >50 and mPAP >30 Dx of ILD	Yes	mPAP=40.2	IV: Increased CO, Decreased mPAP Inhaled: Decreased mPAP (> than IV)
Boeck et al. [221] 2012	Inhaled iloprost 10 µg, 20 µg n=16 Randomized	>40 years COPD 20 py ROB history	Yes	mPAP=51.8±8.6	Unchanged 6MWD Worsened hypoxemia at rest Unchanged peak O2 consumption
Saggar et al. [222] 2014	Treprostinil subcutaneously (one IV) 12 week study n=15	Pulmonary fibrosis	Yes	mPAP=47±8	Increased 6MWD Improved QoL Decrease mPAP, PVR, RAP Decreased BNP

Abbreviations: *PH* pulmonary hypertension, *PASP* pulmonary artery systolic pressure, *n* number, *yrs* years old, *NYHA* New York Heart Association, *CHF* congestive heart failure, *LVEF* left ventricle ejection fraction, *mPAP* mean pulmonary artery pressure, *DLco* diffusion capacity, *VO²* peak oxygen consumption, *tid* three times a day, *mPAP* mean pulmonary arterial pressure, *6MWD* 6 min walk distance, *bid* twice a day, *HFpEF* heart failure with preserved ejection fraction, *mo* months, *RV* right ventricle, *PVR* pulmonary vascular resistance, *FEV1* forced expiratory volume in 1 s, *FVC* forced vital capacity, *RVSP* right ventricular systolic pressure, DLCO, *ILD* interstitial lung disease, *BNP* brain natriuretic peptide, *QoL* quality of life, *RAP* right atrial pressure, *CO* cardiac output

(FGF). INPULSIS-1 & -2 and TOMORROW were randomized controlled trials that demonstrated a decrease in the decline of FVC with nintedanib treatment at 1 year of therapy. The TOMORROW study showed a decrease in exacerbations and quality of life, as well as a dose-dependent trend towards fewer respiratory deaths, though these findings were not confirmed by the INPULSIS studies. Neither trial resulted in a decrease in respiratory or all-cause mortality. The primary adverse event in both trials was gastrointestinal, primarily diarrhea. Nintedanib has also received Breakthrough Therapy Designation by the FDA [184, 234].

Currently, end stage pulmonary patients lack mechanical support to the same extent that LVAD has transformed destination therapy in advanced heart failure. In acute situations of respiratory compromise ECMO has been used to oxygenate the blood when the lungs were damaged. The advent of the *Novalung* may be the first step towards a pulmonary LVAD equivalent. The initial *Novalung* was a pumpless system with a low-resistance diffusion membrane attached to an oxygen source, designed to treat hypercapneic respiratory failure in a spontaneously ventilated patient. The *Novalung* has been successfully used as a bridge to transplant in patients with hypercapneic respiratory failure and respiratory acidosis [235]. This is remarkable because ECMO and mechanical ventilation are both risk factors for post-transplant mortality. Subsequent trials have used a *Novalung* veno-venous pump driven device in patients with hypoxemic respiratory failure with success [236]. The *Novalung* is not without risks, with adverse events including catheter thrombosis and infection. Despite these risks, the use of *Novalung* as bridge to transplant in awake patient allows participation in physical therapy, normal eating habits and ambulation in the pre-transplant period, therefore minimizing several of the known risks for increased mortality after transplant [237]. There are a few projects focused on designing devices as a bridge to transplant for end-stage lung disease. The emergence of an ventilatory therapy for COPD and ILD patients, the most severe of which often develop PH, is an exciting advance as it has the potential to relieve hypoxemia and hypercapnea prior to transplant.

Overlap Syndromes

Systemic Sclerosis (SSc), lymphangioleiomyomatosis (LAM), pulmonary langerhans cell histiocytosis (PLCH) and sarcoidosis have significant overlap between Group 1, 2, and 3 PH as they can develop pulmonary vascular disease, diastolic dysfunction and parenchymal lung destruction. These diseases pose significant PH therapeutic challenges.

Systemic Sclerosis

Systemic sclerosis (SSc), or scleroderma, is a rare autoimmune disorder characterized by diffuse fibrosis, dysimmunity and vasculopathy [238]. Abnormal vascular endothelium and dysregulation of fibroblast activity with excessive collagen deposition culminate in poor blood supply to various organs resulting in a variety of disease manifestations [239]. Clinically, SSc is divided into limited cutaneous and diffuse cutaneous SSc, based on serologic testing and clinical symptoms [240]. Limited systemic sclerosis, previous referred as CREST syndrome, tends have limited organ involvement and has an overall better prognosis [241].

The prevalence of SSc has a wide range from 7 to 489 cases per million population, with the United States prevalence reportedly 240 cases per million [242–244]. At present, 60 % of mortality in patients with SSc is attributed to lung disease [245]. The pulmonary manifestations of SSc include interstitial lung disease (SSc-ILD) and pulmonary hypertension, either in isolation or concomitantly.

Interstitial lung disease is the most common pulmonary manifestation of SSc affecting around 40 % of patients [239]. However, autopsy reports suggest that parenchymal involvement approaches 100 % [246]. Early SSc-ILD often precedes radiographic findings and diffusion impairment is one of earliest detectable signs of lung involvement [247]. The histologic pattern of SSc-ILD is most commonly non-specific interstitial pneumonitis (NSIP), but organizing pneumonia and diffuse alveolar damage have been reported [248]. However, due to the commonality of SSc-ILD, lung biopsies are rarely performed except to rule out other parenchymal processes.

Pulmonary hypertension in SSc (SSc-PH) is also very common and some estimations approach 40 % of patients affected, depending on the PH definition and screening method applied [122, 249, 250]. PH associated with SSc maybe the consequence of SSc-ILD, left heart disease or pulmonary arterial hypertension (SSc-PAH), thus rigorous evaluation must be performed.

Therapy for SSc-ILD has mainly focused on anti-inflammatory medications based on evidence from bronchoalveolar lavage and biopsy suggesting abnormal inflammatory response and fibrosis as the etiology of lung parenchymal destruction [251–253]. Numerous studies have demonstrated limited treatment success but cyclophosphamide is currently considered the mainstay of therapy [254–256]. A large multi-center study suggested therapy with daily oral cyclophosphamide preserved lung function and symptomatology in patients with SSc-ILD with active alveolitis [257]. Other studies have used the combination of cyclophosphamide with systemic steroids with some success as well [258–260]. However, due to the increased risks of renal crisis with systemic steroids, current management attempts to minimize systemic steroid use. Alternative therapies include mycophenolate mofetil and azathioprine, which have been shown to have some benefit in SSc-ILD. Mycophenolate has preserved lung function in small trials but no large randomized trials have been completed [261]. Azathioprine is useful following induction therapy with cyclophosphamide [262, 263]. Current recommendations include initial therapy with cyclophosphamide followed by maintenance therapy with mycophenolate or azithropine [264].

Management of scleroderma-associated diastolic dysfunction, and subsequent Group 2 PH, concentrates on managing comorbidities including blood pressure control with ACEi and encouraging exercise.

Lymphangioleiomyomatosis (LAM)

LAM is a rare disorder mostly seen in women of childbearing age. It commonly presents as an inherited syndrome called the tuberous sclerosis complex. It also occurs alone as isolated or sporadic LAM. Genetic mutations have been described on the in the tuberous sclerosis 1 or 2 genes (*TSC1* or *TSC2*). The *TSC1* and *TSC2* genes regulate the production of proteins hamartin and tuberin, respectively. These two proteins act as tumor suppressors, regulating cell growth and apoptosis. This disease requires both copies of the *TSC1* gene or *TSC2* gene to be mutated with complete loss of functional hamartin or tuberin. The loss of these proteins allows unregulated cell grow and division resulting in smooth muscle cells (LAM cells), which lead to both parenchymal and vascular lung disease.

The dysregulation of smooth muscle proliferation is noted within the airways of the lung, blood vessels, and lymphatic system. Within the lungs, dysregulation of smooth muscle growth in the walls of the airways results in narrowing and clinically relevant obstructive lung disease. Progressive airway obstruction and air trapping lead to cyst formation which is characteristic of this disease. A similar process occurs in the pulmonary vasculature resulting in progressive blood vessel occlusion contributing to the development of PH. Lymphatic occlusion within the lung parenchyma results in fluid filled cysts and pleural effusions.

Patients often present with variable clinical symptoms including shortness of breath, cough, hemoptysis or spontaneous pneumothorax. Thin wall cysts within the lung along with pleural effusions are the classic findings seen on chest imaging, but imaging may be normal as well. The diagnosis of LAM is difficult and should be entertained in any young woman who presents with obstructive lung disease, spontaneous or recurrent pneumothorax or chylous pleural effusion. High resolution CT scan can often assist with the diagnoses but lung biopsy is often required for concrete diagnoses. Variable results have been obtained with transbronchial biopsies and surgical lung biopsy is often needed to diagnoses this disease.

There is currently no universally accepted therapy for LAM [265]. Pulmonary complications such as pneumothorax should be treated conservatively with standard therapies . Chylothorax is often recurrent even in the setting of a low-fat diet, requiring pleurodesis in many cases [266]. There is no specific therapy for the progressive parenchymal destruction noted with LAM. In the past, therapy has focused on treating with hormonal manipulation with some reports of success with anti-estrogen therapy [267]. However, the use of bilateral oophorectomy and progesterone therapies are controversial with a meta-analysis revealing no benefit of progesterone therapy [268]. More recently, sirolimus has shown promise with stabilization of lung function and improved symptomatology and should be consider as therapy once drug toxicities have been discussed [269]. Due to the progressive nature of this disease, lung transplantation is often indicated in patients with advanced disease and has comparable survival versus patients with other lung diseases [270].

Currently, PH associated with LAM is categorized as Group 5 PH [2]. At least in some part, the pathogenesis of PH in LAM is related to hypoxemia and reduced vascular compliance due the cystic lesions and vascular compression [271]. However, surgical biopsies have revealed abnormal pulmonary vasculature with LAM cell invasion and pulmonary blood vessel obstruction. Based on these findings, independent pulmonary vascular disease may also be contributing to the PH noted in LAM patients. PH has been noted in 8 % of patients with LAM based on echocardiography but very little data is available regarding pulmonary hemodynamics [271]. Only two studies have even evaluated the hemodynamic profiles of patients with PH and LAM [272, 273]. Precapillary hypertension was felt to be clinically evident in 20 of 29 patients with six undergoing specific vasodilator therapy approved for PH. The pulmonary vascular resistance and mean pulmonary artery pressures improved in this study suggesting PAH therapies may have a role in selected patients with LAM [273].

Pulmonary Langerhans Cell Histiocytosis

Pulmonary Langerhans cell histiocytosis (PLCH) is a very rare disease characterized by the abnormal infiltration of the lung parenchyma, lymphoid tissue and vasculature with dendritic cells known as Langerhans cells [274]. Langerhans cells are a distinct population of dendritic cells located in the epithelium of the tracheobronchial tree. These Langerhans cells express CD1a and contain Birbeck granules [275, 276]. Normally, these cells actively survey the tracheobronchial tree for antigen deposition and encounters with antigens lead to cellular activation with antigen presentation and migration to lymphoid tissue [277]. In PLCH, this process becomes dysregulated with abnormal accumulation of Langerhans cells. This accumulation clearly plays a role in disease development however the etiology of the disease process and the origin of these cells remains poorly understood.

PLCH occurs almost exclusively in smokers and there does not appear to be a major gender difference [278, 279]. Further epidemiological data are not currently available and the true prevalence is largely unknown. Various studies have attempted to estimate the prevalence of this disease, but due to heterogeneity it is very difficult to study. One study suggested the prevalence to be 0.7–2.7 cases per million in a Japanese population [280]. PLCH tends to affect young adults with a peak age frequency of 20–40 years old [281]. Clinical presentation is highly variable ranging from asymptomatic with incidental chest x-ray diagnosis to respiratory failure. Spontaneous pneumothorax is the initial presenting symptoms in 10–20 % of the cases and tends to be more common in males [279]. Physical examination is usually normal unless a pneumothorax or advance parenchymal disease is noted.

Reticular nodular pattern with or without cysts in the upper and middle lung zones are the most common patterns seen on chest x-ray [282, 283]. As the disease progresses, the parenchymal findings transition to cysts, giving the x-ray an emphysematous pattern. High resolution CT is currently recommended when PLCH is being entertained as a potential diagnosis. The typical pattern seen is small nodules with thick and thin walled cysts surrounded by normal appearing lung parenchyma [279]. Following the CT imaging over time has revealed progression of the lesions from nodules to cavitated nodules, followed by thick walled cyst which subsequently evolve to thin walled nodules [284]. Spirometry often reveals obstructive lung disease but may be normal in early disease [285]. Most commonly, diffusion impairment is noted in 70–90 % of patients [278, 286]. Bronchoscopy is rarely helpful in making the diagnoses but may rule out other diseases such as atypical infections and obtaining lung tissue remains the gold standard for diagnosis. Definitive diagnosis require the identification of Langerhans cell histocytes within a granuloma in the lung parenchyma [279].

Pre-capillary pulmonary hypertension is common in PLCH when patients are referred for transplantation and is commonly attributed to ILD and chronic hypoxemia [287]. However, PH associated with PLCH is often noted in patients with minor ventilation abnormalities which suggest pulmonary vascular dysfunction [285]. Histopathological findings not only reveal parenchymal lung disease but widespread pulmonary vascular involvement has been noted [286, 288]. Langerhans cell granuloma formation has been described in the small and medium sized pulmonary arteries, contributing to the vasculopathy and pulmonary hypertension.

The progression of PLCH disease is highly variable and specific therapies are largely unproven. Spontaneous remission has been described and tobacco cessation may lead to complete resolution of disease as well [289]. Poor prognosis is associated with numerous factors including advanced age, multi-organ involvement, and reduced diffusion capacity, but pulmonary hypertension most reliably predicts a worse prognosis [278, 290]. Pulmonary hypertension has been noted in up to 92 % of patients referred for lung transplantation at a single center but specific PH therapies have not been studied and are unproven [287]. One reason for the lack of data relates to the high incidence of pulmonary venular obstruction and the risk of pulmonary edema with vasodilation. Prior publications have reported clinically relevant pulmonary edema with the use of epoprostenol and suggest it may be hazardous in this group of patients [291]. However, other studies suggest the use of PAH therapies improved hemodynamics without worsening oxygenation. There was also an insignificant trend toward better survival in the 29 patients studied [292]. Currently, there is no consensus about the use of PAH therapies in PLCH associated PAH and clinical judgment should be used until further studies are available.

Sarcoidosis

Sarcoidosis is a granulomatous disease of unknown etiology that may affect the pulmonary parenchyma or vasculature. Current literature suggests this disease is an abnormal response to an unknown antigen resulting in T cell activation, cellular recruitment, proliferation and differentiation leading to non-caseating granuloma formation [293]. Genetic risk factors have been linked to specific HLA alleles along with non-HLA genes, but these associations need further investigation [294, 295]. The reported prevalence of sarcoidosis varies based on sex, racial groups and geographic location [296]. However, due to the variability of disease presentation and symptomatology an accurate prevalence is largely unknown. The diagnosis of sarcoidosis is based on a various clinic symptoms or incidental findings and a documented granulomatous process of unknown etiology. Clinical symptoms are highly variable involving a single organ or widespread inflammation but common pulmonary symptoms include dyspnea, cough, and chest pain.

Pulmonary disease is present in greater than 90 % of patients diagnosed with sarcoidosis and pulmonary function testing is often abnormal [297]. Pulmonary function testing has been reported to reveal restrictive along with obstructive lung disease without a clear diagnostic pattern being described [298, 299]. Chest imaging is also highly variable but classic findings include adenopathy and pulmonary infiltrates, upon which the current staging system is based [300]. Initiating therapy with corticosteroids is subsequently based on chest x-ray staging and symptomatology and not all patients require therapy [293]. Corticosteroid therapy has been linked to chest x-ray improvements and symptoms, however, there is limited evidence of lung function improvement [301]. Anti-TNF agents such as infliximab have been recently looked promising in the therapy of sarcoidosis [302]. These agents tend to be more useful in patients with an forced vital capacity less than 70 % and significant extrapulmonary disease [303]. Spontaneous remission is not uncommon, even in the higher stages of disease, which makes the decision to initiate therapy challenging [304].

The prevalence of pulmonary hypertension related to sarcoidosis (SAPH) SAPH is highly variable and ranges from 4.1 to 79 % with prevalence increasing with disease severity [305–307]. Pathologic studies have reported 69–100 % pulmonary artery involvement with invasion of the vessel walls with granulomas that result in various vascular changes including vessel occlusion [308, 309]. These vascular

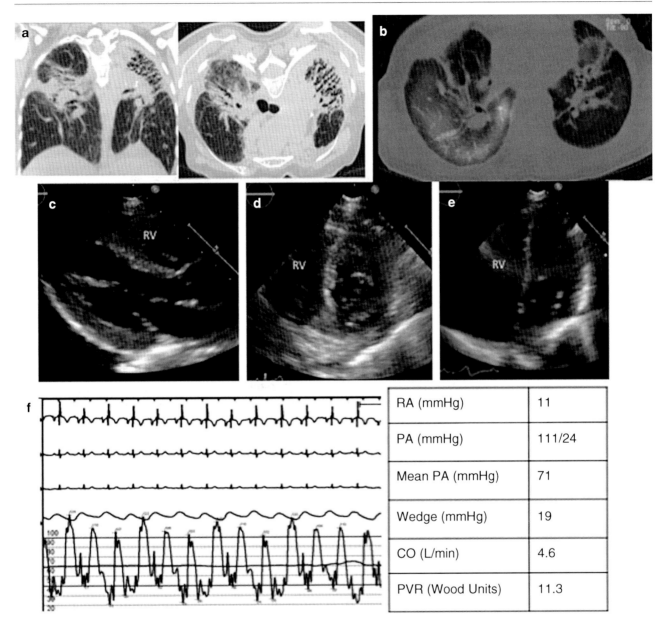

RA (mmHg)	11
PA (mmHg)	111/24
Mean PA (mmHg)	71
Wedge (mmHg)	19
CO (L/min)	4.6
PVR (Wood Units)	11.3

Fig. 3.10 PH from sarcoidosis (Group 2/3 Overlap). (**a**) Chest CT with upper lobe fibrosis, (**b**) Ventilation-Perfusion scan showing matched defects, (**c**) Parasternal long axis showing enlarged RV, (**d**) Parasternal short axis showing enlarged RV and mild septal flattening, (**e**) Apical 4 chamber with large RV, (**f**) RHC tracing of the pulmonary artery pressures, mPAP 71 mmHg

changes are ultimately felt to cause the SAPH found in patients. The resulting PH is thought to be secondary to parenchymal destruction and distortion of lung vasculature (Fig. 3.10) [310]. The optimum therapeutic strategy is largely unknown for SAPH. Vasodilator therapy has been reported to be safe and effective in numerous case reports and case series but large randomized studies have not been conducted. These studies have reported the use of prostacyclin analogs, inhaled NO and PDE5i. However, the largest study to evaluate the use of bosentan was in 35 patients with SAPH [311].

This study revealed significant hemodynamic improvement with bosentan after 16 weeks of therapy. This is the first relatively large study to truly evaluated vasodilator therapy in SAPH and suggests PAH therapies may be a therapeutic option in select patients with SAPH.

Conclusion

PH is often present in cardiac disease and hypoxic lung disease. The diagnostic and therapeutic challenge is to determine what proportion is secondary to Group 2 or

Group 3 PH. Research has yet to confirm that pulmonary vasodilator therapy is beneficial in these conditions and treatment goals currently focus on treating the underlying disease process. The reality of the current classifications of PH is that many of the vascular process overlap and individual patients can often demonstrate characteristics of multiple groups of PH. There is still significant research to be done to determine the efficacy of therapeutically targeting PH in Group 2 and Group 3 PH.

References

1. Strange G, et al. Pulmonary hypertension: prevalence and mortality in the Armadale echocardiography cohort. Heart. 2012;98(24):1805–11.
2. Simonneau G, et al. Updated clinical classification of pulmonary hypertension. J Am Coll Cardiol. 2013;62(25 Suppl):D34–41.
3. Vachiery JL, et al. Pulmonary hypertension due to left heart diseases. J Am Coll Cardiol. 2013;62(25 Suppl):D100–8.
4. Fang JC, DeMarco T, Givertz MM, Borlaug BA, Lewis GD, Rame JE, Gomberg-Maitland M, Murali S, Frantz RP, McGlothlin D, Horn EM and Benza RL. World Health Organization Pulmonary Hypertension group 2: pulmonary hypertension due to left heart disease in the adult–a summary statement from the Pulmonary Hypertension Council of the International Society for Heart and Lung Transplantation. J Heart Lung Transplant. 2012;31:913–33.
5. Seeger W, et al. Pulmonary hypertension in chronic lung diseases. J Am Coll Cardiol. 2013;62(25 Suppl):D109–16.
6. McLaughlin VV, et al. ACCF/AHA 2009 expert consensus document on pulmonary hypertension a report of the American College of Cardiology Foundation Task Force on Expert Consensus Documents and the American Heart Association developed in collaboration with the American College of Chest Physicians; American Thoracic Society, Inc.; and the Pulmonary Hypertension Association. J Am Coll Cardiol. 2009;53(17):1573–619.
7. Perez VA, Haddad F, Zamanian RT. Diagnosis and management of pulmonary hypertension associated with left ventricular diastolic dysfunction. Pulm Circ. 2012;2(2):163–9.
8. Lam CS, et al. Pulmonary hypertension in heart failure with preserved ejection fraction: a community-based study. J Am Coll Cardiol. 2009;53(13):1119–26.
9. Costard-Jackle A, Fowler MB. Influence of preoperative pulmonary artery pressure on mortality after heart transplantation: testing of potential reversibility of pulmonary hypertension with nitroprusside is useful in defining a high risk group. J Am Coll Cardiol. 1992;19(1):48–54.
10. Ghio S, et al. Independent and additive prognostic value of right ventricular systolic function and pulmonary artery pressure in patients with chronic heart failure. J Am Coll Cardiol. 2001;37(1):183–8.
11. Grigioni F, et al. Prognostic implications of serial assessments of pulmonary hypertension in severe chronic heart failure. J Heart Lung Transplant. 2006;25(10):1241–6.
12. Abramson SV, et al. Pulmonary hypertension predicts mortality and morbidity in patients with dilated cardiomyopathy. Ann Intern Med. 1992;116(11):888–95.
13. Butler J, et al. Pre-transplant reversible pulmonary hypertension predicts higher risk for mortality after cardiac transplantation. J Heart Lung Transplant. 2005;24(2):170–7.
14. Galie N, et al. Guidelines for the diagnosis and treatment of pulmonary hypertension: the Task Force for the Diagnosis and Treatment of Pulmonary Hypertension of the European Society of Cardiology (ESC) and the European Respiratory Society (ERS), endorsed by the International Society of Heart and Lung Transplantation (ISHLT). Eur Heart J. 2009;30(20):2493–537.
15. Guazzi M. Alveolar gas diffusion abnormalities in heart failure. J Card Fail. 2008;14(8):695–702.
16. Haddad F, et al. Pulmonary hypertension associated with left heart disease: characteristics, emerging concepts, and treatment strategies. Prog Cardiovasc Dis. 2011;54(2):154–67.
17. West JB, Mathieu-Costello O. Vulnerability of pulmonary capillaries in heart disease. Circulation. 1995;92(3):622–31.
18. Elliott AR, et al. Short-term reversibility of ultrastructural changes in pulmonary capillaries caused by stress failure. J Appl Physiol. 1992;73(3):1150–8.
19. Palestini P, et al. Composition, biophysical properties, and morphometry of plasma membranes in pulmonary interstitial edema. Am J Physiol Lung Cell Mol Physiol. 2002;282(6):L1382–90.
20. Townsley MI, et al. Pulmonary microvascular permeability. Responses to high vascular pressure after induction of pacing-induced heart failure in dogs. Circ Res. 1995;77(2):317–25.
21. Rich S, Rabinovitch M. Diagnosis and treatment of secondary (noncategory 1) pulmonary hypertension. Circulation. 2008;118(21):2190–9.
22. Olson TP, et al. Repeat length polymorphism of the serotonin transporter gene influences pulmonary artery pressure in heart failure. Am Heart J. 2007;153(3):426–32.
23. Du L, et al. Signaling molecules in nonfamilial pulmonary hypertension. N Engl J Med. 2003;348(6):500–9.
24. Loscalzo J, Welch G. Nitric oxide and its role in the cardiovascular system. Prog Cardiovasc Dis. 1995;38(2):87–104.
25. Loscalzo J. Nitric oxide and vascular disease. N Engl J Med. 1995;333(4):251–3.
26. Yu SM, Hung LM, Lin CC. cGMP-elevating agents suppress proliferation of vascular smooth muscle cells by inhibiting the activation of epidermal growth factor signaling pathway. Circulation. 1997;95(5):1269–77.
27. Ooi H, Colucci WS, Givertz MM. Endothelin mediates increased pulmonary vascular tone in patients with heart failure: demonstration by direct intrapulmonary infusion of sitaxsentan. Circulation. 2002;106(13):1618–21.
28. Porter TR, et al. Endothelium-dependent pulmonary artery responses in chronic heart failure: influence of pulmonary hypertension. J Am Coll Cardiol. 1993;22(5):1418–24.
29. Cooper CJ, et al. Role of nitric oxide in the local regulation of pulmonary vascular resistance in humans. Circulation. 1996;93(2):266–71.
30. Cooper CJ, et al. The influence of basal nitric oxide activity on pulmonary vascular resistance in patients with congestive heart failure. Am J Cardiol. 1998;82(5):609–14.
31. Radomski MW, Palmer RM, Moncada S. An L-arginine/nitric oxide pathway present in human platelets regulates aggregation. Proc Natl Acad Sci U S A. 1990;87(13):5193–7.
32. Thenappan T, et al. Clinical characteristics of pulmonary hypertension in patients with heart failure and preserved ejection fraction. Circ Heart Fail. 2011;4(3):257–65.
33. Hoeper MM, et al. Diagnosis, assessment, and treatment of nonpulmonary arterial hypertension pulmonary hypertension. J Am Coll Cardiol. 2009;54(1 Suppl):S85–96.
34. Nagueh SF, et al. Recommendations for the evaluation of left ventricular diastolic function by echocardiography. J Am Soc Echocardiogr. 2009;22(2):107–33.
35. Opotowsky AR, et al. A simple echocardiographic prediction rule for hemodynamics in pulmonary hypertension. Circ Cardiovasc Imaging. 2012;5(6):765–75.
36. Zile MR, Brutsaert DL. New concepts in diastolic dysfunction and diastolic heart failure: Part I: diagnosis, prognosis, and measurements of diastolic function. Circulation. 2002;105(11):1387–93.

37. Paulus WJ, et al. How to diagnose diastolic heart failure: a consensus statement on the diagnosis of heart failure with normal left ventricular ejection fraction by the Heart Failure and Echocardiography Associations of the European Society of Cardiology. Eur Heart J. 2007;28(20):2539–50.

38. Ryan JJ, et al. Current practice for determining pulmonary capillary wedge pressure predisposes to serious errors in the classification of patients with pulmonary hypertension. Am Heart J. 2012;163(4):589–94.

39. Drakos SG, et al. Effect of reversible pulmonary hypertension on outcomes after heart transplantation. J Heart Lung Transplant. 2007;26(4):319–23.

40. Borlaug BA, et al. Exercise hemodynamics enhance diagnosis of early heart failure with preserved ejection fraction. Circ Heart Fail. 2010;3(5):588–95.

41. Tolle JJ, et al. Exercise-induced pulmonary arterial hypertension. Circulation. 2008;118(21):2183–9.

42. Maron BA, et al. The invasive cardiopulmonary exercise test. Circulation. 2013;127(10):1157–64.

43. Hoeper MM, et al. Definitions and diagnosis of pulmonary hypertension. J Am Coll Cardiol. 2013;62(25 Suppl):D42–50.

44. Fox BD, et al. High prevalence of occult left heart disease in scleroderma-pulmonary hypertension. Eur Respir J. 2013;42(4):1083–91.

45. Fujimoto N, et al. Hemodynamic responses to rapid saline loading: the impact of age, sex, and heart failure. Circulation. 2013; 127(1):55–62.

46. Nishimura RA, et al. 2014 AHA/ACC guideline for the management of patients with valvular heart disease: a report of the American College of Cardiology/American Heart Association Task Force on Practice Guidelines. J Am Coll Cardiol. 2014; 63(22):e57–185.

47. Nishimura RA, et al. 2014 AHA/ACC Guideline for the Management of Patients with Valvular Heart Disease: executive summary: a report of the American College of Cardiology/ American Heart Association Task Force on Practice Guidelines. Circulation. 2014;129(23):2440–92.

48. Levine MJ, et al. Progressive improvement in pulmonary vascular resistance after percutaneous mitral valvuloplasty. Circulation. 1989;79(5):1061–7.

49. Zielinski T, et al. Pulmonary hemodynamics at rest and effort, 6 and 12 months after mitral valve replacement: a slow regression of effort pulmonary hypertension. Int J Cardiol. 1993;42(1):57–62.

50. Nishimura RA, Otto C. 2014 ACC/AHA valve guidelines: earlier intervention for chronic mitral regurgitation. Heart. 2014;100(12): 905–7.

51. Barbieri A, et al. Prognostic and therapeutic implications of pulmonary hypertension complicating degenerative mitral regurgitation due to flail leaflet: a multicenter long-term international study. Eur Heart J. 2011;32(6):751–9.

52. Li M, et al. Impact of valve prosthesis-patient mismatch on pulmonary arterial pressure after mitral valve replacement. J Am Coll Cardiol. 2005;45(7):1034–40.

53. Crawford Jr FA. Residual pulmonary artery hypertension after mitral valve replacement: size matters! J Am Coll Cardiol. 2005;45(7):1041–2.

54. Goldstone AB, et al. Incidence, epidemiology, and prognosis of residual pulmonary hypertension after mitral valve repair for degenerative mitral regurgitation. Am J Cardiol. 2011;107(5):755–60.

55. Casaclang-Verzosa G, et al. E/Ea is the major determinant of pulmonary artery pressure in moderate to severe aortic stenosis. J Am Soc Echocardiogr. 2008;21(7):824–7.

56. Johnson LW, et al. Pulmonary hypertension in isolated aortic stenosis. Hemodynamic correlations and follow-up. J Thorac Cardiovasc Surg. 1988;95(4):603–7.

57. Silver K, et al. Pulmonary artery hypertension in severe aortic stenosis: incidence and mechanism. Am Heart J. 1993;125(1):146–50.

58. Faggiano P, et al. Pulmonary artery hypertension in adult patients with symptomatic valvular aortic stenosis. Am J Cardiol. 2000; 85(2):204–8.

59. Kapoor N, Varadarajan P, Pai RG. Echocardiographic predictors of pulmonary hypertension in patients with severe aortic stenosis. Eur J Echocardiogr. 2008;9(1):31–3.

60. Melby SJ, et al. Impact of pulmonary hypertension on outcomes after aortic valve replacement for aortic valve stenosis. J Thorac Cardiovasc Surg. 2011;141(6):1424–30.

61. Malouf JF, et al. Severe pulmonary hypertension in patients with severe aortic valve stenosis: clinical profile and prognostic implications. J Am Coll Cardiol. 2002;40(4):789–95.

62. Sinning JM, et al. Decrease of pulmonary hypertension impacts on prognosis after transcatheter aortic valve replacement. EuroIntervention. 2014;9(9):1042–9.

63. Khandhar S, et al. Survival benefit of aortic valve replacement in patients with severe aortic regurgitation and pulmonary hypertension. Ann Thorac Surg. 2009;88(3):752–6.

64. Naidoo DP, et al. Pulmonary hypertension in aortic regurgitation: early surgical outcome. Q J Med. 1991;80(291):589–95.

65. Guglin M, Khan H. Pulmonary hypertension in heart failure. J Card Fail. 2010;16(6):461–74.

66. Delgado JF, et al. Impact of mild pulmonary hypertension on mortality and pulmonary artery pressure profile after heart transplantation. J Heart Lung Transplant. 2001;20(9):942–8.

67. Mikus E, et al. Reversibility of fixed pulmonary hypertension in left ventricular assist device support recipients. Eur J Cardiothorac Surg. 2011;40(4):971–7.

68. Kiefer TL, Bashore TM. Pulmonary hypertension related to left-sided cardiac pathology. Pulm Med. 2011;2011:381787.

69. Malkowska AM, Waring WS. Constrictive pericarditis is an easily overlooked cause of right heart failure: a case report. Cases J. 2008;1(1):27.

70. Brunner NW, et al. A case of recurrent pericardial constriction presenting with severe pulmonary hypertension. Pulm Circ. 2013;3(2):436–9.

71. Guazzi M, et al. The effects of phosphodiesterase-5 inhibition with sildenafil on pulmonary hemodynamics and diffusion capacity, exercise ventilatory efficiency, and oxygen uptake kinetics in chronic heart failure. J Am Coll Cardiol. 2004;44(12):2339–48.

72. Lewis GD, et al. Sildenafil improves exercise capacity and quality of life in patients with systolic heart failure and secondary pulmonary hypertension. Circulation. 2007;116(14):1555–62.

73. Guazzi M, et al. Long-term use of sildenafil in the therapeutic management of heart failure. J Am Coll Cardiol. 2007;50(22): 2136–44.

74. Lewis GD, et al. Determinants of ventilatory efficiency in heart failure: the role of right ventricular performance and pulmonary vascular tone. Circ Heart Fail. 2008;1(4):227–33.

75. Behling A, et al. Effects of 5′-phosphodiesterase four-week long inhibition with sildenafil in patients with chronic heart failure: a double-blind, placebo-controlled clinical trial. J Card Fail. 2008;14(3):189–97.

76. Guazzi M, et al. Six months of Sildenafil therapy improves heart rate recovery in patients with heart failure. Int J Cardiol. 2009;136(3):341–3.

77. Guazzi M, et al. Pulmonary hypertension in heart failure with preserved ejection fraction: a target of phosphodiesterase-5 inhibition in a 1-year study. Circulation. 2011;124(2):164–74.

78. Guazzi M, et al. PDE5 inhibition with sildenafil improves left ventricular diastolic function, cardiac geometry, and clinical status in patients with stable systolic heart failure: results of a 1-year, prospective, randomized, placebo-controlled study. Circ Heart Fail. 2011;4(1):8–17.

79. Guazzi M, Vicenzi M, Arena R. Phosphodiesterase 5 inhibition with sildenafil reverses exercise oscillatory breathing in chronic

heart failure: a long-term cardiopulmonary exercise testing placebo-controlled study. Eur J Heart Fail. 2012;14(1):82–90.

80. Reichenbach A, Al-Hiti H, Malek I, Pirk J, Goncalvesova E, Kautzner J, Melenovsky V. The effects of phosphodiesterase 5 inhibition on hemodynamics, functional status and survival in advanced heart failure and pulmonary hypertension: A case-control study. Int J Cardiol. 2013;168:60–5.

81. Redfield MM, et al. PhosphdiesteRasE-5 Inhibition to Improve CLinical Status and EXercise Capacity in Diastolic Heart Failure (RELAX) trial: rationale and design. Circ Heart Fail. 2012;5(5):653–9.

82. Givertz MM, et al. Acute endothelin A receptor blockade causes selective pulmonary vasodilation in patients with chronic heart failure. Circulation. 2000;101(25):2922–7.

83. Luscher TF, et al. Hemodynamic and neurohumoral effects of selective endothelin A (ET(A)) receptor blockade in chronic heart failure: the Heart Failure ET(A) Receptor Blockade Trial (HEAT). Circulation. 2002;106(21):2666–72.

84. Perez-Villa F, et al. Initial experience with bosentan therapy in patients considered ineligible for heart transplantation because of severe pulmonary hypertension. Clin Transplant. 2006;20(2):239–44.

85. Kaluski E, et al. Clinical and hemodynamic effects of bosentan dose optimization in symptomatic heart failure patients with severe systolic dysfunction, associated with secondary pulmonary hypertension–a multi-center randomized study. Cardiology. 2008;109(4):273–80.

86. Hefke T, Zittermann A, Fuchs U, Schulte-Eistrup S, Gummert JF, Schulz U. Bosentan effects on hemodynamics and clinical outcome in heart failure patients with pulmonary hypertension awaiting cardiac transplantation. J Thorac Cardiovasc Surg. 2012;60:26–34.

87. Padeletti M, et al. Effect of bosentan on pulmonary hypertension secondary to systolic heart failure. Pharmacology. 2013;92(5–6):281–5.

88. Montalescot G, et al. Effects of prostacyclin on the pulmonary vascular tone and cardiac contractility of patients with pulmonary hypertension secondary to end-stage heart failure. Am J Cardiol. 1998;82(6):749–55.

89. Weston MW, Isaac BF, Crain C. The use of inhaled prostacyclin in nitroprusside-resistant pulmonary artery hypertension. J Heart Lung Transplant. 2001;20(12):1340–4.

90. Sablotzki A, et al. Iloprost improves hemodynamics in patients with severe chronic cardiac failure and secondary pulmonary hypertension. Can J Anaesth. 2002;49(10):1076–80.

91. von Scheidt W, et al. Prostaglandin E1 testing in heart failure-associated pulmonary hypertension enables transplantation: the PROPHET study. J Heart Lung Transplant. 2006;25(9):1070–6.

92. Serra W, et al. Benefit of prostaglandin infusion in severe heart failure: preliminary clinical experience of repetitive administration. Int J Cardiol. 2011;146(1):e10–5.

93. Bonderman D, et al. Riociguat for patients with pulmonary hypertension caused by systolic left ventricular dysfunction: a phase IIb double-blind, randomized, placebo-controlled, dose-ranging hemodynamic study. Circulation. 2013;128(5):502–11.

94. Califf RM, et al. A randomized controlled trial of epoprostenol therapy for severe congestive heart failure: The Flolan International Randomized Survival Trial (FIRST). Am Heart J. 1997;134(1):44–54.

95. Kalra PR, Moon JC, Coats AJ. Do results of the ENABLE (Endothelin Antagonist Bosentan for Lowering Cardiac Events in Heart Failure) study spell the end for non-selective endothelin antagonism in heart failure? Int J Cardiol. 2002;85(2–3):195–7.

96. Nagendran J, et al. Endothelin axis is upregulated in human and rat right ventricular hypertrophy. Circ Res. 2013;112(2):347–54.

97. Cooper TJ, Guazzi M, Al-Mohammad A, Amir O, Bengal T, Cleland JG, Dickstein K. Sildenafil in heart failure (silhf). An investigator-initiated multinational randomized controlled clinical trial: Rationale and design. Eur J Heart Fail. 2013;15:119–22.

98. New England Research Institutes; National Heart, Lung, and Blood Institute Massachusetts General Hospital. Phosphodiesterase type 5 inhibition with tadalafil changes outcomes in heart failure (PITCH-HF). In: Clinicaltrials.gov [Internet]. Bethesda (MD): National Library of Medicine (US) 2013. Available from: http://clinicaltrials.gov/ct2/show/NCT01910389. NLM identifier: NCT01910389.

99. Redfield MM, et al. Effect of phosphodiesterase-5 inhibition on exercise capacity and clinical status in heart failure with preserved ejection fraction: a randomized clinical trial. JAMA. 2013;309(12):1268–77.

100. Nativi-Nicolau J, Ryan JJ, Fang JC. Current therapeutic approach in heart failure with preserved ejection fraction. Heart Fail Clin. 2014;10(3):525–38.

101. Bayer. Phase IIb Safety and Efficacy Study of Four Dose Regimens of BAY1021189 in Patients with Heart Failure and Preserved Ejection Fraction Suffering from Worsening Chronic Heart Failure (SOCRATES-PRESERVED). In: Clinicaltrials.gov [Internet]. Bethesda (MD): National Library of Medicine (US) 2013. Available from: http://clinicaltrials.gov/ct2/show/NCT01951638. NLM identifier: NCT01951638.

102. Actelion. Safety and tolerability of macitentan in subjects with combined pre- and post-capillary pulmonary hypertension due to left ventricular dysfunction (MELODY-1). In: Clinicaltrials.gov [Internet]. Bethesda (MD): National Library of Medicine (US) 2014. Available from: http://clinicaltrials.gov/ct2/show/NCT02070991. NLM identifier: NCT02070991.

103. Benza RL, Raina A, Abraham WT, Adamson PB, Lindenfeld J, Miller AB, Bourge RC, Bauman J, Yadav J. Pulmonary hypertension related to left heart disease: Insight from a wireless implantable hemodynamic monitor. J Heart Lung Transplant. 2015;34(3):329–37.

104. Abraham WT, et al. Wireless pulmonary artery haemodynamic monitoring in chronic heart failure: a randomised controlled trial. Lancet. 2011;377(9766):658–66.

105. Hyduk A, et al. Pulmonary hypertension surveillance – United States, 1980–2002. MMWR Surveill Summ. 2005;54(5):1–28.

106. Chaouat A, Naeije R, Weitzenblum E. Pulmonary hypertension in COPD. Eur Respir J. 2008;32(5):1371–85.

107. Minai OA, Chaouat A, Adnot S. Pulmonary hypertension in COPD: epidemiology, significance, and management: pulmonary vascular disease: the global perspective. Chest. 2010;137(6 Suppl):39S–51.

108. Minai OA, et al. Clinical characteristics and prediction of pulmonary hypertension in severe emphysema. Respir Med. 2014;108(3):482–90.

109. Stark RD, Finnegan P, Bishop JM. Daily requirement of oxygen to reverse pulmonary hypertension in patients with chronic bronchitis. Br Med J. 1972;3(5829):724–8.

110. Oswald-Mammosser M, et al. Prognostic factors in COPD patients receiving long-term oxygen therapy. Importance of pulmonary artery pressure. Chest. 1995;107(5):1193–8.

111. Kessler R, et al. Predictive factors of hospitalization for acute exacerbation in a series of 64 patients with chronic obstructive pulmonary disease. Am J Respir Crit Care Med. 1999;159(1):158–64.

112. Lettieri CJ, et al. Prevalence and outcomes of pulmonary arterial hypertension in advanced idiopathic pulmonary fibrosis. Chest. 2006;129(3):746–52.

113. Nadrous HF, et al. Pulmonary hypertension in patients with idiopathic pulmonary fibrosis. Chest. 2005;128(4):2393–9.

114. Jankowich MD, Rounds SI. Combined pulmonary fibrosis and emphysema syndrome: a review. Chest. 2012;141(1):222–31.

115. Mapel DW, et al. Idiopathic pulmonary fibrosis: survival in population based and hospital based cohorts. Thorax. 1998;53(6):469–76.

116. Corte TJ, Wort SJ, Wells AU. Pulmonary hypertension in idiopathic pulmonary fibrosis: a review. Sarcoidosis Vasc Diffuse Lung Dis. 2009;26(1):7–19.

117. Behr J, Ryu JH. Pulmonary hypertension in interstitial lung disease. Eur Respir J. 2008;31(6):1357–67.

118. Handa T, et al. Incidence of pulmonary hypertension and its clinical relevance in patients with sarcoidosis. Chest. 2006;129(5): 1246–52.

119. Shorr AF, et al. Pulmonary hypertension in advanced sarcoidosis: epidemiology and clinical characteristics. Eur Respir J. 2005; 25(5):783–8.

120. Launay D, et al. Prevalence and characteristics of moderate to severe pulmonary hypertension in systemic sclerosis with and without interstitial lung disease. J Rheumatol. 2007;34(5):1005–11.

121. Trad S, et al. Pulmonary arterial hypertension is a major mortality factor in diffuse systemic sclerosis, independent of interstitial lung disease. Arthritis Rheum. 2006;54(1):184–91.

122. Chang B, et al. Scleroderma patients with combined pulmonary hypertension and interstitial lung disease. J Rheumatol. 2003; 30(11):2398–405.

123. Johnson SR, Granton JT. Pulmonary hypertension in systemic sclerosis and systemic lupus erythematosus. Eur Respir Rev. 2011;20(122):277–86.

124. Bartsch P, Saltin B. General introduction to altitude adaptation and mountain sickness. Scand J Med Sci Sports. 2008;18 Suppl 1:1–10.

125. Xu XQ, Jing ZC. High-altitude pulmonary hypertension. Eur Respir Rev. 2009;18(111):13–7.

126. Sime F, et al. Pulmonary hypertension in children born and living at high altitudes. Am J Cardiol. 1963;11:143–9.

127. Aldashev AA, et al. Characterization of high-altitude pulmonary hypertension in the Kyrgyz: association with angiotensin-converting enzyme genotype. Am J Respir Crit Care Med. 2002;166(10):1396–402.

128. Sime F, Penaloza D, Ruiz L. Bradycardia, increased cardiac output, and reversal of pulmonary hypertension in altitude natives living at sea level. Br Heart J. 1971;33(5):647–57.

129. Kauppert CA, et al. Pulmonary hypertension in obesity-hypoventilation syndrome. Respir Med. 2013;107(12):2061–70.

130. Kessler R, et al. The obesity-hypoventilation syndrome revisited: a prospective study of 34 consecutive cases. Chest. 2001;120(2): 369–76.

131. Minai OA, et al. Frequency and impact of pulmonary hypertension in patients with obstructive sleep apnea syndrome. Am J Cardiol. 2009;104(9):1300–6.

132. Sajkov D, McEvoy RD. Obstructive sleep apnea and pulmonary hypertension. Prog Cardiovasc Dis. 2009;51(5):363–70.

133. Stenmark KR, Fagan KA, Frid MG. Hypoxia-induced pulmonary vascular remodeling: cellular and molecular mechanisms. Circ Res. 2006;99(7):675–91.

134. Desmouliere A, et al. Transforming growth factor-beta 1 induces alpha-smooth muscle actin expression in granulation tissue myofibroblasts and in quiescent and growing cultured fibroblasts. J Cell Biol. 1993;122(1):103–11.

135. Hinz B, et al. Alpha-smooth muscle actin expression upregulates fibroblast contractile activity. Mol Biol Cell. 2001;12(9):2730–41.

136. Howell K, Preston RJ, McLoughlin P. Chronic hypoxia causes angiogenesis in addition to remodelling in the adult rat pulmonary circulation. J Physiol. 2003;547(Pt 1):133–45.

137. Bonnet S, et al. An abnormal mitochondrial-hypoxia inducible factor-1alpha-Kv channel pathway disrupts oxygen sensing and triggers pulmonary arterial hypertension in fawn hooded rats: similarities to human pulmonary arterial hypertension. Circulation. 2006;113(22):2630–41.

138. Marsboom G, et al. Lung (1)(8)F-fluorodeoxyglucose positron emission tomography for diagnosis and monitoring of pulmonary arterial hypertension. Am J Respir Crit Care Med. 2012; 185(6):670–9.

139. Archer SL, et al. Mitochondrial metabolism, redox signaling, and fusion: a mitochondria-ROS-HIF-1alpha-Kv1.5 O2-sensing pathway at the intersection of pulmonary hypertension and cancer. Am J Physiol Heart Circ Physiol. 2008;294(2):H570–8.

140. Hickey MM, et al. The von Hippel-Lindau Chuvash mutation promotes pulmonary hypertension and fibrosis in mice. J Clin Invest. 2010;120(3):827–39.

141. Hu CJ, et al. Differential roles of hypoxia-inducible factor 1alpha (HIF-1alpha) and HIF-2alpha in hypoxic gene regulation. Mol Cell Biol. 2003;23(24):9361–74.

142. Azarov I, et al. Nitric oxide scavenging by red blood cells as a function of hematocrit and oxygenation. J Biol Chem. 2005; 280(47):39024–32.

143. Deem S, et al. Red-blood-cell augmentation of hypoxic pulmonary vasoconstriction: hematocrit dependence and the importance of nitric oxide. Am J Respir Crit Care Med. 1998;157(4 Pt 1):1181–6.

144. MacNee W. Pathophysiology of cor pulmonale in chronic obstructive pulmonary disease. Part two. Am J Respir Crit Care Med. 1994;150(4):1158–68.

145. Shujaat A, Bajwa AA, Cury JD. Pulmonary hypertension secondary to COPD. Pulm Med. 2012;2012:203952.

146. Strange C, Highland KB. Pulmonary hypertension in interstitial lung disease. Curr Opin Pulm Med. 2005;11(5):452–5.

147. Cosgrove GP, et al. Pigment epithelium-derived factor in idiopathic pulmonary fibrosis: a role in aberrant angiogenesis. Am J Respir Crit Care Med. 2004;170(3):242–51.

148. Ebina M, et al. Heterogeneous increase in CD34-positive alveolar capillaries in idiopathic pulmonary fibrosis. Am J Respir Crit Care Med. 2004;169(11):1203–8.

149. Farkas L, et al. VEGF ameliorates pulmonary hypertension through inhibition of endothelial apoptosis in experimental lung fibrosis in rats. J Clin Invest. 2009;119(5):1298–311.

150. He H, et al. Vascular endothelial growth factor signals endothelial cell production of nitric oxide and prostacyclin through flk-1/KDR activation of c-Src. J Biol Chem. 1999;274(35):25130–5.

151. Wang H, Keiser JA. Vascular endothelial growth factor upregulates the expression of matrix metalloproteinases in vascular smooth muscle cells: role of flt-1. Circ Res. 1998;83(8):832–40.

152. Voelkel NF, Vandivier RW, Tuder RM. Vascular endothelial growth factor in the lung. Am J Physiol Lung Cell Mol Physiol. 2006;290(2):L209–21.

153. Xing D, et al. Endothelial cells overexpressing interleukin-8 receptors reduce inflammatory and neointimal responses to arterial injury. Circulation. 2012;125(12):1533–41.

154. Fu J, et al. Targeted delivery of pulmonary arterial endothelial cells overexpressing interleukin-8 receptors attenuates monocrotaline-induced pulmonary vascular remodeling. Arterioscler Thromb Vasc Biol. 2014;34(7):1539–47.

155. Richards TJ, et al. Peripheral blood proteins predict mortality in idiopathic pulmonary fibrosis. Am J Respir Crit Care Med. 2012;185(1):67–76.

156. Yamamoto C, et al. Airway inflammation in COPD assessed by sputum levels of interleukin-8. Chest. 1997;112(2):505–10.

157. Farkas L, et al. Pulmonary hypertension and idiopathic pulmonary fibrosis: a tale of angiogenesis, apoptosis, and growth factors. Am J Respir Cell Mol Biol. 2011;45(1):1–15.

158. Kasahara Y, et al. Endothelial cell death and decreased expression of vascular endothelial growth factor and vascular endothelial growth factor receptor 2 in emphysema. Am J Respir Crit Care Med. 2001;163(3 Pt 1):737–44.

159. Burke DL, et al. Sustained hypoxia promotes the development of a pulmonary artery-specific chronic inflammatory microenvironment. Am J Physiol Lung Cell Mol Physiol. 2009;297(2):L238–50.

160. Frid MG, et al. Hypoxia-induced pulmonary vascular remodeling requires recruitment of circulating mesenchymal precursors of a monocyte/macrophage lineage. Am J Pathol. 2006;168(2): 659–69.

161. Distler JH, et al. Hypoxia-induced increase in the production of extracellular matrix proteins in systemic sclerosis. Arthritis Rheum. 2007;56(12):4203–15.

162. Eddahibi S, et al. Interleukin-6 gene polymorphism confers susceptibility to pulmonary hypertension in chronic obstructive pulmonary disease. Proc Am Thorac Soc. 2006;3(6):475–6.

163. Gourh P, et al. Plasma cytokine profiles in systemic sclerosis: associations with autoantibody subsets and clinical manifestations. Arthritis Res Ther. 2009;11(5):R147.

164. Humbert M, et al. Increased interleukin-1 and interleukin-6 serum concentrations in severe primary pulmonary hypertension. Am J Respir Crit Care Med. 1995;151(5):1628–31.

165. Nishimaki T, et al. Immunological analysis of pulmonary hypertension in connective tissue diseases. J Rheumatol. 1999;26(11):2357–62.

166. Savale L, et al. Impact of interleukin-6 on hypoxia-induced pulmonary hypertension and lung inflammation in mice. Respir Res. 2009;10:6.

167. Giaid A, Saleh D. Reduced expression of endothelial nitric oxide synthase in the lungs of patients with pulmonary hypertension. N Engl J Med. 1995;333(4):214–21.

168. Dinh-Xuan AT, et al. Impairment of endothelium-dependent pulmonary-artery relaxation in chronic obstructive lung disease. N Engl J Med. 1991;324(22):1539–47.

169. Barbera JA, et al. Reduced expression of endothelial nitric oxide synthase in pulmonary arteries of smokers. Am J Respir Crit Care Med. 2001;164(4):709–13.

170. Orte C, et al. Expression of pulmonary vascular angiotensin-converting enzyme in primary and secondary plexiform pulmonary hypertension. J Pathol. 2000;192(3):379–84.

171. Morrell NW, et al. Angiotensin converting enzyme expression is increased in small pulmonary arteries of rats with hypoxia-induced pulmonary hypertension. J Clin Invest. 1995;96(4): 1823–33.

172. Morrell NW, Morris KG, Stenmark KR. Role of angiotensin-converting enzyme and angiotensin II in development of hypoxic pulmonary hypertension. Am J Physiol. 1995;269(4 Pt 2): H1186–94.

173. Nong Z, et al. Inhibition of tissue angiotensin-converting enzyme with quinapril reduces hypoxic pulmonary hypertension and pulmonary vascular remodeling. Circulation. 1996;94(8):1941–7.

174. Al Dabal L, Bahammam AS. Obesity hypoventilation syndrome. Ann Thorac Med. 2009;4(2):41–9.

175. Campo A, et al. Hyperleptinaemia, respiratory drive and hypercapnic response in obese patients. Eur Respir J. 2007;30(2): 223–31.

176. Yee BJ, et al. Treatment of obesity hypoventilation syndrome and serum leptin. Respiration. 2006;73(2):209–12.

177. Raghu G, Brown KK. Interstitial lung disease: clinical evaluation and keys to an accurate diagnosis. Clin Chest Med. 2004;25(3):409–19. v.

178. Matthay RA. Effects of theophylline on cardiovascular performance in chronic obstructive pulmonary disease. Chest. 1985;88(2 Suppl):112S–7.

179. Long term domiciliary oxygen therapy in chronic hypoxic cor pulmonale complicating chronic bronchitis and emphysema. Report of the Medical Research Council Working Party. Lancet. 1981; 1(8222):681–6.

180. Continuous or nocturnal oxygen therapy in hypoxemic chronic obstructive lung disease: a clinical trial. Nocturnal Oxygen Therapy Trial Group. Ann Intern Med. 1980;93(3):391–8.

181. Weitzenblum E, et al. Long-term oxygen therapy can reverse the progression of pulmonary hypertension in patients with chronic obstructive pulmonary disease. Am Rev Respir Dis. 1985;131(4): 493–8.

182. Weg IL, et al. Development of pulmonary hypertension after lung volume reduction surgery. Am J Respir Crit Care Med. 1999; 159(2):552–6.

183. Sciurba FC, et al. Improvement in pulmonary function and elastic recoil after lung-reduction surgery for diffuse emphysema. N Engl J Med. 1996;334(17):1095–9.

184. Richeldi L, et al. Efficacy and safety of nintedanib in idiopathic pulmonary fibrosis. N Engl J Med. 2014;370(22):2071–82.

185. Rodman DM, Lindenfeld J. Successful treatment of sarcoidosis-associated pulmonary hypertension with corticosteroids. Chest. 1990;97(2):500–2.

186. Rafii R, et al. A review of current and novel therapies for idiopathic pulmonary fibrosis. J Thorac Dis. 2013;5(1):48–73.

187. Wells AU, Kokosi M, Karagiannis K. Treatment strategies for idiopathic interstitial pneumonias. Curr Opin Pulm Med. 2014;20(5):442–8.

188. Demedts M, et al. High-dose acetylcysteine in idiopathic pulmonary fibrosis. N Engl J Med. 2005;353(21):2229–42.

189. Idiopathic Pulmonary Fibrosis Clinical Research N, et al. Prednisone, azathioprine, and N-acetylcysteine for pulmonary fibrosis. N Engl J Med. 2012;366(21):1968–77.

190. Idiopathic Pulmonary Fibrosis Clinical Research N, et al. Randomized trial of acetylcysteine in idiopathic pulmonary fibrosis. N Engl J Med. 2014;370(22):2093–101.

191. Antezana AM, et al. Pulmonary hypertension in high-altitude chronic hypoxia: response to nifedipine. Eur Respir J. 1998;12(5): 1181–5.

192. Aldashev AA, et al. Phosphodiesterase type 5 and high altitude pulmonary hypertension. Thorax. 2005;60(8):683–7.

193. Rivera-Ch M, Leon-Velarde F, Huicho L. Treatment of chronic mountain sickness: critical reappraisal of an old problem. Respir Physiol Neurobiol. 2007;158(2–3):251–65.

194. Aaron SD, et al. Effect of weight reduction on respiratory function and airway reactivity in obese women. Chest. 2004;125(6):2046–52.

195. Sutton Jr FD, et al. Progesterone for outpatient treatment of Pickwickian syndrome. Ann Intern Med. 1975;83(4):476–9.

196. Raurich JM, et al. Hypercapnic respiratory failure in obesity-hypoventilation syndrome: CO(2) response and acetazolamide treatment effects. Respir Care. 2010;55(11):1442–8.

197. Gottlieb J. Lung transplantation for interstitial lung diseases. Curr Opin Pulm Med. 2014;20(5):457–462

198. Yusen RD, et al. The Registry of the International Society for Heart and Lung Transplantation: Thirtieth Adult Lung and Heart-Lung Transplant Report – 2013; focus theme: age. J Heart Lung Transplant. 2013;32(10):965–78.

199. Kotloff RM, Thabut G. Lung transplantation. Am J Respir Crit Care Med. 2011;184(2):159–71.

200. Fitton TP, et al. Impact of secondary pulmonary hypertension on lung transplant outcome. J Heart Lung Transplant. 2005;24(9): 1254–9.

201. Selimovic N, Andersson B, Bech-Hanssen O, Lomsky M, Riise GC, Rundqvist B. Right ventricular ejection fraction during exercise as a predictor of mortality in patients awaiting lung transplantation: A cohort study. BMJ open. 2013;3(4): Epub. e002108. doi:10.1136/bmjopen-2012-002108.

202. Kawut SM, et al. Exercise testing determines survival in patients with diffuse parenchymal lung disease evaluated for lung transplantation. Respir Med. 2005;99(11):1431–9.

203. Huerd SS, et al. Secondary pulmonary hypertension does not adversely affect outcome after single lung transplantation. J Thorac Cardiovasc Surg. 2000;119(3):458–65.

204. Ghofrani HA, et al. Sildenafil for treatment of lung fibrosis and pulmonary hypertension: a randomised controlled trial. Lancet. 2002;360(9337):895–900.

205. Madden BP, et al. A potential role for sildenafil in the management of pulmonary hypertension in patients with parenchymal lung disease. Vascul Pharmacol. 2006;44(5):372–6.

206. Collard HR, et al. Sildenafil improves walk distance in idiopathic pulmonary fibrosis. Chest. 2007;131(3):897–9.

207. Corte TJ, et al. The use of sildenafil to treat pulmonary hypertension associated with interstitial lung disease. Respirology. 2010; 15(8):1226–32.

208. Idiopathic Pulmonary Fibrosis Clinical Research N, et al. A controlled trial of sildenafil in advanced idiopathic pulmonary fibrosis. N Engl J Med. 2010;363(7):620–8.

209. Rao RS, et al. Sildenafil improves six-minute walk distance in chronic obstructive pulmonary disease: a randomised, double-blind, placebo-controlled trial. Indian J Chest Dis Allied Sci. 2011;53(2):81–5.

210. Blanco I, et al. Hemodynamic and gas exchange effects of sildenafil in patients with chronic obstructive pulmonary disease and pulmonary hypertension. Am J Respir Crit Care Med. 2010; 181(3):270–8.

211. Zimmermann GS, et al. Haemodynamic changes in pulmonary hypertension in patients with interstitial lung disease treated with PDE-5 inhibitors. Respirology. 2014;19(5):700–6.

212. Sharif-Kashani B, et al. The effect of amlodipine and sildenafil on the NT-ProBNP level of patients with COPD-induced pulmonary hypertension. Iran J Pharm Res. 2014;13(Suppl):161–8.

213. Goudie AR, et al. Tadalafil in patients with chronic obstructive pulmonary disease: a randomised, double-blind, parallel-group, placebo-controlled trial. Lancet Respir Med. 2014;2(4): 293–300.

214. Seibold JR, et al. Randomized, prospective, placebo-controlled trial of bosentan in interstitial lung disease secondary to systemic sclerosis. Arthritis Rheum. 2010;62(7):2101–8.

215. Stolz D, et al. A randomised, controlled trial of bosentan in severe COPD. Eur Respir J. 2008;32(3):619–28.

216. King Jr TE, et al. BUILD-3: a randomized, controlled trial of bosentan in idiopathic pulmonary fibrosis. Am J Respir Crit Care Med. 2011;184(1):92–9.

217. Raghu G, et al. Macitentan for the treatment of idiopathic pulmonary fibrosis: the randomised controlled MUSIC trial. Eur Respir J. 2013;42(6):1622–32.

218. Raghu G, et al. Treatment of idiopathic pulmonary fibrosis with ambrisentan: a parallel, randomized trial. Ann Intern Med. 2013;158(9):641–9.

219. Corte TJ, et al. Bosentan in pulmonary hypertension associated with fibrotic idiopathic interstitial pneumonia. Am J Respir Crit Care Med. 2014;190(2):208–17.

220. Olschewski H, et al. Inhaled prostacyclin and iloprost in severe pulmonary hypertension secondary to lung fibrosis. Am J Respir Crit Care Med. 1999;160(2):600–7.

221. Boeck L, et al. Acute effects of aerosolized iloprost in COPD related pulmonary hypertension – a randomized controlled crossover trial. PLoS One. 2012;7(12), e52248.

222. Saggar R, et al. Changes in right heart haemodynamics and echocardiographic function in an advanced phenotype of pulmonary hypertension and right heart dysfunction associated with pulmonary fibrosis. Thorax. 2014;69(2):123–9.

223. Barbera JA, Peinado VI, Santos S. Pulmonary hypertension in chronic obstructive pulmonary disease. Eur Respir J. 2003;21(5):892–905.

224. Weissmann N, et al. Stimulation of soluble guanylate cyclase prevents cigarette smoke-induced pulmonary hypertension and emphysema. Am J Respir Crit Care Med. 2014;189(11):1359–73.

225. Hoeper MM, et al. Riociguat for interstitial lung disease and pulmonary hypertension: a pilot trial. Eur Respir J. 2013;41(4):853–60.

226. Royal Brompton and Harefield NHS Foundation Trust; Actelion. Bosentan in pulmonary hypertension in interstitial lung disease treatment study (B-PHIT). In: Clinicaltrials.gov [Internet]. Bethesda (MD): National Library of Medicine (US) 2008. Available from: http://clinicaltrials.gov/ct2/show/NCT00637065. NLM identifier: NCT00637065.

227. Maron BA, et al. Study design and rationale for investigating phosphodiesterase type 5 inhibition for the treatment of pulmo-

nary hypertension due to chronic obstructive lung disease: the TADA-PHiLD (TADAlafil for Pulmonary Hypertension associated with chronic obstructive Lung Disease) trial. Pulm Circ. 2013;3(4):889–97.

228. Kojonazarov B, et al. Effects of fasudil in patients with high-altitude pulmonary hypertension. Eur Respir J. 2012;39(2): 496–8.

229. Kojonazarov B, et al. Bosentan reduces pulmonary artery pressure in high altitude residents. High Alt Med Biol. 2012;13(3):217–23.

230. Hotta J, et al. Polymorphisms of renin-angiotensin system genes with high-altitude pulmonary edema in Japanese subjects. Chest. 2004;126(3):825–30.

231. Gan Y, Herzog EL, Gomer RH. Pirfenidone treatment of idiopathic pulmonary fibrosis. Ther Clin Risk Manage. 2011;7:39–47.

232. Noble PW, et al. Pirfenidone in patients with idiopathic pulmonary fibrosis (CAPACITY): two randomised trials. Lancet. 2011;377(9779):1760–9.

233. King Jr TE, et al. A phase 3 trial of pirfenidone in patients with idiopathic pulmonary fibrosis. N Engl J Med. 2014;370(22):2083–92.

234. Richeldi L, et al. Efficacy of a tyrosine kinase inhibitor in idiopathic pulmonary fibrosis. N Engl J Med. 2011;365(12):1079–87.

235. Bartosik W, Egan JJ, Wood AE. The Novalung interventional lung assist as bridge to lung transplantation for self-ventilating patients – initial experience. Interact Cardiovasc Thorac Surg. 2011;13(2):198–200.

236. Fischer S, et al. Bridge to lung transplantation with the extracorporeal membrane ventilator Novalung in the veno-venous mode: the initial Hannover experience. ASAIO J. 2007;53(2):168–70.

237. Hayes Jr D, et al. Ambulatory venovenous extracorporeal respiratory support as a bridge for cystic fibrosis patients to emergent lung transplantation. J Cyst Fibros. 2012;11(1):40–5.

238. Jimenez SA, Derk CT. Following the molecular pathways toward an understanding of the pathogenesis of systemic sclerosis. Ann Intern Med. 2004;140(1):37–50.

239. Hassoun PM. Lung involvement in systemic sclerosis. Presse Med. 2011;40(1 Pt 2):e3–17.

240. Gabrielli A, Avvedimento EV, Krieg T. Scleroderma. N Engl J Med. 2009;360(19):1989–2003.

241. Steen VD, Powell DL, Medsger Jr TA. Clinical correlations and prognosis based on serum autoantibodies in patients with systemic sclerosis. Arthritis Rheum. 1988;31(2):196–203.

242. Valesini G, et al. Geographical clustering of scleroderma in a rural area in the province of Rome. Clin Exp Rheumatol. 1993;11(1): 41–7.

243. Shinkai H. Epidemiology of progressive systemic sclerosis in Japan. In: Black CM, Myers AR, editors. Progressive systemic sclerosis (current topics in rheumatology). New York: Gower; 1985. p. 79–81.

244. Mayes MD, et al. Prevalence, incidence, survival, and disease characteristics of systemic sclerosis in a large US population. Arthritis Rheum. 2003;48(8):2246–55.

245. Steen VD, Medsger TA. Changes in causes of death in systemic sclerosis, 1972–2002. Ann Rheum Dis. 2007;66(7):940–4.

246. D'Angelo WA, et al. Pathologic observations in systemic sclerosis (scleroderma). A study of fifty-eight autopsy cases and fifty-eight matched controls. Am J Med. 1969;46(3):428–40.

247. Wells AU, et al. Serial CT in fibrosing alveolitis: prognostic significance of the initial pattern. AJR Am J Roentgenol. 1993;161(6): 1159–65.

248. Varga J. Systemic sclerosis: an update. Bull NYU Hosp Jt Dis. 2008;66(3):198–202.

249. Murata I, et al. Echocardiographic evaluation of pulmonary arterial hypertension in patients with progressive systemic sclerosis and related syndromes. Jpn Circ J. 1992;56(10):983–91.

250. Battle RW, et al. Prevalence of pulmonary hypertension in limited and diffuse scleroderma. Chest. 1996;110(6):1515–9.

251. Wells AU, et al. Fibrosing alveolitis in systemic sclerosis. Bronchoalveolar lavage findings in relation to computed tomographic appearance. Am J Respir Crit Care Med. 1994;150(2):462–8.

252. Harrison NK, et al. Pulmonary involvement in systemic sclerosis: the detection of early changes by thin section CT scan, bronchoalveolar lavage and 99mTc-DTPA clearance. Respir Med. 1989;83(5):403–14.

253. Fischer A, et al. Clinically significant interstitial lung disease in limited scleroderma: histopathology, clinical features, and survival. Chest. 2008;134(3):601–5.

254. White B, et al. Cyclophosphamide is associated with pulmonary function and survival benefit in patients with scleroderma and alveolitis. Ann Intern Med. 2000;132(12):947–54.

255. Akesson A, et al. Improved pulmonary function in systemic sclerosis after treatment with cyclophosphamide. Arthritis Rheum. 1994;37(5):729–35.

256. Airo P, et al. Intravenous cyclophosphamide therapy for systemic sclerosis. A single-center experience and review of the literature with pooled analysis of lung function test results. Clin Exp Rheumatol. 2004;22(5):573–8.

257. Tashkin DP, et al. Cyclophosphamide versus placebo in scleroderma lung disease. N Engl J Med. 2006;354(25):2655–66.

258. Pakas I, et al. Cyclophosphamide with low or high dose prednisolone for systemic sclerosis lung disease. J Rheumatol. 2002; 29(2):298–304.

259. Griffiths B, et al. Systemic sclerosis and interstitial lung disease: a pilot study using pulse intravenous methylprednisolone and cyclophosphamide to assess the effect on high resolution computed tomography scan and lung function. J Rheumatol. 2002;29(11):2371–8.

260. Silver RM, et al. Cyclophosphamide and low-dose prednisone therapy in patients with systemic sclerosis (scleroderma) with interstitial lung disease. J Rheumatol. 1993;20(5):838–44.

261. Swigris JJ, et al. Mycophenolate mofetil is safe, well tolerated, and preserves lung function in patients with connective tissue disease-related interstitial lung disease. Chest. 2006;130(1):30–6.

262. Berezne A, et al. Therapeutic strategy combining intravenous cyclophosphamide followed by oral azathioprine to treat worsening interstitial lung disease associated with systemic sclerosis: a retrospective multicenter open-label study. J Rheumatol. 2008;35(6):1064–72.

263. Paone C, et al. Twelve-month azathioprine as maintenance therapy in early diffuse systemic sclerosis patients treated for 1-year with low dose cyclophosphamide pulse therapy. Clin Exp Rheumatol. 2007;25(4):613–6.

264. Cappelli S, et al. Immunosuppression for interstitial lung disease in systemic sclerosis. Eur Respir Rev. 2013;22(129):236–43.

265. Harari S, Torre O, Moss J. Lymphangioleiomyomatosis: what do we know and what are we looking for? Eur Respir Rev. 2011;20(119):34–44.

266. Ryu JH, et al. Chylothorax in lymphangioleiomyomatosis. Chest. 2003;123(2):623–7.

267. Eliasson AH, Phillips YY, Tenholder MF. Treatment of lymphangioleiomyomatosis. A meta-analysis. Chest. 1989;96(6):1352–5.

268. Taveira-DaSilva AM, et al. Decline in lung function in patients with lymphangioleiomyomatosis treated with or without progesterone. Chest. 2004;126(6):1867–74.

269. McCormack FX, et al. Efficacy and safety of sirolimus in lymphangioleiomyomatosis. N Engl J Med. 2011;364(17):1595–606.

270. Pechet TT, et al. Lung transplantation for lymphangioleiomyomatosis. J Heart Lung Transplant. 2004;23(3):301–8.

271. Taveira-DaSilva AM, et al. Pulmonary artery pressure in lymphangioleiomyomatosis: an echocardiographic study. Chest. 2007; 132(5):1573–8.

272. Reynaud-Gaubert M, et al. Lung transplantation for lymphangioleiomyomatosis: the French experience. Transplantation. 2008; 86(4):515–20.

273. Cottin V, et al. Pulmonary hypertension in lymphangioleiomyomatosis: characteristics in 20 patients. Eur Respir J. 2012; 40(3):630–40.

274. Favara BE, et al. Contemporary classification of histiocytic disorders. The WHO Committee On Histiocytic/Reticulum Cell Proliferations. Reclassification Working Group of the Histiocyte Society. Med Pediatr Oncol. 1997;29(3):157–66.

275. Nezelof C, Basset F, Rousseau MF. Histiocytosis X histogenetic arguments for a Langerhans cell origin. Biomedicine. 1973;18(5): 365–71.

276. Vermaelen K, Pauwels R. Pulmonary dendritic cells. Am J Respir Crit Care Med. 2005;172(5):530–51.

277. Suri HS, et al. Pulmonary langerhans cell histiocytosis. Orphanet J Rare Dis. 2012;7:16.

278. Vassallo R, et al. Clinical outcomes of pulmonary Langerhans'-cell histiocytosis in adults. N Engl J Med. 2002;346(7):484–90.

279. Tazi A. Adult pulmonary Langerhans' cell histiocytosis. Eur Respir J. 2006;27(6):1272–85.

280. Watanabe R, et al. Clinico-epidemiological features of pulmonary histiocytosis X. Intern Med. 2001;40(10):998–1003.

281. Howarth DM, et al. Langerhans cell histiocytosis: diagnosis, natural history, management, and outcome. Cancer. 1999;85(10):2278–90.

282. Sundar KM, et al. Pulmonary Langerhans cell histiocytosis: emerging concepts in pathobiology, radiology, and clinical evolution of disease. Chest. 2003;123(5):1673–83.

283. Epler GR, et al. Normal chest roentgenograms in chronic diffuse infiltrative lung disease. N Engl J Med. 1978;298(17):934–9.

284. Brauner MW, et al. Pulmonary Langerhans cell histiocytosis: evolution of lesions on CT scans. Radiology. 1997;204(2):497–502.

285. Crausman RS, et al. Pulmonary histiocytosis X: pulmonary function and exercise pathophysiology. Am J Respir Crit Care Med. 1996;153(1):426–35.

286. Travis WD, et al. Pulmonary Langerhans cell granulomatosis (histiocytosis X). A clinicopathologic study of 48 cases. Am J Surg Pathol. 1993;17(10):971–86.

287. Dauriat G, et al. Lung transplantation for pulmonary langerhans' cell histiocytosis: a multicenter analysis. Transplantation. 2006;81(5): 746–50.

288. Colby TV, Lombard C. Histiocytosis X in the lung. Hum Pathol. 1983;14(10):847–56.

289. Mogulkoc N, et al. Pulmonary Langerhans' cell histiocytosis: radiologic resolution following smoking cessation. Chest. 1999;115(5):1452–5.

290. Chaowalit N, et al. Echocardiographic and clinical characteristics of pulmonary hypertension complicating pulmonary Langerhans cell histiocytosis. Mayo Clin Proc. 2004;79(10):1269–75.

291. Fartoukh M, et al. Severe pulmonary hypertension in histiocytosis X. Am J Respir Crit Care Med. 2000;161(1):216–23.

292. Le Pavec J, et al. Pulmonary Langerhans cell histiocytosis-associated pulmonary hypertension: clinical characteristics and impact of pulmonary arterial hypertension therapies. Chest. 2012;142(5):1150–7.

293. Baughman RP, Culver DA, Judson MA. A concise review of pulmonary sarcoidosis. Am J Respir Crit Care Med. 2011;183(5):573–81.

294. Hunninghake GW, et al. ATS/ERS/WASOG statement on sarcoidosis. American Thoracic Society/European Respiratory Society/World Association of Sarcoidosis and other Granulomatous Disorders. Sarcoidosis Vasc Diffuse Lung Dis. 1999;16(2):149–73.

295. Schurmann M, et al. Results from a genome-wide search for predisposing genes in sarcoidosis. Am J Respir Crit Care Med. 2001;164(5):840–6.

296. Thomas KW, Hunninghake GW. Sarcoidosis. JAMA. 2003; 289(24):3300–3.

297. Baughman RP, et al. Clinical characteristics of patients in a case control study of sarcoidosis. Am J Respir Crit Care Med. 2001;164(10 Pt 1):1885–9.

298. Keir G, Wells AU. Assessing pulmonary disease and response to therapy: which test? Semin Respir Crit Care Med. 2010;31(4): 409–18.

299. Handa T, et al. Clinical and radiographic indices associated with airflow limitation in patients with sarcoidosis. Chest. 2006;130(6):1851–6.

300. Scadding JG. Prognosis of intrathoracic sarcoidosis in England. A review of 136 cases after five years' observation. Br Med J. 1961;2(5261):1165–72.

301. Paramothayan NS, Lasserson TJ, Jones PW. Corticosteroids for pulmonary sarcoidosis. Cochrane Database Syst Rev. 2005;2, CD001114.

302. Baughman RP, et al. Infliximab therapy in patients with chronic sarcoidosis and pulmonary involvement. Am J Respir Crit Care Med. 2006;174(7):795–802.

303. Baughman RP, Lower EE, Drent M. Inhibitors of tumor necrosis factor (TNF) in sarcoidosis: who, what, and how to use them. Sarcoidosis Vasc Diffuse Lung Dis. 2008;25(2):76–89.

304. Gibson GJ, et al. British Thoracic Society Sarcoidosis study: effects of long term corticosteroid treatment. Thorax. 1996;51(3): 238–47.

305. Diaz-Guzman E, et al. Pulmonary hypertension caused by sarcoidosis. Clin Chest Med. 2008;29(3):549–63. x.

306. Mayock RL, et al. Manifestations of sarcoidosis. Analysis of 145 patients, with a review of nine series selected from the literature. Am J Med. 1963;35:67–89.

307. Milman N, et al. Pulmonary hypertension in end-stage pulmonary sarcoidosis: therapeutic effect of sildenafil? J Heart Lung Transplant. 2008;27(3):329–34.

308. Rosen Y, et al. Granulomatous pulmonary angiitis in sarcoidosis. Arch Pathol Lab Med. 1977;101(4):170–4.

309. Takemura T, et al. Pulmonary vascular involvement in sarcoidosis: granulomatous angiitis and microangiopathy in transbronchial lung biopsies. Virchows Arch A Pathol Anat Histopathol. 1991;418(4):361–8.

310. Cordova FC, D'Alonzo G. Sarcoidosis-associated pulmonary hypertension. Curr Opin Pulm Med. 2013;19(5):531–7.

311. Baughman RP, et al. Bosentan for sarcoidosis-associated pulmonary hypertension: a double-blind placebo controlled randomized trial. Chest. 2014;145(4):810–7.

Gaurav Choudhary and Corey E. Ventetuolo

Introduction

Pulmonary hypertension (PH) is defined as a mean pulmonary artery pressure (mPAP) ≥ 25 mm Hg at rest and is clinically classified into five groups (World Health Organization [WHO] Groups 1–5) based on the predominant underlying pathology [1]. Registries including largely WHO Group 1 pulmonary arterial hypertension (PAH) and to a lesser extent population-based studies of patients with PH due to primary cardiopulmonary diseases (WHO Group 2 and 3, respectively), have enhanced our understanding of the epidemiology of pulmonary vascular disease. Less is known about chronic thromboembolic disease (WHO Group 4), and the miscellaneous systemic conditions included in WHO Group 5. Finding common epidemiologic trends across the classes may enhance our understanding of pathophysiology and ultimately enhance our approach to treatment. In modern practice, patients often have a mix of features from several sub-groups, and require comprehensive diagnostic testing. Given this overlap, this review will begin with a broad overview of what is known about the epidemiology of PH in the general adult population and common clinical risk factors that may play a role in PH pathogenesis, and then the discussion will be focused on the epidemiology of individual WHO Groups as a means for reviewing recent registry data and ongoing gaps in knowledge.

G. Choudhary, MD (✉)
Division of Cardiology, Department of Medicine,
Providence VA Medical Center,
Alpert Medical School of Brown University,
830 Chalkstone Ave, Providence, RI 02908, USA
e-mail: Gaurav_Choudhary@brown.edu

C.E. Ventetuolo, MD, MS
Division of Pulmonary, Critical Care and Sleep Medicine,
Departments of Medicine and Health Services Policy and Practice,
Rhode Island Hospital, Alpert Medical School of Brown University, 593 Eddy Street, Providence, RI 02903, USA
e-mail: corey_ventetuolo@brown.edu

Defining Pulmonary Hypertension in Population-Based Studies

While the diagnosis of PH requires direct measurement of mPAP by right heart catheterization, the initial test that suggests the presence of PH is often echocardiography. Echocardiography is non-invasive and can be used in population-based studies to ascertain the prevalence of PH. About 2/3 of subjects in the general population have measurable tricuspid regurgitant (TR) velocity, which can be used to estimate pulmonary artery systolic pressures (PASP) [2, 3]. However, use of echocardiography in the assessment and management of PH remains an area of much controversy and right heart catheterization remains the *sine qua non* of PAH diagnosis [4, 5]. While echocardiography derived PASP has been shown to lack precision when compared to right heart catheterization-derived PASP [6, 7], the sensitivity and specificity of echo derived PASP (>39 mmHg) has been reported as 87 % and 81 %, respectively [8]. In a meta-analysis, the sensitivity and specificity of echocardiographically derived PASP (using variable cut-offs) in diagnosing PH was reported as 83 % and 72 %, respectively. Hence, despite its inherent limitations, echocardiography remains a useful tool for screening for PH and in large-scale epidemiological studies.

Prevalence of Pulmonary Hypertension in the General Population

Only a handful of studies have looked at the prevalence of PH in the general adult population. In a community-based cohort, Lam et al. [2] reported that median PASP (assuming a right atrial pressure [RAP] of 5 mmHg) in a random sample of the Olmsted County population ≥ 45 years of age (n = 1413, white, 43 % male) was 26 mmHg (IQ Range 6 mmHg) corresponding to an estimated PH prevalence of 2–3 % (PASP ≥ 40 mmHg, assumed RAP = 5 mmHg). In contrast, in an African American (AA) cohort from Jackson Heart Study

© Springer International Publishing Switzerland 2016
B.A. Maron et al. (eds.), *Pulmonary Hypertension: Basic Science to Clinical Medicine*, DOI 10.1007/978-3-319-23594-3_4

Fig. 4.1 Group specific prevalence of pulmonary hypertension

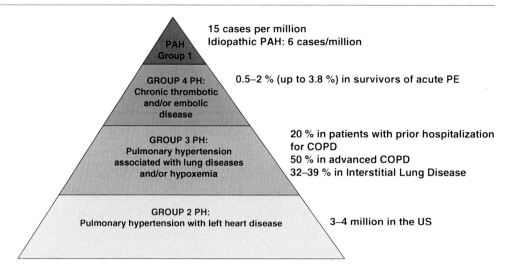

15 cases per million
Idiopathic PAH: 6 cases/million

0.5–2 % (up to 3.8 %) in survivors of acute PE

20 % in patients with prior hospitalization for COPD
50 % in advanced COPD
32–39 % in Interstitial Lung Disease

3–4 million in the US

(n = 3282, 32.5 % male), the median PASP was 27 mmHg (IQ range 18 mmHg) and the prevalence of PH (PASP ≥ 40 mmHg, assumed RA pressure = 5 mmHg) was 6.8 % [3]. Large data base studies looking at patients referred for echocardiograms have reported the prevalence of PH as 6.6 % (n = 21,483, TR gradient ≥ 36 mmHg) [9], 9.1 % (n = 10,314, PASP > 40 assuming RAP as 10 mmHg) [10] and 14 % (n = 10,471, PASP ≥ 40) [11]. The variability in prevalence in these cohorts is likely related to different population demographic characteristics, co-morbidities, and assumptions related to estimation of right atrial pressure.

Among patients that have PH, the most prevalent group is Group 2 PH (i.e., PH related to left heart disease). It is estimated that about three to four million adults in the US may have group 2 PH [12]. This is followed by PH associated with parenchymal lung diseases and/or hypoxemia (Group 3 PH), which affects up to 20 % of patients with a prior hospitalization for chronic obstructive pulmonary disease (COPD) exacerbation and 32–39 % of patients with interstitial lung disease [12]. Compared to Groups 2 and 3, PH associated with chronic thromboembolic disease (Group 4) and PAH (Group 1 PAH, prevalence ~15 cases/ million) is rare (Fig. 4.1).

Temporal trends in mortality and hospitalization where PH was listed as any contributing cause of death or any-listed hospital diagnosis in the National Vital Statistic System and hospital discharge data from the National Hospital Discharge Survey for 1980–2002 show stability in PH-related mortality (per 100,000: 5.2 in 1980 to 5.4 in 2002), but an increase in hospitalizations (per 100,000: 40.8 in 1980 to 90.1 in 2002) over the same two decade time period [13]. However, the mortality rates increased among women but decreased among men during this period. In Medicare enrollees aged >65 years, the annual number of hospitalizations for pulmonary hypertension as any-listed diagnosis tripled from 1990 to 2002. The age-standardized hospitalization rate per 100,000 in this group was 197.8 in 1990 and 649.7 in 2002

[13]. Since these data are dependent on appropriate ICD coding, it is unclear if the increase is due to an increased awareness of the diagnosis versus an actual increase in the number of incident PH cases. However, ageing and an attendant increase in the burden of heart failure in the general population suggests that PH might continue to be a more frequent diagnosis associated with hospitalizations and mortality.

Pulmonary Hypertension: Demographics and Comorbidities

Age

The PASP and prevalence of PH increases with age [2, 3, 14]. This relationship is independent of other comorbidities and cardiopulmonary function [3]. The prevalence ratio of having PH in subjects >65 years of age is tenfold higher compared to those younger than 45 years of age. The higher prevalence of PH in older people may be related to decreasing vascular compliance of the pulmonary arteries with age, which also occurs in the systemic arteries [2, 3].

Sex

Studies reporting on the relationship between PASP and PH and sex in the general population have yielded conflicting results. In the AA population, women have an increased age-adjusted prevalence of PH compared to men that is independent of other comorbidities. Fifteen percent of AA women over 65 years of age have PH compared to 9 % of AA men [3] (Fig. 4.2). In contrast, studies performed in a general population of young adults [15], and in normal echocardiograms performed over a decade at Massachusetts General Hospital [14] showed higher PASP in males, while in the

Fig. 4.2 Prevalence of pulmonary hypertension in African-American men and women across age groups [3]

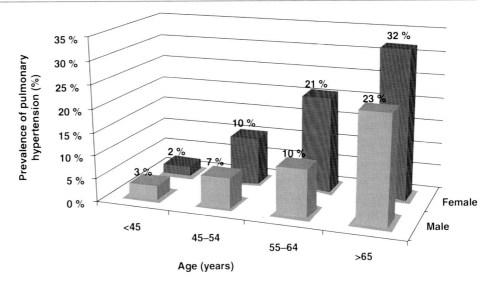

Olmstead County population cohort [2] no relationship between sex and PA pressure was observed. Determining whether the relationship between sex and PH is race-specific and relates to specific biologic factors such as estrogen and estrogen metabolites needs further validation in additional population-based cohorts [16–20].

Race/Ethnicity

Little data is available comparing PASP or PH prevalence according to race. In the CARDIA (Coronary Artery Risk Development in Young Adults) study, AAs were found to have higher mPAP (assessed by pulmonary artery acceleration time on echocardiography) independent of age, sex, body mass index (BMI), smoking status, and presence of diastolic dysfunction [15]. Similarly, in one community-based cohort, PH prevalence was 6.8 % in AA compared to an estimated prevalence of ~2–3 % in whites based on the cumulative frequency of PASP [2, 3]. However, these cohorts had differences in cardiopulmonary co-morbidities, and it remains to be determined if race is an independent risk factor for developing PH after adjusting for age and other chronic conditions.

Obesity

Obesity or higher BMI is positively associated with PH prevalence and PASP [2, 3, 14, 15]. For example, in AA, the presence of obesity increases the adjusted prevalence of PH by 66 % compared to individuals with normal BMI [3]. A similar relationship between obesity and PASP > 30 mmHg (odds ratio of 1.67) was observed by McQuillan and colleagues [14]. The pathophysiological mechanisms are not delineated clearly, but may be related to the presence of left ventricular

diastolic dysfunction, sleep disordered breathing, obesity-hypoventilation syndrome or insulin resistance/adipose leading to vascular inflammation.

Cardiovascular Comorbidities

Considering that the most common cause of PH is related to left ventricular (LV) dysfunction and left atrial (LA) hypertension, it is not surprising that the presence of PH is related to changes in LV systolic and diastolic function and left sided valvular diseases. Hypertension, coronary artery disease, diabetes, congestive heart failure and severe mitral and aortic valvular disease are more common in subjects with PH [2, 3]. The underlying mechanism(s) to account for these relationships are likely related to presence of diastolic dysfunction and elevated LA pressures. Indeed, echocardiographic markers of systolic dysfunction and LV diastolic function (LV hypertrophy, LA size and Doppler indices of diastolic function) are correlated with PASP and PH [2, 3, 14, 15].

Pulmonary Comorbidities

COPD is associated with PH [21] and the underlying mechanism(s) are multifactorial. Hypoxia, vascular remodeling, destruction of capillaries in emphysema, hyperinflation, and LV diastolic dysfunction constitute likely mechanisms responsible for increased PASP in the settings of parenchymal lung diseases. The prevalence of chronic lung diseases increases with increasing PASP in the general population [2, 3]. Also, airway obstruction assessed by spirometry is associated with a twofold increase in the adjusted risk for PH independent of other co-morbidities [3]. A significant association between a restrictive spirometry pattern

[22–26] and the presence of PH was also observed in the Jackson Heart Study Cohort [3]. A restrictive spirometry pattern can be caused by fibrotic lung disease, obesity, diabetes, heart disease, and hypertension [22, 25]. However, the relationship between restriction and PH was independent of these co-morbidities suggesting other as yet unrecognized factors contribute to these associations.

Pulmonary Hypertension: Prognosis

Elevated PASP has been shown to result in higher mortality in the general population. This was demonstrated in the both Caucasian (Adjusted HR: 1.46 per 10 mmHg) [2] and AA cohorts (Adjusted HR: 1.38 per 10 mmHg) [27]. Also, elevated PASP is an independent predictor of admissions for congestive heart failure in the general population (Adjusted HR: 2.03 per 10 mmHg). Higher mortality has been noted in patient cohorts with multiple cardiopulmonary morbidities such as the U.S. military Veteran population in which 44.1 % of patients with echocardiographically-determined PASP > 60 mmHg were deceased at a median follow up of 832 days [9].

World Health Organization Group 1 Pulmonary Arterial Hypertension

The epidemiology of WHO Group 1 PAH is the most well defined among the five WHO groups. The earliest prospective multicenter registry from the National Institutes of Health, which included patients with idiopathic PAH (IPAH), heritable PAH (HPAH), and PAH associated with anorexigen use, reported a mean age of 36 ± 15 years and a female:male ratio of 1.7:1 overall (Table 4.1). Before the advent of targeted PAH therapy, 1-, 3-, and 5-year survival for this cohort was 68 %, 48 %, and 34 %, respectively, with an estimated median survival of 2.8 years (95 % confidence interval 1.9–3.7 years) [28] (Table 4.2). This early snapshot of what was then known as "primary pulmonary hypertension", a rare disease affecting young females of child-bearing age, has evolved in recent years as we have come to understand more about WHO Group 1 disease including PAH associated with conditions such as connective tissue disease (CTD).

Prevalence and Incidence

A number of population-based registries have offered insight into PAH prevalence and incidence. In several countries in Europe, the centralization of PAH care has allowed for widescale estimates of pulmonary vascular disease burden. The network of French centers (n = 17) described a prevalence of 15 cases/million for WHO Group 1 PAH (5.9 cases/million for IPAH), although significant regional variation was noted (5–25 cases/million French adults), and an incidence of 2.4 cases/million/year in 2002–2003 [35]. The prevalence of IPAH, HPAH, and anorexigen-associated PAH was 6.6 cases/million in 2009, with an estimated incidence of 1.1 cases/million/year in the United Kingdom (UK) and Ireland [34]. Across Spain, the prevalence of PAH has been reported to be 16 cases per million and the incidence 3.7 cases/million/year [38]. The overall population prevalence of PAH in Scotland was 52 cases per million population; prevalence estimates were higher when compared to an expert referral center (the Scottish Pulmonary Vascular Unit), raising the question of whether registries from expert centers adequately capture the true population impact of pulmonary vascular disease. The overall annual incidence of PAH over a 16 year study period as estimated from the Scottish Morbidity Record was 7.1 cases per million population; the incidence of IPAH, CTD-associated PAH and congenital heart disease (CHD) associated PAH respectively was 3.3, 2.1 and 1.7 cases per million population [31].

Survival

Multiple registries have captured survival in both the pre- and post-PAH treatment eras (Table 4.2) [28, 32–34, 38–43]. Comparing these estimates, it appears that short-term survival has improved over time and is approximately 90 % at 1 year and 75 % at 3 years. Longer-term survival remains poor, however, with registries reporting survival rates between 21 and 75 % at 5 years. Of course, registries are susceptible to survivor bias and outcome estimates may be heavily influenced by mixing of prevalent versus incident cases.

Demographics: Age, Sex, and Race

Single center US-based registries including various WHO Group 1 etiologies have reported slightly older average age (4th–5th decade of life) than that reported in the NIH registry, but confirmed 70 % female predominance, as have other national reports [30–32, 35, 40]. In 2006, the Registry to Evaluate Early And Long-term pulmonary arterial hypertension disease management (REVEAL) began enrolling patients with WHO Group 1 PAH as traditionally defined as well as patients with PH and elevated left heart filling pressures (pulmonary capillary wedge pressure 16–18 mmHg) from 54 US-based community and academic sites [36, 44]. In patients with IPAH, the average age at enrollment was 53 ± 15 years of age and 80 % were female, signaling a possible shift in demographics as compared to earlier PAH registries.

Table 4.1 Major PAH registries and characteristics of patients enrolled

Registry	Years	Type	N	Age, yrs	Female sex, %	FC III/IV, %	6MWD, m	RAP, mmHg	mPAP, mmHg	CI, L/min/m^2	PVRI (mmHg/L/min·m^2) or PVR (Wood units)
NIH [28, 29]	1981–1985	IPAH, HPAH anorexigen	187	36 ± 15	1:7:1	–	–	10 ± 6	60 ± 18	2.3 ± 0.9	26 ± 14
PHC [30]	1982–2007	Mixed, 42 % IPAH	576	48 ± 14	77	80	–	11 ± 6	52 ± 14	2.2 ± 0.9	12 ± 7
SMR [31]	1986–2001	Mixed, 47 % IPAH	374	–	70	–	–	–	–	–	–
Mayo [32]	1995–2004	Mixed, 56 % IPAH	484	52 ± 15	75	71	329 ± 125	13 ± 6	53 ± 13	2.5 ± 0.8	–
Chinese [33]	1999–2004	IPAH, HPAH	72	36 ± 12	71	61	–	8 ± 3	59 ± 15	–	20 ± 9
UK/Ireland [34]	2001–2009	Mixed, 93 % IPAH	482	50 ± 17	70	84	292 ± 123	10 ± 6	54 ± 14	2.1 ± 0.7	13 ± 6
French [35]	2002–2003	Mixed, 39 % IPAH	674	50 ± 15	65	75	329 ± 109	8 ± 5	55 ± 15	2.5 ± 0.8	21 ± 10
REVEAL [36]	2006–2007	Mixed, 46 % IPAH	2525	53 ± 14	80	51	366 ± 126	9 ± 6	51 ± 14	2.4 ± 0.8	21 ± 13
COMPERA [37]	2007–	Mixed, 62 % IPAH	1283	68 (55–75)	64	87	303 ± 132	8 ± 5	44 ± 12	2.3 ± 0.8	10 ± 6
Spain [38]	2007–2008	Mixed, 36 % IPAH	866	45 ± 17	71	69	363 ± 120	9 ± 5	54 ± 16	2.6 ± 0.9	12 ± 6
Chinese [39]	2007–2009	63 % IPAH, 37 % CTD	276	33 ± 15[a]	70[a]	52[a]	394 ± 114[a]	12 ± 6[a]	63 ± 18[a]	2.5 ± 0.9[a]	17 ± 10[a]

PAH pulmonary arterial hypertension, *IPAH* idiopathic PAH, *HPAH* heritable PAH, *CTD* connective tissue disease, *PHC* pulmonary hypertension connection, *SMR* Scottish Morbidity Record, *REVEAL* Registry to Evaluate Early and Long-term PAH disease management, *COMPERA* Comparative, Prospective Registry of Newly Initiated Therapies for Pulmonary Hypertension, *FC* functional class, *6MWD* 6-min walk distance, *RAP* right atrial pressure, mmHg, *mPAP* mean pulmonary artery pressure, mmHg, *CI* cardiac index
[a]IPAH

Table 4.2 Survival rates at 1, 3, and 5 years among patients enrolled in registries

Registry	Years	1 year, %	3 year, %	5 year, %
NIH [28]	1981–1985	68	48	34
PHC [40]	1982–2007	86	69	61
Mayo [32]	1995–2004	81	61	48
Chinese [33]	1999–2004	68	39	21
UK/Ireland [34]	2001–2009	93	73	61
French [41]	2002–2003	83	67	58
REVEAL [42]	2006–2007	91	74	65
COMPERA [43]	2007	93	84[b]	–
Spain [38]	2007–2008	89	77	66[a]
Chinese [39]	2007–2009	92	80	75[a]

PHC pulmonary hypertension connection, *REVEAL* Registry to Evaluate Early and Long-term PAH disease management, *COMPERA* Comparative, Prospective Registry of Newly Initiated Therapies for Pulmonary Hypertension
[a]Idiopathic pulmonary arterial hypertension
[b]In anticoagulation group

Whether the observations from REVEAL signal a true change in disease biology (e.g., via epigenetic influences), greater disease awareness in an aging population, and/or that the "pure" idiopathic PAH pathophenotype has been diluted to include overlapping forms of PH in modern clinical practice is not known. Similar trends were observed in the UK and Ireland registry, where patients enrolled later (2007–2009) tended to be older, more obese, and have more comorbid diabetes and ischemic heart disease as compared to PAH patients enrolled earlier (2001–2003) [34]. The Comparative Prospective Registry of Newly Initiated Therapies for Pulmonary Hypertension (COMPERA) database, which commenced in 2007 and included patients from multinational European centers, reported an average age at diagnosis of 71 ± 16 years among incident IPAH cases [37]. Patients diagnosed at a younger age appear to have worse hemodynamic burden, yet better functional tolerance and survival as compared to older aged patients, who have more comorbidities and are more commonly obese [34, 37]. In addition, survival with modern PAH treatment had improved. This has been shown in a retrospective evaluation of cohort of patients from 2007 to 2009 in China, where targeted PAH therapy was introduced in 2006 [39]. While baseline characteristics for incident IPAH patients remained similar to the NIH registry, survival with modern PAH treatment had improved, as has been observed in other cohorts [45].

Female sex has long been established as the major clinical risk factor for PAH, but recent epidemiologic data has suggested that males have poorer survival than females and that age may be an important modifier of the relationship between sex and outcomes [13, 38, 41–43, 46]. Lifetime hormonal fluctuations (e.g., menarche, menopause, androgen fluctuations at puberty and in older age) that differentially regulate cardiopulmonary function as well as sex-specific responses

to therapy have been proposed as possible explanations for these observations [20, 47–49]. In fact, among older patients, sex-based differences in PAH prevalence appear to be diminished [34, 37, 46]. Males have greater hemodynamic burden at diagnosis as compared to females, but these differences are attenuated after age 45 in a cohort of clinical trial participants [46]. Similarly, in the REVEAL registry, men had higher RAP and mPAP at diagnosis (as well as worse survival especially in those older than 60 years of age) [42, 50]. These observations have not been consistent across all registries, however, and further work is needed to refine the sex-age interaction in pulmonary vascular disease [34, 39].

Less is known about the role of race/ethnicity in disease prevalence and outcomes. In the NIH registry, the distribution of race/ethnicity observed in patients was similar to that of the general US population, although there was a greater female:male predominance among blacks (4.3:1) [28]. This observation was also made in the UK and Ireland, where 12.3 % of 424 patients were nonwhite, 85 % of whom were female (as compared to 70 % female in white patients) and in the US, where a 5.4:1 female to male ratio was observed in AA from the REVEAL registry [34, 36]. AA have higher rates of hospitalization and death as compared to whites, and appear to have a less robust response to treatment with endothelin receptor antagonists in PAH clinical trials [13, 47, 51, 52]. Han Chinese patients appear to have similar characteristics to white patients at baseline; in a small cohort from a single US center, Asian descent was an independent predictor of death [33, 52]. While neither sex nor race/ethnicity were associated with delay in diagnosis (>2 years between symptom onset and evaluation for PAH) in the REVEAL registry, it is unknown whether these possible differences in outcomes are due to true differences in disease biology, variable therapeutic responses, and/or confounding by socioeconomic status such as limited access to care as has been noted in other cardiopulmonary diseases [53]. Irrespective of the precise reason, it is important to note that lower socioeconomic status (assessed as a composite of level of education, medical reimbursement, employment status, and household income) was strongly associated with mortality after adjustment for age, sex, disease factors, and PAH treatments in the Chinese cohort [54].

Group 1 Pulmonary Arterial Hypertension Subtypes and Associated Conditions

Heritable Pulmonary Hypertension

Mutations in the bone morphogenic protein receptor type 2 (BMPR2), a member of the transforming growth factor [TGF]-β family, are present in 70–80 % of families with PAH and roughly 25 % of patients with IPAH [55, 56]. These mutations are transmitted in an autosomal dominant fashion with

Table 4.3 Conditions associated with pulmonary hypertension and considerations for screening

WHO group	Associated condition	Estimated prevalence, %	Screening
I.	Systemic sclerosis and scleroderma spectrum disorders	~12 % [83, 84]	Yes; annually with echocardiogram, DLCO, NT-proBNP [86, 87]
	Human immunodeficiency virus infection	0.5 % [88–90]	None recommended
	Portopulmonary hypertension	2 % [91–95], higher in those referred for orthotopic liver transplant	Pre-transplant evaluation
	Congenital heart disease	~30 % [96–98]	At diagnosis
V.	Sickle cell disease	10 % PAH, higher using tricuspid jet velocity [99]	Adults > 18 years of age, echocardiography every 1–3 years [100]

incomplete penetrance. TGF-β signaling including the BMPR2 pathway is felt to play a major role in disease pathogenesis. Further evidence is provided by rarer mutations in TGF-β receptor components activin-like receptor kinase-1 (ALK-1) and endoglin (ENG), both of which have been implicated in hereditary hemorrhagic telangiectasia and PAH [57, 58]. Variants in other genes, including mothers against decapentaplegic homologue (SMADs), proteins in the TGF-β signaling pathway, and more recently caviolin 1 (CAV1) and the potassium channel subfamily K member 3 (KCNK3) (neither of which directly relate to TGF-β) have also been implicated in heritable disease although are less common than BMPR2 mutations [59–62]. BMPR2 mutation carriers tend to present at a younger age and with more severe hemodynamic compromise and ALK-1 carriers may have a worse overall prognosis as compared to other idiopathic and heritable patients [63, 64]. Patients with HPAH otherwise have similar features to those with IPAH, and as such many registries and clinical trials have approached these two entities as one sub-group.

Drug- and Toxin-Induced Pulmonary Hypertension

A number of drugs and toxins have been implicated in the development of pulmonary vascular disease, some with more definitive epidemiologic links than others [65]. A comprehensive list and ranking of definite, possible, likely, and unlikely agents was updated during the 5th World Symposium in Nice, France in 2013 [65]. The most classic example of drug-induced PAH are the anorexigens such as fenfluramine, in which risk appears to be exposure duration-dependent (particularly beyond several months), although fatal cases have been reported from just short-term use [66–72]. Fenfluramine products were withdrawn from the market worldwide in the 1990s, but a related available compound, benfluorex, has been linked to PH as well as to valvular disease [71]. Although tyrosine kinase inhibitors have been studied to treat PAH, the use of dasatinib for chronic myelogenous leukemia has been associated with the development of

PAH [73–75]. Treatment with interferon has also been identified as a possible risk factor after case reports emerged of patients treated with interferon for hepatitis C, multiple sclerosis, and oncologic conditions developed PAH [65, 76–81]. Drug- and toxin-associated PAH accounted for 2 % of PAH patients in the UK and Ireland, 7 % of incident and 13 % of prevalent cases in France, and 11 % of patients in REVEAL, with similar baseline characteristics to those patients with IPAH [36, 41, 82].

Connective Tissue Disease

A number of systemic diseases are associated with the development of pulmonary vasculopathy, although the mechanisms by which PAH develops in these varied conditions are generally poorly understood. In patients with CTD, those with systemic sclerosis are at greatest risk. Roughly 12 % of CTD patients develop PAH and it is a major cause of death in systemic sclerosis [83–85]. To that end, current recommendations are to screen patients with systemic sclerosis or scleroderma spectrum disorders for PAH using noninvasive testing (echocardiogram, diffusion capacity of the lungs for carbon monoxide) and biomarkers (N-terminal pro-brain natriuretic peptide) annually [86, 87] (Table 4.3). Additional CTDs such as systemic lupus erythematosus, mixed connective tissue disease, and rheumatoid arthritis have been linked to pulmonary vascular disease, and while the true prevalence of PAH in these conditions is unknown PAH appears to occur less commonly and is associated with better outcomes than when associated with systemic sclerosis [101, 102].

After IPAH, CTD-PAH patients tend to be the second most represented subgroup in registries, allowing for comparisons between these groups [31, 35, 36, 38]. CTD-PAH patients tend to be older, have less hemodynamic impairment, and may have left-sided abnormalities such as left atrial enlargement and increased left-ventricular end-diastolic diameter, signaling the potential role of pulmonary venous hypertension in some patients [36, 39]. Survival is poorer in CTD-PAH as compared to idiopathic disease and, among CTD-PAH, lowest in patients with systemic sclerosis [29, 39, 102, 103].

Human Immunodeficiency Virus

Non-rheumatologic systemic diseases that are associated with the development of PAH include human immunodeficiency virus (HIV) infection [65, 104]. Over the past several decades, multiple studies have estimated the prevalence of pulmonary vascular disease in HIV infected patients to be approximately 0.5 % [88–90]. While rare, PAH complicating HIV infection has not decreased appreciably in frequency despite the advent of antiretroviral therapy, and the mechanistic link between PAH and HIV has not been clearly established [89]. HIV ribonucleic acid has not been isolated in the pulmonary vasculature, but HIV proteins such as Tat and Nef cause endothelial dysfunction [105–111]. Disease characteristics are similar to IPAH patients, although female sex does not appear to be a risk factor for the development of PAH in HIV [35, 112]. While HIV-associated PAH has historically had the least favorable prognosis among PAH subtypes, patients may respond well to targeted PAH therapy and contemporary survival rates compared to those with IPAH (88 % at 1 year and 72 % at 3 years) [38, 113, 114].

Portopulmonary Hypertension

The presence of portal hypertension without other clinical risk factors or associated conditions in a patient with PAH is designated as portopulmonary hypertension [115]. Between 3 and 6 % of patients referred for liver transplantation have associated PAH; the prevalence of pulmonary arteriopathy was lower in an autopsy study of unselected patients with cirrhosis [91–95]. Neither degree of cirrhosis nor portal hypertension appears to be related to the risk of portopulmonary hypertension, whereas female sex and autoimmune hepatitis are independent risk factors for the development of PAH in these patients [92, 116, 117]. While the pathogenesis of portopulmonary hypertension has not been entirely elucidated, abnormalities to endothelin-, sex hormone-, and nitric oxide biology have been implicated in disease development [118, 119]. In pulmonary vascular disease registries, portopulmonary hypertension accounts for 4–11 % of Group 1 patients [35–37, 53]. Although the degree of hemodynamic impairment appears to be milder, survival was poorer in portopulmonary hypertension as compared to IPAH/HPAH (67 % vs. 85 % at 2 years and 40 % vs. 64 % at 5 years, respectively) in a US-based registry [120]. Because of the very high rate of peri-operative mortality in patients with portpulmonary hypertension undergoing liver transplantation (100 % in those with mPAP>50 mmHg), all patients

undergoing evaluation for liver transplant should be screened for the presence of pulmonary vascular disease (Table 4.3) [121].

Congenital Heart Disease

Adults constitute a significant and increasing proportion of patients with CHD [122]. Depending on the nature of the defect (closed vs. open) and the population studied, PAH has been reported in 4–34 % of adults with CHD and confers a worse outcome when present [96–98]. Chronic left-to-right shunting that increases pulmonary blood flow results in pulmonary vascular changes and, depending on the nature of the defect, increased right heart volume and pressure to induce endothelial damage, cytotoxicity, and, ultimately, precapillary pulmonary vascular disease [123]. Because of the high prevalence of PAH associated with CHD, all congenital patients should be assessed and followed for the development of PAH. Modern PAH registries have reported CHD-associated PAH in 11–24 % of Group 1 disease [34–36, 38, 124] The most recent consensus guidelines from the 5th World Symposium in Nice, France included a more detailed sub-classification of PAH associated with CHD (in both children and adults) as well as an approach to correction of open shunts [1].

Schistosomiasis

Chronic schistosomiasis is perhaps the most common cause of PAH owing to the widespread prevalence of *schistosomiasis mansoni* infection worldwide. However, since parasite exposure tends to occur in developing countries, this PAH subtype remains incompletely studied. Cardiopulmonary complications including PAH are believed to occur when embolized worm eggs become trapped in the presinusoidal vasculature and result in portal hypertension and portosystemic shunt. Whereas direct pulmonary vascular exposure to egg antigens does not appear to underlie the pathobiology of schistosomiasis-PAH, many of the mechanistic pathways implicated in IPAH (e.g., TGF-β and inflammatory cytokines) have been implicated in the development of schistosoma-related pulmonary vascular injury experimentally *in vivo* [125–127]. In a prospective screening study of 65 patients with the hepatosplenic form of disease in Brazil, the prevalence of hemodynamic PAH was 4.6 % [128]. Untreated patients with schistosoma-related PAH may have less severe hemodynamic changes (i.e., lower mPAP and pulmonary vascular resistance, higher cardiac output) as compared to treated idiopathic patients, with similar rates of survival [129]. Although the role of targeted PAH therapy is undefined in this population, a small uncontrolled study of schistosomiasis-associated PAH demonstrated improvements in exercise tolerance and hemodynamics with oral PAH therapy [130].

WHO Group 2 Pulmonary Hypertension with Left Heart Disease

Pulmonary hypertension with left heart disease is observed in patients with heart failure (preserved and reduced LV ejection fraction) and mitral/aortic valvular disease [131]. The true prevalence of PH in this population is difficult to ascertain because of heterogeneity of study cohorts, comorbidities, different methods of defining PH and use of either echocardiographic or invasive hemodynamics. In a community based heart failure population in Olmstead county (n = 1049), the overall prevalence of PH (PASP >=35 mmHg) was noted to be 79 % [132] while a prevalence of 50 % was noted in a sub-population of Danish patients with heart failure (n = 388, PASP > 39 mmHg) [133].

Little data is available for community-based populations with heart failure with reduced ejection fraction (HFrEF) and prevalence of PH. Using a cut-off of 20 mmHg of mPAP measured during right heart catheterization, Ghio and colleagues estimated a prevalence of 62 % in patients with left ventricular ejection fraction (LVEF) <35 % [134]. In selected populations, a prevalence of 40 % was noted using a mPAP cut-off of 25 mmHg in patients with Class III and IV heart failure and a mean EF of 27 ± 9 % [135] and 47 % of patients in ESCAPE trial (EF ≤ 30 %, NYHA Class IV) had PH (mPAP ≥25, PCWP > 15 and PVR ≥ 3WU) [136].

Pulmonary hypertension is appears to be more prevalent in heart failure with preserved ejection fraction (HFpEF) than in HFrEF. In a community-based cohort at Olmstead county, the prevalence of PH (PASP > 35 mmHg) was present in about 83 % of patients [137] with HFpEF. In hospitalized patients with HFpEF, the prevalence estimates have been 43 % (moderate PH, mean RVSP 47 ± 17 mmHg) [138], while in a large cardiac catheterization database the prevalence was reported as 52.5 % (mean PAP > 25 and LVEDP > 15) [139]. Also, PH (TR velocity >2.9 m/s) was present in 36 % of patients enrolled in the TOPCAT study that evaluated the role of aldosterone antagonism in HFpEF [140]. The high prevalence of PH in HFpEF is likely related to high burden of cardiopulmonary comorbidities and advanced age in this population [141]. Up to 73 % of patients with severe mitral valve disorders may have PH [142]. Also, patients with severe aortic stenosis may have a prevalence of 30–50 % [143–145].

Presence of PH in left heart disease is associated with a worse prognosis compared to those without PH. Elevated PASP was associated with high morbidity and mortality in heart failure patients with either reduced or preserved ejection fraction [133, 135, 137, 146]. Presence of PH on right heart catheterization in functional class III and IV heart failure patients increased the relative risk of acute heart failure or cardiovascular death by 2.6 fold [135], and the hazards of mortality increased by 30 % with every 10 mmHg increase in PASP in the community based HFpEF cohort [137]. Similarly, presence of PH increases operative mortality and decreases long-term survival (Relative risk: 1.7) in patients undergoing aortic valve replacement for severe aortic stenosis [143].

WHO Group 3 Pulmonary Hypertension Associated with Lung diseases and/or Hypoxemia

Hypoxia causes vasoconstriction in the pulmonary circulation and, if prolonged, results in irreversible pulmonary vascular remodeling that increases pulmonary vascular resistance and pressure. In addition, chronic lung diseases such as emphysema are associated with hyperinflation and alveolar capillary destruction and chronic alveolar hypoventilation (as can occur in sleep disordered breathing and other neuromuscular disorders) that further contribute to the development of PH in this population. In a cohort of 998 patients admitted with COPD as the only risk factor for PH, Chaouat and colleagues reported that about 50 % of patients had a mPAP > 20 mmHg and 1.1 % with mPAP ≥ 40 mmHg [21]. In patients with more severe lung disease, such as those with severe COPD and referred for lung volume reduction surgery or transplantation, the prevalence may range from 50 to 90 % [147, 148]. However, PH in COPD patients is mostly mild-moderate in severity [21, 149]. PH is more prevalent and is hemodynamically severe (mPAP >40 mmHg) in about half of patients with combined pulmonary fibrosis and emphysema [150].

In patients with idiopathic pulmonary fibrosis, the prevalence of PH as assessed by right heart catheterization has been reported in two retrospective studies as 31.6 % [151] and 33.9 % [152]. Shorr and colleagues reported that of the 3457 patients that were listed for lung transplant over a 10 year period 46.1 % had PH by right heart catheterization [153]. The presence of PH correlates linearly with mortality in patients with IPF [151], a PASP > 50 mmHg by echocardiography [154] and mPAP > 17 [155], in particular, predict mortality in IPF. The prevalence of PH in other types of interstitial lung disease and in pulmonary fibrosis patients with less severe disease is not well established.

The presence of PH in patients with COPD [156–158] and pulmonary fibrosis [153–155, 159] portends poor prognosis. In patients with COPD that were started on long term oxygen therapy (n = 84), co-morbid PH (mPAP > 25 mmHg) was associated with 36 % survival at 5 years compared to

62 % in those without PH [158] and was a better predictor of survival than the forced expiratory volume in 1 s (FEV1), hypoxemia or hypercapnia. Also, presence of elevated mPAP (>18 mmHg) was independently associated with risk of COPD exacerbation in cohort of moderate to severe COPD patients [160]. Similarly dilated pulmonary artery (ratio of the diameter of the pulmonary artery to the diameter of the aorta > 1), a marker of elevated PAP was associated with severe exacerbations of COPD [161].

While several studies have reported that the prevalence of PH in sleep disordered breathing ranges from 17 to 52 %, many investigators used a cut-off of mPAP > 20 mmHg and did not control for concomitant heart and lung disease that are associated with PH [162]. The presence of PH in sleep disordered breathing has been shown to correlate with age, BMI, pO_2, pCO_2 pulmonary capillary wedge pressure, FEV1 and forced vital capacity [162].

Exposure to chronic hypoxia at high altitude results in pulmonary vasoconstriction and vascular remodeling leading to PH that is associated with chronic mountain sickness [163]. However, there are limited number of studies evaluating the true prevalence of PH in general high altitude residents using echocardiography or right heart catheterization [164].

WHO Group 4 Chronic Thromboembolic Pulmonary Hypertension

Chronic thromboembolic pulmonary hypertension (CTEPH) is distinct from the other WHO groups as a potentially curable form of pulmonary vascular disease. Despite advances in our understanding of best practices for diagnosis and treatment of CTEPH, less is known about the epidemiology of this form of PH [165]. Although some series have suggested that up to 42 % of patients diagnosed with CTEPH had no known history of venous thromboembolism, current evidence supports a thromboembolic mechanism even in cases without known prior acute VTE, although the pathogenesis of vascular remodeling may be more complex than a failure to resorb acute thrombi alone [166–169].

In patients with prior pulmonary embolus (PE) the published incidence rate of CTEPH varies widely, but does not exceed 10 % [167, 170–173]. In one prospective cohort of unselected patients with PE routinely screened 1 year after their index event, the incidence of CTEPH was 0.57 % (95 % confidence interval 0.02–1.2 %) [173]. A second study that screened for CTEPH only in the presence of symptoms documented CTEPH in ~1 % of the study sample [171]. The incidence of symptomatic (persistent dyspnea after unselected PE) CTEPH was 1 % and 4 % at 1 and 2 years, respectively, in a study that used gold standard diagnostic testing (ventilation-perfusion lung scanning, pulmonary

angiogram, and right heart catheterization) and followed patients prospectively for a median of 94 months [170]. In Spain, CTEPH burden was evaluated as part of a country-wide registry for pulmonary vascular disease; the prevalence of CTEPH was 3.2 cases/million adults and the incidence was 0.9 cases/million/year, with reported 1-, 3-, and 5-year survival rates of 93 %, 75 %, and 65 % [38].

Observational studies have identified various risk factors for the development of CTEPH. These include a history of prior or recurrent VTE, prior splenectomy, and the presence of shunt or indwelling foreign bodies (such as pacemakers) [170, 174]. Some but not all clotting diatheses, such as the presence of lupus anticoagulant or antiphospholipid antibodies in 10–20 % of patients and higher factor VIII levels, increase the risk of CTEPH [175–177]. While many studies have examind unselected cohorts of PE patients not enriched for right ventricular dysfunction or high-risk features, size of perfusion defect on presentation has been shown to confer an increased risk of CTEPH, although there are currently no recommendations to screen such patients for the development of chronic disease after their acute event [170].

WHO Group 5 Pulmonary Hypertension with Unclear or Multifactorial Mechanisms

The etiology of PH in Group 5 is either unclear or as a result of pathophysiological mechanisms observed in Groups 1 to 4 (For detailed review see [178]). The underlying mechanism of PH in this group varies and includes vasoconstriction, pulmonary vascular remodeling, vascular occlusion with thrombi/ tumors, external compression, increased cardiac output, pulmonary venous hypertension or veno-occlusion.

The hematologic disorders associated with PH include myeloproliferative disorders, splenectomy, and hemoglobinopathies. It has been estimated that PH defined by echocardiography (RVSP > 35 mm Hg) complicates 13–50 % of patients with polycythemia vera, essential thrombocythemia, and primary myelofibrosis [179–184]. The underlying mechanism may be related to thromboembolic disease, precapillary PH (similar to IPAH), or extra-medullary hematopoiesis in the lung [178, 179]. Anagrelide and dasatinib used in the treatment of certain myeloproliferative disorders have been shown to promote PH as well [74, 185, 186]. A history of splenectomy has been reported in 2.5–11.5 % of patients with IPAH and 8.5 % of patients with CTEPH [187, 188]. The most likely mechanism of PH in asplenic patients is due to hypercoagulopathy resulting in in situ thrombosis and delayed thrombus resolution [178, 189].

Approximately 30 % of adult sickle cell (SC) patients have abnormal TR velocities, but only 10 % of patients meet hemodynamic criteria for PAH, as other cardiopulmonary effects in

SC may cause PH (e.g., left heart/valvular disease, high-output failure related to hemolysis) [99]. For these reasons, PH related to the chronic hemolytic anemia (including SC, thalassemia, spherocytosis, and stomatacytosis) was reclassified during the World Symposium in Nice from WHO Group 1 to WHO Group 5 (and has also transiently been in Group 4) [1]. Pulmonary vascular disease complicated SC disease has been associated with increased mortality [190, 191]. Higher TR velocity on Doppler echocardiography is a correlate for pulmonary pressures and has been shown to identify patients at risk for death [192]. As such, the American Thoracic Society recommends all adults with SS disease > 18 years of age be screened with echocardiography every 1–3 years, although this is an area of considerable controversy [100, 193]. Older age and markers of poorer disease control (e.g., more severe anemia, hemolysis, and renal dysfunction) have been associated with a higher risk of PH in some studies [99, 190, 191]. Treatment of PH (without confirmation of PAH by RHC) with phosphodiesterase-type 5 inhibitors led to increased morbidity in a clinical trial of SC patients, highlighting the complexities of this PH phenotype [194].

Other systemic disorders associated with PH include sarcoidosis, pulmonary Langerhans cell histiocytosis (PLCH), lymphangioleiomyomatosis (LAM), neurofibromatosis, vasculitis, Whipple disease, and POEMS (Polyneuropathy, Organomegaly, Endocrinopathy, Monoclonal protein, Skin changes) syndrome. The development in PH in such conditions portends a poor prognosis [178]. The overall prevalence of PH in sarcoidosis is 5–15 % [195, 196], in PLCH is 11 % [197] and LAM is 7 % [198]. However the prevalence is much higher in patients referred for transplantation with these diseases (74–79 % in sarcoidosis [199, 200], 92–100 % in PLCH [201, 202] and 45 % in LAM [203]).

Metabolic disorders such as glycogen storage disorders, Gaucher disease, thyroid disorders and Hurler syndrome/Hurler-Scheie syndrome have been shown to be associated with PH. The data on prevalence of PH in these diseases is limited and is discussed in detail in a recent review by Lahm et al. [178]. Other associated conditions with PH include those related to the compression of pulmonary vessels (fibrosing mediastinitis, lymphadenopathy, tumor) and obstruction of the pulmonary vessels (endovascular tumor, tumor emboli, pulmonary tumor thrombotic microangiopathy, pulmonary vein stenosis).

Chronic renal failure patients may develop PH due to underlying pulmonary venous hypertension from volume overload and/or intrinsic left heart disease, true pulmonary arterial vasculopathy, or high-output cardiac failure related to long-standing fistulas. Impaired endothelial function, metabolic and hormonal changes, vascular calcification and calcium/phosphate imbalance have been proposed as potential additional mechanisms [204, 205] Small retrospective studies have demonstrated a high prevalence of echocardiographic PH among patients with end-stage renal disease, ranging from 19 % to as high at 56 % [204–210]. Advanced chronic kidney disease and hemodialysis via arteriovenous access appear to be independent risk factors for the development and progression of PH [205, 206]. Pre-transplantation echocardiographic PH may also be a predictor of post-transplant allograft failure and survival [204]. Further studies are needed to better characterize PH in renal failure as well as other etiologies in WHO Group 5.

Summary and Conclusions

Considerable progress has been made in our understanding of the epidemiology of pulmonary vascular disease. To this point, predominantly center-based registries have informed our knowledge of current PAH characteristics and population-based observational studies have provided a snapshot of PH complicating chronic cardiopulmonary disease. Modern therapy has no doubt improved prognosis in PAH. Yet, how basic demographic characteristics such as age and sex modify risk (regardless of clinical sub-type) and survival in PH or PAH remain poorly understood. A comprehensive and multi-faceted approach that captures patients across settings, time, and geography will likely be required to address further the unsolved epidemiologic issues of pulmonary vascular disease.

References

1. Simonneau G, Gatzoulis MA, Adatia I, Celermajer D, Denton C, Ghofrani A, et al. Updated clinical classification of pulmonary hypertension. J Am Coll Cardiol. 2013;62(25 Suppl):029.
2. Lam CS, Borlaug BA, Kane GC, Enders FT, Rodeheffer RJ, Redfield MM. Age-associated increases in pulmonary artery systolic pressure in the general population. Circulation. 2009;119(20):2663–70.
3. Choudhary G, Jankowich M, Wu W-C. Prevalence and clinical characteristics associated with pulmonary hypertension in African-Americans. PLoS One. 2013;8(12), e84264.
4. Rudski LG. Point: can Doppler echocardiography estimates of pulmonary artery systolic pressures be relied upon to accurately make the diagnosis of pulmonary hypertension? Yes. Chest. 2013;143(6):1533–6.
5. Rich JD. Counterpoint: can Doppler echocardiography estimates of pulmonary artery systolic pressures be relied upon to accurately make the diagnosis of pulmonary hypertension? No. Chest. 2013;143(6):1536–9.
6. Rich JD, Shah SJ, Swamy RS, Kamp A, Rich S. Inaccuracy of Doppler echocardiographic estimates of pulmonary artery pressures in patients with pulmonary hypertension: implications for clinical practice. Chest. 2011;139(5):988–93.
7. Farber HW, Foreman AJ, Miller DP, McGoon MD. REVEAL Registry: correlation of right heart catheterization and echocardiography in patients with pulmonary arterial hypertension. Congest Heart Fail. 2011;17(2):56–64.
8. Bech-Hanssen O, Karason K, Rundqvist B, Bollano E, Lindgren F, Selimovic N. Can pulmonary hypertension and increased

pulmonary vascular resistance be ruled in and ruled out by echocardiography? J Am Soc Echocardiogr. 2013;26(5):469–78.

9. Enea I, Ghio S, Bongarzoni A, Casazza F, D'Armini AM et al. (2010) Echocardiographic alterations suggestive of pulmonary hypertension in the Italian ultrasonography laboratories. Epidemiological data from the INCIPIT study (INCidence of Pulmonary Hypertension in Italian ulTrasonography laboratories). G Ital Cardiol (Rome). 11:402–7.

10. Strange G, Playford D, Stewart S, Deague JA, Nelson H, Kent A, et al. Pulmonary hypertension: prevalence and mortality in the Armadale echocardiography cohort. Heart. 2012;98(24):1805–11.

11. Maron B, Choudhary G, Khan U, Jankowich M, McChesney H, Ferrazzani P, et al. The clinical profile and under-diagnosis of pulmonary hypertension in U.S. Veteran patients. Circ Heart Fail. 2013;6(5):906–12.

12. Shah SJ. Pulmonary hypertension. JAMA. 2012;308(13):1366–74.

13. Hyduk A, Croft JB, Ayala C, Zheng K, Zheng ZJ, Mensah GA. Pulmonary hypertension surveillance – United States, 1980-2002. MMWR Surveill Summ. 2005;54(5):1–28.

14. McQuillan BM, Picard MH, Leavitt M, Weyman AE. Clinical correlates and reference intervals for pulmonary artery systolic pressure among echocardiographically normal subjects. Circulation. 2001;104(23):2797–802.

15. Guglin M, Kolli S, Chen R. Determinants of pulmonary hypertension in young adults. Int J Clin Pract Suppl. 2012;177:13–9.

16. Setiawan VW, Haiman CA, Stanczyk FZ, Le Marchand L, Henderson BE. Racial/ethnic differences in postmenopausal endogenous hormones: the multiethnic cohort study. Cancer Epidemiol Biomarkers Prev. 2006;15(10):1849–55.

17. Sweeney L, Voelkel NF. Estrogen exposure, obesity and thyroid disease in women with severe pulmonary hypertension. Eur J Med Res. 2009;14(10):433–42.

18. Taraseviciute A, Voelkel NF. Severe pulmonary hypertension in postmenopausal obese women. Eur J Med Res. 2006;11(5):198–202.

19. Bogaard HJ, Al Husseini A, Farkas L, Farkas D, Gomez-Arroyo J, Abbate A, et al. Severe pulmonary hypertension: the role of metabolic and endocrine disorders. Pulm Circ. 2012;2(2):148–54.

20. Ventetuolo C, Ouyang P, Bluemke D, Tandri H, Barr R, Bagiella E, et al. Sex hormones and the right ventricle: the MESA-right ventricle study. Am J Respir Crit Care Med. 2009;179(1_Meeting Abstracts):A4150.

21. Chaouat A, Naeije R, Weitzenblum E. Pulmonary hypertension in COPD. Eur Respir J. 2008;32(5):1371–85.

22. Mannino DM, McBurnie MA, Tan W, Kocabas A, Anto J, Vollmer WM, et al. Restricted spirometry in the Burden of Lung Disease Study. Int J Tuberc Lung Dis. 2012;16(10):1405–11.

23. Fimognari FL, Pasqualetti P, Moro L, Franco A, Piccirillo G, Pastorelli R, et al. The association between metabolic syndrome and restrictive ventilatory dysfunction in older persons. J Gerontol A Biol Sci Med Sci. 2007;62(7):760–5.

24. Scarlata S, Pedone C, Fimognari FL, Bellia V, Forastiere F, Incalzi RA. Restrictive pulmonary dysfunction at spirometry and mortality in the elderly. Respir Med. 2008;102(9):1349–54.

25. Mannino DM, Holguin F, Pavlin BI, Ferdinands JM. Risk factors for prevalence of and mortality related to restriction on spirometry: findings from the First National Health and Nutrition Examination Survey and follow-up. Int J Tuberc Lung Dis. 2005;9(6):613–21.

26. Burney PG, Hooper R. Forced vital capacity, airway obstruction and survival in a general population sample from the USA. Thorax. 2011;66(1):49–54.

27. Choudhary G, Jankowich M, Wu WC. Elevated pulmonary artery systolic pressure predicts heart failure admissions in African Americans: Jackson Heart Study. Circ Heart Fail. 2014;7(4):558–64.

28. D'Alonzo GE, Barst RJ, Ayres SM, Bergofsky EH, Brundage BH, Detre KM, et al. Survival in patients with primary pulmonary hypertension. Results from a national prospective registry. Ann Intern Med. 1991;115(5):343–9.

29. Rich S, Dantzker DR, Ayres SM, Bergofsky EH, Brundage BH, Detre KM, et al. Primary pulmonary hypertension. A national prospective study. Ann Intern Med. 1987;107(2):216–23.

30. Thenappan T, Shah SJ, Rich S, Gomberg-Maitland M. A USA-based registry for pulmonary arterial hypertension: 1982-2006. Eur Respir J. 2007;30(6):1103–10.

31. Peacock AJ, Murphy NF, McMurray JJ, Caballero L, Stewart S. An epidemiological study of pulmonary arterial hypertension. Eur Respir J. 2007;30(1):104–9.

32. Kane GC, Maradit-Kremers H, Slusser JP, Scott CG, Frantz RP, McGoon MD. Integration of clinical and hemodynamic parameters in the prediction of long-term survival in patients with pulmonary arterial hypertension. Chest. 2011;139(6):1285–93.

33. Jing ZC, Xu XQ, Han ZY, Wu Y, Deng KW, Wang H, et al. Registry and survival study in Chinese patients with idiopathic and familial pulmonary arterial hypertension. Chest. 2007;132(2):373–9.

34. Ling Y, Johnson MK, Kiely DG, Condliffe R, Elliot CA, Gibbs JS, et al. Changing demographics, epidemiology, and survival of incident pulmonary arterial hypertension: results from the pulmonary hypertension registry of the United Kingdom and Ireland. Am J Respir Crit Care Med. 2012;186(8):790–6.

35. Humbert M, Sitbon O, Chaouat A, Bertocchi M, Habib G, Gressin V, et al. Pulmonary arterial hypertension in France: results from a National Registry. Am J Respir Crit Care Med. 2006;173(9):1023–30.

36. Badesch DB, Raskob GE, Elliott CG, Krichman AM, Farber HW, Frost AE, et al. Pulmonary arterial hypertension: baseline characteristics from the REVEAL Registry. Chest. 2010;137(2):376–87.

37. Hoeper MM, Huscher D, Ghofrani HA, Delcroix M, Distler O, Schweiger C, et al. Elderly patients diagnosed with idiopathic pulmonary arterial hypertension: results from the COMPERA registry. Int J Cardiol. 2013;168(2):871–80.

38. Escribano-Subias P, Blanco I, Lopez-Meseguer M, Lopez-Guarch CJ, Roman A, Morales P, et al. Survival in pulmonary hypertension in Spain: insights from the Spanish registry. Eur Respir J. 2012;40(3):596–603.

39. Zhang R, Dai LZ, Xie WP, Yu ZX, Wu BX, Pan L, et al. Survival of Chinese patients with pulmonary arterial hypertension in the modern treatment era. Chest. 2011;140(2):301–9.

40. Thenappan T, Shah SJ, Rich S, Tian L, Archer SL, Gomberg-Maitland M. Survival in pulmonary arterial hypertension: a reappraisal of the NIH risk stratification equation. Eur Respir J. 2010;35(5):1079–87.

41. Humbert M, Sitbon O, Chaouat A, Bertocchi M, Habib G, Gressin V, et al. Survival in patients with idiopathic, familial, and anorexigen-associated pulmonary arterial hypertension in the modern management era. Circulation. 2010;122(2):156–63.

42. Benza RL, Miller DP, Gomberg-Maitland M, Frantz RP, Foreman AJ, Coffey CS, et al. Predicting survival in pulmonary arterial hypertension: insights from the Registry to Evaluate Early and Long-Term Pulmonary Arterial Hypertension Disease Management (REVEAL). Circulation. 2010;122(2):164–72.

43. Olsson KM, Delcroix M, Ghofrani HA, Tiede H, Huscher D, Speich R, et al. Anticoagulation and survival in pulmonary arterial hypertension: results from the Comparative, Prospective Registry of Newly Initiated Therapies for Pulmonary Hypertension (COMPERA). Circulation. 2014;129(1):57–65.

44. McGoon MD, Krichman A, Farber HW, Barst RJ, Raskob GE, Liou TG, et al. Design of the REVEAL registry for US patients with pulmonary arterial hypertension. Mayo Clin Proc. 2008;83(8):923–31.

45. Benza RL, Miller DP, Barst RJ, Badesch DB, Frost AE, McGoon MD. An evaluation of long-term survival from time of diagnosis in pulmonary arterial hypertension from the REVEAL Registry. Chest. 2012;142(2):448–56.

46. Ventetuolo CE, Praestgaard A, Palevsky HI, Klinger JR, Halpern SD, Kawut SM. Sex and haemodynamics in pulmonary arterial hypertension. Eur Respir J. 2014;43(2):523–30.

47. Gabler NB, French B, Strom BL, Liu Z, Palevsky HI, Taichman DB, et al. Race and sex differences in response to endothelin receptor antagonists for pulmonary arterial hypertension. Chest. 2012;141(1):20–6.

48. Mathai SC, Hassoun PM, Puhan MA, Zhou Y, Wise RA. Gender differences in response to tadalafil in pulmonary arterial hypertension. Chest. 2014;14(10):14–0263.

49. Kawut SM, Al-Naamani N, Agerstrand C, Rosenzweig EB, Rowan C, Barst RJ, et al. Determinants of right ventricular ejection fraction in pulmonary arterial hypertension. Chest. 2009; 135(3):752–9.

50. Shapiro S, Traiger GL, Turner M, McGoon MD, Wason P, Barst RJ. Sex differences in the diagnosis, treatment, and outcome of patients with pulmonary arterial hypertension enrolled in the registry to evaluate early and long-term pulmonary arterial hypertension disease management sex differences in pulmonary arterial hypertension. Chest J. 2012; 141(2):363–73.

51. Davis KK, Lilienfeld DE, Doyle RL. Increased mortality in African Americans with idiopathic pulmonary arterial hypertension. J Natl Med Assoc. 2008;100(1):69–72.

52. Kawut SM, Horn EM, Berekashvili KK, Garofano RP, Goldsmith RL, Widlitz AC, et al. New predictors of outcome in idiopathic pulmonary arterial hypertension. Am J Cardiol. 2005;95(2):199–203.

53. Brown LM, Chen H, Halpern S, Taichman D, McGoon MD, Farber HW, et al. Delay in recognition of pulmonary arterial hypertension: factors identified from the REVEAL Registry. Chest. 2011;140(1):19–26.

54. Wu WH, Yang L, Peng FH, Yao J, Zou LL, Liu D, et al. Lower socioeconomic status is associated with worse outcomes in pulmonary arterial hypertension. Am J Respir Crit Care Med. 2013;187(3):303–10.

55. Deng Z, Morse JH, Slager SL, Cuervo N, Moore KJ, Venetos G, et al. Familial primary pulmonary hypertension (gene PPH1) is caused by mutations in the bone morphogenetic protein receptor-II gene. Am J Hum Genet. 2000;67(3):737–44.

56. Soubrier F, Chung WK, Machado R, Grunig E, Aldred M, Geraci M, et al. Genetics and genomics of pulmonary arterial hypertension. J Am Coll Cardiol. 2013;62(25 Suppl):035.

57. Chaouat A, Coulet F, Favre C, Simonneau G, Weitzenblum E, Soubrier F, et al. Endoglin germline mutation in a patient with hereditary haemorrhagic telangiectasia and dexfenfluramine associated pulmonary arterial hypertension. Thorax. 2004;59(5):446–8.

58. Harrison RE, Flanagan JA, Sankelo M, Abdalla SA, Rowell J, Machado RD, et al. Molecular and functional analysis identifies ALK-1 as the predominant cause of pulmonary hypertension related to hereditary haemorrhagic telangiectasia. J Med Genet. 2003;40(12):865–71.

59. Shintani M, Yagi H, Nakayama T, Saji T, Matsuoka R. A new nonsense mutation of SMAD8 associated with pulmonary arterial hypertension. J Med Genet. 2009;46(5):331–7.

60. Ma L, Roman-Campos D, Austin ED, Eyries M, Sampson KS, Soubrier F, et al. A novel channelopathy in pulmonary arterial hypertension. N Engl J Med. 2013;369(4):351–61.

61. Austin ED, Ma L, LeDuc C, Berman Rosenzweig E, Borczuk A, Phillips 3rd JA, et al. Whole exome sequencing to identify a novel gene (caveolin-1) associated with human pulmonary arterial hypertension. Circ Cardiovasc Genet. 2012;5(3):336–43.

62. Nasim MT, Ogo T, Ahmed M, Randall R, Chowdhury HM, Snape KM, et al. Molecular genetic characterization of SMAD signaling molecules in pulmonary arterial hypertension. Hum Mutat. 2011;32(12):1385–9.

63. Sztrymf B, Coulet F, Girerd B, Yaici A, Jais X, Sitbon O, et al. Clinical outcomes of pulmonary arterial hypertension in carriers of BMPR2 mutation. Am J Respir Crit Care Med. 2008; 177(12):1377–83.

64. Girerd B, Montani D, Coulet F, Sztrymf B, Yaici A, Jais X, et al. Clinical outcomes of pulmonary arterial hypertension in patients carrying an ACVRL1 (ALK1) mutation. Am J Respir Crit Care Med. 2010;181(8):851–61.

65. Simonneau G, Gatzoulis MA, Adatia I, Celermajer D, Denton C, Ghofrani A, et al. Updated clinical classification of pulmonary hypertension. J Am Coll Cardiol. 2013;62(25 Suppl):D34–41.

66. Abenhaim L, Moride Y, Brenot F, Rich S, Benichou J, Kurz X, et al. Appetite-suppressant drugs and the risk of primary pulmonary hypertension. International Primary Pulmonary Hypertension Study Group. N Engl J Med. 1996;335(9):609–16.

67. Douglas JG, Munro JF, Kitchin AH, Muir AL, Proudfoot AT. Pulmonary hypertension and fenfluramine. Br Med J (Clin Res Ed). 1981;283(6296):881–3.

68. Mark EJ, Patalas ED, Chang HT, Evans RJ, Kessler SC. Fatal pulmonary hypertension associated with short-term use of fenfluramine and phentermine. N Engl J Med. 1997;337(9):602–6.

69. Rich S, Rubin L, Walker AM, Schneeweiss S, Abenhaim L. Anorexigens and pulmonary hypertension in the United States: results from the surveillance of North American pulmonary hypertension. Chest. 2000;117(3):870–4.

70. Walker AM, Langleben D, Korelitz JJ, Rich S, Rubin LJ, Strom BL, et al. Temporal trends and drug exposures in pulmonary hypertension: an American experience. Am Heart J. 2006; 152(3):521–6.

71. Savale L, Chaumais MC, Cottin V, Bergot E, Frachon I, Prevot G, et al. Pulmonary hypertension associated with benfluorex exposure. Eur Respir J. 2012;40(5):1164–72.

72. Boutet K, Frachon I, Jobic Y, Gut-Gobert C, Leroyer C, Carlhant-Kowalski D, et al. Fenfluramine-like cardiovascular side-effects of benfluorex. Eur Respir J. 2009;33(3):684–8.

73. Rasheed W, Flaim B, Seymour JF. Reversible severe pulmonary hypertension secondary to dasatinib in a patient with chronic myeloid leukemia. Leuk Res. 2009;33(6):861–4.

74. Montani D, Bergot E, Gunther S, Savale L, Bergeron A, Bourdin A, et al. Pulmonary arterial hypertension in patients treated by dasatinib. Circulation. 2012;125(17):2128–37.

75. Sano M, Saotome M, Urushida T, Katoh H, Satoh H, Ohnishi K, et al. Pulmonary arterial hypertension caused by treatment with dasatinib for chronic myeloid leukemia – critical alert. Intern Med. 2012;51(17):2337–40.

76. Caravita S, Secchi MB, Wu SC, Pierini S, Paggi A. Sildenafil therapy for interferon-beta-1a-induced pulmonary arterial hypertension: a case report. Cardiology. 2011;120(4):187–9.

77. Dhillon S, Kaker A, Dosanjh A, Japra D, VanThiel DH. Irreversible pulmonary hypertension associated with the use of interferon alpha for chronic hepatitis C. Dig Dis Sci. 2010;55(6):1785–90.

78. Savale L, Gunther S, Chaumais MC, Jais X, Sattler C, Macari EA, et al. Pulmonary arterial hypertension in patients treated with interferon. Eur Respir J. 2014;44(6):1627–34.

79. Jochmann N, Kiecker F, Borges AC, Hofmann MA, Eddicks S, Sterry W, et al. Long-term therapy of interferon-alpha induced pulmonary arterial hypertension with different PDE-5 inhibitors: a case report. Cardiovasc Ultrasound. 2005;3:26.

80. Fruehauf S, Steiger S, Topaly J, Ho AD. Pulmonary artery hypertension during interferon-alpha therapy for chronic myelogenous leukemia. Ann Hematol. 2001;80(5):308–10.

81. Sangal RB, Taylor LE, Gillani F, Poppas A, Klinger JR, Ventetuolo CE. Risk of echocardiographic pulmonary hypertension in individuals with human immunodeficiency virus-hepatitis C virus coinfection. Ann Am Thorac Soc. 2014;11(10):1553–9.

82. Souza R, Humbert M, Sztrymf B, Jais X, Yaici A, Le Pavec J, et al. Pulmonary arterial hypertension associated with fenfluramine exposure: report of 109 cases. Eur Respir J. 2008;31(2):343–8.

83. Hachulla E, Gressin V, Guillevin L, Carpentier P, Diot E, Sibilia J, et al. Early detection of pulmonary arterial hypertension in systemic sclerosis: a French nationwide prospective multicenter study. Arthritis Rheum. 2005;52(12):3792–800.

84. Mukerjee D, St George D, Coleiro B, Knight C, Denton CP, Davar J, et al. Prevalence and outcome in systemic sclerosis associated pulmonary arterial hypertension: application of a registry approach. Ann Rheum Dis. 2003;62(11):1088–93.

85. Steen VD, Medsger TA. Changes in causes of death in systemic sclerosis, 1972-2002. Ann Rheum Dis. 2007;66(7):940–4.

86. Khanna D, Gladue H, Channick R, Chung L, Distler O, Furst DE, et al. Recommendations for screening and detection of connective tissue disease-associated pulmonary arterial hypertension. Arthritis Rheum. 2013;65(12):3194–201.

87. Humbert M, Yaici A, de Groote P, Montani D, Sitbon O, Launay D, et al. Screening for pulmonary arterial hypertension in patients with systemic sclerosis: clinical characteristics at diagnosis and long-term survival. Arthritis Rheum. 2011;63(11):3522–30.

88. Opravil M, Pechere M, Speich R, JollerJemelka HI, Jenni R, Russi EW, et al. HIV-associated primary pulmonary hypertension – a case control study. Am J Respir Crit Care Med. 1997;155(3):990–5.

89. Sitbon O, Lascoux-Combe C, Delfraissy JF, Yeni PG, Raffi F, De Zuttere D, et al. Prevalence of HIV-related pulmonary arterial hypertension in the current antiretroviral therapy era. Am J Respir Crit Care Med. 2008;177(1):108–13.

90. Speich R, Jenni R, Opravil M, Pfab M, Russi EW. Primary pulmonary-hypertension in HIV infection. Chest. 1991;100(5):1268–71.

91. Krowka MJ, Swanson KL, Frantz RP, McGoon MD, Wiesner RH. Portopulmonary hypertension: results from a 10-year screening algorithm. Hepatology. 2006;44(6):1502–10.

92. Colle IO, Moreau R, Godinho E, Belghiti J, Ettori F, Cohen-Solal A, et al. Diagnosis of portopulmonary hypertension in candidates for liver transplantation: a prospective study. Hepatology. 2003;37(2):401–9.

93. Castro M, Krowka MJ, Schroeder DR, Beck KC, Plevak DJ, Rettke SR, et al. Frequency and clinical implications of increased pulmonary artery pressures in liver transplant patients. Mayo Clin Proc. 1996;71(6):543–51.

94. Yang YY, Lin HC, Lee WC, Hou MC, Lee FY, Chang FY, et al. Portopulmonary hypertension: distinctive hemodynamic and clinical manifestations. J Gastroenterol. 2001;36(3):181–6.

95. McDonnell PJ, Toye PA, Hutchins GM. Primary pulmonary hypertension and cirrhosis: are they related? Am Rev Respir Dis. 1983;127(4):437–41.

96. Lowe BS, Therrien J, Ionescu-Ittu R, Pilote L, Martucci G, Marelli AJ. Diagnosis of pulmonary hypertension in the congenital heart disease adult population impact on outcomes. J Am Coll Cardiol. 2011;58(5):538–46.

97. Duffels MG, Engelfriet PM, Berger RM, van Loon RL, Hoendermis E, Vriend JW, et al. Pulmonary arterial hypertension in congenital heart disease: an epidemiologic perspective from a Dutch registry. Int J Cardiol. 2007;120(2):198–204.

98. Engelfriet PM, Duffels MG, Moller T, Boersma E, Tijssen JG, Thaulow E, et al. Pulmonary arterial hypertension in adults born with a heart septal defect: the Euro Heart Survey on adult congenital heart disease. Heart. 2007;93(6):682–7.

99. Parent F, Bachir D, Inamo J, Lionnet F, Driss F, Loko G, et al. A hemodynamic study of pulmonary hypertension in sickle cell disease. N Engl J Med. 2011;365(1):44–53.

100. Klings ES, Machado RF, Barst RJ, Morris CR, Mubarak KK, Gordeuk VR, et al. An official American Thoracic Society clinical practice guideline: diagnosis, risk stratification, and management of pulmonary hypertension of sickle cell disease. Am J Respir Crit Care Med. 2014;189(6):727–40.

101. Condliffe R, Kiely DG, Peacock AJ, Corris PA, Gibbs JS, Vrapi F, et al. Connective tissue disease-associated pulmonary arterial hypertension in the modern treatment era. Am J Respir Crit Care Med. 2009;179(2):151–7.

102. Chung L, Liu J, Parsons L, Hassoun PM, McGoon M, Badesch DB, et al. Characterization of connective tissue disease-associated pulmonary arterial hypertension from REVEAL: identifying systemic sclerosis as a unique phenotype. Chest. 2010;138(6):1383–94.

103. Chung L, Farber HW, Benza R, Miller DP, Parsons L, Hassoun PM, et al. Unique predictors of mortality in patients with pulmonary arterial hypertension associated with systemic sclerosis in the reveal registry. Chest. 2014;3(10):13–3014.

104. Mehta NJ, Khan IA, Mehta RN, Sepkowitz DA. HIV related pulmonary hypertension: analytic review of 131 cases. Chest. 2000;118(4):1133–41.

105. Cool CD, Voelkel NF, Bull T. Viral infection and pulmonary hypertension: is there an association? Expert Rev Respir Med. 2011;5(2):207–16.

106. Hofman FM, Wright AD, Dohadwala MM, Wongstaal F, Walker SM. Exogenous TAT protein activated human endothelial cells. Blood. 1993;82(9):2774–80.

107. Humbert M, Monti G, Brenot F, Sitbon O, Portier A, Grangeotkeros L, et al. Increased interleukin-1 and interleukin-6 serum concentrations in severe primary pulmonary hypertension. Am J Respir Crit Care Med. 1995;151(5):1628–31.

108. James CO, Huang MB, Khan M, Garcia-Barrio M, Powell MD, Bond VC. Extracellular Nef protein targets CD4(+) T cells for apoptosis by interacting with CXCR4 surface receptors. J Virol. 2004;78(6):3099–109.

109. Almodovar S, Hsue PY, Morelli J, Huang L, Flores SC. Pathogenesis of HIV-associated pulmonary hypertension: potential role of HIV-1 Nef. Proc Am Thorac Soc. 2011;8(3):3 08–12.

110. Marecki JC, Cool CD, Parr JE, Beckey VE, Luciw PA, Tarantal AF, et al. HIV-1 Nef is associated with complex pulmonary vascular lesions in SHIV-nef-infected macaques. Am J Respir Crit Care Med. 2006;174(4):437–45.

111. Almodovar S, Knight R, Allshouse AA, Roemer S, Lozupone C, McDonald D, et al. Human Immunodeficiency Virus nef signature sequences are associated with pulmonary hypertension. AIDS Res Hum Retroviruses. 2012;28(6):607–18.

112. Petitpretz P, Brenot F, Azarian R, Parent F, Rain B, Herve P, et al. Pulmonary hypertension in patients with human immunodeficiency virus infection. Comparison with primary pulmonary hypertension. Circulation. 1994;89(6):2722–7.

113. McLaughlin VV, Presberg KW, Doyle RL, Abman SH, McCrory DC, Fortin T, et al. Prognosis of pulmonary arterial hypertension: ACCP evidence-based clinical practice guidelines. Chest. 2004;126(1 Suppl):78S–92.

114. Degano B, Guillaume M, Savale L, Montani D, Jais X, Yaici A, et al. HIV-associated pulmonary arterial hypertension: survival and prognostic factors in the modern therapeutic era. AIDS. 2010;24(1):67–75.

115. Fritz JS, Fallon MB, Kawut SM. Pulmonary vascular complications of liver disease. Am J Respir Crit Care Med. 2013; 187(2):133–43.

116. Hadengue A, Benhayoun MK, Lebrec D, Benhamou JP. Pulmonary hypertension complicating portal hypertension: prevalence and relation to splanchnic hemodynamics. Gastroenterology. 1991;100(2):520–8.

117. Kawut SM, Krowka MJ, Trotter JF, Roberts KE, Benza RL, Badesch DB, et al. Clinical risk factors for portopulmonary hypertension. Hepatology. 2008;48(1):196–203.

118. Roberts KE, Fallon MB, Krowka MJ, Brown RS, Trotter JF, Peter I, et al. Genetic risk factors for portopulmonary hypertension in patients with advanced liver disease. Am J Respir Crit Care Med. 2009;179(9):835–42.

119. Neuhofer W, Gulberg V, Gerbes AL. Endothelin and endothelin receptor antagonism in portopulmonary hypertension. Eur J Clin Invest. 2006;3:54–61.

120. Krowka MJ, Miller DP, Barst RJ, Taichman D, Dweik RA, Badesch DB, et al. Portopulmonary hypertension: a report from the US-based REVEAL Registry. Chest. 2012;141(4):906–15.

121. Krowka MJ, Plevak DJ, Findlay JY, Rosen CB, Wiesner RH, Krom RA. Pulmonary hemodynamics and perioperative cardiopulmonary-related mortality in patients with portopulmonary hypertension undergoing liver transplantation. Liver Transpl. 2000;6(4):443–50.

122. Marelli AJ, Mackie AS, Ionescu-Ittu R, Rahme E, Pilote L. Congenital heart disease in the general population: changing prevalence and age distribution. Circulation. 2007;115(2):163–72.

123. Hopkins WE, Waggoner AD. Severe pulmonary hypertension without right ventricular failure: the unique hearts of patients with Eisenmenger syndrome. Am J Cardiol. 2002;89(1):34–8.

124. Barst RJ, Ivy DD, Foreman AJ, McGoon MD, Rosenzweig EB. Four- and seven-year outcomes of patients with congenital heart disease-associated pulmonary arterial hypertension (from the REVEAL Registry). Am J Cardiol. 2014;113(1):147–55.

125. Graham BB, Chabon J, Bandeira A, Espinheira L, Butrous G, Tuder RM. Significant intrapulmonary Schistosoma egg antigens are not present in schistosomiasis-associated pulmonary hypertension. Pulm Circ. 2011;1(4):456–61.

126. Graham BB, Chabon J, Gebreab L, Poole J, Debella E, Davis L, et al. Transforming growth factor-beta signaling promotes pulmonary hypertension caused by Schistosoma mansoni. Circulation. 2013;128(12):1354–64.

127. Graham BB, Chabon J, Kumar R, Kolosionek E, Gebreab L, Debella E, et al. Protective role of IL-6 in vascular remodeling in Schistosoma pulmonary hypertension. Am J Respir Cell Mol Biol. 2013;49(6):951–9.

128. Lapa M, Dias B, Jardim C, Fernandes CJ, Dourado PM, Figueiredo M, et al. Cardiopulmonary manifestations of hepatosplenic schistosomiasis. Circulation. 2009;119(11):1518–23.

129. dos Santos Fernandes CJ, Jardim CV, Hovnanian A, Hoette S, Dias BA, Souza S, et al. Survival in schistosomiasis-associated pulmonary arterial hypertension. J Am Coll Cardiol. 2010;56(9):715–20.

130. Fernandes CJ, Dias BA, Jardim CV, Hovnanian A, Hoette S, Morinaga LK, et al. The role of target therapies in schistosomiasis-associated pulmonary arterial hypertension. Chest. 2012;141(4):923–8.

131. Guazzi M, Borlaug BA. Pulmonary hypertension due to left heart disease. Circulation. 2012;126(8):975–90.

132. Bursi F, McNallan SM, Redfield MM, Nkomo VT, Lam CS, Weston SA, et al. Pulmonary pressures and death in heart failure: a community study. J Am Coll Cardiol. 2012;59(3):222–31.

133. Kjaergaard J, Akkan D, Iversen KK, Kjoller E, Kober L, Torp-Pedersen C, et al. Prognostic importance of pulmonary hypertension in patients with heart failure. Am J Cardiol. 2007;99(8):1146–50.

134. Ghio S, Gavazzi A, Campana C, Inserra C, Klersy C, Sebastiani R, et al. Independent and additive prognostic value of right ventricular systolic function and pulmonary artery pressure in patients with chronic heart failure. J Am Coll Cardiol. 2001;37(1):183–8.

135. Grigioni F, Potena L, Galie N, Fallani F, Bigliardi M, Coccolo F, et al. Prognostic implications of serial assessments of pulmonary hypertension in severe chronic heart failure. J Heart Lung Transplant. 2006;25(10):1241–6.

136. Khush KK, Tasissa G, Butler J, McGlothlin D, De Marco T, Investigators E. Effect of pulmonary hypertension on clinical outcomes in advanced heart failure: analysis of the Evaluation Study of Congestive Heart Failure and Pulmonary Artery Catheterization Effectiveness (ESCAPE) database. Am Heart J. 2009;157(6):1026–34.

137. Lam CS, Roger VL, Rodeheffer RJ, Borlaug BA, Enders FT, Redfield MM. Pulmonary hypertension in heart failure with preserved ejection fraction: a community-based study. J Am Coll Cardiol. 2009;53(13):1119–26.

138. Klapholz M, Maurer M, Lowe AM, Messineo F, Meisner JS, Mitchell J, et al. Hospitalization for heart failure in the presence of a normal left ventricular ejection fraction: results of the New York Heart Failure Registry. J Am Coll Cardiol. 2004;43(8):1432–8.

139. Leung CC, Moondra V, Catherwood E, Andrus BW. Prevalence and risk factors of pulmonary hypertension in patients with elevated pulmonary venous pressure and preserved ejection fraction. Am J Cardiol. 2010;106(2):284–6.

140. Shah AM, Claggett B, Sweitzer NK, Shah SJ, Anand IS, O'Meara E, et al. Cardiac structure and function and prognosis in heart failure with preserved ejection fraction: findings from the echocardiographic study of the Treatment of Preserved Cardiac Function Heart Failure with an Aldosterone Antagonist (TOPCAT) Trial. Circ Heart Fail. 2014;7(5):740–51.

141. Thenappan T, Shah SJ, Gomberg-Maitland M, Collander B, Vallakati A, Shroff P, et al. Clinical characteristics of pulmonary hypertension in patients with heart failure and preserved ejection fraction. Circ Heart Fail. 2011;4(3):257–65.

142. Hart SA, Krasuski RA, Wang A, Kisslo K, Harrison JK, Bashore TM. Pulmonary hypertension and elevated transpulmonary gradient in patients with mitral stenosis. J Heart Valve Dis. 2010;19(6):708–15.

143. Melby SJ, Moon MR, Lindman BR, Bailey MS, Hill LL, Damiano Jr RJ. Impact of pulmonary hypertension on outcomes after aortic valve replacement for aortic valve stenosis. J Thorac Cardiovasc Surg. 2011;141(6):1424–30.

144. Johnson LW, Hapanowicz MB, Buonanno C, Bowser MA, Marvasti MA, Parker Jr FB. Pulmonary hypertension in isolated aortic stenosis. Hemodynamic correlations and follow-up. J Thorac Cardiovasc Surg. 1988;95(4):603–7.

145. Silver K, Aurigemma G, Krendel S, Barry N, Ockene I, Alpert J. Pulmonary artery hypertension in severe aortic stenosis: incidence and mechanism. Am Heart J. 1993;125(1):146–50.

146. Abramson SV, Burke JF, Kelly Jr JJ, Kitchen 3rd JG, Dougherty MJ, Yih DF, et al. Pulmonary hypertension predicts mortality and morbidity in patients with dilated cardiomyopathy. Ann Intern Med. 1992;116(11):888–95.

147. Scharf SM, Iqbal M, Keller C, Criner G, Lee S, Fessler HE, et al. Hemodynamic characterization of patients with severe emphysema. Am J Respir Crit Care Med. 2002;166(3):314–22.

148. Thabut G, Dauriat G, Stern JB, Logeart D, Levy A, Marrash-Chahla R, et al. Pulmonary hemodynamics in advanced COPD candidates for lung volume reduction surgery or lung transplantation. Chest. 2005;127(5):1531–6.

149. Hoeper MM, Barbera JA, Channick RN, Hassoun PM, Lang IM, Manes A, et al. Diagnosis, assessment, and treatment of nonpulmonary arterial hypertension pulmonary hypertension. J Am Coll Cardiol. 2009;54(1 Suppl):S85–96.

150. Cottin V, Le Pavec J, Prevot G, Mal H, Humbert M, Simonneau G, et al. Pulmonary hypertension in patients with combined pulmonary fibrosis and emphysema syndrome. Eur Respir J. 2010;35(1):105–11.

151. Lettieri CJ, Nathan SD, Barnett SD, Ahmad S, Shorr AF. Prevalence and outcomes of pulmonary arterial hypertension in advanced idiopathic pulmonary fibrosis. Chest. 2006;129(3):746–52.

152. Zisman DA, Ross DJ, Belperio JA, Saggar R, Lynch 3rd JP, Ardehali A, et al. Prediction of pulmonary hypertension in idiopathic pulmonary fibrosis. Respir Med. 2007;101(10):2153–9.

153. Shorr AF, Wainright JL, Cors CS, Lettieri CJ, Nathan SD. Pulmonary hypertension in patients with pulmonary fibrosis awaiting lung transplant. Eur Respir J. 2007;30(4):715–21.

154. Nadrous HF, Pellikka PA, Krowka MJ, Swanson KL, Chaowalit N, Decker PA, et al. Pulmonary hypertension in patients with idiopathic pulmonary fibrosis. Chest. 2005;128(4):2393–9.

155. Hamada K, Nagai S, Tanaka S, Handa T, Shigematsu M, Nagao T, et al. Significance of pulmonary arterial pressure and diffusion capacity of the lung as prognosticator in patients with idiopathic pulmonary fibrosis. Chest. 2007;131(3):650–6.

156. Weitzenblum E, Hirth C, Ducolone A, Mirhom R, Rasaholinjanahary J, Ehrhart M. Prognostic value of pulmonary artery pressure in chronic obstructive pulmonary disease. Thorax. 1981;36(10):752–8.

157. Traver GA, Cline MG, Burrows B. Predictors of mortality in chronic obstructive pulmonary disease. A 15-year follow-up study. Am Rev Respir Dis. 1979;119(6):895–902.

158. Oswald-Mammosser M, Weitzenblum E, Quoix E, Moser G, Chaouat A, Charpentier C, et al. Prognostic factors in COPD patients receiving long-term oxygen therapy. Importance of pulmonary artery pressure. Chest. 1995;107(5):1193–8.

159. Cottin V, Nunes H, Brillet PY, Delaval P, Devouassoux G, Tillie-Leblond I, et al. Combined pulmonary fibrosis and emphysema: a distinct underrecognised entity. Eur Respir J. 2005;26(4):586–93.

160. Kessler R, Faller M, Fourgaut G, Mennecier B, Weitzenblum E. Predictive factors of hospitalization for acute exacerbation in a series of 64 patients with chronic obstructive pulmonary disease. Am J Respir Crit Care Med. 1999;159(1):158–64.

161. Wells JM, Washko GR, Han MK, Abbas N, Nath H, Mamary AJ, et al. Pulmonary arterial enlargement and acute exacerbations of COPD. N Engl J Med. 2012;367(10):913–21.

162. Atwood Jr CW, McCrory D, Garcia JG, Abman SH, Ahearn GS, American College of Chest P. Pulmonary artery hypertension and sleep-disordered breathing: ACCP evidence-based clinical practice guidelines. Chest. 2004;126(1 Suppl):72S–7.

163. Penaloza D, Arias-Stella J. The heart and pulmonary circulation at high altitudes: healthy highlanders and chronic mountain sickness. Circulation. 2007;115(9):1132–46.

164. Xu XQ, Jing ZC. High-altitude pulmonary hypertension. Eur Respir Rev. 2009;18(111):13–7.

165. Kim NH, Delcroix M, Jenkins DP, Channick R, Dartevelle P, Jansa P, et al. Chronic thromboembolic pulmonary hypertension. J Am Coll Cardiol. 2013;62(25 Suppl):024.

166. Condliffe R, Kiely DG, Gibbs JS, Corris PA, Peacock AJ, Jenkins DP, et al. Prognostic and aetiological factors in chronic thromboembolic pulmonary hypertension. Eur Respir J. 2009;33(2):332–8.

167. Fedullo PF, Auger WR, Kerr KM, Rubin LJ. Chronic thromboembolic pulmonary hypertension. N Engl J Med. 2001;345(20):1465–72.

168. Morris TA, Marsh JJ, Chiles PG, Auger WR, Fedullo PF, Woods Jr VL. Fibrin derived from patients with chronic thromboembolic pulmonary hypertension is resistant to lysis. Am J Respir Crit Care Med. 2006;173(11):1270–5.

169. Egermayer P, Peacock AJ. Is pulmonary embolism a common cause of chronic pulmonary hypertension? Limitations of the embolic hypothesis. Eur Respir J. 2000;15(3):440–8.

170. Pengo V, Lensing AW, Prins MH, Marchiori A, Davidson BL, Tiozzo F, et al. Incidence of chronic thromboembolic pulmonary hypertension after pulmonary embolism. N Engl J Med. 2004;350(22):2257–64.

171. Becattini C, Agnelli G, Pesavento R, Silingardi M, Poggio R, Taliani MR, et al. Incidence of chronic thromboembolic pulmonary hypertension after a first episode of pulmonary embolism. Chest. 2006;130(1):172–5.

172. Dentali F, Donadini M, Gianni M, Bertolini A, Squizzato A, Venco A, et al. Incidence of chronic pulmonary hypertension in patients with previous pulmonary embolism. Thromb Res. 2009;124(3):256–8.

173. Klok FA, van Kralingen KW, van Dijk AP, Heyning FH, Vliegen HW, Huisman MV. Prospective cardiopulmonary screening program to detect chronic thromboembolic pulmonary hypertension in patients after acute pulmonary embolism. Haematologica. 2010;95(6):970–5.

174. Bonderman D, Wilkens H, Wakounig S, Schafers HJ, Jansa P, Lindner J, et al. Risk factors for chronic thromboembolic pulmonary hypertension. Eur Respir J. 2009;33(2):325–31.

175. Bonderman D, Turecek PL, Jakowitsch J, Weltermann A, Adlbrecht C, Schneider B, et al. High prevalence of elevated clotting factor VIII in chronic thromboembolic pulmonary hypertension. Thromb Haemost. 2003;90(3):372–6.

176. Auger WR, Permpikul P, Moser KM. Lupus anticoagulant, heparin use, and thrombocytopenia in patients with chronic thromboembolic pulmonary hypertension: a preliminary report. Am J Med. 1995;99(4):392–6.

177. Wolf M, Boyer-Neumann C, Parent F, Eschwege V, Jaillet H, Meyer D, et al. Thrombotic risk factors in pulmonary hypertension. Eur Respir J. 2000;15(2):395–9.

178. Lahm T, Chakinala MM. World Health Organization group 5 pulmonary hypertension. Clin Chest Med. 2013;34(4):753–78.

179. Adir Y, Humbert M. Pulmonary hypertension in patients with chronic myeloproliferative disorders. Eur Respir J. 2010;35(6):1396–406.

180. Reisner SA, Rinkevich D, Markiewicz W, Tatarsky I, Brenner B. Cardiac involvement in patients with myeloproliferative disorders. Am J Med. 1992;93(5):498–504.

181. Garypidou V, Vakalopoulou S, Dimitriadis D, Tziomalos K, Sfikas G, Perifanis V. Incidence of pulmonary hypertension in patients with chronic myeloproliferative disorders. Haematologica. 2004;89(2):245–6.

182. Altintas A, Karahan Z, Pasa S, Cil T, Boyraz T, Iltumur K, et al. Pulmonary hypertension in patients with essential thrombocythemia and reactive thrombocytosis. Leuk Lymphoma. 2007;48(10):1981–7.

183. Gupta R, Perumandla S, Patsiornik Y, Niranjan S, Ohri A. Incidence of pulmonary hypertension in patients with chronic myeloproliferative disorders. J Natl Med Assoc. 2006;98(11):1779–82.

184. Cortelezzi A, Gritti G, Del Papa N, Pasquini MC, Calori R, Gianelli U, et al. Pulmonary arterial hypertension in primary myelofibrosis is common and associated with an altered angiogenic status. Leukemia. 2008;22(3):646–9.

185. Willems E, Canivet JL, Ghaye B, de Leval L, Radermecker M, Preiser JC, et al. Pulmonary veno-occlusive disease in myeloproliferative disorder. Eur Respir J. 2009;33(1):213–6.

186. Hennigs JK, Keller G, Baumann HJ, Honecker F, Kluge S, Bokemeyer C, et al. Multi tyrosine kinase inhibitor dasatinib as novel cause of severe pre-capillary pulmonary hypertension? BMC Pulm Med. 2011;11:30.

187. Jais X, Ioos V, Jardim C, Sitbon O, Parent F, Hamid A, et al. Splenectomy and chronic thromboembolic pulmonary hypertension. Thorax. 2005;60(12):1031–4.

188. Hoeper MM, Niedermeyer J, Hoffmeyer F, Flemming P, Fabel H. Pulmonary hypertension after splenectomy? Ann Intern Med. 1999;130(6):506–9.

189. Frey MK, Alias S, Winter MP, Redwan B, Stubiger G, Panzenboeck A, et al. Splenectomy is modifying the vascular remodeling of thrombosis. J Am Heart Assoc. 2014;3(1), e000772.

190. Mehari A, Gladwin MT, Tian X, Machado RF, Kato GJ. Mortality in adults with sickle cell disease and pulmonary hypertension. JAMA. 2012;307(12):1254–6.

191. Fonseca GH, Souza R, Salemi VM, Jardim CV, Gualandro SF. Pulmonary hypertension diagnosed by right heart catheterisation in sickle cell disease. Eur Respir J. 2012;39(1):112–8.

192. Gladwin MT, Sachdev V, Jison ML, Shizukuda Y, Plehn JF, Minter K, et al. Pulmonary hypertension as a risk factor for death in patients with sickle cell disease. N Engl J Med. 2004;350(9):886–95.

193. Yawn BP, Buchanan GR, Afenyi-Annan AN, Ballas SK, Hassell KL, James AH, et al. Management of sickle cell disease: summary of the 2014 evidence-based report by expert panel members. JAMA. 2014;312(10):1033–48.

194. Machado RF, Barst RJ, Yovetich NA, Hassell KL, Kato GJ, Gordeuk VR, et al. Hospitalization for pain in patients with sickle cell disease treated with sildenafil for elevated TRV and low exercise capacity. Blood. 2011;118(4):855–64.

195. Handa T, Nagai S, Miki S, Fushimi Y, Ohta K, Mishima M, et al. Incidence of pulmonary hypertension and its clinical relevance in patients with sarcoidosis. Chest. 2006;129(5):1246–52.

196. Bourbonnais JM, Samavati L. Clinical predictors of pulmonary hypertension in sarcoidosis. Eur Respir J. 2008;32(2):296–302.

197. Chaowalit N, Pellikka PA, Decker PA, Aubry MC, Krowka MJ, Ryu JH, et al. Echocardiographic and clinical characteristics of pulmonary hypertension complicating pulmonary Langerhans cell histiocytosis. Mayo Clin Proc. 2004;79(10):1269–75.

198. Cottin V, Harari S, Humbert M, Mal H, Dorfmuller P, Jais X, et al. Pulmonary hypertension in lymphangioleiomyomatosis: characteristics in 20 patients. Eur Respir J. 2012;40(3):630–40.

199. Shorr AF, Helman DL, Davies DB, Nathan SD. Pulmonary hypertension in advanced sarcoidosis: epidemiology and clinical characteristics. Eur Respir J. 2005;25(5):783–8.

200. Milman N, Burton CM, Iversen M, Videbaek R, Jensen CV, Carlsen J. Pulmonary hypertension in end-stage pulmonary sarcoidosis: therapeutic effect of sildenafil? J Heart Lung Transplant. 2008;27(3):329–34.

201. Fartoukh M, Humbert M, Capron F, Maitre S, Parent F, Le Gall C, et al. Severe pulmonary hypertension in histiocytosis X. Am J Respir Crit Care Med. 2000;161(1):216–23.

202. Dauriat G, Mal H, Thabut G, Mornex JF, Bertocchi M, Tronc F, et al. Lung transplantation for pulmonary langerhans' cell histiocytosis: a multicenter analysis. Transplantation. 2006;81(5):746–50.

203. Reynaud-Gaubert M, Mornex JF, Mal H, Treilhaud M, Dromer C, Quetant S, et al. Lung transplantation for lymphangioleiomyomatosis: the French experience. Transplantation. 2008;86(4): 515–20.

204. Issa N, Krowka MJ, Griffin MD, Hickson LJ, Stegall MD, Cosio FG. Pulmonary hypertension is associated with reduced patient survival after kidney transplantation. Transplantation. 2008;86(10):1384–8.

205. Abassi Z, Nakhoul F, Khankin E, Reisner SA, Yigla M. Pulmonary hypertension in chronic dialysis patients with arteriovenous fistula: pathogenesis and therapeutic prospective. Curr Opin Nephrol Hypertens. 2006;15(4):353–60.

206. Tarrass F, Benjelloun M, Medkouri G, Hachim K, Benghanem MG, Ramdani B. Doppler echocardiograph evaluation of pulmonary hypertension in patients undergoing hemodialysis. Hemodial Int. 2006;10(4):356–9.

207. Havlucu Y, Kursat S, Ekmekci C, Celik P, Serter S, Bayturan O, et al. Pulmonary hypertension in patients with chronic renal failure. Respiration. 2007;74(5):503–10.

208. Abdelwhab S, Elshinnawy S. Pulmonary hypertension in chronic renal failure patients. Am J Nephrol. 2008;28(6):990–7.

209. Kumbar L, Fein PA, Rafiq MA, Borawski C, Chattopadhyay J, Avram MM. Pulmonary hypertension in peritoneal dialysis patients. Adv Perit Dial. 2007;23:127–31. Conference on Peritoneal Dialysis.

210. Bozbas SS, Akcay S, Altin C, Bozbas H, Karacaglar E, Kanyilmaz S, et al. Pulmonary hypertension in patients with end-stage renal disease undergoing renal transplantation. Transplant Proc. 2009;41(7):2753–6.

The Effects of Chronic Hypoxia on Inflammation and Pulmonary Vascular Function

Kurt R. Stenmark, Steven C. Pugliese, Jens Poth,
Maria G. Frid, Evgenia Gerasimovskaya, Eva Nozik-Grayck,
and Karim C. El Kasmi

Introduction

Inflammation is increasingly recognized as an important pathogenetic element in PH [1–4]. Expanding on initial observations of accumulation of inflammatory cells in PH, it has recently been documented by members of our investigative team that the amount of perivascular inflammatory infiltrate correlates with parameters of vascular remodeling and hemodynamics in PH [5–8]. Thus, it is increasingly clear that early (animal models) and persistent inflammation (animals and humans) is present and contributes to pulmonary vascular disease [3, 9]. Importantly, inflammatory cell infiltrates in nearly all experimental animal models of PH and human PH are largely adventitial and/or perivascular in nature [9–12]. Accordingly, these and other observations support a paradigm of vascular inflammation in which cells in the adventitia form a suitable niche to promote inflammation, which progresses inward toward the media and intima [9, 12–15]. In support of this so called "outside-in" hypothesis of adventitial regulation of inflammation are observations that in a wide variety of vascular injuries, notably those associated with PH, there is a rapid influx of leukocytes into the adventitial compartment [10, 16]. Both adventitial fibroblasts and recruited macrophages, in response to a variety of stimuli (including hypoxia, cytokines, and vascular injury)

activate, in a time-dependent and pulmonary artery specific manner, expression of cytokines and chemokines, their receptors and adhesion molecules making it possible for these cells to initiate and perpetuate inflammatory responses in an "outside-in" fashion. Studies have also demonstrated that abrogating mononuclear phagocyte accumulation in the vessel wall completely attenuated the pulmonary vascular remodeling process [16, 17]. These observations therefore support the idea that temporal/spatial dysregulation and/or failure of the normal switch-off signal in resident vascular cells and/or macrophages may directly contribute to the persistence of a chronic inflammatory immune response and ultimately to vascular remodeling.

It has been proposed that a positive feedback loop between the resident stromal/mesenchymal cells and resident/infiltrating macrophages is a key candidate mechanism for persistence of inflammation in a variety of diseases ranging from cancer to PH [18–21]. Moreover, growing evidence has indicated that epigenetic marks may "lock" innate immune cells into distinct functional phenotypes with loss of functional plasticity and failure to respond to regulatory signals. The inflammatory microenvironment in the pulmonary vascular circulation could therefore promote epigenetic marks in fibroblasts and macrophages, locking their functional phenotype into a pro-fibrogenic and pro-remodeling phenotypes [22–26]. Different signaling processes mediated largely by STAT1, STAT3, and STAT6 may drive macrophage gene expression patterns that promote remodeling [27].

The focus of this review will be specifically on the cellular and molecular mechanisms leading to the development of inflammation and pulmonary vascular remodeling in the context of hypoxia and chronic lung disease herein known as hypoxic PH or World Health Organization (WHO) Group 3 PH. While we focus on mesenchymal-macrophage interactions, which occur during the development of PH, our primary goal is to elucidate new concepts involving the intertwining roles of hypoxia, inflammation, and their effects on recruited immune and progenitor cells in the setting of hypoxic PH. It is our belief that a better understanding of

K.R. Stenmark, MD (✉) • J. Poth, MD, PhD • M.G. Frid, PhD
E. Gerasimovskaya, PhD • E. Nozik-Grayck, MD
Department of Pediatrics, University of Colorado Denver,
12700 E.19th Ave, Research 2, Box B131, Aurora,
CO 80045, USA
e-mail: kurt.stenmark@ucdenver.edu

S.C. Pugliese, MD
Division of Pulmonary Sciences and Critical Care Medicine,
Department of Medicine, University of Colorado Denver,
Aurora, CO, USA

K.C. El Kasmi, MD, PhD
Department of Pediatrics, Children's Hospital Colorado,
Aurora, CO, USA

© Springer International Publishing Switzerland 2016
B.A. Maron et al. (eds.), *Pulmonary Hypertension: Basic Science to Clinical Medicine*, DOI 10.1007/978-3-319-23594-3_5

disease mechanisms in hypoxia-related lung diseases will lead to improved targeted therapies at least for patients with WHO Group 3 PH.

The Effect of Acute and Chronic Hypoxia on the Inflammatory Status of Resident Pulmonary Vascular Cells

In an effort to better understand the pathophysiologic mechanisms involved in forms of PH related to lung disease and/or global hypoxia (WHO Group 3 PH), several animal models have been used; namely the hypoxic mouse, rat, calf, lamb, and pig models [9, 28]. While there are differences between humans with Group 3 PH and animal models, several key conserved pathologic features exist that characterize the changes observed in the three compartments of the vascular wall (intima, media, adventitia) and their respective resident cells (endothelial, smooth muscle, and fibroblasts). It should be noted that the degree of pulmonary vascular remodeling in response to hypoxia increases with phylogenic order of species (cow > rat > mouse) and directly correlates to the amount of perivascular inflammation [12]. We discuss below the effects of chronic hypoxia on the pathology of the vascular wall as well as on resident cells both in vivo and in vitro and underscore the importance of these cells with respect to the initiation and perpetuation of remodeling and inflammation.

The Intima: Endothelial Cells

Hypoxia has significant effects on the regulation of synthesis and secretion of vasoactive factors and inflammatory cytokines in PAECs. Hypoxia causes PAECs to induce a vasoconstrictive environment through decreased production and/ or activity of prostacyclin and nitric oxide (NO) as well as increased production of endothelin, serotonin, leukotrienes, and other mediators [29–35]. In vitro studies also demonstrate that exposure of PAECs to hypoxia causes the synthesis and release of pro-inflammatory (IL1, IL6, IL8), pro-mitogenic (VEGF-1, endothelin-1, thromboxane, PDGF-B, CX3CL1) and anti-thrombic mediators, (increased tissue factor, decreased thrombomodulin) as well as increased expression of inflammatory cell adhesion molecules (VCAM, ICAM, P-selectin) [29, 36–40]. These findings support a PAEC contribution to the observation that hypoxic forms of PH have a consistent and important inflammatory component and that the endothelium likely plays a role. However, they do not fully explain the observations that inflammatory cells aggregate mostly in the adventitia of chronically hypoxic animals [9, 10, 12, 13, 16, 25]. It is possible that ECs of the vasa vasorum exhibit specific upregulation of

adhesion molecules and cytokines that could facilitate it acting as a conduit for leukocyte delivery to the hypoxic vessel. This possibly should be explored as emerging evidence points to distinct EC-inflammatory cell interactions in EC's of different organs [41, 42]. The role of the vasa in hypoxia-induced pulmonary vascular remodeling and inflammation is discussed in detail below.

The Media: Smooth Muscle Cells

The sine qua non of vessel remodeling in hypoxic PH is thickening of the media at all levels of the pulmonary arterial bed and the appearance of cells expressing alpha-smooth muscle actin (α-SMA) in partially muscular or non-muscular small pulmonary arteries. Because the small pulmonary arteries account for the majority of total cross sectional area in the pulmonary vascular bed, it is these changes in the distal pulmonary arteries that account for the greatest changes in pulmonary vascular resistance [8, 43–46]. The thickening of muscular and large elastic vessels can include both hyperplastic and hyperproliferative responses as well changes as changes in extracellular matrix composition. These changes likely contribute to decreases in compliance of the large vessels, a functional change increasingly thought to be important in PH disease progression [47].

The data regarding SMC proliferation under hypoxic conditions has recently been extensively reviewed [48]. To summarize, there is evidence of a modest increase in SMC proliferation in rodents and large animals in response to chronic hypoxia. In vivo studies in large animal models suggest that there are subsets of undifferentiated resident cells with high proliferative potential in proximal PAs and undifferentiated resident and perhaps non-resident cells in distal PAs that proliferate in response to hypoxia. Regarding in vitro studies, our work in large animal models demonstrate that in proximal PAs there are different SMC populations, with a continuum of proliferative potential whereby the least differentiated cells have the highest proliferative potential. In SMCs isolated from distal PAs of normal animals, there exists a uniform population of well differentiated non proliferative cells, while a second population of highly proliferative non resident cells can be isolated from hypoxic animals. Regarding the vast literature of whether SMCs proliferate in response to hypoxia in vitro, it becomes nearly impossible to be concrete in the answer to this question. This is because the differences in any of the following factors can influence the results of the experiment: species, location of PA from which cells are isolated, cell population within specific location of PA used, severity of hypoxia, seeding density, presence or absence of co-mitogens (e.g. presence of serum or even low concentrations of growth factors), and duration of hypoxia [49]. A review by Pak et al notes conflicting reports on 16 studies that try to answer this very question and elucidates how each of these conditions can alter the results of the experiment [49]. While SMC proliferation cannot be studied in vivo in humans, more recent work has demonstrated distal well- differentiated PASMCs, characterized by α-SMA and SMMHC expression, isolated from humans with PAH appear to be hyperproliferative at baseline compared to SMCs from control patients [50]. Questions remain regarding whether in vitro culture selects for a subset of cells that are hyperproliferative and may only represent a small number of cells in vivo. Nonetheless, this data suggests that there are important differences between SMCs isolated from hypoxic animal models and humans with PAH with regard to their ability to proliferate without exogenous growth factors and mitogens.

Medial smooth muscle cells may also have important functions with regard to recruitment of circulating inflammatory and progenitor cells as well as in the activation of resident progenitor cells. Horita et al reported mice with an inducible smooth muscle-specific PTEN deletion develop severe PH with intimal obliteration after 4 weeks of chronic hypoxia [51]. Furthermore, there was increased whole lung expression of inflammatory mediators (SDF-1, IL6) and increased perivascular macrophage recruitment. Interestingly, hypoxia induced perivascular proliferation in the SMC-specific PTEN knockout mice was most dramatically increased in α-SMA negative cells. While the authors show decreased PASMC PTEN expression in patients with IPAH, we do not know whether this leads to increased perivascular inflammation in humans, especially in those with hypoxic PH. It is therefore possible that in patients with hypoxic PH, the combination of hypoxia plus a second hit (PTEN deletion) can transform resident SMC's into cells that are capable of inflammatory cell recruitment, local endothelial cell proliferation and proliferation and migration to distal previously non-muscularized vessels. Also of possible relevance are studies showing that decreases in myocardin related transcription factor-A (MRTF-A) in SMCs, which can occur when BMPR2 signaling is impaired as has been reported to occur in response to chronic hypoxia, may lead to a pro-inflammatory SMC [52, 53].

Interestingly, MRTF-A inhibits RelA/p65 in a BMP-dependent manner [53]. Similarly Yeager et al has shown that endothelin-1 (ET-1)-stimulated pulmonary artery SMCs, via the unfolded protein response, release pro-inflammatory and chemotactic mediators [54]. While this experiment was not performed in a hypoxic model of PH, given local endothelin-1 production in response to hypoxia by endothelial cells, this process likely occurs in hypoxic models of PH as well. There is evidence that hypoxia induces PASMC ET-1 in a HIF1 dependent manner which induces a feed forward loop whereby ET-1 further stimulates HIF1α protein and HIF1 gene expression [55]. On the other hand, at least in hypoxic animal models, there is evidence that recruited pro-inflammatory cells exert mitogenic effects on medial pulmonary artery SMCs in vitro [56, 57]. These data above raise the possibility that resident SMCs have the potential to induce a feed-forward loop whereby they induce a pro-inflammatory and pro-mitogenic environment and in turn respond with increased proliferation.

The Adventitia: Resident Fibroblasts and Immune Cells

The outermost portion of the vessel wall, the adventitia, serves the vessel as an extracellular matrix (ECM) scaffold that contains conduits for nutrient supply and removal, that is the vasa vasorum, lymphatic vessels and trophic nerves, as well as resident cells such as fibroblasts, progenitor cells, immune cells (macrophages and dendritic cells). Due to this cellular and structural complexity the adventitia is the most heterogeneous compartment of the vessel wall. In response to hypoxia in humans and in animal models of PH, the adventitia undergoes substantial thickening due to a significant increase in collagen and ECM protein deposition, marked expansion of the vasa vasorum, proliferation of resident fibroblasts and possibly macrophages, activation of resident progenitor cells, as well as recruitment of circulating immune and progenitor cells [12]. Accumulating experimental data suggest that, in response to vascular stresses, including hypoxia and over-distention, the resident adventitial fibroblast, in the function of a sentinel cell, is the first to become activated and to respond through proliferation, upregulation of contractile and extracellular matrix proteins, and to release factors that can directly affect medial SMC tone and growth as well as stimulate the recruitment of inflammatory and progenitor cells [25, 58, 59]. This has led to the idea that as opposed to the usual paradigm of inflammation and remodeling being driven from the inside-out that an alternative paradigm of an "outside-in" hypothesis, in which vascular inflammation is initiated in the adventitia and progresses inward toward the media and intima driving with it the remodeling process [12, 13, 15]. In support of the "outside-in" hypothesis of adventitial regulation of inflammation are observations that, in a wide variety of vascular injuries, there is a rapid influx of leukocytes into the adventitial compartment [14, 60–63]. In experimental models of PH, both chronic hypoxic exposure and monocrotaline treatment lead to the early appearance and persistence of inflammatory/progenitor cells in the adventitia of both large and small pulmonary arteries, followed by prominent vascular remodeling [9, 11, 16, 25, 64–66]. Studies in the hypoxic pulmonary circulation have demonstrated a complex, time-dependent and pulmonary artery-specific upregulation of several cytokines/chemokines, their receptors, and adhesion molecules, which appear to be produced/expressed by adventitial fibroblasts and recruited monocytes, and are likely involved in the initiation and perpetuation of the inflammatory response in a "outside-in" fashion [10, 11, 67].

The adventitia can therefore be regarded as playing a critical role in initial steps of the pathogenesis of vascular inflammation and remodeling [63]. The adventitia comprises canonical innate immune cells, specifically macrophages and dendritic cells (DCs), but also cells that have only recently been regarded capable of exerting immune functions, such as the adventitial fibroblast [25]. Macrophages and DCs are diffusely scattered in the pulmonary arteries of man and animals [10, 68]. Increases in their numbers are observed in Pulmonary Arteries (PA) in the setting of PH raising the possibility for a role in perpetuating inflammation just as in the systemic circulation [10, 68]. Additionally, in a variety of pathological conditions such as asthma [69], COPD [70], and PH [3, 4, 7], DCs demonstrate a marked proclivity to reside in the adventitia, likely modulating inflammatory, immunological, and vascular cell proliferative processes. The presence of dendritic cells (DCs) in the lung has been known for over 25 years [71]. The principal job of pulmonary DCs is to encounter putative self and non-self/environmental antigens, primarily at epithelial surfaces, and coordinate appropriate innate and acquired immunity responses [72]. Circulating or tissue-resident, DCs are normally immature until triggered by a multitude of signals, including ingestion of apoptotic cells, to express DC-SIGN, CD83, and additional markers of maturation [73].

Macrophages, DCs, and adventitial fibroblasts are all equipped with the necessary machinery, (e.g. toll-like receptors [TLRs], inflammasome components [NLRs], to potently respond to a variety of exogenous and endogenous danger signals. Such activation results in generation of a host of cytokines, chemokines, as well as mediators of oxidative stress (ROS, NOS) and tissue remodeling (TIMPS, MMPs) by macrophages/DCs and also fibroblasts [25, 74–76]. Interestingly, the pattern of expression of TLRs appears to be vessel specific, which contributes to vessel-specific risk for inflammatory vasculopathies [77]. Monocytes/macrophages and classical and plasmacytoid DCs originate from hematopoietic stem cells and are replaced continually from a common macrophage and DC precursor [78, 79]. It has now become evident that certain tissue resident macrophages such as liver Kupffer cells, epidermal Langerhans cells, microglia, and pleural macrophages are able to proliferate and renew independently from the bone marrow. These cells represent a lineage of tissue macrophages that derive from the yolk sac and are genetically distinct from bone marrow derived macrophages [79]. Therefore, certain populations of tissue resident macrophages and DCs may be present in the adventitia and may constitute a distinct population with the ability to self renew and to exert distinct functional phenotypes. Functional plasticity and diversity is increasingly recognized to be an essential feature of the mononuclear phagocyte system and may be regarded a condition sine qua non for the coordinated initiation, propagation and resolution of local immune responses [74, 80, 81]. A diverse set of macrophage functional phenotypes has thus been demonstrated to be involved in a wide variety of pathologies: macrophages can promote or resolve fibrosis, promote insulin resistance and obesity, are essential in thermoregulation through generation of catecholamines, are essential for wound healing, can promote and restrict T cell responses, promote angiogenesis, promote or suppress tumor growth, fight pathogens, and control homeostasis in local immune networks such as the gut [22, 74, 80–84].

One recently discussed idea is that macrophages and DCs, based on the fact that no surface or functional marker definitively distinguishes macrophages from dendritic cells, do not represent separate entities but rather two extremes of regulated functional activation states on a continuum of a yet unknown number of functional activities [85]. Chief among these are the capability of macrophages to mount strong pro-inflammatory cytokine responses (initiating innate immune responses) and DCs to be strong antigen presenters and inducers of T cell responses (initiating adaptive immune response). However, as pointed out, both cell types can perform both functions in response to adequate stimulation [85].

For a long period of time, fibroblast activation was regarded as relatively insignificant in regulating immune responses and focus was placed primarily on immune interactions between lymphocytes, macrophages and dendritic cells. It is now becoming clear that many danger signals are not antigen-specific, and, currently, focus is shifting toward an extended immune system in which fibroblasts play an important role in innate immune responses. Importantly, there is convincing evidence that fibroblasts taken from diseased tissue display a fundamentally different phenotype compared with fibroblasts taken from normal tissues at the same anatomical site [20, 25, 26, 86, 87].

The activated adventitial fibroblast appears to exert a functional plasticity reminiscent of that of macrophages/DCs in that they have been shown to express a combination of functional phenotypes including generation of pro-inflammatory cytokines and molecules necessary for antigen presentation and T-cell stimulation [25]. This functional plasticity of the activated adventitial fibroblast may therefore play a key role in initiating and propagating adventitial inflammation through generation of numerous cytokines and chemokines that create a microenvironment tailored to fine-tuning the activation of tissue resident macrophages and DCs as well as promoting recruitment of blood derived inflammatory monocytes [15, 25].

Therefore, in inflammatory responses in the adventitia of the PA, macrophage, DC and fibroblast activation can be fine-tuned over a large scale of functional phenotypes, including switching from pro-inflammatory to pro-fibrotic or pro-resolving functional phenotypes or complete deactivation. In the absence of a specific antigen, as could be the case in initiating stages of hypoxia induced or idiopathic PH initially a functional phenotype characterized by generation of pro-inflammatory mediators may be displayed by macrophages, DCs and fibroblasts. Over time this phenotype maybe fine-tuned toward generation of pro-remodeling and pro-fibrogenic mediators generated by macrophages and fibroblasts. In contrast, in the presence of specific antigen, an antigen processing and T cell activating functional phenotype (dendritic cell phenotype) may prevail [15, 22, 23, 74, 80, 81].

Importantly, there is growing evidence that epigenetic marks may "lock" innate immune cells into a distinct functional phenotype, which may result in loss of functional plasticity and failure to respond to regulatory signals, such that adventitial fibroblasts retain a pro-inflammatory phenotype driving recruitment of inflammatory monocytes and DC precursors and promoting epigenetic marks in macrophages locking their functional phenotype into a pro-fibrogenic and pro-remodeling macrophage [22–24, 88, 89]. The molecular basis for this persistently activated fibroblast phenotype at sites of chronic inflammation remains unclear, although findings suggest that NF-κB signaling pathway plays a critical role in perpetuating chronic persistent inflammatory responses [90, 91]. Therefore, temporal-spatial dysregulation and/or failure in the normal "switch-off signal" in fibroblasts and/or macrophages/DCs may directly contribute to the persistence of a chronic inflammatory immune response.

The transition to a chronic inflammatory phenotype also requires changes in the adhesion molecule and chemokine receptor expression on fibroblasts and recruited hematopoetic cells respectively. Fibroblasts express and upregulate adhesion molecules, including ICAM-1 and VCAM-1 that cause adhesion of leukocytes in response to a variety of stimuli. Secretion of cytokines, including Transforming growth factor-β (TGF-β), by the activated fibroblast cause activation and upregulation of receptors such as CXCR4 on newly recruited hematopoetic cells, as well as secretion of SDF-1, the cognate ligand for CXCR4 [92]. Thus, an environment is created in chronically inflamed tissues, whereby the adventitia acts as a "foster home" for leukocytes leading to their inappropriate/pathologic retention and survival [90].

Cell and Molecular Mechanisms Involved in Hypoxia-Induced Vascular Remodeling

Alveolar Macrophages

In rodent and large animal models of PH, acute exposure to hypoxia leads to increased expression of inflammatory mediators and increased numbers of inflammatory cells in both the alveolar space and around the pulmonary artery [10, 93–95]. Mice exposed to acute hypoxia (8–10 % FIO_2) show increased expression of MCP1, macrophage inflammatory protein (MIP)-2, IL1a, and IL6 in whole lung [93]. Similarly, in rats exposed to acute hypoxia, there are increased numbers of alveolar macrophages and inflammatory mediators including HIF1 in bronchoalveolar lavage (BAL) fluid [96]. Importantly, depletion of alveolar macrophages using clodronate liposomes attenuates alveolar inflammation suggesting a role in either the initiation or maintenance of hypoxia-induced inflammation [96]. Wood and Gonzalez have elegantly described the role of alveolar macrophages as hypoxia sensors that secrete MCP1 and induce both local (alveolar compartment) and systemic inflammation in the mesentery and skeletal muscle through local mast cell degranulation [97]. In hypoxic rats, by artificially maintaining normoxia in the mesentery and skeletal muscle (while the alveolar compartment is hypoxic), they demonstrate these effects are mediated through MCP1 and not regional hypoxemia. While they did not determine the effect on mast cells in the pulmonary vasculature, many other groups have confirmed the importance of mast cells in hypoxic PH, IPAH, and other forms of PH [98–102].

Unfortunately, in the aforementioned experiments [96], the effect of alveolar macrophage depletion on hypoxia-induced PH was not examined and thus the role of alveolar macrophages in the pathogenesis of hypoxic PH remains unclear. However, Vergadi et al showed that early recruitment and alternative activation of alveolar macrophages is important for the later development of hypoxic PH [57]. Furthermore, soluble factors generated by alveolar macrophages were able to induce smooth muscle proliferation in vitro [57]. Finally, transgenic and inducible overexpression of lung specific heme oxygenase (HO)-1, an anti-inflammatory mediator, resulted in down regulation of alveolar compartment inflammatory cytokines, and conversion of the alternatively activated macrophage phenotype into anti-inflammatory IL-10 producing phenotype [57]. These studies suggest that HO-1 plays a critical role in regulating cellular phenotypes. Inflammatory cytokines/mediators, including leukotrienes in the alveolar compartment have also been reported in the monocrotaline rat model of PH and in infants with persistent PH of the newborn [103–105]. These studies suggest that the alveolar macrophage and mediators derived thereof affect cellular phenotypes in the pulmonary vascular wall thorough paracrine signaling pathways.

Resident and Recruited Perivascular Macrophages

The role of resident and recruited perivascular macrophages in shaping pulmonary vascular remodeling also remains largely unknown. Due to the inherent difficulty associated with isolating perivascular macrophages, very little is known regarding the importance of these cells in hypoxic PH. However, recent work supports the hypothesis that resident tissue macrophages play important roles in maintaining tissue homeostasis by communicating with the local parenchymal and non-parenchymal cells (i.e. "client" cells) [106]. It is believed that under tissue stress, resident macrophages instruct their client cells to mount an appropriate response, including the recruitment of blood monocytes to complement the resident macrophage pool (e.g. recruitment of CCR2+ cells) [106]. Recruitment of CCR2+ inflammatory macrophages has been shown to be critical in a wide variety of acute and chronic inflammatory disease models [107–110]. Consistent with this hypothesis, Frid et al, have demonstrated that ablation of circulating blood monocytes in a rat model of hypoxic PH prevented both remodeling and PH [16]. It can be hypothesized further that 'client cells' play a critical role in providing turn off signals to both resident and recruited macrophages and resident cells, like fibroblasts, in order to promote resolution of inflammation. Thus, intricate cross-talk between resident and recruited macrophages with their client cells is key in maintaining tissue homeostasis, coordinating an appropriate inflammatory response tailored to the inciting noxious agent and finally providing signals that allow for resolution when the inflammatory trigger has been removed. Malfunctioning of this cross-talk is thus hypothesized to result in aberrant permanent activation of macrophages and "client cells" with subsequent progression to chronic non-resolving inflammation as the driver of pathologic tissue remodeling. Consistent with this hypothesis, El Kasmi et al recently published that activated adventitial fibroblasts, derived from humans with IPAH and animal models of PH, polarize naïve macrophages via paracrine IL6 and induce a pro-inflammatory, pro-fibrotic phenotype regulated by STAT3-HIF1-C/EBPβ and independent of IL4/IL13-STAT6 signaling [20]. More importantly, this paper brings to light important macrophage signaling pathways (IL6-STAT3-HIF1-C/EBPβ) which have previously been implicated in PH and hypoxia-induced inflammation, and challenge the current paradigm of IL-4/IL-13–STAT6–mediated alternative activation of macrophages hypoxic PH. It should be mentioned that this work was largely done using fibroblasts from a hypoxic calf model of PH and from patients with IPAH, establishing conserved signaling pathways between the two forms of PH. This study also raises important questions about the role of resident macrophages in instructing adventitial fibroblasts (i.e. client cell) into an activated phenotype. Evidence of macrophage stromal cell inflammatory crosstalk has been reported in adipose tissue, cancer, and rheumatoid arthritis [111–113].

In the study mentioned earlier, Vergadi et al show early alveolar macrophage recruitment (day 4) and elevated IL4 and IL13 in BAL fluid in hypoxic mice [57]. This macrophage phenotype was characterized by expression of Arg 1, Fizz1, Ym1 and CD206, canonical IL4/IL13-STAT6 target genes. Overexpression of lung specific HO-1, an anti-inflammatory anti-oxidant enzyme, resulted in attenuation of hypoxic PH, down regulation of inflammatory cytokines, and a change in macrophage phenotype to an "anti-inflammatory" IL-10 producing cell. While this paper supports the role of IL4/IL13 –STAT6 signaling in hypoxic PH, the target genes examined can also be induced by hypoxia/HIF signaling and metabolites involved in aerobic glycolysis such as lactate and thus more rigorous characterization is warranted in future studies to define the functional phenotype of macrophages in mouse models of hypoxic PH [18]. Nevertheless, this work and prior studies by the Kourembanas group highlight the therapeutic potential of HO-1 signaling as a novel anti-inflammatory pathway and specifically in modulating macrophage programming [93, 114].

Molecular Mediators of Hypoxia-Induced Inflammation: RELM

Work from the John's laboratory has implicated hypoxia-induced mitogenic factor (HIMF, also known as FIZZ1 or RELM), a member of the resistin family of proteins, in the pathogenesis of hypoxic PH. They have demonstrated both alveolar epithelium and perivascular expression of HIMF in the hypoxic mouse model of PH [115]. Additionally, RELM-b, the closest human homolog to HIMF, is expressed in the endothelium and vascular smooth muscle of remodeled vessels, as well as in plexiform lesions, macrophages, T cells, and myofibroblast-like cells in humans with scleroderma PH [116]. Because HIMF expression in macrophages has been involved in canonical TH2 responses mediated through IL4 and STAT6, it is noteworthy that HIMF expression in hypoxic mice is not attenuated in IL4 or STAT6 knockout mice. These data suggests that other pathways, such as hypoxia/HIF1 signaling can induce HIMF expression [115]. Interestingly, intravenous injection of HIMF results in PH and pulmonary vascular remodeling in wild type but not IL4 knockout mice mediated, at least in part, by inducing endothelial cell apoptosis [117]. Exactly how IL4 facilitates HIMF induced pulmonary vascular remodeling independent of the canonical IL4-STAT6 pathway remains to be determined. Intriguingly, recent work by Colegio et al shows that tumor-derived lactic acid can lead to FIZZ1 expression in tumor-associated macrophages in a HIF1 dependent and IL4/IL13 independent manner [18]. This work supports the idea that mediators produced downstream of glycolysis, which occurs in hypoxic PH and PAH, are able to directly affect pulmonary vascular remodeling [118].

NF-κB is important in the initiation of inflammation especially with regard to hypoxia, but little is known about NF-κB signaling in macrophages and fibroblasts in hypoxic PH. NF-κB expression is increased in the lungs in animal models of PH, including hypoxic PH, and chemical inhibitors attenuate experimental PH [119–122]. NF-κB is also activated in macrophages, perivascular lymphocytes, smooth muscle cells and endothelial cells the vessel wall of patients with IPAH [123]. Unpublished data from our lab using RNAseq in adventitial fibroblasts from calves with hypoxic PH show the NF-κB pathway to be significantly up-regulated compared to control fibroblasts. This is consistent with increased fibroblast NF-κB signaling in other inflammatory diseases [90, 124]. We have also demonstrated that these fibroblasts produce large amounts of MCP1 and in turn can induce naïve monocytes to produce MCP1 [25]. A similar feed forward loop of human mesenchymal stromal cell (MSC) activation of naïve macrophages that in turn induce MSC migration has previously been described [125]. MCP1 has been shown to induce smooth muscle cell proliferation and increased IL6 production in an NF-κB dependent fashion [126]. We suspect that the NF-κB pathway is necessary for IL6 production in adventitial fibroblasts and is also up-regulated in activated perivascular macrophages in response to paracrine MCP1, although more work is necessary to prove this hypothesis.

While more work needs to be done regarding IL6, STAT3, and HIF1 signaling in macrophage polarization and pulmonary vascular remodeling in PH, numerous recently published papers suggest these pathways are essential for immune cell recruitment, hypoxia-induced inflammation, and chronic non-resolving inflammation in other diseases. Using a wire-induced femoral artery injury model in mice with macrophage-specific deletion (LysMcre) of HIF1α, Nakayama et al found a reduction in vascular remodeling, macrophage recruitment, and perivascular inflammation (IL6, TNF-α) [127]. Fielding et al recently used a mouse model of acute peritoneal inflammation to demonstrate that IL6 was required to switch from acute inflammation to a chronic pro-fibrotic state and the development of peritoneal fibrosis [128]. Lastly, in human rheumatoid arthritis synovial fibroblasts, STAT3 was required for hypoxia-induced inflammation [129]. Although not yet demonstrated in macrophages with regard to inflammation, cooperative signaling between STAT3 and HIF1 modulates hypoxia induced signaling in cancer cells [130]. Future studies need to be designed to dissect and define the role of IL6, STAT3, and HIF1 in regulating the transition from acute to chronic inflammation and promoting "arrest" of vascular cells in a pro-fibrotic phenotype that propagates pulmonary vascular remodeling.

In summary, several signaling pathways (HIF1, IL6-STAT3, NF-κB, HIMF, IL4/IL13-STAT6) with regard to macrophage activation have been implicated in hypoxic PH. We believe that fibroblast-macrophage crosstalk is essential for chronic non-resolving inflammation in hypoxic PH and through epigenetic mechanisms discussed in detail below, involves an epigenetically "locked in" activated mesenchymal cells that stimulate macrophage activation. We acknowledge that macrophages constantly survey local tissue status and alter their phenotype based on the changing tissue microenvironment [131]. Therefore, it is more than likely that an activated pro-inflammatory macrophage phenotype has a reversible transcriptional program that can be transformed into an anti-inflammatory pro-resolution macrophage based on local stimuli. This may have important therapeutic implications in reversing chronic non-resolving inflammatory processes (Fig. 5.1).

Role of Extracellular Purine Nucleotides and Adenosine as Regulators of Pulmonary Arterial Inflammation and Remodeling

Extracellular ATP and other nucleotides (ADP, UTP, UDP) and adenosine have long been known as regulators of vascular function, particularly involved in control of blood flow, vascular cell proliferation, migration, chemotaxis, and inflammatory responses [132–134]. Although extracellular nucleotides are the most ubiquitous, they remain the least investigated endogenous signaling molecules. Evidence is accumulating that vascular EC, as well as smooth muscle, epithelial, hematopoietic and other cells, can release ATP in response to hypoxia, inflammation, fluid shear stress, neurotransmission, and other stress-related stimuli and trigger diverse cell-specific responses through metabotropic (P2Y) and ligand-gated (P2X) receptors [134, 135] Most of these environmental stimuli may play a role in controlling extracellular ATP levels in vascular wall adventitia.

A number of studies support the idea that extracellular nucleotides could contribute to the development of vascular disease [136–139]. Extracellular ATP has been implicated in the hyperplasia and hypertrophy of arterial walls in spontaneously hypertensive rats, in regulation of vascular permeability [140, 141], and in control of proliferation and migration of vascular and hematopoietic cells including monocytes [136, 139, 142–144]. Importantly, in stimulating cell proliferation and migration, ATP acts synergistically with cytokines and integrins [136, 143–146] thereby supporting the physiological relevance of extracellular ATP under hypoxic and inflammatory conditions.

Previously, we demonstrated that pulmonary artery adventitial fibroblasts and vasa vasorum endothelial cells (VVECs) are a potent source of extracellular ATP, which acts as an autocrine/paracrine factor augmenting hypoxia-induced VVEC angiogenesis [147, 148]. These angiogenic

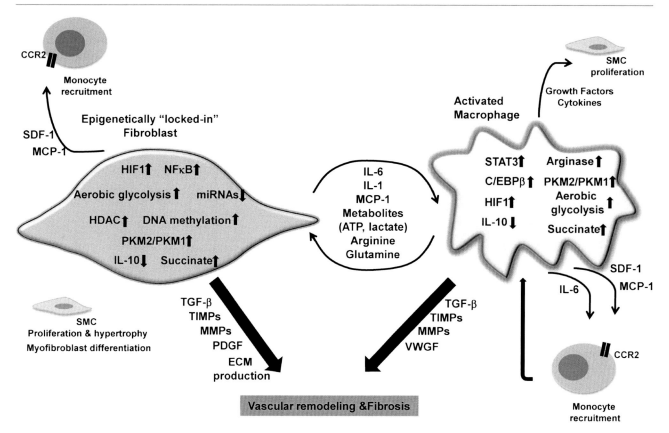

Fig. 5.1 Proposed intra- and inter-cellular signaling mechanisms involved in fibroblast-macrophage crosstalk in chronic non-resolving perivascular inflammation underlying irreversible pulmonary vascular remodeling. In this process, the adventitial fibroblast undergoes epigenetic changes that "lock" this cell into a pro-inflammatory and pro-mitogenic phenotype. Central drivers of this phenotypic arrest are continuously increased NF-κB and HIF signaling, increased PKM2 to PKM1 ratio, increased aerobic glycolysis, suppression of micro-RNAs (*mIRs*), increased histone deacetylase (*HDAC*) activity and DNA methylation, and suppressed anti-inflammatory IL-10 generation. The functional consequences are promotion of SMC hypertrophy and proliferation, and activation of resident and recruited macrophages/monocytes into a pro-inflammatory and pro-remodeling phenotype. Activation of the transcription factors STAT3, C/EBPβ, HIF1 alters PKM2 to PKM1 ratio, drives increases in aerobic glycolysis and promotes succinate accumulation. Activation of Arginase1 and decreased IL-10 are additional features of this macrophage phenotype. In a feed-forward loop, pro-inflammatory cytokines and chemokines (IL-6, IL-1, MCP1), metabolites (ATP and lactate), and tissue availability of Arginine and Glutamine, enables the fibroblast-macrophage signaling unit to persist in an activated state and perpetuate vascular remodeling and fibrosis. *TIMPs* tissue inhibitors of metalloproteinases, *MMPs* matrix metalloproteinases, *SDF-1*, stromal cell-derived factor 1, *MCP-1* monocyte chemoattractant protein-1, *CCR2* C-C chemokine receptor type 2, *VWGF* vascular endothelial growth factor, *HIF1* hypoxia inducible factor 1, *HDAC* histone deacetylase, *STAT3* Signal transducer and activator of transcription 3, *PKM1/2* Pyruvate kinase isozymes M1/M2

effects of ATP in VVECs are mediated through P2Y1, and P2Y13 purinergic receptors, prolonged/dramatic activation of PI3K/mTOR and ERK1/2 pathways, and the elevation of cytoplasmic and nucleoplasmic Ca2+ [149]. The responses to extracellular ATP might be particularly important in the hypoxic and inflamed adventitial microenvironment where increased extracellular ATP level can be expected.

In addition to endogenous ATP release, the concentrations of extracellular nucleotides near purinergic receptor are regulated by ecto-nucleoside triphosphate diphospho-hydrolase-1 (NTPDase1/CD39) and ecto-5′-nucleotidase/CD73 [150–152] responsible for extracellular adenosine production from ATP and ADP. However, it is unresolved whether ecto-nucleotidase expression and activities are altered in EC from vessels undergoing hypoxia-induced remodeling. In the

vascular system, endothelial E-NTPDase1/CD39 in conjunction with ecto-5′-nucleotidase/CD73, have been implicated in playing a critical role through the termination of pro-thrombotic and pro-inflammatory effects of circulating ATP and ADP and their conversion into adenosine. This keeps the haemostatic process tightly regulated by preventing excessive clot formation and vessel occlusion [152–154]. Data on disordered cellular migration, vascular inflammation, enhanced leakiness, pathological angiogenesis and neo-intima formation in mice deficient in NTPDase1 (*Cd39/Entpd⁻/⁻*) [150, 155] or ecto-5′-nucleotidase/CD73 [156] demonstrated the importance of coordinated purine homeostasis for proper vascular endothelial functions.

It was demonstrated that significant down-regulation of ecto-nucleotidase activities on vascular endothelium and other cell types during chronic hypoxia and oxidative stress was accompanied by elevated ATP and ADP levels, increased endothelial activation, and concomitant development of vascular disorders [136, 156, 157]. On the other hand, other investigators have shown endothelial nucleotide-inactivating ectoenzymes NTPDase1/CD39 and ecto-5'-nucleotidase/CD73 can be upregulated during acute hypoxia and inflammation. This increases the intravascular adenosine concentrations and dampens excessive inflammatory responses by affecting endothelial barrier function, adhesion and transmigration of lymphoid cells, and expression of other molecules involved in the adhesion cascade [158–160]. Using a direct enzymatic approach, we found that NTPDase1/CD39 and ecto-5'-nucleotidase/CD73 are impaired in VVECs from chronically hypoxic calves, which may serve as an important pre-requisite for consistently elevated ATP and ADP levels at sites of vasa vasorum angiogenesis, enhanced EC proliferation and, eventually, the exacerbation of pathological vascular remodeling [161].

Another important consequence of hypoxia-induced pulmonary vascular remodeling observed in chronically hypoxic animals is infiltration and homing of circulating inflammatory and progenitor cells to the PA adventitia and around the expanding VV, ultimately leading to adventitial inflammation and pathologic vascular remodeling [16, 56]. Although endothelial dysfunction and permeability changes have been intensively investigated in pulmonary artery endothelial cells, the mechanisms that control the pulmonary vasa vasorum permeability remain largely unexplored.

Extracellular adenosine, a product of ATP hydrolysis, has been shown to play a protective role against vascular leak under conditions associated with hypoxia and inflammation [158, 162–166]. Studies from CD73 (−/−) mice provided evidence that extracellular adenosine reverses hypoxia-induced vascular leakage in different organs, especially in the lung [165]. Adenosine binds to A_{2A} and A_{2B} receptors that function by activating adenylyl cyclase and generation of cAMP, or to A_1 and A_3 receptors that function by inhibiting adenylyl cyclase and increasing intracellular Ca^{2+} levels by a pathway involving phospholipase C [135, 165, 167–169]. Previous studies demonstrated a protective role of A2B adenosine receptors in hypoxia-induced vascular leak in adenosine receptor-knockout mice [164, 165]. Consistent with this observation, a recent report indicated permeability of pulmonary artery endothelial cells is regulated by A2A and A2B adenosine receptors and an adenosine transporter, pointing out an importance of both the extracellular and intracellular adenosine [170]. However the role of individual adenosine receptor subtypes in vasa vasorum permeability was unknown.

In agreement with previous findings, our recent study revealed a potent barrier protective effect of extracellular adenosine on the VVEC. The response was observed in VVEC isolated from both control and chronically hypoxic animals, but the cells from control animals exhibited more prominent response. Using pharmacological and genetic approaches, we found that the effect of adenosine on VVEC permeability is mediated mostly by A1R, while A2AR, A2BR and A3R are not likely to be involved. Importantly, a decrease in expression of A1R in VVEC of hypoxic animals correlates with a lower Trans Endothelial Resistance (TER) compared to VVEC of controls. The evidence of A1R involvement in barrier protection is also consistent with an anti-inflammatory role of A1R in several tissues [171–173] and may explain both anti-inflammatory and barrier-protective functions of A1R in vasa vasorum. For example, recent studies reported that A1R in lung microvascular endothelial cells participates in microvascular permeability and leukocyte transmigration [173] and in anti-inflammatory preconditioning [174]. Data from animal models also indicate the involvement of A1R in attenuation of endotoxin-induced lung injury, pulmonary edema, and alveolar destruction. Activation of adenosine A1 and A2 receptors have also been shown to reduce endotoxin-induced cellular energy depletion and edema formation in the lung [175]. However, our findings are different from the results in human lung microvascular endothelial cells, which demonstrated a role of A2AR in adenosine-induced barrier enhancement [175–177]. In contrast to studies showing cAMP-dependent regulation of endothelial barrier function, our studies revealed a role of Gαi/PI3K/Akt pathway actin cytoskeleton remodeling in mediating the effects of A1R activation, suggesting a non-canonical (possibly cAMP–independent) pathway of VVEC barrier regulation [178].

TNF-α and Vasa Vasorum Permeability

TNF-α, one of the most potent pro-inflammatory factors, regulates vascular endothelial cell permeability through stress fiber formation and interruption of cellular junctions [179–181]. TNF-α expression level and activity can be up-regulated under hypoxia, inflammation, and PH [182–185]. It has been shown that among several cell types, macrophages and perivascular adipocytes are potent sources of TNF-α [185, 186]. As the presence of macrophages was observed in pulmonary artery adventitia of chronically hypoxic animals [16], it can be expected that TNF-α, may have a paracrine effect on adventitial vasa vasorum in the pulmonary artery wall. The data from our recent study also show that TNF-α decrease the TER in control VVECs (VVEC-Co), and this effect of TNF-α was blunted by adenosine [178]. Interestingly, TNF-α failed to decrease TER in VVEC isolated from hypoxic animals. This suggests a possibility of persistent phenotypical changes in VVEC in response to chronic hypoxia that could involve TNF-α and adenosine receptors, as well as components of intracellular signaling pathways. We demonstrated that TNF-α was unable to further impair barrier function in VVEC-Hyp, (contrary to VVEC-Co), suggesting that exposure of VVEC to chronic hypoxia impairs these cells' permeability. Finally, we showed a significant attenuation of TNF-α-induced VVEC permeability upon adenosine treatment, indicative of the barrier-protective effect of adenosine.

In a view of pathologic consequence of hypoxia-induced vasa vasorum neovascularization and its function as a conduit for circulating inflammatory cells to the vascular wall, our data indicate that down-regulation of A1R in chronic hypoxia may represent a pathological mechanism of dysregulation of vasa vasorum barrier function. This may lead to pulmonary vascular remodeling and inflammation, such as that observed in hypoxic PH. We propose that A1Rs can be recognized as a vascular bed-specific and novel therapeutic target to regulate vasa vasorum barrier function and pathologic vascular remodeling in chronic hypoxia.

Regulation of Inflammatory Cells in Adventitia by Extracellular Nucleotides and Adenosine

As mentioned above, hypoxia-induced pulmonary vascular remodeling observed in chronically hypoxic animals is accompanied by extravasation and homing of circulating inflammatory and progenitor cells to the PA adventitia and around the expanding VV network [16, 56]. A number of studies have demonstrated that monocyte/macrophage inflammation functions are tightly regulated by extracellular nucleotides and adenosine. Extracellular ATP exerts pro-inflammatory and cytotoxic effects on monocytes/macrophages via regulation of cytokine and chemokine production including IL-1α, IL-6, IL-18, and TNFα, α9δ eicosanoids, including leukotrienes LTB$_4$ and LTC$_4$ and prostaglandins PGE$_2$ and PGD$_2$ [132]. Therefore, it is expected that in the adventitial microenvironment, extracellular ATP endogenously released by adventitial fibroblasts and vasa vasorum in response to local hypoxia and oxidative stress, functions as an inflammatory mediator via activation of macrophages and another type of inflammatory cells. In contrast, extracellular adenosine may prevent excessive accumulation and the activation of inflammatory cells in the adventitia via modulation of cytokine production and inhibition of chemotactic response to ATP [132] (Fig. 5.2).

Chronic Hypoxia, Inflammation, and Pulmonary Vascular Function: Relationship to Oxidative Stress

To fully understand the impact of chronic hypoxia and unresolved inflammation on the pathogenesis of pulmonary vascular disease, it is essential to also recognize the relationship of inflammation to oxidative stress and altered redox regulated signaling. Accumulating evidence indicates that reactive oxygen species (ROS) are increased in PH, including chronic hypoxia-induced PH, contributing to both vasoconstriction and pulmonary vascular remodeling [187–193]. ROS are generated as a result of inflammation, and conversely, ROS activate inflammatory pathways, thus both processes are closely linked and central to pulmonary vascular dysfunction.

The primary ROS implicated in cell signaling in the vasculature are superoxide and hydrogen peroxide. Superoxide is rapidly catalyzed to hydrogen peroxide and oxygen by the superoxide dismutase (SOD) family of antioxidant enzymes, or, in the face of inadequate SOD, reacts with nitric oxide, inactivating its bioactivity and forming toxic products like peroxynitrite. Hydrogen peroxide has been implicated in both normal cell signaling and pathologic signaling. It is scavenged by antioxidant enzymes including catalase and glutathione peroxidases, or in the presence of iron, can form the highly reactive hydroxyl radical.

The main sources of superoxide and hydrogen peroxide in the vasculature are the NAPDH oxidases, uncoupled eNOS, mitochondrial electron transport chain, and xanthine oxidase [194, 195]. The NADPH oxidases are a family of transmembrane multimeric proteins that are comprised of 7 different homologs with various regulatory subunits; Nox1, Nox2, Nox4 and Nox5 are expressed in the pulmonary vasculature. The Nox2 isoform of NADPH oxidase is abundantly expressed and induced in inflammatory cells present in the vessel wall, in particular in the PA adventitial compartment. In addition, the PA adventitial fibroblasts contain predominantly Nox4, as well as Nox2, and are a major source of ROS contributing to the "outside-in" effects of the PA adventitia on pulmonary vasoconstriction and remodeling [12, 196, 197]. Nox2 and Nox4 are also expressed in endothelial cells and PASMC, and collectively, the NADPH oxidases have been shown to promote vascular dysfunction. While endothelial nitric oxide synthase (eNOS) generates nitric oxide under physiologic conditions, in disease states, the two enzymatic domains of eNOS become uncoupled, resulting in release of superoxide. The uncoupling of eNOS can occur with deficiencies in L-arginine substrate; increased ADMA, an L-arginine analog; increased arginase activity; or BH$_4$ deficiency due to low production or oxidation. The mitochondrial electron transport chain is also well established to be a major source of ROS generation and numerous studies implicate mitochondrial dysfunction and mitochondrial-derived ROS in pulmonary vascular disease [198–200]. However, the role of the mitochondria in pulmonary vascular disease is complicated by the opposing observations that mitochondrial ROS production decreases in fawn hooded rats with spontaneous PH and mitochondrial ROS are decreased in the setting of hypoxia. Using new tools, there is

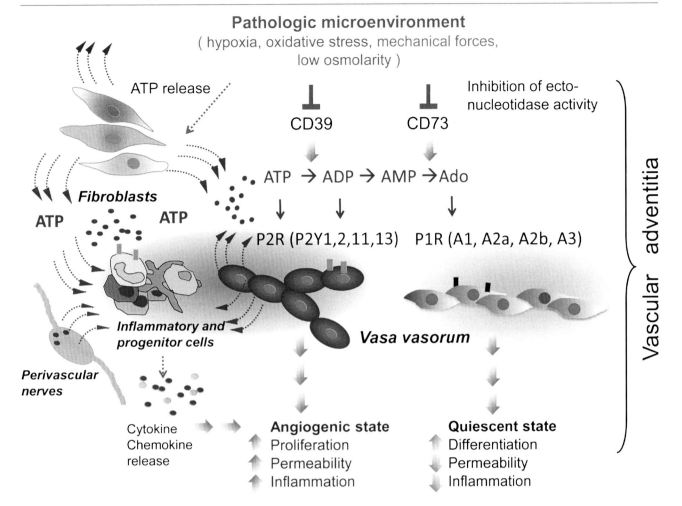

Fig. 5.2 Schematic view of the role of extracellular nucleotides in pulmonary artery adventitia. Stress conditions such as hypoxia, inflammation, oxidative stress, and mechanical forces stimulate ATP release from adventitial fibroblasts, vasa vasorum endothelial cells, perivascular nerves, and inflammatory cells. In addition, extracellular ATP stimulates monocytes/macrophages to release multiple inflammatory mediators that creates a pathologic microenvironment in the pulmonary artery adventitia. Endogenously released ATP, by acting on P2 purinergic receptors (*P2R*) results in angiogenic activation of the vasa vasorum, characterized by increased proliferation and dysregulated barrier properties. Elevated extracellular ATP is subsequently hydrolyzed by ecto-enzymes, NTPDase1/CD39 to ADP and AMP and by ecto-5′-nucleotidase/CD73 to Adenosine (*Ado*). In turn, extracellular adenosine by acting on P1 purinergic receptors (*P1R*) induces a phenotypic switch of the vasa vasorum endothelial cell to a more quiescent state, characterized by low proliferation rate and improved barrier function. Inhibition of NTPDase1/CD39 and ecto-5′-nucleotidase/CD73 activities by hypoxia and oxidative stress results in consistently elevated levels of extracellular ATP and lower levels of adenosine that eventually exacerbate pathological vascular remodeling

evidence that ROS production may even be regulated differently in the mitochondrial matrix compared to the mitochondrial intermembrane space [195, 201]. Xanthine dehydrogenase can be oxidized to xanthine oxidase (XO, also known as xanthine oxidoreductase, XOR), which then catalyzes the conversion of hypoxanthine and xanthine to uric acid with concurrent release of superoxide. XO has been shown to be an important source of oxidative stress in hypoxia induced PH and the lamb model of PH associated with elevated pulmonary blood flow [195, 202–205]. Furthermore, XO-derived ROS contribute to injury in a number of processes associated with inflammation including ischemia-reperfusion injury, acute lung injury, COPD and cigarette exposure, and cancer [188, 196, 205–216]. Our

recent work demonstrates that XO promotes the inflammatory state of pulmonary mononuclear phagocytes through effects on HIF-1α, further supporting the close link between ROS and inflammation [217]. The production of ROS by these important sources can be activated by pro-inflammatory cytokines, including interleukins and tumor necrosis factor-α, and conversely, the ROS generated in the vessel wall can augment inflammation by activating redox sensitive targets including key transcription factors, NF-κβ, AP-1, and HIF. In addition, ROS can modulate a wide range of other signaling molecules that impact inflammation, proliferation, migration, differentiation, and matrix production [194]. The best described redox sensitive targets include receptor and nonreceptor tyrosine kinases, serine/threonine kinases, protein

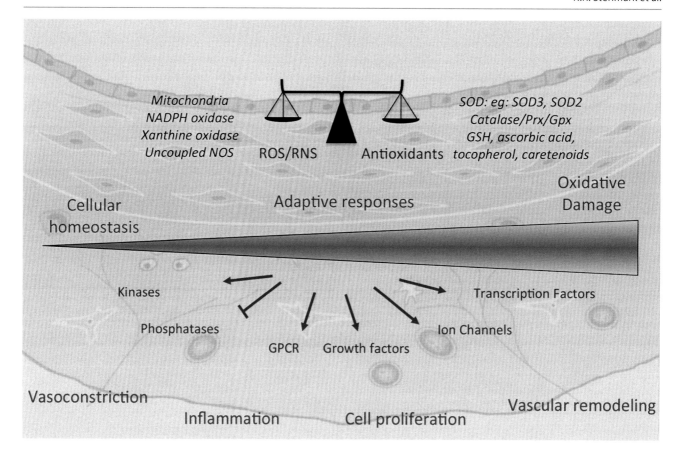

Fig. 5.3 Redox regulated signaling in pulmonary vascular remodeling. ROS/RNS are important in cellular homeostasis and their levels are tightly controlled by enzymatic and non enzymatic antioxidant systems. In the setting of disease, an increase in ROS due to increased production or decreased antioxidant defenses may initially enable adaptive responses but eventually leads to oxidative stress. ROS can directly activate key redox sensitive targets that lead ultimately to pulmonary vasoconstriction, inflammation, cell proliferation and vascular remodeling. *ROS* reactive oxygen species, *RNS* reactive nitrogen species, *NADPH* nicotinamide adenine dinucleotide phosphate, *NOS* nitric oxide synthase, *SOD* superoxide dismutase, *SOD3* extracellular SOD, *SOD2* mitochondrial SOD, *Prx* peroxireductases, *Gpx* glutathione peroxidase, *GSH* glutathione, *GPCR* G-protein coupled receptor

tyrosine phosphatases, growth factors, adhesion molecules and ion channels [194–196, 218].

The importance of ROS in inflammation and pulmonary vascular dysfunction is further evidenced by the critical role of antioxidant enzymes. The major vascular antioxidant enzymes are SOD, catalase and glutathione peroxidase [195]. The extracellular isoform of SOD, extracellular superoxide dismutase (EC-SOD or SOD3) is the dominant SOD isoform in the vasculature and is highly localized to the vascular adventitia [219, 220]. In multiple models of vascular disease, including chronic hypoxic PH, loss of SOD3 enhances inflammation and vascular dysfunction, while overexpression of SOD3 protects [194, 221–223]. Mice lacking SOD1 also exhibit exaggerated chronic hypoxic PH [224] and SOD2 has been shown to be decreased in the lungs of fawn hooded rats, and the pulmonary arteries of patients with IPAH [225–229]. Though catalase or glutathione peroxidase have not been shown to be consistently altered in PH, loss of catalase can lead to hydrogen peroxide mediated inactivation of SOD3 and glutathione peroxidase may increase to compensate for oxidative stress but remain overall insufficient [195, 230].

Collectively, these studies strongly support the premise that generation of ROS contribute to the chronic inflammation and pulmonary vascular dysfunction in the setting of hypoxia by further augmenting inflammation as well as other redox sensitive signaling pathways involved in disease pathogenesis (Fig. 5.3).

Contribution of Epigenetics to Chronic Hypoxia-Induced Lung Vascular Inflammation and Remodeling in PH

It is increasingly appreciated that chronic inflammatory microenvironments lead to stable heritable changes in gene expression and cell function without modification of the underlying DNA base composition; i.e. epigenetic change [231, 232]. There are at least three distinct mechanisms of epigenetic regulation, DNA methylation, histone modifications, and gene silencing, mediated by microRNAs (miRs). These pathways of gene regulation are often altered in human diseases such as cancer and are well recognized to contribute to uncontrolled cell growth, migration, and invasion [233–235]. Further, it is also important to note that there are substantial interactions between these epigenetic pathways involved in gene regulation. Studies in a wide variety of cells, mostly cancerous, have demonstrated that hypoxia can regulate changes in all of these epigenetic regulatory pathways [236, 237].

Changes in epigenetic modifications have recently been associated with PH, a disease characterized not only by chronic inflammation but also by mesenchymal cell (SMC and fibroblast) proliferation, resistance to apoptosis, and fibrosis as noted above [15, 238]. For instance, recent studies have demonstrated that superoxide dismutase (SOD) 2 expression is decreased in pulmonary arteries and plexiform lesions because of hypermethylation of CpG islands in the SOD2 gene [227]. Reversal of the methylation was shown to rescue SOD2 expression and to inhibit proliferation and to increase cell apoptosis of PASMCs from the Fawn Hooded rat [227]. Histone acetylation has also been shown to play an important role in the development of PH, and specifically hypoxic PH. Increased HDAC expression has been reported in lung tissues of patients with IPAH as well as in tissues from hypoxia induced PH rats and calves [239]. Specific increases in Class I HDACs were observed in the fibroblast from hypoxic animals as well as in cells from IPAH patients. Treatment with Class I HDAC inhibitors markedly decreased cytokine/chemokine mRNA expression levels in fibroblasts as well as in their ability to induce monocyte migration and pro-inflammatory activation. Most interestingly studies with several HDAC inhibitors, including the Class I specific HDAC inhibitor were shown to both suppress and reverse hypoxia induced cardiopulmonary remodeling in rats [88, 239].

Increases in HDAC expression, and thus histone acetylation, also were shown to contribute to the abnormalities of mesenchymal cell proliferation in rats, calves, and sheep [26, 88, 239, 240]. Studies in cells derived from the hypertensive pulmonary circulation of all three species have demonstrated that HDAC inhibition results in a decrease in proliferation mediated in part because regulation cell cycle regulatory genes, including p16^{INK}, p21, and p27. In PASMCs of hypoxic sheep fetuses, HDAC inhibition also decreased PDGF-induced cell migration and ERK activation as well as modulating global DNA methylation, again consistent with the idea that interactions among the epigenetic mechanisms are important in controlling cell phenotypes [239, 240]. It is also interesting to note that chromatin immunoprecipitation analysis experiments have shown that TGF-β which is thought to play an important role in hypoxic and other forms of PH, increases binding of Smad2/3, Smad4, and the transcriptional co-repressor HDAC-1 to the PPAR-γ promoter. This reduces PPAR-γ, which has been shown to be associated with heightened proliferation and other abnormal activities in cells from the PH animals. Treatment with the PPAR-γ agonist, rosiglitazone, prevented this interaction again implicating the role of HDACs in chronic hypoxia induced remodeling [241].

Recent studies have also implicated miRs in the development of PH. miR204 expression has been shown to be decreased in animal models of PH and in human patient samples and rescue of miR204 reverses PH in rats [242]. miR17 has also been shown to be upregulated in hypoxia and monocrotaline-induced PH and inhibition of miR17 improved mitigated PH in both species [243]. miR17 has also been shown to be upregulated by hypoxia in cultured human PASMCs. In addition, it was shown that inhibiting miR17-5P expression decreased hypoxia-induced arginase protein levels in human PASMCs, which has been shown to be involved in promoting proliferation [244]. Several other miRs and miR targets have been shown to be involved in the development of hypoxic PH. Studies by Gou et al. found that miR210 is the predominant miR induced by hypoxia in human PASMCs [245]. Others have called miR210 the master hypoxamir [246]. Transcriptional induction of miR210 is HIF1α dependent. Inhibition of miR210 in human PASMCs causes significant decrease in cell number under hypoxic conditions due to increased apoptosis probably via regulation of the transcription factor E2F3 [245]. Another interesting study has demonstrated that hypoxia and miR210 increase proliferation in idiopathic pulmonary fibrosis (IPF) fibroblasts [247]. miR210 expression markedly increases in IPF fibroblasts in response to hypoxia and knockdown of miR210 decreases hypoxia induced IPF-fibroblast proliferation. Importantly, the investigators showed that silencing HIF2α inhibits the hypoxia mediated increase in miR210 expression, indicating that in certain cells HIF2 is upstream of miR210 [247]. Importantly, in situ analysis of IPF lung tissue demonstrated that miR210 expression was distributed similarly with HIF2α and the hypoxic marker CA-1X in cells within the IPF fibrotic reticulum. Thus, the authors raised the possibility that a pathologic feed-forward loop could exist in fibrotic lungs in which hypoxia promotes fibroblast proliferation via stimulation of miR210 expression, which in turn worsens hypoxia. Other miRs including miR-145, 21, and 206 have been implicated in hypoxic forms of PH [248–251]. miR 21 expression is increased in the distal PA's of hypoxia exposed mice and putative targets of miR 21 including BMPR2 were increased [252]. Sequestration of miR21 diminished chronic hypoxia-induced PH and vascular remodeling. miR145 is also of particular interest as it was shown that miR145 was increased in hypoxic mouse lungs and that miR145 deficiency (KO mice) and anti-miR145 both resulted in significant protection from hypoxia-induced PH.

Another recent study has demonstrated the complex relationship between gene regulation and gene expression with regard to epigenetic mechanisms. Wang et al. demonstrated in adventitial fibroblasts from neonatal calves with severe hypoxia induced PH that miR124 expression was decreased and that miR124 directly regulated MCP1 expression and indirectly regulated proliferation through the alternative splicing factor PTBP1 [26]. Further, it was shown that down-regulation of miR124 was mediated through Class I specific HDACs. The authors discovered that treatment of PH fibroblasts with HDAC inhibitors, including SAHA, apicidin, and OSU42 led to significant increases in miR124 while decreasing direct targets of miR124, including the alternative splicing factor PTBP1 and the pro-inflammatory cytokine MCP1. Thus, miR expression itself, under hypoxic conditions, is regulated by epigenetic modifications, specifically the removal of acetylation marks on histone resulting in more condensed chromatin structure and inhibition of transcription. Collectively, these epigenetic changes, which occur in the setting of hypoxia and inflammation, begin to explain the constitutively activated phenotype of PH fibroblasts [26].

The aforementioned studies demonstrate that, while positive adaptive responses to acute hypoxia in the lung are probably crucial for maintaining homeostatic responses, long-term chronic hypoxia can result in responses that are detrimental to the lung and the lung vasculature. The classical adaptive responses to hypoxia, that aim to restore oxygen homeostasis in tissues, including the lung, are regulated by the HIF family of proteins. It is thus not surprising that in addition to work specifically in the lung that there is much current research, which implicates epigenetic mechanisms in modulating the cellular response to hypoxic environments [237, 253, 254]. There is increasing evidence supporting the idea that the activity of hypoxia induced transcription factors, including HIF is superimposed on a background of epigenetic changes that are essential for determining the cellular or tissues specific hypoxic response. For instance, interesting work demonstrates that epigenetic modifications at the DNA and histone level have the ability to dictate HIF binding to target gene promoters and thus to regulating hypoxic gene expression. Further, hypoxia itself is a potent inducer of chromatin remodeling via the regulation of enzymes that modulate DNA methylation and histone modifications. Long-term adaptation to chronic hypoxia involves significant modification of chromatin structure in order to maintain the hypoxic phenotype, even in the absence of HIF1. It is important to note that data in the pulmonary circulation, along with many other organs, suggest that chronic hypoxia is capable of inducing changes in gene expression that are independent of classical HIF pathway. Again, this is probably due to alterations in the methylation status of gene sequence or modification of the histone code, which are likely mediated through prolonged alterations in epigenetic modifying enzymes.

There are four current opinions on the interactions of epigenetics and hypoxia:

1. HIF stabilization is influenced by the epigenetically controlled expression of Von Hippel Lindau (VHL) and PHD3.
2. Epigenetic mechanisms regulate HIF binding by maintaining a transcriptionally active chromatin confirmation within and around HIF binding site regions. This may occur through the action of the HIF1α co-activation complex or through direct modifications of HR rebinding sites, which prevent HIF binding.
3. A significant number of histone dimethylase enzymes are direct HIF1 target genes and therefore play a role in the regulation of transcription during hypoxic responses.
4. Significant global changes in histone modifications and DNA methylation occur in response to hypoxic exposure.

Investigation of all these possibilities in the setting of chronic hypoxia in the lung will be important as it will likely dictate new therapeutic approaches to ameliorate chronic hypoxia induced lung tissue responses. At present, current data points to the possibility that HDAC inhibitors are important in controlling hypoxic generated proliferative inflammatory and fibrotic responses. Clearly, other possibilities that will be aimed at DNA methylation and/or histone methylation will be tested in the not too distant future.

Conclusion

Hypoxic, or WHO Group 3, PH comprises a heterogeneous group of diseases sharing the common feature of chronic hypoxia-induced pulmonary vascular remodeling, which is usually mild to moderate in nature and which can be largely reversible as compared with the progressive irreversible disease seen in WHO Group I disease. Despite the fact that patients with WHO Group 3 PH are much more likely to die as a result of their underlying lung disease than from complications of PH, the presence of PH in these patients is the most important marker of morbidity and mortality. Furthermore, this patient population is exponentially larger than that of patients with PAH, yet numerous clinical trials involving pulmonary vasodilators proven efficacious for PAH have either failed or shown harm in patients with hypoxic PH. Further, there is a subset of hypoxic PH patients that develop severe "out-of-proportion" PH characterized by pulmonary vascular remodeling that is irreversible and similar to that in WHO Group 1 disease. In both mild to moderate as well as severe forms of the disease, inflammation appears to play an important role in the disease process. In this review, we highlight the mechanisms involved in both the initiation and perpetuation of inflammation in the vessel wall as well as the interplay between hypoxia, inflammation and their effects on resident pulmonary vascular cells and recruited immune and progenitor cells. We hypothesize that those patients with severe, "out of proportion" and irreversible hypoxic PH, experience an as yet undefined "second hit" whereby the mechanisms involved go beyond those related to hypoxia alone, leading to chronic non-resolving inflammation. We propose that important epigenetic changes, at least in mesenchymal cells, and possibly in perivascular macrophages, are paramount in "locking" cells into a pro-remodeling, pro-inflammatory, and pro-mitogenic phenotype. Furthermore, these fibroblast/macrophage-stromal cell interactions are necessary for the maintenance of chronic non-resolving inflammation and persistent pulmonary vascular remodeling. After nearly 20 years of vasodilator therapies that have reduced morbidity in patients with PAH, mortality remains unacceptably high, forcing the field to move toward treatments targeting the underlying pathogenesis of pulmonary vascular remodeling. Similarly, the persistent failure of pulmonary vasodilators in hypoxic PH urges us to shift away from recycling pulmonary vasodilator therapies proven to be beneficial in PAH to those that aim to disrupt and repair the basic pathologic inflammatory mechanisms responsible for the initiation and perpetuation of disease.

References

1. Morrell NW, Archer SL, Defelice A, Evans S, Fiszman M, Martin T, et al. Anticipated classes of new medications and molecular targets for pulmonary arterial hypertension. Pulm Circ. 2013;3: 226–44.
2. Price LC, Wort SJ, Perros F, Dorfmuller P, Huertas A, Montani D, et al. Inflammation in pulmonary arterial hypertension. Chest. 2012;141:210–21.
3. Tuder RM, Archer SL, Dorfmuller P, Erzurum SC, Guignabert C, Michelakis E, et al. Relevant issues in the pathology and pathobiology of PH. J Am Coll Cardiol. 2013;62:D4–12.
4. Rabinovitch M, Guignabert C, Humbert M, Nicolls MR. Inflammation and immunity in the pathogenesis of pulmonary arterial hypertension. Circ Res. 2014;115:165–75.
5. Tuder RM, Voelkel NF. PH and inflammation. J Lab Clin Med. 1998;132:16–24.
6. Stacher E, Graham BB, Hunt JM, Gandjeva A, Groshong SD, McLaughlin VV, et al. Modern age pathology of pulmonary arterial hypertension. Am J Respir Crit Care Med. 2012;186:261–72.
7. Savai R, Pullamsetti SS, Kolbe J, Bieniek E, Voswinckel R, Fink L, et al. Immune and inflammatory cell involvement in the pathology of idiopathic pulmonary arterial hypertension. Am J Respir Crit Care Med. 2012;186:897–908.
8. Tuder RM, Stacher E, Robinson J, Kumar R, Graham BB. Pathology of PH. Clin Chest Med. 2013;34:639–50.
9. Stenmark KR, Meyrick B, Galie N, Mooi WJ, McMurtry IF. Animal models of pulmonary arterial hypertension: the hope for etiological discovery and pharmacological cure. Am J Physiol Lung Cell Mol Physiol. 2009;297:L1013–32.
10. Burke DL, Frid MG, Kunrath CL, Karoor V, Anwar A, Wagner BD, et al. Sustained hypoxia promotes the development of a pulmonary artery-specific chronic inflammatory microenvironment. Am J Physiol Lung Cell Mol Physiol. 2009;297:L238–50.
11. Stenmark KR, Davie NJ, Reeves JT, Frid MG. Hypoxia, leukocytes, and the pulmonary circulation. J Appl Physiol. 2005;98: 715–21.
12. Stenmark KR, Yeager ME, El Kasmi KC, Nozik-Grayck E, Gerasimovskaya EV, Li M, et al. The adventitia: essential regulator of vascular wall structure and function. Annu Rev Physiol. 2013;75:23–47.
13. Stenmark KR, Nozik-Grayck E, Gerasimovskaya E, Anwar A, Li M, Riddle S, et al. The adventitia: essential role in pulmonary vascular remodeling. Compr Physiol. 2011;1:141–61.
14. Hassoun PM, Mouthon L, Barbera JA, Eddahibi S, Flores SC, Grimminger F, et al. Inflammation, growth factors, and pulmonary vascular remodeling. J Am Coll Cardiol. 2009;54:S10–9.
15. Stenmark KR, Frid MG, Yeager M, Li M, Riddle S, McKinsey T, et al. Targeting the adventitial microenvironment in PH: a potential approach to therapy that considers epigenetic change. Pulm Circ. 2012;2:3–14.
16. Frid MG, Brunetti JA, Burke DL, Carpenter TC, Davie NJ, Reeves JT, et al. Hypoxia-induced pulmonary vascular remodeling requires recruitment of circulating mesenchymal precursors of a monocyte/macrophage lineage. Am J Pathol. 2006;168:659–69.
17. Thenappan T, Goel A, Marsboom G, Fang YH, Toth PT, Zhang HJ, et al. A central role for CD68(+) macrophages in hepatopulmonary syndrome. Reversal by macrophage depletion. Am J Respir Crit Care Med. 2011;183:1080–91.
18. Colegio OR, Chu NQ, Szabo AL, Chu T, Rhebergen AM, Jairam V, et al. Functional polarization of tumour-associated macrophages by tumour-derived lactic acid. Nature. 2014;513:559–63.
19. Nathan C, Ding A. Nonresolving inflammation. Cell. 2010; 140:871–82.
20. El Kasmi KC, Pugliese SC, Riddle SR, Poth JM, Anderson AL, Frid MG, et al. Adventitial fibroblasts induce a distinct proinflammatory/profibrotic macrophage phenotype in PH. J Immunol. 2014;193:597–609.
21. Schmall A, Al-Tamari HM, Herold S, Kampschulte M, Weigert A, Wietelmann A, et al. Macrophage and cancer cell crosstalk via CCR2 and CX3CR1 is a fundamental mechanism driving lung cancer. Am J Respir Crit Care Med. 2014.
22. Daley JM, Brancato SK, Thomay AA, Reichner JS, Albina JE. The phenotype of murine wound macrophages. J Leukoc Biol. 2010; 87:59–67.
23. Ishii M, Wen H, Corsa CA, Liu T, Coelho AL, Allen RM, et al. Epigenetic regulation of the alternatively activated macrophage phenotype. Blood. 2009;114:3244–54.
24. Liao X, Sharma N, Kapadia F, Zhou G, Lu Y, Hong H, et al. Kruppel-like factor 4 regulates macrophage polarization. J Clin Invest. 2011;121:2736–49.
25. Li M, Riddle SR, Frid MG, El Kasmi KC, McKinsey TA, Sokol RJ, et al. Emergence of fibroblasts with a proinflammatory epigenetically altered phenotype in severe hypoxic PH. J Immunol. 2011;187:2711–22.
26. Wang D, Zhang H, Li M, Frid MG, Flockton AR, McKeon BA, et al. MicroRNA-124 controls the proliferative, migratory, and inflammatory phenotype of pulmonary vascular fibroblasts. Circ Res. 2014;114:67–78.
27. Wynn TA, Chawla A, Pollard JW. Macrophage biology in development, homeostasis and disease. Nature. 2013;496:445–55.
28. Lawrie A. A report on the use of animal models and phenotyping methods in PH research. Pulm Circ. 2014;4:2–9.
29. Aaronson PI, Robertson TP, Ward JP. Endothelium-derived mediators and hypoxic pulmonary vasoconstriction. Respir Physiol Neurobiol. 2002;132:107–20.
30. Faller DV. Endothelial cell responses to hypoxic stress. Clin Exp Pharmacol Physiol. 1999;26:74–84.

31. Badesch DB, Orton EC, Zapp LM, Westcott JY, Hester J, Voelkel NF, et al. Decreased arterial wall prostaglandin production in neonatal calves with severe chronic PH. Am J Respir Cell Mol Biol. 1989;1:489–98.

32. Herget J, Wilhelm J, Novotna J, Eckhardt A, Vytasek R, Mrazkova L, et al. A possible role of the oxidant tissue injury in the development of hypoxic PH. Physiol Res/Academia Scientiarum Bohemoslovaca. 2000;49:493–501.

33. Preston IR, Hill NS, Warburton RR, Fanburg BL. Role of 12-lipoxygenase in hypoxia-induced rat pulmonary artery smooth muscle cell proliferation. Am J Physiol Lung Cell Mol Physiol. 2006;290:L367–74.

34. Kourembanas S, Bernfield M. Hypoxia and endothelial-smooth muscle cell interactions in the lung. Am J Respir Cell Mol Biol. 1994;11:373–4.

35. Chen YF, Oparil S. Endothelin and PH. J Cardiovasc Pharmacol. 2000;35:S49–53.

36. Stenmark KR, Fagan KA, Frid MG. Hypoxia-induced pulmonary vascular remodeling: cellular and molecular mechanisms. Circ Res. 2006;99:675–91.

37. Ali MH, Schlidt SA, Chandel NS, Hynes KL, Schumacker PT, Gewertz BL. Endothelial permeability and IL-6 production during hypoxia: role of ROS in signal transduction. Am J Physiol. 1999;277:L1057–65.

38. Strukova S. Blood coagulation-dependent inflammation. Coagulation-dependent inflammation and inflammation-dependent thrombosis. Front Biosci: J Virtual Libr. 2006;11:59–80.

39. Ten VS, Pinsky DJ. Endothelial response to hypoxia: physiologic adaptation and pathologic dysfunction. Curr Opin Crit Care. 2002;8:242–50.

40. Zhang J, Hu H, Palma NL, Harrison JK, Mubarak KK, Carrie RD, et al. Hypoxia-induced endothelial CX3CL1 triggers lung smooth muscle cell phenotypic switching and proliferative expansion. Am J Physiol Lung Cell Mol Physiol. 2012;303:L912–22.

41. Cao Z, Ding BS, Guo P, Lee SB, Butler JM, Casey SC, et al. Angiocrine factors deployed by tumor vascular niche induce B cell lymphoma invasiveness and chemoresistance. Cancer Cell. 2014;25:350–65.

42. Sandler VM, Lis R, Liu Y, Kedem A, James D, Elemento O, et al. Reprogramming human endothelial cells to haematopoietic cells requires vascular induction. Nature. 2014;511:312–8.

43. Welsh DJ, Peacock AJ. Cellular responses to hypoxia in the pulmonary circulation. High Alt Med Biol. 2013;14:111–6.

44. Arias-Stella J, Kruger H, Recavarren S. Pathology of chronic mountain sickness. Thorax. 1973;28:701–8.

45. Arias-Stella J, Saldana M. The terminal portion of the pulmonary arterial tree in people native to high altitudes. Circulation. 1963;28:915–25.

46. Heath D, Smith P, Rios Dalenz J, Williams D, Harris P. Small pulmonary arteries in some natives of La Paz. Bolivia Thorax. 1981;36:599–604.

47. Hunter KS, Lammers SR, Shandas R. Pulmonary vascular stiffness: measurement, modeling, and implications in normal and hypertensive pulmonary circulations. Compr Physiol. 2011;1:1413–35.

48. Pugliese SC, Poth JM, Fini MA, Olschewski A, El Kasmi KC, Stenmark KR. The role of inflammation in hypoxic PH: from cellular mechanisms to clinical phenotypes. Am J Physiol Lung Cell Mol Physiol. 2015;308(3):L229–52, ajplung 00238 2014.

49. Pak O, Aldashev A, Welsh D, Peacock A. The effects of hypoxia on the cells of the pulmonary vasculature. Eur Respir J. 2007;30:364–72.

50. Falcetti E, Hall SM, Phillips PG, Patel J, Morrell NW, Haworth SG, et al. Smooth muscle proliferation and role of the prostacyclin (IP) receptor in idiopathic pulmonary arterial hypertension. Am J Respir Crit Care Med. 2010;182:1161–70.

51. Horita H, Furgeson SB, Ostriker A, Olszewski KA, Sullivan T, Villegas LR, et al. Selective inactivation of PTEN in smooth muscle cells synergizes with hypoxia to induce severe PH. J Am Heart Assoc. 2013;2, e000188.

52. Lagna G, Ku MM, Nguyen PH, Neuman NA, Davis BN, Hata A. Control of phenotypic plasticity of smooth muscle cells by bone morphogenetic protein signaling through the myocardin-related transcription factors. J Biol Chem. 2007;282:37244–55.

53. Wang D, Prakash J, Nguyen P, Davis-Dusenbery BN, Hill NS, Layne MD, et al. Bone morphogenetic protein signaling in vascular disease: anti-inflammatory action through myocardin-related transcription factor A. J Biol Chem. 2012;287:28067–77.

54. Yeager ME, Belchenko DD, Nguyen CM, Colvin KL, Ivy DD, Stenmark KR. Endothelin-1, the unfolded protein response, and persistent inflammation: role of pulmonary artery smooth muscle cells. Am J Respir Cell Mol Biol. 2012;46:14–22.

55. Pisarcik S, Maylor J, Lu W, Yun X, Undem C, Sylvester JT, et al. Activation of hypoxia-inducible factor-1 in pulmonary arterial smooth muscle cells by endothelin-1. Am J Physiol Lung Cell Mol Physiol. 2013;304:L549–61.

56. Frid MG, Li M, Gnanasekharan M, Burke DL, Fragoso M, Strassheim D, et al. Sustained hypoxia leads to the emergence of cells with enhanced growth, migratory, and promitogenic potentials within the distal pulmonary artery wall. Am J Physiol Lung Cell Mol Physiol. 2009;297:L1059–72.

57. Vergadi E, Chang MS, Lee C, Liang OD, Liu X, Fernandez-Gonzalez A, et al. Early macrophage recruitment and alternative activation are critical for the later development of hypoxia-induced PH. Circulation. 2011;123:1986–95.

58. Orton EC, LaRue SM, Ensley B, Stenmark K. Bromodeoxyuridine labeling and DNA content of pulmonary arterial medial cells from hypoxia-exposed and nonexposed healthy calves. Am J Vet Res. 1992;53:1925–30.

59. Wilcox JN, Okamoto EI, Nakahara KI, Vinten-Johansen J. Perivascular responses after angioplasty which may contribute to postangioplasty restenosis: a role for circulating myofibroblast precursors? Ann N Y Acad Sci. 2001;947:68–90; dicussion -2.

60. Best PJ, Hasdai D, Sangiorgi G, Schwartz RS, Holmes DR, Jr Simari RD, et al. Apoptosis. Basic concepts and implications in coronary artery disease. Arterioscler Thromb Vasc Biol. 1999;19:14–22.

61. Okamoto E, Couse T, De Leon H, Vinten-Johansen J, Goodman RB, Scott NA, et al. Perivascular inflammation after balloon angioplasty of porcine coronary arteries. Circulation. 2001;104: 2228–35.

62. Scott NA, Cipolla GD, Ross CE, Dunn B, Martin FH, Simonet L, et al. Identification of a potential role for the adventitia in vascular lesion formation after balloon overstretch injury of porcine coronary arteries. Circulation. 1996;93:2178–87.

63. Maiellaro K, Taylor WR. The role of the adventitia in vascular inflammation. Cardiovasc Res. 2007;75:640–8.

64. Dorfmuller P, Perros F, Balabanian K, Humbert M. Inflammation in pulmonary arterial hypertension. Eur Respir J. 2003;22: 358–63.

65. Sahara M, Sata M, Morita T, Nakamura K, Hirata Y, Nagai R. Diverse contribution of bone marrow-derived cells to vascular remodeling associated with pulmonary arterial hypertension and arterial neointimal formation. Circulation. 2007;115:509–17.

66. Tuder RM, Marecki JC, Richter A, Fijalkowska I, Flores S. Pathology of PH. Clin Chest Med. 2007;28:23–42, vii.

67. Davie NJ, Crossno Jr JT, Frid MG, Hofmeister SE, Reeves JT, Hyde DM, et al. Hypoxia-induced pulmonary artery adventitial remodeling and neovascularization: contribution of progenitor cells. Am J Physiol Lung Cell Mol Physiol. 2004;286:L668–78.

68. Perros F, Dorfmuller P, Souza R, Durand-Gasselin I, Mussot S, Mazmanian M, et al. Dendritic cell recruitment in lesions of human and experimental PH. Eur Respir J. 2007;29:462–8.

69. Lambrecht BN, Hammad H. Taking our breath away: dendritic cells in the pathogenesis of asthma. Nat Rev Immunol. 2003;3:994–1003.

70. Demedts IK, Bracke KR, Van Pottelberge G, Testelmans D, Verleden GM, Vermassen FE, et al. Accumulation of dendritic cells and increased CCL20 levels in the airways of patients with chronic obstructive pulmonary disease. Am J Respir Crit Care Med. 2007;175:998–1005.

71. Sertl K, Takemura T, Tschachler E, Ferrans VJ, Kaliner MA, Shevach EM. Dendritic cells with antigen-presenting capability reside in airway epithelium, lung parenchyma, and visceral pleura. J Exp Med. 1986;163:436–51.

72. Hammad H, Lambrecht BN. Dendritic cells and airway epithelial cells at the interface between innate and adaptive immune responses. Allergy. 2011;66:579–87.

73. Banchereau J, Briere F, Caux C, Davoust J, Lebecque S, Liu YJ, et al. Immunobiology of dendritic cells. Annu Rev Immunol. 2000;18:767–811.

74. Murray PJ, Wynn TA. Protective and pathogenic functions of macrophage subsets. Nat Rev Immunol. 2011;11:723–37.

75. Hume DA. Differentiation and heterogeneity in the mononuclear phagocyte system. Mucosal Immunol. 2008;1:432–41.

76. Woollard KJ, Geissmann F. Monocytes in atherosclerosis: subsets and functions. Nat Rev Cardiol. 2010;7:77–86.

77. Pryshchep O, Ma-Krupa W, Younge BR, Goronzy JJ, Weyand CM. Vessel-specific toll-like receptor profiles in human medium and large arteries. Circulation. 2008;118:1276–84.

78. Geissmann F, Manz MG, Jung S, Sieweke MH, Merad M, Ley K. Development of monocytes, macrophages, and dendritic cells. Science. 2010;327:656–61.

79. Schulz C, Gomez Perdiguero E, Chorro L, Szabo-Rogers H, Cagnard N, Kierdorf K, et al. A lineage of myeloid cells independent of Myb and hematopoietic stem cells. Science. 2012;336:86–90.

80. Sica A, Mantovani A. Macrophage plasticity and polarization: in vivo veritas. J Clin Invest. 2012;122:787–95.

81. Gordon S, Mantovani A. Diversity and plasticity of mononuclear phagocytes. Eur J Immunol. 2011;41:2470–2.

82. Pesce JT, Ramalingam TR, Mentink-Kane MM, Wilson MS, El Kasmi KC, Smith AM, et al. Arginase-1-expressing macrophages suppress Th2 cytokine-driven inflammation and fibrosis. PLoS Pathog. 2009;5, e1000371.

83. El Kasmi KC, Qualls JE, Pesce JT, Smith AM, Thompson RW, Henao-Tamayo M, et al. Toll-like receptor-induced arginase 1 in macrophages thwarts effective immunity against intracellular pathogens. Nat Immunol. 2008;9:1399–406.

84. Nguyen KD, Qiu Y, Cui X, Goh YP, Mwangi J, David T, et al. Alternatively activated macrophages produce catecholamines to sustain adaptive thermogenesis. Nature. 2011;480:104–8.

85. Hume DA. Macrophages as APC and the dendritic cell myth. J Immunol. 2008;181:5829–35.

86. Brouty-Boye D, Pottin-Clemenceau C, Doucet C, Jasmin C, Azzarone B. Chemokines and CD40 expression in human fibroblasts. Eur J Immunol. 2000;30:914–9.

87. Pap T, Muller-Ladner U, Gay RE, Gay S. Fibroblast biology. Role of synovial fibroblasts in the pathogenesis of rheumatoid arthritis. Arthritis Res. 2000;2:361–7.

88. Cavasin MA, Demos-Davies K, Horn TR, Walker LA, Lemon DD, Birdsey N, et al. Selective class I histone deacetylase inhibition suppresses hypoxia-induced cardiopulmonary remodeling through an antiproliferative mechanism. Circ Res. 2012;110:739–48.

89. Satoh T, Takeuchi O, Vandenbon A, Yasuda K, Tanaka Y, Kumagai Y, et al. The Jmjd3-Irf4 axis regulates M2 macrophage polarization and host responses against helminth infection. Nat Immunol. 2010;11:936–44.

90. Buckley CD, Pilling D, Lord JM, Akbar AN, Scheel-Toellner D, Salmon M. Fibroblasts regulate the switch from acute resolving to chronic persistent inflammation. Trends Immunol. 2001;22:199–204.

91. Lo D, Feng L, Li L, Carson MJ, Crowley M, Pauza M, et al. Integrating innate and adaptive immunity in the whole animal. Immunol Rev. 1999;169:225–39.

92. Buckley CD, Amft N, Bradfield PF, Pilling D, Ross E, Arenzana-Seisdedos F, et al. Persistent induction of the chemokine receptor CXCR4 by TGF-beta 1 on synovial T cells contributes to their accumulation within the rheumatoid synovium. J Immunol. 2000;165:3423–9.

93. Minamino T, Christou H, Hsieh CM, Liu Y, Dhawan V, Abraham NG, et al. Targeted expression of heme oxygenase-1 prevents the pulmonary inflammatory and vascular responses to hypoxia. Proc Natl Acad Sci U S A. 2001;98:8798–803.

94. Voelkel NF, Mizuno S, Bogaard HJ. The role of hypoxia in pulmonary vascular diseases: a perspective. Am J Physiol Lung Cell Mol Physiol. 2013;304:L457–65.

95. Kwapiszewska G, Wilhelm J, Wolff S, Laumanns I, Koenig IR, Ziegler A, et al. Expression profiling of laser-microdissected intrapulmonary arteries in hypoxia-induced PH. Respir Res. 2005;6:109.

96. Madjdpour C, Jewell UR, Kneller S, Ziegler U, Schwendener R, Booy C, et al. Decreased alveolar oxygen induces lung inflammation. Am J Physiol Lung Cell Mol Physiol. 2003;284:L360–7.

97. Chao J, Wood JG, Gonzalez NC. Alveolar macrophages initiate the systemic microvascular inflammatory response to alveolar hypoxia. Respir Physiol Neurobiol. 2011;178:439–48.

98. Banasova A, Maxova H, Hampl V, Vizek M, Povysilova V, Novotna J, et al. Prevention of mast cell degranulation by disodium cromoglycate attenuates the development of hypoxic PH in rats exposed to chronic hypoxia. Respiration; Int Rev Thoracic Dis. 2008;76:102–7.

99. Hoffmann J, Yin J, Kukucka M, Yin N, Saarikko I, Sterner-Kock A, et al. Mast cells promote lung vascular remodelling in PH. Eur Respir J. 2011;37:1400–10.

100. Dahal BK, Kosanovic D, Kaulen C, Cornitescu T, Savai R, Hoffmann J, et al. Involvement of mast cells in monocrotaline-induced PH in rats. Respir Res. 2011;12:60.

101. Bartelds B, van Loon RL, Mohaupt S, Wijnberg H, Dickinson MG, Boersma B, et al. Mast cell inhibition improves pulmonary vascular remodeling in PH. Chest. 2012;141:651–60.

102. Farha S, Sharp J, Asosingh K, Park M, Comhair SA, Tang WH, et al. Mast cell number, phenotype, and function in human pulmonary arterial hypertension. Pulm Circ. 2012;2:220–8.

103. Miyata M, Sakuma F, Yoshimura A, Ishikawa H, Nishimaki T, Kasukawa R. PH in rats. 1. Role of bromodeoxyuridine-positive mononuclear cells and alveolar macrophages. Int Arch Allergy Immunol. 1995;108:281–6.

104. Stenmark KR, Morganroth ML, Remigio LK, Voelkel NF, Murphy RC, Henson PM, et al. Alveolar inflammation and arachidonate metabolism in monocrotaline-induced PH. Am J Physiol. 1985;248:H859–66.

105. Stenmark KR, James SL, Voelkel NF, Toews WH, Reeves JT, Murphy RC. Leukotriene C4 and D4 in neonates with hypoxemia and PH. N Engl J Med. 1983;309:77–80.

106. Epelman S, Lavine KJ, Randolph GJ. Origin and functions of tissue macrophages. Immunity. 2014;41:21–35.

107. Chen YF, Zhou D, Metzger T, Gallup M, Jeanne M, Gould DB, et al. Spontaneous development of autoimmune uveitis Is CCR2 dependent. Am J Pathol. 2014;184:1695–705.

108. Majmudar MD, Keliher EJ, Heidt T, Leuschner F, Truelove J, Sena BF, et al. Monocyte-directed RNAi targeting CCR2 improves infarct healing in atherosclerosis-prone mice. Circulation. 2013;127:2038–46.

109. Osterholzer JJ, Olszewski MA, Murdock BJ, Chen GH, Erb-Downward JR, Subbotina N, et al. Implicating exudate macrophages and Ly-6C(high) monocytes in CCR2-dependent lung fibrosis following gene-targeted alveolar injury. J Immunol. 2013;190:3447–57.

110. Arai M, Ikawa Y, Chujo S, Hamaguchi Y, Ishida W, Shirasaki F, et al. Chemokine receptors CCR2 and CX3CR1 regulate skin fibrosis in the mouse model of cytokine-induced systemic sclerosis. J Dermatol Sci. 2013;69:250–8.

111. Ceppo F, Berthou F, Jager J, Dumas K, Cormont M, Tanti JF. Implication of the Tpl2 kinase in inflammatory changes and insulin resistance induced by the interaction between adipocytes and macrophages. Endocrinology. 2014;155:951–64.

112. Comito G, Giannoni E, Segura CP, Barcellos-de-Souza P, Raspollini MR, Baroni G, et al. Cancer-associated fibroblasts and M2-polarized macrophages synergize during prostate carcinoma progression. Oncogene. 2014;33:2423–31.

113. Donlin LT, Jayatilleke A, Giannopoulou EG, Kalliolias GD, Ivashkiv LB. Modulation of TNF-induced macrophage polarization by synovial fibroblasts. J Immunol. 2014;193(5):2373–83.

114. Yet SF, Perrella MA, Layne MD, Hsieh CM, Maemura K, Kobzik L, et al. Hypoxia induces severe right ventricular dilatation and infarction in heme oxygenase-1 null mice. J Clin Invest. 1999;103:R23–9.

115. Yamaji-Kegan K, Su Q, Angelini DJ, Myers AC, Cheadle C, Johns RA. Hypoxia-induced mitogenic factor (HIMF/FIZZ1/RELMalpha) increases lung inflammation and activates pulmonary microvascular endothelial cells via an IL-4-dependent mechanism. J Immunol. 2010;185:5539–48.

116. Angelini DJ, Su Q, Yamaji-Kegan K, Fan C, Teng X, Hassoun PM, et al. Resistin-like molecule-beta in scleroderma-associated PH. Am J Respir Cell Mol Biol. 2009;41:553–61.

117. Yamaji-Kegan K, Takimoto E, Zhang A, Weiner NC, Meuchel LW, Berger AE, et al. Hypoxia-induced mitogenic factor (FIZZ1/RELMalpha) induces endothelial cell apoptosis and subsequent interleukin-4-dependent PH. Am J Physiol Lung Cell Mol Physiol. 2014;306:L1090–103.

118. Tuder RM, Davis LA, Graham BB. Targeting energetic metabolism: a new frontier in the pathogenesis and treatment of PH. Am J Respir Crit Care Med. 2012;185:260–6.

119. Sawada H, Mitani Y, Maruyama J, Jiang BH, Ikeyama Y, Dida FA, et al. A nuclear factor-kappaB inhibitor pyrrolidine dithiocarbamate ameliorates PH in rats. Chest. 2007;132:1265–74.

120. Huang J, Kaminski PM, Edwards JG, Yeh A, Wolin MS, Frishman WH, et al. Pyrrolidine dithiocarbamate restores endothelial cell membrane integrity and attenuates monocrotaline-induced pulmonary artery hypertension. Am J Physiol Lung Cell Mol Physiol. 2008;294:L1250–9.

121. Sarada SKS, Himadri P, Veeramohan PH, Mathew T, Saumya S, Chitharanjan M. Nifedipine inhibits hypoxia induced transvascular leakage through down regulation of NFkB. Respir Physiol Neurobiol. 2012;183:26–34.

122. Li J, Rao J, Liu Y, Cao Y, Zhang Y, Zhang Q, et al. 15-Lipoxygenase promotes chronic hypoxia-induced pulmonary artery inflammation via positive interaction with nuclear factor-kappaB. Arterioscler Thromb Vasc Biol. 2013;33:971–9.

123. Price LC, Caramori G, Perros F, Meng C, Gambaryan N, Dorfmuller P, et al. Nuclear factor kappa-B is activated in the pulmonary vessels of patients with end-stage idiopathic pulmonary arterial hypertension. PLoS One. 2013;8, e75415.

124. Deng X, Xu M, Yuan C, Yin L, Chen X, Zhou X, et al. Transcriptional regulation of increased CCL2 expression in pulmonary fibrosis involves nuclear factor-kappaB and activator protein-1. Int J Biochem Cell Biol. 2013;45:1366–76.

125. Anton K, Banerjee D, Glod J. Macrophage-associated mesenchymal stem cells assume an activated, migratory, pro-inflammatory phenotype with increased IL-6 and CXCL10 secretion. PLoS One. 2012;7, e35036.

126. Viedt C, Vogel J, Athanasiou T, Shen W, Orth SR, Kubler W, et al. Monocyte chemoattractant protein-1 induces proliferation and interleukin-6 production in human smooth muscle cells by differential activation of nuclear factor-kappaB and activator protein-1. Arterioscler Thromb Vasc Biol. 2002;22:914–20.

127. Nakayama T, Kurobe H, Sugasawa N, Kinoshita H, Higashida M, Matsuoka Y, et al. Role of macrophage-derived hypoxia-inducible factor (HIF)-1alpha as a mediator of vascular remodelling. Cardiovasc Res. 2013;99:705–15.

128. Fielding CA, Jones GW, McLoughlin RM, McLeod L, Hammond VJ, Uceda J, et al. Interleukin-6 signaling drives fibrosis in unresolved inflammation. Immunity. 2014;40:40–50.

129. Gao W, McCormick J, Connolly M, Balogh E, Veale DJ, Fearon U. Hypoxia and STAT3 signalling interactions regulate pro-inflammatory pathways in rheumatoid arthritis. Ann Rheum Dis. 2014.

130. Pawlus MR, Wang L, Hu CJ. STAT3 and HIF1alpha cooperatively activate HIF1 target genes in MDA-MB-231 and RCC4 cells. Oncogene. 2014;33:1670–9.

131. Okabe Y, Medzhitov R. Tissue-specific signals control reversible program of localization and functional polarization of macrophages. Cell. 2014;157:832–44.

132. Bours MJ, Swennen EL, Di Virgilio F, Cronstein BN, Dagnelie PC. Adenosine 5'-triphosphate and adenosine as endogenous signaling molecules in immunity and inflammation. Pharmacol Ther. 2006;112:358–404.

133. Burnstock G. Pathophysiology and therapeutic potential of purinergic signaling. Pharmacol Rev. 2006;58:58–86.

134. Erlinge D, Burnstock G. P2 receptors in cardiovascular regulation and disease. Purinergic Signal. 2008;4:1–20.

135. Ralevic V, Burnstock G. Receptors for purines and pyrimidines. Pharmacol Rev. 1998;50:413–92.

136. Gerasimovskaya EV, Ahmad S, White CW, Jones PL, Carpenter TC, Stenmark KR. Extracellular ATP is an autocrine/paracrine regulator of hypoxia-induced adventitial fibroblast growth. Signaling through extracellular signal-regulated kinase-1/2 and the Egr-1 transcription factor. J Biol Chem. 2002;277:44638–50.

137. Abbracchio MP, Burnstock G, Boeynaems JM, Barnard EA, Boyer JL, Kennedy C, et al. International Union of Pharmacology LV3: update on the P2Y G protein-coupled nucleotide receptors: from molecular mechanisms and pathophysiology to therapy. Pharmacol Rev. 2006;58:281–341.

138. Di Virgilio F, Solini A. P2 receptors: new potential players in atherosclerosis. Br J Pharmacol. 2002;135:831–42.

139. Satterwhite CM, Farrelly AM, Bradley ME. Chemotactic, mitogenic, and angiogenic actions of UTP on vascular endothelial cells. Am J Physiol. 1999;276:H1091–7.

140. Jacobson JR, Dudek SM, Singleton PA, Kolosova IA, Verin AD, Garcia JG. Endothelial cell barrier enhancement by ATP is mediated by the small GTPase Rac and cortactin. Am J Physiol Lung Cell Mol Physiol. 2006;291:L289–95.

141. Kolosova IA, Mirzapoiazova T, Adyshev D, Usatyuk P, Romer LH, Jacobson JR, et al. Signaling pathways involved in adenosine triphosphate-induced endothelial cell barrier enhancement. Circ Res. 2005;97:115–24.

142. Kaczmarek E, Erb L, Koziak K, Jarzyna R, Wink MR, Guckelberger O, et al. Modulation of endothelial cell migration by extracellular nucleotides: involvement of focal adhesion kinase and phosphatidylinositol 3-kinase-mediated pathways. Thromb Haemost. 2005;93:735–42.

143. Lemoli RM, Ferrari D, Fogli M, Rossi L, Pizzirani C, Forchap S, et al. Extracellular nucleotides are potent stimulators of human hematopoietic stem cells in vitro and in vivo. Blood. 2004;104:1662–70.

144. Rossi L, Manfredini R, Bertolini F, Ferrari D, Fogli M, Zini R, et al. The extracellular nucleotide UTP is a potent inducer of hematopoietic stem cell migration. Blood. 2006.

145. Erlinge D, Hou M, Webb TE, Barnard EA, Moller S. Phenotype changes of the vascular smooth muscle cell regulate P2 receptor expression as measured by quantitative RT-PCR. Biochem Biophys Res Commun. 1998;248:864–70.

146. Huang N, Wang DJ, Heppel LA. Extracellular ATP is a mitogen for 3T3, 3T6, and A431 cells and acts synergistically with other growth factors. Proc Natl Acad Sci U S A. 1989;86:7904–8.

147. Gerasimovskaya EV, Woodward HN, Tucker DA, Stenmark KR. Extracellular ATP is a pro-angiogenic factor for pulmonary artery vasa vasorum endothelial cells. Angiogenesis. 2008;11:169–82.

148. Woodward HN, Anwar A, Riddle S, Taraseviciene-Stewart L, Fragoso M, Stenmark KR, et al. PI3K, Rho, and ROCK play a key role in hypoxia-induced ATP release and ATP-stimulated angiogenic responses in pulmonary artery vasa vasorum endothelial cells. Am J Physiol Lung Cell Mol Physiol. 2009;297:L954–64.

149. Lyubchenko T, Woodward H, Veo KD, Burns N, Nijmeh H, Liubchenko GA, et al. P2Y1 and P2Y13 purinergic receptors mediate Ca2+ signaling and proliferative responses in pulmonary artery vasa vasorum endothelial cells. Am J Physiol Cell Physiol. 2011;300:C266–75.

150. Yegutkin GG. Nucleotide- and nucleoside-converting ectoenzymes: Important modulators of purinergic signalling cascade. Biochim Biophys Acta. 1783;2008:673–94.

151. Kaczmarek E, Koziak K, Sevigny J, Siegel JB, Anrather J, Beaudoin AR, et al. Identification and characterization of CD39/vascular ATP diphosphohydrolase. J Biol Chem. 1996;271:33116–22.

152. Robson SC, Sevigny J, Zimmermann H. The E-NTPDase family of ectonucleotidases: structure function relationships and pathophysiological significance. Purinergic Signal. 2006;2:409–30.

153. Marcus AJ, Broekman MJ, Drosopoulos JH, Islam N, Pinsky DJ, Sesti C, et al. Metabolic control of excessive extracellular nucleotide accumulation by CD39/ecto-nucleotidase-1: implications for ischemic vascular diseases. J Pharmacol Exp Ther. 2003;305:9–16.

154. Meghji P, Pearson JD, Slakey LL. Kinetics of extracellular ATP hydrolysis by microvascular endothelial cells from rat heart. Biochem J. 1995;308(Pt 3):725–31.

155. Goepfert C, Sundberg C, Sevigny J, Enjyoji K, Hoshi T, Csizmadia E, et al. Disordered cellular migration and angiogenesis in cd39-null mice. Circulation. 2001;104:3109–15.

156. Zernecke A, Bidzhekov K, Ozuyaman B, Fraemohs L, Liehn EA, Luscher-Firzlaff JM, et al. CD73/ecto-5'-nucleotidase protects against vascular inflammation and neointima formation. Circulation. 2006;113:2120–7.

157. Robson SC, Kaczmarek E, Siegel JB, Candinas D, Koziak K, Millan M, et al. Loss of ATP diphosphohydrolase activity with endothelial cell activation. J Exp Med. 1997;185:153–63.

158. Eltzschig HK, Ibla JC, Furuta GT, Leonard MO, Jacobson KA, Enjyoji K, et al. Coordinated adenine nucleotide phosphohydrolysis and nucleoside signaling in posthypoxic endothelium: role of ectonucleotidases and adenosine A2B receptors. J Exp Med. 2003;198:783–96.

159. Koszalka P, Ozuyaman B, Huo Y, Zernecke A, Flogel U, Braun N, et al. Targeted disruption of cd73/ecto-5'-nucleotidase alters thromboregulation and augments vascular inflammatory response. Circ Res. 2004;95:814–21.

160. Van Linden A, Eltzschig HK. Role of pulmonary adenosine during hypoxia: extracellular generation, signaling and metabolism by surface adenosine deaminase/CD26. Expert Opin Biol Ther. 2007;7:1437–47.

161. Humbert M, Morrell NW, Archer SL, Stenmark KR, MacLean MR, Lang IM, et al. Cellular and molecular pathobiology of pulmonary arterial hypertension. J Am Coll Cardiol. 2004;43:13S–24.

162. Henttinen T, Jalkanen S, Yegutkin GG. Adherent leukocytes prevent adenosine formation and impair endothelial barrier function by Ecto-5'-nucleotidase/CD73-dependent mechanism. J Biol Chem. 2003;278:24888–95.

163. Hasegawa T, Bouis D, Liao H, Visovatti SH, Pinsky DJ. Ecto-5' nucleotidase (CD73)-mediated adenosine generation and signaling in murine cardiac allograft vasculopathy. Circ Res. 2008; 103:1410–21.

164. Eckle T, Faigle M, Grenz A, Laucher S, Thompson LF, Eltzschig HK. A2B adenosine receptor dampens hypoxia-induced vascular leak. Blood. 2008;111:2024–35.

165. Thompson LF, Eltzschig HK, Ibla JC, Van De Wiele CJ, Resta R, Morote-Garcia JC, et al. Crucial role for ecto-5'-nucleotidase (CD73) in vascular leakage during hypoxia. J Exp Med. 2004; 200:1395–405.

166. Paty PS, Sherman PF, Shepard JM, Malik AB, Kaplan JE. Role of adenosine in platelet-mediated reduction in pulmonary vascular permeability. Am J Physiol. 1992;262:H771–7.

167. Fredholm BB, IJzerman AP, Jacobson KA, Klotz KN, Linden J. International Union of Pharmacology. XXV. Nomenclature and classification of adenosine receptors. Pharmacol Rev. 2001;53: 527–52.

168. Merighi S, Mirandola P, Varani K, Gessi S, Leung E, Baraldi PG, et al. A glance at adenosine receptors: novel target for antitumor therapy. Pharmacol Ther. 2003;100:31–48.

169. Jacobson KA, Gao ZG. Adenosine receptors as therapeutic targets. Nat Rev Drug Discov. 2006;5:247–64.

170. Lu Q, Harrington EO, Newton J, Casserly B, Radin G, Warburton R, et al. Adenosine protected against pulmonary edema through transporter- and receptor A2-mediated endothelial barrier enhancement. Am J Physiol Lung Cell Mol Physiol. 2010;298: L755–67.

171. Tsutsui S, Schnermann J, Noorbakhsh F, Henry S, Yong VW, Winston BW, et al. A1 adenosine receptor upregulation and activation attenuates neuroinflammation and demyelination in a model of multiple sclerosis. J Neurosc: Off J Soc Neurosci. 2004; 24:1521–9.

172. Park SW, Chen SW, Kim M, Brown KM, D'Agati VD, Lee HT. Protection against acute kidney injury via A(1) adenosine receptor-mediated Akt activation reduces liver injury after liver ischemia and reperfusion in mice. J Pharmacol Exp Ther. 2010;333:36–47.

173. Yildiz G, Demiryurek AT, Gumusel B, Lippton H. Ischemic preconditioning modulates ischemia-reperfusion injury in the rat lung: role of adenosine receptors. Eur J Pharmacol. 2007;556: 44–50.

174. Nakav S, Chaimovitz C, Sufaro Y, Lewis EC, Shaked G, Czeiger D, et al. Anti-inflammatory preconditioning by agonists of adenosine A1 receptor. PLoS One. 2008;3, e2107.

175. Heller AR, Rothermel J, Weigand MA, Plaschke K, Schmeck J, Wendel M, et al. Adenosine A1 and A2 receptor agonists reduce endotoxin-induced cellular energy depletion and oedema formation in the lung. Eur J Anaesthesiol. 2007;24:258–66.

176. Umapathy NS, Zemskov EA, Gonzales J, Gorshkov BA, Sridhar S, Chakraborty T, et al. Extracellular beta-nicotinamide adenine dinucleotide (beta-NAD) promotes the endothelial cell barrier integrity via PKA- and EPAC1/Rac1-dependent actin cytoskeleton rearrangement. J Cell Physiol. 2010;223:215–23.

177. Sayner SL. Emerging themes of cAMP regulation of the pulmonary endothelial barrier. Am J Physiol Lung Cell Mol Physiol. 2011;300:L667–78.

178. Siddaramappa Umapathy N, Kaczmarek E, Fatteh N, Burns N, Lucas R, Stenmark KR, et al. Adenosine A1 receptors promote vasa vasorum endothelial cell barrier integrity via Gi and Akt-dependent actin cytoskeleton remodeling. PLoS One. 2013;8, e59733.

179. Petrache I, Birukova A, Ramirez SI, Garcia JG, Verin AD. The role of the microtubules in tumor necrosis factor-alpha-induced endothelial cell permeability. Am J Respir Cell Mol Biol. 2003;28:574–81.

180. Kiemer AK, Weber NC, Furst R, Bildner N, Kulhanek-Heinze S, Vollmar AM. Inhibition of p38 MAPK activation via induction of MKP-1: atrial natriuretic peptide reduces TNF-alpha-induced actin polymerization and endothelial permeability. Circ Res. 2002;90:874–81.

181. Friedl J, Puhlmann M, Bartlett DL, Libutti SK, Turner EN, Gnant MF, et al. Induction of permeability across endothelial cell monolayers by tumor necrosis factor (TNF) occurs via a tissue factor-dependent mechanism: relationship between the procoagulant and permeability effects of TNF. Blood. 2002;100:1334–9.

182. Taylor CT, Dzus AL, Colgan SP. Autocrine regulation of epithelial permeability by hypoxia: role for polarized release of tumor necrosis factor alpha. Gastroenterology. 1998;114:657–68.

183. Yu X, Deng L, Wang D, Li N, Chen X, Cheng X, et al. Mechanism of TNF-alpha autocrine effects in hypoxic cardiomyocytes: initiated by hypoxia inducible factor 1alpha, presented by exosomes. J Mol Cell Cardiol. 2012;53:848–57.

184. Soon E, Holmes AM, Treacy CM, Doughty NJ, Southgate L, Machado RD, et al. Elevated levels of inflammatory cytokines predict survival in idiopathic and familial pulmonary arterial hypertension. Circulation. 2010;122:920–7.

185. Liu FQ, Liu Y, Lui VC, Lamb JR, Tam PK, Chen Y. Hypoxia modulates lipopolysaccharide induced TNF-alpha expression in murine macrophages. Exp Cell Res. 2008;314:1327–36.

186. Rajsheker S, Manka D, Blomkalns AL, Chatterjee TK, Stoll LL, Weintraub NL. Crosstalk between perivascular adipose tissue and blood vessels. Curr Opin Pharmacol. 2010;10:191–6.

187. Fresquet F, Pourageaud F, Leblais V, Brandes RP, Savineau JP, Marthan R, et al. Role of reactive oxygen species and gp91phox in endothelial dysfunction of pulmonary arteries induced by chronic hypoxia. Br J Pharmacol. 2006;148:714–23.

188. Hoshikawa Y, Ono S, Suzuki S, Tanita T, Chida M, Song C, et al. Generation of oxidative stress contributes to the development of PH induced by hypoxia. J Appl Physiol. 2001;90:1299–306.

189. Jackson IL, Chen L, Batinic-Haberle I, Vujaskovic Z. Superoxide dismutase mimetic reduces hypoxia-induced O2*-, TGF-beta, and VEGF production by macrophages. Free Radic Res. 2007;41:8–14.

190. Jernigan NL, Resta TC, Walker BR. Contribution of oxygen radicals to altered NO-dependent pulmonary vasodilation in acute and chronic hypoxia. Am J Physiol Lung Cell Mol Physiol. 2004;286:L947–55.

191. Liu JQ, Zelko IN, Erbynn EM, Sham JS, Folz RJ. Hypoxic PH: role of superoxide and NADPH oxidase (gp91phox). Am J Physiol Lung Cell Mol Physiol. 2006;290:L2–10.

192. Nozik-Grayck E, Huang YC, Carraway MS, Piantadosi CA. Bicarbonate-dependent superoxide release and pulmonary artery tone. Am J Physiol Heart Circ Physiol. 2003;285:H2327–35.

193. Weissmann N, Zeller S, Schafer RU, Turowski C, Ay M, Quanz K, et al. Impact of mitochondria and NADPH oxidases on acute and sustained hypoxic pulmonary vasoconstriction. Am J Respir Cell Mol Biol. 2006;34:505–13.

194. Nozik-Grayck E, Stenmark KR. Role of reactive oxygen species in chronic hypoxia-induced PH and vascular remodeling. Adv Exp Med Biol. 2007;618:101–12.

195. Aggarwal S, Gross CM, Sharma S, Fineman JR, Black SM. Reactive oxygen species in pulmonary vascular remodeling. Compr Physiol. 2013;3:1011–34.

196. Al Ghouleh I, Khoo NK, Knaus UG, Griendling KK, Touyz RM, Thannickal VJ, et al. Oxidases and peroxidases in cardiovascular and lung disease: new concepts in reactive oxygen species signaling. Free Radic Biol Med. 2011;51:1271–88.

197. Frazziano G, Champion HC, Pagano PJ. NADPH oxidase-derived ROS and the regulation of pulmonary vessel tone. Am J Physiol Heart Circ Physiol. 2012;302:H2166–77.

198. Paulin R, Michelakis ED. The metabolic theory of pulmonary arterial hypertension. Circ Res. 2014;115:148–64.

199. Maron BA, Loscalzo J. PH: pathophysiology and signaling pathways. Handb Exp Pharmacol. 2013;218:31–58.

200. Cottrill KA, Chan SY. Metabolic dysfunction in PH: the expanding relevance of the Warburg effect. Eur J Clin Invest. 2013;43: 855–65.

201. Waypa GB, Marks JD, Guzy R, Mungai PT, Schriewer J, Dokic D, et al. Hypoxia triggers subcellular compartmental redox signaling in vascular smooth muscle cells. Circ Res. 2010;106:526–35.

202. Granger DN. Role of xanthine oxidase and granulocytes in ischemia-reperfusion injury. Am J Physiol. 1988;255: H1269–75.

203. Hartney T, Birari R, Venkataraman S, Villegas L, Martinez M, Black SM, et al. Xanthine oxidase-derived ROS upregulate Egr-1 via ERK1/2 in PA smooth muscle cells; model to test impact of extracellular ROS in chronic hypoxia. PLoS One. 2011;6, e27531.

204. Sharma S, Kumar S, Wiseman DA, Kallarackal S, Ponnala S, Elgaish M, et al. Perinatal changes in superoxide generation in the ovine lung: alterations associated with increased pulmonary blood flow. Vascul Pharmacol. 2010;53:38–52.

205. Jankov RP, Kantores C, Pan J, Belik J. Contribution of xanthine oxidase-derived superoxide to chronic hypoxic PH in neonatal rats. Am J Physiol Lung Cell Mol Physiol. 2008;294:L233–45.

206. Adkins WK, Taylor AE. Role of xanthine oxidase and neutrophils in ischemia-reperfusion injury in rabbit lung. J Appl Physiol. 1990;69:2012–8.

207. Boueiz A, Damarla M, Hassoun PM. Xanthine oxidoreductase in respiratory and cardiovascular disorders. Am J Physiol Lung Cell Mol Physiol. 2008;294:L830–40.

208. Chinnaiyan AM, Huber-Lang M, Kumar-Sinha C, Barrette TR, Shankar-Sinha S, Sarma VJ, et al. Molecular signatures of sepsis: multiorgan gene expression profiles of systemic inflammation. Am J Pathol. 2001;159:1199–209.

209. Ichinose M, Sugiura H, Yamagata S, Koarai A, Tomaki M, Ogawa H, et al. Xanthine oxidase inhibition reduces reactive nitrogen species production in COPD airways. Eur Respir J. 2003;22: 457–61.

210. Kim BS, Serebreni L, Hamdan O, Wang L, Parniani A, Sussan T, et al. Xanthine oxidoreductase is a critical mediator of cigarette smoke-induced endothelial cell DNA damage and apoptosis. Free Radic Biol Med. 2013;60:336–46.

211. Mangerich A, Dedon PC, Fox JG, Tannenbaum SR, Wogan GN. Chemistry meets biology in colitis-associated carcinogenesis. Free Radic Res. 2013;47:958–86.

212. Nanduri J, Vaddi DR, Khan SA, Wang N, Makerenko V, Prabhakar NR. Xanthine oxidase mediates hypoxia-inducible factor-2alpha degradation by intermittent hypoxia. PLoS One. 2013;8, e75838.

213. Riaz AA, Schramm R, Sato T, Menger MD, Jeppsson B, Thorlacius H. Oxygen radical-dependent expression of CXC chemokines regulate ischemia/reperfusion-induced leukocyte adhesion in the mouse colon. Free Radic Biol Med. 2003;35:782–9.

214. Riaz AA, Wan MX, Schafer T, Dawson P, Menger MD, Jeppsson B, et al. Allopurinol and superoxide dismutase protect against leucocyte-endothelium interactions in a novel model of colonic ischaemia-reperfusion. Br J Surg. 2002;89:1572–80.

215. Shibata K, Cregg N, Engelberts D, Takeuchi A, Fedorko L, Kavanagh BP. Hypercapnic acidosis may attenuate acute lung injury by inhibition of endogenous xanthine oxidase. Am J Respir Crit Care Med. 1998;158:1578–84.

216. Xiang L, Klintman D, Thorlacius H. Allopurinol inhibits CXC chemokine expression and leukocyte adhesion in endotoxemic liver injury. Inflamm Res: Off J Eur Histamine Res Soc … [et al]. 2003;52:353–8.

217. Gibbings S, Elkins ND, Fitzgerald H, Tiao J, Weyman ME, Shibao G, et al. Xanthine oxidoreductase promotes the inflammatory state of mononuclear phagocytes through effects on chemokine

expression, peroxisome proliferator-activated receptor-{gamma} sumoylation, and HIF-1{alpha}. J Biol Chem. 2011;286:961–75.

218. Freund-Michel V, Guibert C, Dubois M, Courtois A, Marthan R, Savineau JP, et al. Reactive oxygen species as therapeutic targets in PH. Ther Adv Respir Dis. 2013;7:175–200.

219. Fukai T, Ushio-Fukai M. Superoxide dismutases: role in redox signaling, vascular function, and diseases. Antioxid Redox Signal. 2011;15:1583–606.

220. Ushio-Fukai M. Compartmentalization of redox signaling through NADPH oxidase-derived ROS. Antioxid Redox Signal. 2009;11: 1289–99.

221. Van Rheen Z, Fattman C, Domarski S, Majka S, Klemm D, Stenmark KR, et al. Lung extracellular superoxide dismutase overexpression lessens bleomycin-induced PH and vascular remodeling. Am J Respir Cell Mol Biol. 2011;44:500–8.

222. Ahmed MN, Zhang Y, Codipilly C, Zaghloul N, Patel D, Wolin M, et al. Extracellular superoxide dismutase overexpression can reverse the course of hypoxia-induced PH. Mol Med. 2012;18:38–46.

223. Xu D, Guo H, Xu X, Lu Z, Fassett J, Hu X, et al. Exacerbated pulmonary arterial hypertension and right ventricular hypertrophy in animals with loss of function of extracellular superoxide dismutase. Hypertension. 2011;58:303–9.

224. Ramiro-Diaz JM, Nitta CH, Maston LD, Codianni S, Giermakowska W, Resta TC, et al. NFAT is required for spontaneous PH in superoxide dismutase 1 knockout mice. Am J Physiol Lung Cell Mol Physiol. 2013;304:L613–25.

225. Redout EM, Wagner MJ, Zuidwijk MJ, Boer C, Musters RJ, van Hardeveld C, et al. Right-ventricular failure is associated with increased mitochondrial complex II activity and production of reactive oxygen species. Cardiovasc Res. 2007;75:770–81.

226. Bowers R, Cool C, Murphy RC, Tuder RM, Hopken MW, Flores SC, et al. Oxidative stress in severe PH. Am J Respir Crit Care Med. 2004;169:764–9.

227. Archer SL, Marsboom G, Kim GH, Zhang HJ, Toth PT, Svensson EC, et al. Epigenetic attenuation of mitochondrial superoxide dismutase 2 in pulmonary arterial hypertension: a basis for excessive cell proliferation and a new therapeutic target. Circulation. 2010;121:2661–71.

228. Fijalkowska I, Xu W, Comhair SA, Janocha AJ, Mavrakis LA, Krishnamachary B, et al. Hypoxia inducible-factor1alpha regulates the metabolic shift of pulmonary hypertensive endothelial cells. Am J Pathol. 2010;176:1130–8.

229. Bonnet S, Michelakis ED, Porter CJ, Andrade-Navarro MA, Thebaud B, Bonnet S, et al. An abnormal mitochondrial-hypoxia inducible factor-1alpha-Kv channel pathway disrupts oxygen sensing and triggers pulmonary arterial hypertension in fawn hooded rats: similarities to human pulmonary arterial hypertension. Circulation. 2006;113:2630–41.

230. Wedgwood S, Lakshminrusimha S, Fukai T, Russell JA, Schumacker PT, Steinhorn RH. Hydrogen peroxide regulates extracellular superoxide dismutase activity and expression in neonatal PH. Antioxid Redox Signal. 2011;15:1497–506.

231. Klein K, Gay S. Epigenetic modifications in rheumatoid arthritis, a review. Curr Opin Pharmacol. 2013;13:420–5.

232. Shanmugam MK, Sethi G. Role of epigenetics in inflammation-associated diseases. Subcell Biochem. 2013;61:627–57.

233. You JS, Jones PA. Cancer genetics and epigenetics: two sides of the same coin? Cancer Cell. 2012;22:9–20.

234. Timp W, Feinberg AP. Cancer as a dysregulated epigenome allowing cellular growth advantage at the expense of the host. Nat Rev Cancer. 2013;13:497–510.

235. McCarthy N. Epigenetics: worth another look? Nat Rev Cancer. 2012;12:2.

236. Perez-Perri JI, Acevedo JM, Wappner P. Epigenetics: new questions on the response to hypoxia. Int J Mol Sci. 2011;12: 4705–21.

237. Brigati C, Banelli B, di Vinci A, Casciano I, Allemanni G, Forlani A, et al. Inflammation, HIF-1, and the epigenetics that follows. Mediators Inflamm. 2010;2010:263914.

238. Soubrier F, Chung WK, Machado R, Grunig E, Aldred M, Geraci M, et al. Genetics and genomics of pulmonary arterial hypertension. J Am Coll Cardiol. 2013;62:D13–21.

239. Zhao L, Chen CN, Hajji N, Oliver E, Cotroneo E, Wharton J, et al. Histone deacetylation inhibition in PH: therapeutic potential of valproic acid and suberoylanilide hydroxamic acid. Circulation. 2012;126:455–67.

240. Yang Q, Lu Z, Ramchandran R, Longo LD, Raj JU. Pulmonary artery smooth muscle cell proliferation and migration in fetal lambs acclimatized to high-altitude long-term hypoxia: role of histone acetylation. Am J Physiol Lung Cell Mol Physiol. 2012;303:L1001–10.

241. Gong K, Xing D, Li P, Aksut B, Ambalavanan N, Yang Q, et al. Hypoxia induces downregulation of PPAR-gamma in isolated pulmonary arterial smooth muscle cells and in rat lung via transforming growth factor-beta signaling. Am J Physiol Lung Cell Mol Physiol. 2011;301:L899–907.

242. Courboulin A, Paulin R, Giguere NJ, Saksouk N, Perreault T, Meloche J, et al. Role for miR-204 in human pulmonary arterial hypertension. J Exp Med. 2011;208:535–48.

243. Pullamsetti SS, Doebele C, Fischer A, Savai R, Kojonazarov B, Dahal BK, et al. Inhibition of microRNA-17 improves lung and heart function in experimental PH. Am J Respir Crit Care Med. 2012;185:409–19.

244. Jin Y, Jin Y, Chen B, Tipple TE, Nelin LD. Arginase II is a target of miR-17-5p and regulates miR-17-5p expression in human pulmonary artery smooth muscle cells. Am J Physiol Lung Cell Mol Physiol. 2014;307:L197–204.

245. Gou D, Ramchandran R, Peng X, Yao L, Kang K, Sarkar J, et al. miR-210 has an antiapoptotic effect in pulmonary artery smooth muscle cells during hypoxia. Am J Physiol Lung Cell Mol Physiol. 2012;303:L682–91.

246. Chan YC, Banerjee J, Choi SY, Sen CK. miR-210: the master hypoxamir. Microcirculation. 2012;19:215–23.

247. Bodempudi V, Hergert P, Smith K, Xia H, Herrera J, Peterson M, et al. miR-210 promotes IPF fibroblast proliferation in response to hypoxia. Am J Physiol Lung Cell Mol Physiol. 2014;307(4): L283–94.

248. Caruso P, Dempsie Y, Stevens HC, McDonald RA, Long L, Lu R, et al. A role for miR-145 in pulmonary arterial hypertension: evidence from mouse models and patient samples. Circ Res. 2012;111:290–300.

249. Sarkar J, Gou D, Turaka P, Viktorova E, Ramchandran R, Raj JU. MicroRNA-21 plays a role in hypoxia-mediated pulmonary artery smooth muscle cell proliferation and migration. Am J Physiol Lung Cell Mol Physiol. 2010;299:L861–71.

250. Yue J, Guan J, Wang X, Zhang L, Yang Z, Ao Q, et al. MicroRNA-206 is involved in hypoxia-induced PH through targeting of the HIF-1alpha/Fhl-1 pathway. Lab Invest: J Tech Meth Pathol. 2013;93:748–59.

251. Caruso P, MacLean MR, Khanin R, McClure J, Soon E, Southgate M, et al. Dynamic changes in lung microRNA profiles during the development of PH due to chronic hypoxia and monocrotaline. Arterioscler Thromb Vasc Biol. 2010;30:716–23.

252. Yang S, Banerjee S, Freitas A, Cui H, Xie N, Abraham E, et al. miR-21 regulates chronic hypoxia-induced pulmonary vascular remodeling. Am J Physiol Lung Cell Mol Physiol. 2012;302: L521–9.

253. Watson JA, Watson CJ, McCann A, Baugh J. Epigenetics, the epicenter of the hypoxic response. Epigenetics: Off J DNA Methylation Soc. 2010;5:293–6.

254. Chen S, Sang N. Histone deacetylase inhibitors: the epigenetic therapeutics that repress hypoxia-inducible factors. J Biomed Biotechnol. 2011;2011:197946.

Genetics of Pulmonary Vascular Disease

Lijiang Ma and Wendy K. Chung

Abbreviations

ACD/MPV	Alveolar capillary dysplasia with misalignment of the pulmonary veins
AK	Adenylate kinase
ALK1	Activin-like Kinase-Type I
ALK6	Activin Receptor-like Kinase-6
ANCAs	Anti-neutrophil cytoplasmic antibodies
AT-III	Antithrombin III ATS: Arterial tortuosity syndrome
BAX	BCL-2 associated X-protein
BMPR2	Bone Morphogenetic Protein Receptor type 2 gene
BMPRIB	BMP receptor type IB
CAV1	Caveolin 1
CBLN2	Cerebellin 2
CCB	Calcium channel blockade
CHD	Congenital heart disease
COL3A1	Type III collagen
COPD	Chronic obstructive pulmonary disease
CSS	Churg-strauss syndrome
CTEPH	Chronic thrombotic embolic pulmonary hypertension
EIF2AK4	Eukaryotic Translation Initiation Factor 2 Alpha Kinase 4

ENG	Endoglin
F5	Coagulation factor V
FOXF1	Forkhead box F1
G-6-PD	Glucose-6-phosphate dehydrogenase
GCA	Giant cell arteritis
GLUT10	Glucose transporter 10
HDACs	Histone deacetylases
HHT	Hereditary hemorrhagic telangiectasia
HIF-1α	Hypoxia inducible factor 1α
HIV	Human immunodeficiency virus
HK	Hexokinase
HLA	Human leukocyte antigen
HPAH	Hereditary pulmonary arterial hypertension
HPS	Hepatopulmonary syndrome
IL12B	Interleukin 12B
IPAH	Idiopathic pulmonary arterial hypertension
KCNK3	Potassium Channel subfamily K, member 3
MTHFR	Methylenetetrahydrofolate reductase
NT5C3A	uridine 5-prime monophosphate hydrolase
PAH	Pulmonary arterial hypertension
PAVMs	Pulmonary arteriovenous malformations
PCH	Pulmonary capillary hemangiomatosis
PE	Pulmonary emboli
PFK	Phosphofructokinase
PGK1	Phosphoglycerate kinase 1
PK	Pyruvate kinase
PON1	Paraoxonase 1
PPHN	Persistent pulmonary hypertension of the newborn
PTPN22	protein tyrosine phosphatases nonreceptor-type 22
PVH	Pulmonary venous hypertension
PVOD	Pulmonary veno-occlusive disease
RBC	Red blood cell
SCD	Sickle cell disease
SERPINA1	Serpin peptidase inhibitor clade A, member 1
SLC2A10	Solute carrier family 2 member 10
SMAD1	Mothers against decapentaplegic 1
SMAD2	Mothers against decapentaplegic 2

L. Ma, MD, PhD
Molecular Genetics in Department of Pediatrics,
Columbia University Medical Center,
1150 St. Nicholas Avenue, Room 620,
New York 10032, NY, USA

Pediatrics, Columbia University Medical Center,
New York, NY, USA

W.K. Chung, MD, PhD (✉)
Molecular Genetics in Departments of Pediatrics and Medicine,
Columbia University Medical Center,
1150 St. Nicholas Avenue, Room 620,
New York 10032, NY, USA
e-mail: wkc15@columbia.edu

© Springer International Publishing Switzerland 2016
B.A. Maron et al. (eds.), *Pulmonary Hypertension: Basic Science to Clinical Medicine*, DOI 10.1007/978-3-319-23594-3_6

SMAD3	Mothers against decapentaplegic 3
SMAD4	Mothers against decapentaplegic 4
SMAD8	Mothers against decapentaplegic 8
SOD2	Superoxide dismutase 2
SSc	Systemic sclerosis
TBX2	T-box transcription factor-2
TBX4	T-box transcription factor-4
TGFβ	Transforming growth factor β
TGFBR2	TGF-β receptor II
TMEM70	Transmembrane protein 70
VTE	Venous thromboembolism
GWAS	Genome-wide association study

Introduction

The pulmonary circulation is composed of large conduit arteries, small muscular arteries, a thin-walled capillary bed and pulmonary veins. Small intrapulmonary arteries control regional distribution of pulmonary blood flow and determine pulmonary vascular resistance. The major function of the pulmonary circulation is gas exchange that occurs in the capillary bed. Pulmonary vascular disease for which genetic data are available includes pulmonary arterial hypertension, pulmonary veno-occlusive disease, pulmonary embolism, chronic thromboembolic and luminal pulmonary embolic disease, and arteriovenous malformations. This chapter reviews the genetic bases of pulmonary vascular diseases. Our increasing knowledge of these diseases has provided new opportunities for earlier diagnosis and treatment.

Pulmonary Arterial Hypertension

Pulmonary arterial hypertension (PAH) is a rare disease characterized by distinctive changes in pulmonary arterioles that lead to progressive elevation of pulmonary artery pressure, pulmonary vascular resistance, right sided heart failure, and a high mortality rate. According to the Fourth World Symposium on Pulmonary Hypertension held in 2008 in Dana Point, California, pulmonary arterial hypertension can be categorized into five groups including idiopathic pulmonary arterial hypertension, hereditary pulmonary arterial hypertension, drug-induced or toxin-induced pulmonary arterial hypertension, PAH with identifiable causes, (such as connective tissue disease), and persistent pulmonary hypertension of the newborn [105]. The incidence of idiopathic or familial pulmonary arterial hypertension is approximately seven to ten cases per million individuals. The incidence of pulmonary vascular disease in patients with other diseases is not known, but approximately 0.5–2 % of patients with portal hypertension or HIV infection have pulmonary vascular

disease [97]. The etiology of PAH is heterogeneous and incompletely understood. In the prospective National Institutes of Health registry, 6 % of PAH was familial, characterized by autosomal dominant transmission with incomplete penetrance [8, 91]. Much of PAH is of unknown cause and termed idiopathic PAH (IPAH). Heritable PAH and idiopathic PAH have similar clinical courses. The disease is more frequent in adult women, with a range of 2:1 to 4:1 women to men affected [40, 54].

Genetics of PAH

Genes play an important role in the pathogenesis of idiopathic and heritable PAH. Germline mutations in bone morphogenetic protein receptor 2 (*BMPR2*), a member of the transforming growth factor β (TGFβ) superfamily of receptors, were identified in 2000 as the major genetic cause for hereditary and idiopathic PAH. Mutations in *BMPR2* have been identified in 70 % of cases of familial PAH, as well as in 10–40 % of cases of idiopathic PAH [2]. The wide range in prevalence of *BMPR2* mutations in IPAH is due to differences in study sample sizes, but, overall, approximately 20 % of IPAH patients carry *BMPR2* mutations. A total of 298 *BMPR2* unique mutations in PAH have been reported [70]. Patients with *BMPR2* mutations are less likely to respond to acute vasodilators or benefit from calcium channel blockade (CCB) treatment than mutation-negative patients, and appear to have more severe disease at diagnosis [96].

The mechanism by which these mutations contribute to the pathogenesis of PAH has been elucidated only partially. Mutations in *BMPR2* are all likely to be partial or complete loss of function [11, 68]. To investigate how heterozygous mutations in *BMPR2* cause PAH, mice with mutant *Bmpr2* alleles were generated [10]. *Bmpr2* homozygous mutant mice die early before embryonic day 9.5. Mice carrying one mutant allele of *Bmpr2* survive and reproduce normally [11]. However, these mice have increased mean pulmonary arterial pressure and pulmonary vascular resistance compared with wild type littermates yet have no evidence of systemic hypertension. Histologically, the wall thickness of muscularized pulmonary arteries (<100 μm in diameter) and the number of alveolar-capillary units are increased in *Bmpr2* heterozygous mice, which occurs in the absence of systemic vascular remodeling. However, pathological changes are specific to the pulmonary vasculature. Pathological features of severe PAH such as intimal fibrosis, arterial occlusion, or plexiform lesions are not observed in heterozygous mice [115]. *BMPR2* expression is almost completely absent in the endothelial cells of plexiform or concentric vascular lesions of familial PAH patients with heterozygous *BMPR2* mutations [7]. In *Bmpr2* R899X heterozygous mice, one-third have pulmonary hypertension in association with extensive pruning, muscularization of small pulmonary vessels, and development of large structural pulmonary vascular changes [116]. To investigate the role of BMPR2 signaling in pulmonary vascular endothelium, *Bmpr2* was deleted in pulmonary endothelial cells using *Bmpr2* conditional knockout mice [52]. A subset of mice with heterozygous (20 %) and homozygous (40 %) conditional deletion of *Bmpr2* in pulmonary endothelial cells developed pulmonary arterial hypertension. These mice have high right ventricular systolic pressure, excessive thickening of small arteries, occluded arteries, *in situ* thrombotic lesion, and higher proliferation index in endothelial cells and smooth muscle cells. Homozygous conditional *Bmpr2* mutants had more severe histological features than the heterozygous animals. This study indicated that *Bmpr2* deficiency in the endothelium alone is sufficient to predispose to PAH histopathological features [52]. Smooth muscle-specific transgenic mice expressing a dominant-negative *Bmpr2* genotype (c.504 insT, L168FfsX12) also developed pulmonary hypertension with no increase in systemic arterial pressure [115].

The penetrance of *BMPR2* mutations for PAH is low with an estimated lifetime risk of 20 % [65]. Alterations in BMPR2 isoform ratios or amount of *BMPR2* expression for the normal allele may provide an explanation of the reduced penetrance among *BMPR2* mutation carriers. On the other hand, a 'second hit' that involves other genetic and/or environmental modifiers of *BMPR2* may be necessary to induce development of PAH, as suggested by a linkage study indicating that *BMPR2* and a 3q22 locus interact epistatically [94]. Candidates for modifiers include sex hormones with altered androgen to estrogen balance, given the increased penetrance of PAH in female *BMPR2* carriers, and the observation that the majority of women with PAH are postmenopausal [28, 66, 100]. Other somatic mutations of genes relevant to BMPR2 signaling and microsatellite instability have been demonstrated in the pulmonary arteries of PAH patients, including loss of chromosome 13 that, in turn, deletes *SMAD8* [3, 69].

Mutations in other TGFβ family members are additional rare causes of PAH. Mutations in *ALK1* [111], *ENG* [24] and *SMAD4* cause hereditary hemorrhagic telangiectasia (HHT) and associated PAH (see arterial venous malformation section). HHT is a systemic disease characterized by the presence of multiple arteriovenous malformations (AVMs) that lack intervening capillaries and results in direct connections between arteries and veins. The most frequent manifestations of HHT are epistaxis and mucocutaneous telangiectases, although a smaller percentage of patients develop clinically significant AVMs, including pulmonary AVMs. Rarely, patients with HHT (<1 %) develop PAH that is histopathologically indistinguishable from other forms of PAH [30].

Homozygous *Endoglin* knockout mice die at gestational day 10.0–10.5 due to defects in vessel and heart development [15]. In this transgenic model, abnormal vascular smooth muscle cell formation and internal bleeding was seen in the peritoneal cavity due to fragile vessels, indicating endoglin is critical for angiogenesis. Mice heterozygous for a loss-of-function mutation in *Alk1* develop age-dependent dilation of thin-walled blood vessels of the skin, extremities, oral cavity, and solid internal organs (e.g., lung, liver, intestine, spleen, and brain), as well as occult gastrointestinal bleeding [108]. A missense mutation (K43E) and two nonsense mutations (C202X, R294X) in *SMAD8* are implicated as rare genetic causes of PAH [35, 84, 104]. The BMP receptor type IB (*BMPR1B*), also called activin receptor-like kinase-6 (*ALK6*) is rarely associated with PAH, and two missense variants in *BMPR1B* were found in IPAH patients [26].

Caveolin 1 (CAV1) regulates Mothers against decapentaplegic 2/3 (SMAD2/3) phosphorylation. Two frameshift mutations (P158P fsX22 and P158H fxX22) were identified in both familial cases (frequency 1/62) and in IPAH (frequency 1/198) [9]. The expression of *CAV1* is necessary for the formation of caveolae, which are 50–100 nm diameter plasma membrane invaginations and cytoplasmic vesicles present in numerous cell types including endothelial and smooth muscle cells of the systemic and pulmonary vasculature, and type I alveolar cells of the lung. CAV1 downregulates Smad2/3 phosphorylation directly and loss of CAV1 enhances Smad2/3 signaling, which has been observed in the lungs of patients with PAH, providing a mechanistic link to the TGFβ receptor superfamily abnormalities. KCNK3 is a member of the two pore domain potassium channels expressed in pulmonary artery smooth muscle cells, and mutations in *KCNK3* are a rare cause of both familial PAH and IPAH [66]. KCNK3 is believed to be responsible for setting the resting membrane potential, responding to hypoxia, and regulating pulmonary vascular tone [47, 50, 83, 86, 87]. A novel heterozygous missense variant c.608 G>A, p. G203D in *KCNK3* was identified by whole exome sequencing in a familial PAH case. Five additional heterozygous missense variants (E182K, T8K, Y192C, G97R, and V221L) in 2 of 82 unrelated familial PAH patients and 3 of 230 idiopathic PAH patients were identified by further screening for *KCNK3* genetic abnormalities. All six rare variants are novel, located in highly conserved protein domains, predicted to be damaging and were shown functionally to result in loss-of-function *in vitro*. Application of a phospholipase A2 inhibitor was capable of rescuing channel activity in some but not all disease associated mutants, suggesting a potential novel mechanism for therapeutic intervention through KCNK3 in patients with pulmonary arterial hypertension [66]. Figure 6.1 summarizes the molecular pathogenesis and molecular genetics of HPAH.

In addition to rare mutations as a monogenic cause of HPAH, GWAS performed in a cohort of idiopathic and familial PAH patients identified an association of common

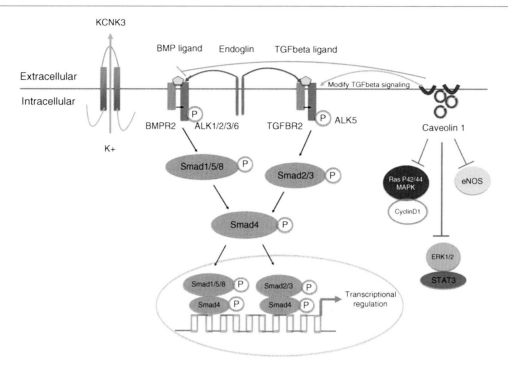

Fig. 6.1 Molecular pathogenesis of hereditary PAH. BMP binds to BMPR2. Upon ligand binding, the type II receptor phosphorylates a type I receptor, including ALK1, ALK2, ALK3 or ALK6. This leads to phosphorylation of Smad1/5/8 and phosphorylation of Smad4 with translocation of the phosphorylated Smads to the nucleus to modulate the expression of target genes. Upon TGFβ ligand binding, the TGFβ type II receptor phosphorylates a type I receptor, ALK5. This leads to phosphorylation of Smad2/3 which phosphorylate Smad4 and translocate to the nucleus. Endoglin is an accessory membrane glycoprotein that interacts with signaling receptor complexes for the BMP and TGF-β superfamily. Caveolin-1 normally dampens BMP signaling by inhibiting receptors or their signaling downstream to prevent vascular proliferation. Lack of caveolin-1 causes activation of STAT3 and ERK1/2 signaling, activation of Ras/p42/44/MAP kinase and upregulation of cyclin D1. Caveolin-1 functions as a tonic inhibitor of eNOS to facilitate NO mediated relaxation. Caveolin-1 modifies TGF beta signaling at the plasma membrane which may provide a mechanistic link between *Caveolin-1* and *BMPR2* mutations in the pathogenesis of PAH. KCNK3 is a potassium channel protein in pulmonary artery smooth muscle cells. Activation of K+ channel causes K+ efflux, membrane hyper polarization, and vasodilatation [67]. *PAH* pulmonary arterial hypertension, *BMP* bone morphogenetic protein, *BMPR2* bone morphogenetic protein receptor 2, *ALK* activin-like kinase, *TGFβ* transforming growth factor beta, *STAT3* signal transducer and activator of transcription 3, *ERK* extracellularly-regulated kinase, *MAP* mitogen activated kinase, *NO* nitric oxide, *KCNK3* Potassium channel subfamily K, member 3

variants in *CBLN2* with a twofold increased risk of disease expression [43]. *CBLN2* is expressed in the lung, with higher expression in explanted lungs from individuals with PAH and in endothelial cells cultured from explanted PAH lungs.

In addition to germ line mutations, somatic changes may also play a role in the pathogenesis of PAH. In normal pulmonary arteries, endothelial cells grow in a monolayer. In the lungs of patients with severe pulmonary hypertension, there is dysregulation of endothelial cell growth, forming intravascular plexiform lesions [121]. Endothelial cells within the plexiform lesions are clonal and arise from a single cell. These cells are genetically unstable and exhibit microsatellite instability and contain mutations in the TGF-β receptor II (*TGFBR2*) and BCL-2 associated X-protein (*BAX*) genes. Additionally, protein expression of TGF-BRII (6 of 19 lesions) and BAX (4 of 19 lesions) proteins was reduced in endothelial cells within plexiform lesions [121]. Chromosome abnormalities were identified in five out of nine pulmonary artery endothelial cells and smooth muscle cells analyzed by chromosome microarray from PAH patients [3]. Four of these were whole chromosome losses; the X chromosome was deleted in three female subjects, one patient harbored a germline *BMPR2* mutation and somatic loss of chromosome 13, which constitutes a second genetic hit in the same pathway by deleting *SMAD8*. The fifth abnormality was an interstitial deletion of the short arm of chromosome-8, 8p23.1-p12. These chromosome abnormalities may confer a growth advantage, and, thus, contribute to disease progression [3].

Germline chromosome copy number changes and microdeletion/duplications associated with pulmonary hypertension have not been studied extensively. A germline micro deletion of 17q22q23.2, encompassing T-box transcription factor-2 and 4 (*TBX2* and *TBX4*), was, however, identified in a patient with a syndromic disorder that included pulmonary hypertension [85].

Epigenetic changes do not alter the DNA sequence [17]. Changes in the methylation of superoxide dismutase were found in cells from the pulmonary vasculature in PAH patients [5]. Down regulation of superoxide dismutase 2 (SOD2) and normoxic activation of hypoxia inducible factor (HIF-1α) were found in pulmonary arteries and plexiform lesions in PAH [14, 16]. Decrease in SOD2 results from methylation of CpG islands in *SOD2* by lung DNA methyltransferases. The partial silencing of *SOD2* alters redox signaling, activates HIF-1α and leads to excessive cell proliferation.

Histone deacetylases (HDACs) catalyze removal of acetyl groups from lysine residues in a variety of proteins. HDACs regulate gene transcription by deacetylating nucleosomal histones. Expression of Class I HDACs is elevated dramatically in pulmonary arteries of PAH patients [122], and recent studies have demonstrated that Class I specific HDAC inhibitors can prevent hypoxia-induced pulmonary arteriole remodeling to preserve right ventricular function [22].

Pediatric PAH

PAH in children is much more heterogeneous than in adults and can be associated with congenital heart disease (CHD), bronchopulmonary dysplasia, vascular disease, pediatric lung disease, hepatic disease, pediatric thromboembolic disease and hematological disorders. The prevalence of IPAH/ HPAH in children was estimated to be ~2.2 cases per million with a lower female/male ratio (1.8:1) compared to adults [95]. The natural history of IPAH in children is poor, with a median untreated survival after diagnosis of 10 months compared to 2.8 years for adults [32]. In children, *BMPR2* mutations have been evaluated with variable results. One study identified no *BMPR2* mutations in 13 children with IPAH [46] while in a study reported by Harrison and colleagues, 22 % of children with IPAH or pulmonary hypertension associated with CHD had *ALK1*, *ENG* or *BMPR2* mutations [49]. *BMPR2* mutation positive children appeared less likely to respond to acute vasodilators than mutation negative children [95].

Other genes are likely to play an important role in childhood PAH. Two novel missense mutations (c.479 G>A S160N, c.1176 C>A F392L) in *BMPR1B* were identified in pediatric IPAH [26]. The F392L variant was inherited from unaffected father and S160N was not tested in proband's parents because their samples were not available. These two variants are located in highly conserved *BMPR1B* protein regions. Functional studies showed the transcriptional activation of the BMPR1B F392L protein with SMAD8 increased above that of wild-type BMPR1B with SMAD8, and those of BMPR1B S160N and F392L with SMAD8 and SMAD4 were each increased above those of the wild-type BMPR1B with SMAD8 and SMAD4.

Two novel missense mutations (c.2519 G>A p.G840E, c.2698 A>C p.T900P) in *NOTCH3* were identified in two PAH patients. Whether these two variants are inherited or *de novo* is unknown because samples from probands' parents were not available. These variants are located in highly conserved *NOTCH3* protein regions, and functional studies indicated these mutations were involved in cell proliferation and viability [27].

Persistent Pulmonary Hypertension of the Newborn

Persistent pulmonary hypertension of the newborn (PPHN) is characterized by severe hypoxemia shortly after birth, absence of cyanotic congenital heart disease, marked pulmonary hypertension, and vasoreactivity with extrapulmonary right-to-left shunting of blood across the ductus arteriosus and/or foramen ovale. A recent study suggested PPHN is a frequent and life-threatening complication in patients with mutations in *TMEM70* which causes a rare nuclear ATP synthase deficiency in pulmonary vascular endothelial cells [21].

Pulmonary Hypertension Secondary to CHD

Pulmonary arterial hypertension is a complication of CHD, most commonly occurring in patients who have systemic-to-pulmonary shunts with increased pulmonary blood flow. With increasing survival of patients with CHD after early surgical repair, PAH associated with CHD is now more common: approximately 5 % of adults with CHD develop PAH. Among adults with PAH, 11.3 % have PAH-CHD, whereas in children, almost half of all PAH cases are linked to CHD [42]. The pathophysiology of PAH with CHD varies according to the underlying structural heart defect, presence and size of intra- or extra-cardiac shunt, and status of the right ventricle. There are cases in which the PAH-CHD cannot be explained fully by the associated cardiac defect alone, and in these cases other mechanisms are likely to be responsible for pulmonary vascular dysfunction. Examples include patients with PAH and small atrial or ventricular septal defects. Interestingly, in one study *BMPR2* mutations were identified in 6 % of adults and children with PAH-CHD [92], although this mutation is not known to associate with the pathogenesis of structural heart disease *per se*. In a different study, one *BMPR2* mutation and one *Endoglin* mutation were identified in 11 children with CHD-PAH [88].

Pulmonary Hypertension Associated with Chronic Obstructive Pulmonary Disease

Chronic obstructive pulmonary disease (COPD) is a group of obstructive lung diseases, primarily emphysema and chronic bronchitis, which can lead to pulmonary hypertension and cor pulmonale. Alpha-1-antitrypsin deficiency, caused by mutations in the serpin peptidase inhibitor, clade A, member 1 (*SERPINA1*) gene is inherited as an autosomal recessive disorder characterized by increased risk for the development of severe destructive lung disease, such as emphysema, at an early age [99]. Pulmonary hypertension occurs in one-third of these patients.

Co-morbidities Associated with PAH

Several coexisting medical conditions have been associated with pulmonary arterial hypertension including connective tissue disease, infection with the human immunodeficiency virus (HIV), human herpes virus, portal hypertension, thrombocytosis, hemoglobinopathies, and hereditary hemorrhagic telangiectasia [38]. Hepatopulmonary syndrome (HPS) affects 10–30 % of patients with cirrhosis and portal hypertension. One study showed that polymorphisms in eight genes (*Caveolin 3, ENG, NADPH Oxidase 4, Estrogen receptor 2, von Willebrand factor, Runt-related transcription factor 1, Tyrosine kinase with immunoglobulin and EGF factor homology domains factor 1*) were associated with disease expression, possibly through the regulation of angiogenesis modulating the risk of HPS [93]. Connective tissue disease-associated PAH may be observed in systemic sclerosis (SSc), mixed connective tissue disease and systemic lupus erythematosus, and is most commonly seen in systemic sclerosis (with reported prevalence varying from 4.9 to 26.7 %). Human leukocyte antigen (HLA) DRw52 and DRw6 are associated with significantly increased risks of SSc-PAH [62]. However, sequencing has not identified mutations in TGFβ receptor genes, including *BMPR2, ALK1, TGFBR2* and *ENG*, in SSc-PAH patients [60, 82, 101].

Pulmonary Venous Hypertension

Pulmonary venous hypertension (PVH) is a well-described cause of pulmonary hypertension in patients with left heart disease associated with elevated left heart filling pressure from a number of processes, including left ventricular systolic dysfunction, left-sided valvular disease, constrictive pericardial disease, and restrictive cardiomyopathies. Traditionally, PVH has been defined as a mean pulmonary artery pressure ≥25 mmHg, pulmonary capillary wedge pressure ≥15 mmHg, and transpulmonic gradient <10 mmHg. Risk factors associated with pulmonary venous hypertension are age ≥80 years, left ventricular end diastolic pressure ≥25 mmHg, atrial arrhythmias, chronic obstructive pulmonary disease, and dyspnea on exertion. The spectrum of vascular remodeling seen in PVH varies widely among patients.

Pulmonary Veno-Occlusive Disease

Pulmonary veno-occlusive disease (PVOD) is a rare cause of pulmonary hypertension. Annual incidence of PVOD is approximately 0.1–0.2 cases per million persons in the general population [97]. Unlike IPAH, there does not appear to be a clear gender imbalance among patients with PVOD [73]. Pathologically, PVOD is characterized by the extensive and diffuse obliteration of small pulmonary veins or venules by fibrous tissue. Pulmonary parenchymal abnormalities are common: interstitial edema, pleural effusions and areas of pulmonary hemorrhage are often present [73]. In PVOD, the pressure gradient between the pulmonary capillary wedge and left ventricular compartments at end-diastole is generally increased in affected vascular beds compared to normal lung vascular regions.

The etiology of PVOD remains largely unknown. Infection, toxic exposure, thrombophilia and autoimmune diseases are associated with development of the disease. PVOD presents both sporadically and as familial cases, indicating a genetic cause for at least some forms of PVOD. Mutations in *BMPR2* have been reported in patients with PVOD [81]. Recently, mutations in Eukaryotic Translation Initiation Factor 2 Alpha Kinase 4 (*EIF2AK4*) were identified in multiple independent families with an autosomal recessive form of PVOD [13, 36]. All affected individuals in 13 familial cases carried deleterious homozygous or compound-heterozygous rare variants in *EIF2AK4*. Additional mutation screening demonstrated *EIF2AK4* mutations in 5/20 (25 %) of idiopathic cases of pulmonary capillary hemangiomatosis (PCH) /PVOD [13, 36]. The protein product of *EIF2AK4* belongs to a family of kinases that regulates angiogenesis, and the alpha subunit of this protein plays a critical role in the induction of angiogenesis, proliferation, and resistance to apoptosis in stressful environments. Moreover, EIF2AK4 interacts with SMAD4, SMAD1, ALK-1, ENG, and TGFBR2, thereby interacting with the BMPR2-associated signaling network.

When hemoptysis or hemorrhagic pulmonary effusion, interstitial lung infiltrates, or signs of post capillary pulmonary hypertension are present in the setting of pulmonary hypertension, both PCH and pulmonary veno-occlusive disease should be considered [4]. PCH is caused by the proliferation of pulmonary capillaries infiltrating vascular, bronchial, and interstitial pulmonary structures. Most PCH cases are sporadic, but hereditary forms of PCH consistent with autosomal-recessive transmission have been reported. PCH occurs in young adults and is often only diagnosed after death on autopsy. Pathology demonstrates thickened inter alveolar septae infiltrated by numerous thin-walled vessels and infiltration by capillaries into the walls of pulmonary vessels and bronchi. Signs of post capillary pulmonary hypertension (Kerley B lines, transudative pleural effusion, or a high pulmonary artery wedge pressure) are absent in pulmonary hypertension.

The classification of pulmonary hypertension proposed in the new Dana Point Classification was to maintain European Respiratory Society guidelines, which combined PCH and PVOD into a single subcategory within PAH because of specific similarities in their diagnosis, prognosis, and management. Genetic studies have identified compound heterozygous mutations in *EIF2AK4* in familial PCH and in 2/10 cases of sporadic PCH. Thus, *EIF2AK4* mutations are associated with both PCH and PVOD, which suggests there is a common underlying molecular etiology for PVOD and PCH. [13].

Pulmonary Hypertension due to Luminal Embolism or Chronic Thrombotic Embolic Disease

Pulmonary Embolism

Pulmonary embolism (PE) is common, with an incidence of one to two cases per 1000 person per year [123], which usually occurs in association with deep vein thrombosis. Both inherited and environmental risk factors such as immobility or estrogens predispose to venous thromboemboli (VTE). Approximately 20 % of patients with VTE are believed to have identifiable genetic risk factors, including factor V (F5) Leiden, prothrombin gene mutation G20210A, or deficiencies of protein C, protein S or antithrombin III (AT-III) [12, 29, 45, 89]. The prevalence of factor V Leiden mutations is 9.1 % (272/2977) in patients with isolated PE and 19.4 % (1576/8140) in patients with VTE with or without concomitant PE [34]. The most frequent point mutation in *F5* is R506Q. It occurs at one of three cleavage sites for activated protein C and renders factor V relatively resistant to degradation. This mutation is carried by approximately 2–7 % of Caucasians [72] and present in 1–2 % of African Americans [23, 44]. Several other missense mutations and small insertion/deletions have been identified in F5. Heterozygous carriers of Factor V Leiden have a fivefold increased risk of venous thromboembolism, and that risk is increased 10- to 80-fold in homozygotes [61]. According to American College of Medical Genetics, genetic testing should be performed in patients presenting with idiopathic VTE at age <50 or in recurrent VTE irrespective of age. Patients found to have the factor V Leiden mutation may require prolonged oral anticoagulation.

The prothrombin 20210G>A variant in the 3' untranslated region of the prothrombin gene is present in 2 % of the general population, 6–9 % of individuals with a single VTE, and up to 18 % of individuals with a personal and family history of thrombosis [33, 63, 75, 89]. Carriers of both Factor V

Leiden and the *Prothrombin* 20210G>A variant are found in approximately 0.1 % of the Caucasian population. Mutations in *Protein C* and *Protein S* are approximately tenfold less common than Factor V Leiden mutation, with a combined prevalence of 1 % of the population and are found in 1–3 % of individuals with VTE [77]. The 677C>T variant in the Methylenetetrahydrofolate reductase (*MTHFR*) gene results in a variant thermolabile enzyme with reduced activity for the remethylation of homocysteine. Homozygosity for 677C>T occurs in 10–20 % of the general population and predisposes to mild hyperhomocysteinemia, usually in the setting of suboptimal folate levels [119]. One or more of the genetic variants described above was present in 62.2 % (56/90) of patients with PE [106].

Pulmonary Hypertension due to Chronic Thrombotic Embolic Disease

Patients with recurrent pulmonary emboli are at risk of developing chronic thrombotic embolic pulmonary hypertension (CTEPH), although <1 % of patients with antecedent luminal PE later develop this form of pulmonary vascular disease. Patients with CTEPH have progressive dyspnea, and often present with normal chest radiographs and pulmonary function tests. The diagnosis is suggested when a ventilation perfusion scan shows large perfusion defects with relatively normal ventilation. Pulmonary endarterectomy remains the primary treatment for CTEPH, although recently the soluble guanylyl cyclase stimulator riociguat was demonstrated to significantly improve exercise tolerance and survival in the patient population. Importantly, CTEPH can develop in the setting of chronic PE and is associated with some of the same genetic thromboembolic risk factors reviewed above including factor VIII [55, 59].

Pulmonary Embolism and Pulmonary Hypertension in Sickle Cell Disease, Thalassemia and Other Hemolytic Anemia

Hemolytic anemia includes several genetic diseases such as sickle cell disease, thalassemia, Glucose-6-phosphate dehydrogenase (G6PD) deficiency, pyruvate kinase deficiency, congenital hereditary spherocytosis and paroxysmal nocturnal hemoglobinuria, as well as autoimmune diseases, infection, transfusion and medication induced hemolytic anemia. Patients with hemolytic anemia express a hypercoagulable state [6], and are thus at risk for developing thrombotic complications, including VTE and *in situ* pulmonary vascular thrombosis.

Sickle cell disease (SCD) is an autosomal recessive genetic disorder due to the E6V mutation in the β-globin gene. Rigidity of erythrocytes leads to hemolysis and veno-occlusion. Heterozygous sickle cell disease increases the risk of PE by approximately fourfold, which is among the most frequent cause of death in this patient population [1]. Indeed, pulmonary hypertension has emerged as a major chronic cardiopulmonary complication of SCD, afflicting 20–30 % of SCD patients. The pathogenesis of PH-SCD is complex and may involve hemolysis that depletes nitric oxide synthesis, prothrombotic state/ thromboembolic disease, iron overload, chronic liver disease, HIV infection, nocturnal hypoxemia, left ventricular diastolic dysfunction, and loss of splenic function [71].

Thalassemia is caused by a partial or complete deficiency of either α or β-globin chain synthesis. Beta-thalassemia is one of the most common autosomal recessive disorders worldwide. Thromboembolic events and pulmonary hypertension are more common in β-thalassemia intermedia [58].

Hemolytic anemia caused by red blood cell (RBC) enzymopathies often occur due to congenital enzyme deficiencies in erythrocyte metabolic pathways. The most common hemolytic anemia is G6PD deficiency caused by X-linked mutations in the *G6PD* gene that normally provides defense against oxidative damage [80]. Red cell pyruvate kinase (PK) deficiency is the most common cause of hereditary nonspherocytic hemolytic anemia and is caused by recessively inherited mutations in the gene encoding pyruvate kinase [112]. Other hemolytic anemias due to RBC enzymopathies include recessively inherited mutations in adenylate kinase (*AK*) [79], uridine 5-prime monophosphate hydrolase (*NT5C3A*) [76], hexokinase (*HK*) and phosphofructokinase (*PFK*) [78]. Phosphoglycerate kinase 1 (PGK1) deficiency is an X-linked recessive hemolytic anemia caused by mutations in *PGK1* [25].

Pulmonary Vascular Malformation

Pulmonary vascular malformations are congenital anomalies that occur in pulmonary arteries, veins and capillaries. It is a group of diseases that includes pulmonary arterial and venous malformations, hereditary hemorrhagic telangiectasia, alveolar capillary dysplasia, Ehlers-Danlos syndrome and arterial tortuosity syndrome. Although these syndromes are rare, they are associated with the development of clinically significant pulmonary hypertension.

Pulmonary Arterial Venous Malformations

Pulmonary arteriovenous malformations (PAVMs) are low-resistance, high flow-through vascular structures that connect pulmonary arteries to pulmonary veins abnormally, bypassing the normal pulmonary capillary bed and resulting in an intrapulmonary right to left shunt. As a consequence, PAVMs predispose to hypoxemia and paradoxical emboli. PAVMs are rare (incidence of 2–3 per 100,000), affect females preferentially (male-to-female ratio ~1:1.5–1.8), and hereditary, occurring predominately in association with HHT. Hereditary PAVMs tend to increase in size over time, usually expanding and becoming more evident in the second and third decades of life. Sporadic cases can be caused by infections (such as schistosomiasis and actinomycosis), trauma, and Fanconi syndrome, or occur secondary to hepatopulmonary syndrome or bidirectional cavopulmonary shunts [19].

Hereditary Hemorrhagic Telangiectasia

Hereditary hemorrhagic telangiectasia, or Rendu-Osler-Weber syndrome, is a rare autosomal dominantly inherited disease with a prevalence of 1 or 2 per 100,000. The disease is characterized by vascular dysplasia leading to telangiectasias and arteriovenous malformations of the skin, mucosa, and viscera. Between 20 and 23 % of HHT patients have pulmonary arteriovenous malformations (PAVMs), and, thus, are at risk for pulmonary hypertension [90, 114, 107]. Mutations in *ENG* or *ALK1* are the predominant genetic causes of HHT (62.5 %), although a small percentage of cases (1–2 %) express mutations in *SMAD4* in association with juvenile polyposis. Overall, however, *ALK-1* mutations are the most common genetic cause of HHT-associated PAH [48, 64, 111] and pulmonary arterio-venous malformations [113].

Alveolar Capillary Dysplasia

Alveolar capillary dysplasia with misalignment of the pulmonary veins (ACD/MPV) is a rare childhood disorder that carries a mortality rate approaching 100 %. The pathogenesis of both ACD/MPV and its association with pulmonary hypertension are not well understood. ACD/MPV usually presents with minimal or no parenchymal lung disease and diagnosis is based upon the pathology of immature lobular development, decreased number of pulmonary capillaries located away from the alveolar, epithelium thickened alveolar septae, medial hypertrophy of small pulmonary arteries, muscularization of distal arterioles and malposition of pulmonary vein branches adjacent to pulmonary arteries [20]. Most of ACD/MPV cases are sporadic, but approximately 10 % are familial. Pedigrees suggest both autosomal dominant and recessive patterns of inheritance. Heterozygous point mutations and microdeletions in forkhead box F1 (*FOXF1*) were identified in 40 % ACD/MPV patients [102, 109].

Ehlers-Danlos Vascular Disease

Ehlers-Danlos syndrome is a group of inherited connective tissue disorders of collagen synthesis. Type IV Ehlers-Danlos syndrome (vascular type) is due to autosomal dominantly inherited defects of type III collagen (*COL3A1*) synthesis and is characterized by abnormal fragility of blood vessels leading to spontaneous rupture or dissection of blood vessels. Respiratory complications include hemoptysis and hemopneumothorax. In extreme cases the lungs demonstrate diffuse hemorrhage with hemosiderin-laden alveolar macrophages or old/organized thrombi in the small bronchi [51].

Arterial Tortuosity Syndrome

Arterial tortuosity syndrome (ATS) is a rare autosomal recessive disorder characterized by tortuosity, elongation, stenosis and aneurysm formation in the systemic and pulmonary arteries. Disruption of elastic fibers in the medial layer of the arterial wall is observed. ATS is caused by mutations in the solute carrier family 2, member 10 (*SLC2A10*) gene, encoding the facilitative glucose transporter 10 (GLUT10) [18, 31, 37]. Deficiency of GLUT10 is associated with up regulation of the TGF-beta pathway in the arterial wall, which is responsible for the angiopathy.

Lung Vasculitis

Pulmonary vasculitis occurs with collagen vascular diseases and in granulomatous pulmonary disease. In the collagen vascular group, vasculitis causes diffuse interstitial inflammation and fibrosis. The typical collagen vascular diseases include rheumatoid arthritis, systemic lupus erythematosus, systemic sclerosis and dermatomyositis. Granulomatous pulmonary disease typically produces focal inflammation and manifests as nodules and masses. The most common vasculitis granulomatosis is Wegener's granulomatosis.

Wegener's Granulomatosis

Wegener's granulomatosis (WG) is characterized by necrosis, vasculitis and granulomatous inflammation involving the respiratory tract and kidney. In the lung, granulomatous inflammation produces solitary or multiple discrete parenchymal nodules, which may be bronchocentric, angiocentric or interstitial. The vasculitis may or may not be granulomatous in nature, and larger vessels often have only focal involvement. Polymorphisms in *PTPN22* (R620W) [56], *HLA-DPA1* (rs9277341), *HLA-DPB1* (rs9277554), and semaphorin 6A (*SEMA6A*) (rs26595) [120] are associated with Wegener's granulomatosis.

Churg-Strauss Syndrome

Churg-strauss syndrome (CSS) is a rare small- and medium-sized-vessel vasculitis associated with asthma and eosinophilia. Findings in the lung include a combination of extravascular granulomas, vasculitis and eosinophilic pneumonia. CSS is often preceded by allergic rhinitis, frequently complicated by nasal polyposis and sinusitis. Three SNPs in the *IL10* promotor were significantly associated with ANCA-negative CSS [118].

Giant Cell Arteritis

Giant cell arteritis (GCA) is a granulomatous vasculitis of the aorta and its major branches. GCA can affect the main pulmonary arteries as well as large and medium sized pulmonary elastic arteries in 9–31 % of cases. The vasculitic process is characterized by medial and adventitial chronic inflammation with giant cells and causes elastic laminae destruction, sometimes associated with focal fibrinoid medial necrosis. The most common respiratory symptom is non-productive, persistent cough. Polymorphisms in protein tyrosine phosphatases nonreceptor- type 22 (*PTPN22*) and HLA-DRB1 have been reported with GCA [74, 103, 117].

Takayasu Arteritis

Takayasu arteritis (TA) is a rare granulomatous vasculitis that mainly involves the aorta and its major branches. Incidence of pulmonary artery involvement detected by angiography ranges widely in the literature from 14 to 100 %. Clinical presentations include cough, dyspnea, and/or hemoptysis [110]. The adventitia, media, and intima are infiltrated by mononuclear and giant cells that contribute to the formation of necrotizing or non-necrotizing granulomas. Fragmentation of elastic fibers (elasticophagia) and destruction of the smooth muscle cells in the media leads to weakening of the vessel wall and lumen dilatation. Later, diffuse or nodular fibrosis may predominate and result in stenosis or obliteration of the vascular lumen [39]. The disease usually affects young women and familial cases have been reported, suggesting hereditary factors. Polymorphisms in paraoxonase 1 (*PON1*) and Interleukin-12B (*IL12B*) have been associated with Takayasu arteritis [53, 98].

Impact of Genetics of Pulmonary Vascular Diseases on Clinical Research

The identification of genes that cause pulmonary vascular remodeling and dysfunction has elucidated the molecular underpinnings of pulmonary vascular disease pathogenesis. Although many disease-causing genes have been identified, a significant portion of clinical cases throughout the spectrum of pulmonary vascular diseases are not explained by known genetic mutations. The application of novel genomic sequencing methods, including exome and genome sequencing, to clinical research involving PAH (in particular) is anticipated to expose additional genetic markers of disease expression and help crystalize molecular mechanisms involved in the pathogenesis of this highly morbid condition. Identifying the genetic basis of pulmonary vascular disease, however, represents one of many critical steps towards improved treatment.

Impact of Genetics of Pulmonary Vascular Diseases on Clinical Medicine

Generally, genetic testing in clinical practice is available for either single genes or a panel of disease-specific genes. The cost of genetic testing has decreased significantly in the United States with the introduction of gene panels and increasing acceptance of genetic testing by health insurance parties. Clinical genetic testing in PAH is available for PAH for a panel of genes including *BMPR2*, *ALK1*, *ENG*, *SMAD8*, *CAV1*, and *KCNK3*, and includes both sequencing and deletion/duplication testing. Genetic testing is often sought by parents in pediatric PAH to explain the etiology of the disease, assess risk in other family members, and determine the risk of recurrence in future children. The most commonly cited reason for genetic testing for PAH is to provide information regarding disease risk to offspring [57], and pre-implantation genetic diagnosis has been used to avoid vertical transmission of a familial mutation [41].

Although the utility of genetic testing is primarily for unaffected family members, genetic testing should begin on the affected member of the family to provide critical information regarding whether there is a genetic basis for PAH in the affected family member, and, if present, the specific mutation. Genetic testing is valuable for both familial PAH and IPAH since 20 % of IPAH patients will have an identifiable PAH mutation due to incomplete penetrance and *de novo* mutations. Using the combined approaches of sequencing and deletion duplication analysis, the clinical sensitivity of genetic testing panels for PAH is approximately 75 % with mutations most commonly identified in *BMPR2* [68].

The cost of genetic testing is usually covered in part or in full by insurance with results generally available in 8 weeks. Once the mutation in a family has been identified, testing other family members for a family-specific mutation is relatively inexpensive, accurate, and fast. As a consequence of the incomplete penetrance and variable age of onset, identi-

fication of a *BMPR2* mutation may have complex psychosocial implications on the potentially affected family members and can be associated with feelings of guilt in the proband parent. Thus, genetic counseling should precede genetic testing in PAH.

Genetic testing is helpful when a familial mutation is identified in a symptomatic patient, and predictive testing is able to identify asymptomatic family members who have negative genetic test result. On the other hand, negative genetic test results are informative only when a familial mutation has been identified in a disease-expressing individual, but not in asymptomatic family members. In this scenario, mutation-negative members of the affected family are not at increased risk for PAH, and can then forgo the otherwise recommended serial clinical evaluations and echocardiograms to screen for development of PAH. Conversely, high-risk individuals carrying a familial PAH mutation, or first-degree relatives of individuals with PAH who have not had genetic testing should have regular surveillance tests. For at-risk individuals, regular screening by echocardiogram every 3 years and awareness of disease symptoms should enable early diagnosis and treatment which may improve outcomes [66]. If a mutation is not identified in a patient with familial PAH after testing for a comprehensive panel of PAH genes, clinical exome sequencing may be considered. Clinical exome sequencing should involve consultation with a clinical geneticist due to the complexities of this particular genetic test. Approaches to genetic testing are illustrated in Fig. 6.2.

If an asymptomatic family member of a patient with PAH desires predictive genetic testing and an affected family member is unavailable or unwilling to undergo genetic testing, the asymptomatic family member may pursue genetic testing for a panel of PAH genes. A positive result is straightforward to interpret; however, a variant of uncertain clinical significance may be identified, leaving the patient with uncertainty unless genetic testing of additional family members can be performed to clarify the significance of the detected genetic variant. Finally, a negative genetic test in the asymptomatic family member is not fully informative since that negative genetic test result could either be due to not inheriting a mutation in a gene included in the testing panel or due to being positive for an unidentified PAH gene that was not included in the testing panel. This asymptomatic patient's risk of PAH is reduced with the negative genetic test result, but there is still an increased risk of developing PAH if the PAH is familial unless and until a familial mutation is identified.

Future interventions in pulmonary vascular genetic disorders may involve correcting the underlying genetic defects. As new methods are developed for gene editing, there may be new opportunities for treatment of genetic disorders

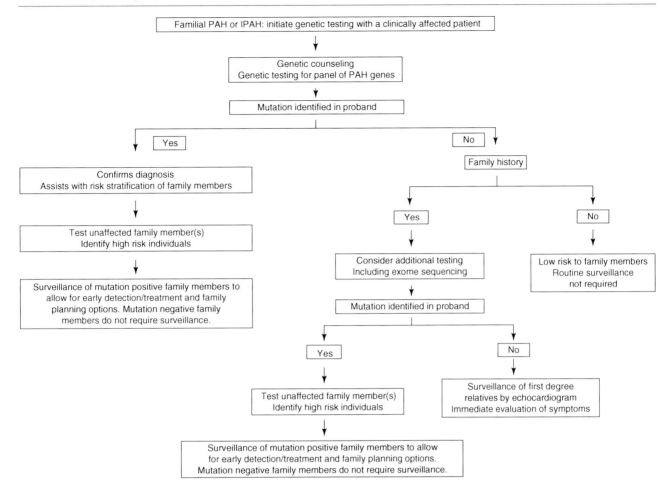

Fig. 6.2 Rational for genetic testing in clinical practice. Patients who have either familial or idiopathic pulmonary arterial hypertension should be offered genetic testing. Genetic counseling should be provided prior to genetic testing. Genetic testing should include a comprehensive panel of PAH genes and should start with an affected individual (proband). If a mutation is identified in a proband, the diagnosis of PAH is confirmed. Unaffected family members of the proband can then be accurately risk stratified by genetic testing for the familial mutation only. Regular surveillance of mutation positive family members will allow early detection and treatment of PAH and family planning. Mutation-negative family members do not require surveillance. For clinically affected PAH patients who have no mutation identified after testing a comprehensive panels of genes, family history is important in determining next steps. If the family history is negative for PAH, family members of the proband are at low risk of PAH and routine surveillance is not required. If the family history is positive for PAH, additional genetic testing, such as whole exome sequencing may be used to identify the genetic basis for the PAH in the family. If no mutation is identified with whole exome sequencing, first-degree relatives should be monitored for PAH with serial echocardiograms. If a mutation is identified by additional genetic testing, unaffected family members can be tested for the familial mutation to identify mutation positive asymptomatic family members at high risk to enable disease surveillance and early detection and treatment of PAH

Summary

The genetics of pulmonary vascular diseases are complex. With recent advances in genetic technology, our knowledge of the genetics of pulmonary vascular diseases is expanding. Novel single gene mutations have been identified in pulmonary arterial hypertension, pulmonary veno-occlusive disease, pulmonary embolism, chronic pulmonary thromboembolic disease and arteriovenous malformations (Table 6.1). While loss-of-function mutations of some genes, such as *BMPR2*, have been established as major monogenetic risk factor for PAH, the disease penetrance is modest, suggesting other genetic or environmental modifiers. Genetic testing is available for PAH and most other pulmonary vascular diseases with a genetic basis, and should be considered for identifying individuals at increased risk of developing disease. Whenever possible, genetic testing within a family should begin with the affected individual to identify a potential familial mutation, and thereby allow for informative, predictive testing of asymptomatic relatives subsequently. Mutation positive individuals should then be evaluated serially to identify the earliest disease manifestations. The efficacy of primary prevention and early initiation of treatment in carriers of PAH-causing mutations has not yet been systematically studied, and is likely to vary according

Table 6.1 Genes and genetic factors identified in pulmonary vascular diseases

Pulmonary vascular diseases	Genes	Frequency	Inheritance
Pulmonary arterial hypertension	BMPR2 SMAD8 ENG ALK1 SMAD4 ALK6 CAV1 KCNK3 NOTCH3 TMEM70	70 % of HPAH, 20 % of IPAH 0.9 % (2/211) of IPAH Unknown for HHT associated PAH 72.7 % of HHT and associated PAH 1.1 % (2/188) of IPAH 4.7 % (2/43) of IPAH 0.8 % (1/119) of HPAH, 0.5 % (1/198) of IPAH 2 % (3/149) of HPAH, 1.3 % (3/230) of IPAH Unknown Unknown	Autosomal dominant with incomplete penetrance
Pulmonary veno-occlusive disease	BMPR2 EIF2AK4	Unknown Unknown	Autosomal dominant Autosomal recessive
Pulmonary embolism	F5 PROTHRMBIN PROTEIN C & PROTEIN S MTHFR	9.1 % of PE, 19.4 % of VTE 6–9 % of VTE Combined prevalence of 1–3 % of VTE Susceptibility to thrombosis	Autosomal dominant
Chronic pulmonary thromboembolic disease	β-globin G-6-PD NT5C3A PK HK PFK PGK1	Mutation frequency in PE is unknown	Autosomal recessive, X linked
Arteriovenous malformations	ALK1	40–46 % of HHT	Autosomal dominant, autosomal recessive
	ENG	22.5–54 % of HHT	
	FOXF1	40 % of ACD/MPV	
	COL3A1	61.4 % of Ehlers-Danlos syndrome type IV	
	SLC2A10	10–92 % of familial ATS	
Pulmonary vasculitis	IL10 PTPN22 PON1 IL12B HLA-DPA1 HLA-DPB1 SEMA6A	Complex trait	Complex trait, multifactorial inheritance

HPAH hereditary pulmonary arterial hypertension, *IPAH* idiopathic pulmonary arterial hypertension, *PE* pulmonary embolism, *VTE* venous thromboembolism, *HHT* hereditary hemorrhagic telangiectasia, *ACD/MPV* alveolar capillary dysplasia with misalignment of the pulmonary veins

to the underlying disease and, possibly, by associated gene. Families may also use the genetic information to make reproductive decisions based upon an increased risk of disease transmission to offspring, recurrence although this is not commonly performed presently.

Glossary

Autosomal dominant A gene on one of the autosomes that is always expressed when one mutation is present.

Deletion/duplication testing Genetic testing that identifies deletions/duplications of part or all of a gene not readily detectable by sequence analysis

De novo An alteration in a gene that is the result of a new mutation

Exome sequencing A technique for sequencing all the protein-coding regions in a genome (known as the exome)

Genetic testing panel Genetic testing of a set of genes associated with a specific disease

Genome wide association study An approach that involves testing for disease association with a large number of genetic markers across the genomes

Incomplete penetrance The genetic trait is expressed in only a fraction of the individuals carrying the genetic predispoisition

Preimplantation genetic diagnosis A procedure used prior to implantation of an embryo created with in vitro fertilization to help identify genetic mutations to prevent the disease from being passed on to the child.

References

1. Adedeji MO, Cespedes J, Allen K, Subramony C, Hughson MD. Pulmonary thrombotic arteriopathy in patients with sickle cell disease. Arch Pathol Lab Med. 2001;125:1436–41.
2. Aldred MA, Vijayakrishnan J, James V, Soubrier F, Gomez-Sanchez MA, Martensson G, Galie N, Manes A, Corris P, Simonneau G, Humbert M, Morrell NW, Trembath RC. BMPR2 gene rearrangements account for a significant proportion of mutations in familial and idiopathic pulmonary arterial hypertension. Hum Mutat. 2006;27(2):212–3.
3. Aldred MA, Comhair SA, Varella-Garcia M, Asosingh K, Xu W, Noon GP, Thistlethwaite PA, Tuder RM, Erzurum SC, Geraci MW, Coldren CD. Somatic chromosome abnormalities in the lungs of patients with pulmonary arterial hypertension. Am J Respir Crit Care Med. 2010;182(9):1153–60.
4. Almagro P, Julià J, Sanjaume M, González G, Casalots J, Heredia JL, Martínez J, Garau J. Pulmonary capillary hemangiomatosis associated with primary pulmonary hypertension: report of 2 new cases and review of 35 cases from the literature. Medicine (Baltimore). 2002;81(6):417–24.
5. Archer SL, Marsboom G, Kim GH, Zhang HJ, Toth PT, Svensson EC, Dyck JR, Gomberg-Maitland M, Thébaud B, Husain AN, Cipriani N, Rehman J. Epigenetic attenuation of mitochondrial superoxide dismutase 2 in pulmonary arterial hypertension: a basis for excessive cell proliferation and a new therapeutic target. Circulation. 2010;121(24):2661–71.
6. Ataga KI, Cappellini MD, Rachmilewitz EA. B-thalassemia and sickle cell anaemia as paradigms of hypercoagulability. Br J Haematol. 2007;139:3–13.
7. Atkinson C, Stewart S, Upton PD, Machado R, Thomson JR, Trembath RC, Morrell NW. Primary pulmonary hypertension is associated with reduced pulmonary vascular expression of type II bone morphogenetic protein receptor. Circulation. 2002;105:1672–8.
8. Austin ED, Loyd JE, Phillips 3rd JA. Genetics of pulmonary arterial hypertension. Semin Respir Crit Care Med. 2009;30:386–98.
9. Austin ED, Ma L, LeDuc C, Berman Rosenzweig E, Borczuk A, Phillips 3rd JA, Palomero T, Sumazin P, Kim HR, Talati MH, West J, Loyd JE, Chung WK. Whole exome sequencing to identify a novel gene (caveolin-1) associated with human pulmonary arterial hypertension. Circ Cardiovasc Genet. 2012;5(3):336–43.
10. Beppu H, Kawabata M, Hamamoto T, Chytil A, Minowa O, Noda T, Miyazono K. BMP type II receptor is required for gastrulation and early development of mouse embryos. Dev Biol. 2000;221:249–58.
11. Beppu H, Ichinose F, Kawai N, Jones RC, Yu PB, Zapol WM, Miyazono K, Li E, Bloch KD. BMPR-II heterozygous mice have mild pulmonary hypertension and an impaired pulmonary vascular remodeling response to prolonged hypoxia. Am J Physiol Lung Cell Mol Physiol. 2004;287(6):L1241–7.
12. Bertina RM, Koeleman BP, Koster T, Rosendaal FR, Dirven RJ, de Ronde H, van der Velden PA, Reitsma PH. Mutation in blood coagulation factor V associated with resistance to activated protein C. Nature. 1994;369:64–7.
13. Best DH, Sumner KL, Austin ED, Chung WK, Brown LM, Borczuk AC, Rosenzweig EB, Bayrak-Toydemir P, Mao R, Cahill BC, Tazelaar HD, Leslie KO, Hemnes AR, Robbins IM, Elliott CG. EIF2AK4 mutations in pulmonary capillary hemangiomatosis. Chest. 2014;145(2):231–6.
14. Bonnet S, Michelakis ED, Porter CJ, Andrade-Navarro MA, Thébaud B, Bonnet S, et al. An abnormal mitochondrial-hypoxia

15. Bourdeau A, Dumont DJ, Letarte M. A murine model of hereditary hemorrhagic telangiectasia. J Clin Invest. 1999;104:1343–51.
16. Bowers R, Cool C, Murphy RC, Tuder RM, Hopken MW, Flores SC, Voelkel NF. Oxidative stress in severe pulmonary hypertension. Am J Respir Crit Care Med. 2004;169:764–9.
17. Bruneau BG. Epigenetic regulation of the cardiovascular system: introduction to a review series. Circ Res. 2010;107(3):324–6.
18. Callewaert BL, Willaert A, Kerstjens-Frederikse WS, De Backer J, Devriendt K, Albrecht B, Ramos-Arroyo MA, Doco-Fenzy M, Hennekam RCM, Pyeritz RE, Krogmann ON, Gillessen-Kaesbach G, Wakeling EL, Nik-zainal S, Francannet C, Mauran P, Booth C, Barrow M, Dekens R, Loeys BL, Coucke PJ, De Paepe AM. Arterial tortuosity syndrome: clinical and molecular findings in 12 newly identified families. Hum Mutat. 2008;29:150–8.
19. Cartin-Ceba R, Swanson KL, Krowka MJ. Pulmonary arteriovenous malformations. Chest. 2013;144(3):1033–44.
20. Castilla-Fernandez Y, Copons-Fernández C, Jordan-Lucas R, Linde-Sillo Á, Valenzuela-Palafoll I, Ferreres Piñas JC, Moreno-Galdó A, Castillo-Salinas F. Alveolar capillary dysplasia with misalignment of pulmonary [corrected] veins: concordance between pathological and molecular diagnosis. J Perinatol. 2013;33(5):401–3.
21. Catteruccia M, Verrigni D, Martinell D, Torraco A, Agovino T, Bonafe L, D'Amico A, Donati MA, Adorisio R, Santorelli FM, Carrozzo R, Bertini E, Dionisi-Vici C. Persistent pulmonary arterial hypertension in the newborn (PPHN): a frequent manifestation of TMEM70 defective patients. Mol Genet Metab. 2014; 111(3):353–9.
22. Cavasin MA, Demos-Davies K, Horn TR, Walker LA, Lemon DD, Birdsey N, Weiser-Evans MC, Harral J, Irwin DC, Anwar A, Yeager ME, Li M, Watson PA, Nemenoff RA, Buttrick PM, Stenmark KR, McKinsey TA. Selective class I histone deacetylase inhibition suppresses hypoxia-induced cardiopulmonary remodeling through an antiproliferative mechanism. Circ Res. 2012;110(5): 739–48.
23. Chan WP, Lee CK, Kwong YL, Lam CK, Liang R. A novel mutation of arg306 of factor V gene in Hong Kong Chinese. Blood. 1998;91:1135–9.
24. Chaouat A, Coulet F, Favre C, Simonneau G, Weitzenblum E, Soubrier F, Humbert M. Endoglin germline mutation in a patient with hereditary haemorrhagic telangiectasia and dexfenfluramine associated pulmonary arterial hypertension. Thorax. 2004;59(5): 446–8.
25. Chiarelli LR, Morera SM, Bianchi P, Fermo E, Zanella A, Galizzi A, Valentini G. Molecular insights on pathogenic effects of mutations causing phosphoglycerate kinase deficiency. PLoS One. 2012;7(2), e32065.
26. Chida A, Shintani M, Nakayama T, Furutani Y, Hayama E, Inai K, Saji T, Nonoyama S, Nakanishi T. Missense mutations of the BMPR1B (ALK6) gene in childhood idiopathic pulmonary arterial hypertension. Circ J. 2012;76(6):1501–8.
27. Chida A, Shintani M, Matsushita Y, Sato H, Eitoku T, Nakayama T, Furutani Y, Hayama E, Kawamura Y, Inai K, Ohtsuki S, Saji T, Nonoyama S, Nakanishi T. Mutations of NOTCH3 in childhood pulmonary arterial hypertension. Mol Genet Genomic Med. 2014;2(3):229–39.
28. Cogan J, Austin E, Hedges L, Womack B, West J, Loyd J, Hamid R. Role of BMPR2 alternative splicing in heritable pulmonary arterial hypertension penetrance. Circulation. 2012;126(15): 1907–16.
29. Comp PC, Esmon CT. Recurrent venous thromboembolism in patients with a partial deficiency of protein S. N Engl J Med. 1984;311:1525–8.

30. Cottin V, Dupuis-Girod S, Lesca G, Cordier JF. Pulmonary vascular manifestations of hereditary hemorrhagic telangiectasia (rendu-osler disease). Respiration. 2007;74(4):361–78.

31. Coucke PJ, Willaert A, Wessels MW, Callewaert B, Zoppi N, De Backer J, Fox JE, Mancini GMS, Kambouris M, Gardella R, Facchetti F, Willems PJ, Forsyth R, Dietz HC, Barlati S, Colombi M, Loeys B, De Paepe A. Mutations in the facilitative glucose transporter GLUT10 alter angiogenesis and cause arterial tortuosity syndrome. Nat Genet. 2006;38:452–7.

32. D'Alonzo GE, Barst RJ, Ayres SM, Bergofsky EH, Brundage BH, Detre KM, Fishman AP, Goldring RM, Groves BM, Kernis JT, Levy PS, Pietra GG, Reid LM, Reeves JT, Rich S, Vreim CE, Williams GW, Wu M. Survival in patients with primary pulmonary hypertension. Results from a national prospective registry. Ann Intern Med. 1991;115:343–9.

33. De Stefano V, Chiusolo P, Paciaroni K, Casorelli I, Di Mario A, Rossi E, Leone G. Prevalence of the factor II G20210A mutation in symptomatic patients with inherited thrombophilia. Thromb Haemost. 1998;80:342–3.

34. Dentali F, Ageno W, Bozzato S, Malato A, Gianni M, Squizzato A, Prisco D. Role of factor V Leiden or G20210A prothrombin mutation in patients with symptomatic pulmonary embolism and deep vein thrombosis: a meta-analysis of the literature. J Thromb Haemost. 2012;10(4):732–7.

35. Drake KM, Zygmunt D, Mavrakis L, Harbor P, Wang L, Comhair SA, Erzurum SC, Aldred MA. Altered MicroRNA processing in heritable pulmonary arterial hypertension: an important role for Smad-8. Am J Respir Crit Care Med. 2011;184(12):1400–8.

36. Eyries M, Montani D, Girerd B, Perret C, Leroy A, Lonjou C, Chelghoum N, Coulet F, Bonnet D, Dorfmüller P, Fadel E, Sitbon O, Simonneau G, Tregouët DA, Humbert M, Soubrier F. EIF2AK4 mutations cause pulmonary veno-occlusive disease, a recessive form of pulmonary hypertension. Nat Genet. 2014;46(1):65–9.

37. Faiyaz-Ul-Haque M, Zaidi SHE, Wahab AA, Eltohami A, Al-Mureikhi MS, Al-Thani G, Peltekova VD, Tsui L-C, Teebi AS. Identification of a pSer81Arg encoding mutation in SLC2A10 gene of arterial tortuosity syndrome patients from 10 Qatari families. (Letter) Clin Genet. 2008;74:189–93.

38. Farber HW, Loscalzo J. Pulmonary arterial hypertension. N Engl J Med. 2004;351(16):1655–65.

39. Fishbein GA, Fishbein MC. Lung vasculitis and alveolar hemorrhage: pathology. Semin Respir Crit Care Med. 2011;32(3):254–63.

40. Frost AE, Badesch DB, Barst RJ, Benza RL, Elliott CG, Farber HW, Krichman A, Liou TG, Raskob GE, Wason P, Feldkircher K, Turner M, McGoon MD. The changing picture of patients with pulmonary arterial hypertension in the United States: how REVEAL differs from historic and non-US Contemporary Registries. Chest. 2011;139(1):128–37.

41. Frydman N, Steffann J, Girerd B, Frydman R, Munnich A, Simonneau G, Humbert M. Pre-implantation genetic diagnosis in pulmonary arterial hypertension due to BMPR2 mutation. Eur Respir J. 2012;39(6):1534–5.

42. Gatzoulis MA, Alonso-Gonzalez R, Beghetti M. Pulmonary arterial hypertension in paediatric and adult patients with congenital heart disease. Eur Respir Rev. 2009;18(113):154–61.

43. Germain M, Eyries M, Montani D, Poirier O, Girerd B, Dorfmüller P, Coulet F, Nadaud S, Maugenre S, Guignabert C, Carpentier W, Vonk-Noordegraaf A, Lévy M, Chaouat A, Lambert JC, Bertrand M, Dupuy AM, Letenneur L, Lathrop M, Amouyel P, de Ravel TJ, Delcroix M, Austin ED, Robbins IM, Hemnes AR, Loyd JE, Berman-Rosenzweig E, Barst RJ, Chung WK, Simonneau G, Trequouet DA, Humbert M, Soubrier F. Genome-wide association analysis identifies a susceptibility locus for pulmonary arterial hypertension. Nat Genet. 2013;45(5):518–21.

44. Gregg JP, Yamane AJ, Grody WW. Prevalence of the factor V-Leiden mutation in four distinct American ethnic populations. Am J Med Genet. 1997;73:334–6.

45. Griffin JH, Evatt B, Zimmerman TS, Kleiss AJ, Wideman C. Deficiency of protein C in congenital thrombotic disease. J Clin Invest. 1981;68:1370–3.

46. Grunig E, Koehler R, Miltenberger-Miltenyi G, Zimmermann R, Gorenflo M, Mereles D, Arnold K, Naust B, Wilkens H, Benz A, von Hippel A, Ulmer HE, Kübler W, Katus HA, Bartram CR, Schranz D, Janssen B. Primary pulmonary hypertension in children may have a different genetic background than in adults. Pediatr Res. 2004;56:571–8.

47. Gurney AM, Osipenko ON, MacMillan D, McFarlane KM, Tate RJ, Kempsill FE. Two-pore domain K channel, TASK-1, in pulmonary artery smooth muscle cells. Circ Res. 2003;93(10):957–64.

48. Harrison RE, Flanagan JA, Sankelo M, Abdalla SA, Rowell J, Machado RD, Elliott CG, Robbins IM, Olschewski H, McLaughlin V, Gruenig E, Kermeen F, Halme M, Räisänen-Sokolowski A, Laitinen T, Morrell NW, Trembath RC. Molecular and functional analysis identifies ALK-1 as the predominant cause of pulmonary hypertension related to hereditary haemorrhagic telangiectasia. J Med Genet. 2003;40(12):865–71.

49. Harrison RE, Berger R, Haworth SG, Tulloh R, Mache CJ, Morrell NW, Aldred MA, Trembath RC. Transforming growth factor-beta receptor mutations and pulmonary arterial hypertension in childhood. Circulation. 2005;111:435–41.

50. Hartness ME, Lewis A, Searle GJ, O'Kelly I, Peers C, Kemp PJ. Combined antisense and pharmacological approaches implicate hTASK as an airway O(2) sensing K(+) channel. J Biol Chem. 2001;276(28):26499–508.

51. Hatake K, Morimura Y, Kudo R, Kawashima W, Kasuda S, Kuniyasu H. Respiratory complications of Ehlers-Danlos syndrome type IV. Leg Med (Tokyo). 2013;15(1):23–7.

52. Hong KH, Lee YJ, Lee E, Park SO, Han C, Beppu H, Li E, Raizada MK, Bloch KD, Oh SP. Genetic ablation of the BMPR2 gene in pulmonary endothelium is sufficient to predispose to pulmonary arterial hypertension. Circulation. 2008;118(7):722–30.

53. Huesca-Gómez C, Soto ME, Castrejón-Téllez V, Pérez-Méndez O, Gamboa R. PON1 gene polymorphisms and plasma PON1 activities in Takayasu's arteritis disease. Immunol Lett. 2013;152(1):77–82.

54. Humbert M, Sitbon O, Chaouat A, Bertocchi M, Habib G, Gressin V, Yaici A, Weitzenblum E, Cordier JF, Chabot F, Dromer C, Pison C, Reynaud-Gaubert M, Haloun A, Laurent M, Hachulla E, Simonneau G. Pulmonary arterial hypertension in France: results from a national registry. Am J Respir Crit Care Med. 2006;173(9):1023–30.

55. Humbert M. Pulmonary arterial hypertension and chronic thromboembolic pulmonary hypertension: pathophysiology. Eur Respir Rev. 2010;19:59–63.

56. Jagiello P, Aries P, Arning L, Wagenleiter SE, Csernok E, Hellmich B, Gross WL, Epplen JT. The PTPN22 620W allele is a risk factor for Wegener's granulomatosis. Arthritis Rheum. 2005;52(12):4039–43.

57. Jones DL, Sandberg JC, Rosenthal MJ, Saunders RC, Hannig VL, Clayton EW. What patients and their relatives think about testing for BMPR2. J Genet Couns. 2008;17(5):452–8.

58. Karimi M, Musallam KM, Cappellini MD, Daar S, El-Beshlawy A, Belhoul K, Saned MS, Temraz S, Koussa S, Taher AT. Risk factors for pulmonary hypertension in patients with β thalassemia intermedia. Eur J Intern Med. 2011;22(6):607–10.

59. Kim NH, Lang IM. Risk factors for chronic thromboembolic pulmonary hypertension. Eur Respir Rev. 2012;21(123):27–31.

60. Koumakis E, Wipff J, Dieudé P, Ruiz B, Bouaziz M, Revillod L, Guedj M, Distler JH, Matucci-Cerinic M, Humbert M,

Riemekasten G, Airo P, Melchers I, Hachulla E, Cusi D, Wichmann HE, Hunzelmann N, Tiev K, Caramaschi P, Diot E, Kowal-Bielecka O, Cuomo G, Walker U, Czirják L, Damjanov N, Lupoli S, Conti C, Müller-Nurasyid M, Müller-Ladner U, Riccieri V, Cracowski JL, Cozzi F, Bournia VK, Vlachoyiannopoulos P, Chiocchia G, Boileau C, Allanore Y. TGFβ receptor gene variants in systemic sclerosis-related pulmonary arterial hypertension: results from a multicentre EUSTAR study of European Caucasian patients. Ann Rheum Dis. 2012;71(11):1900–3.

61. Kujovich JL, Factor V. Leiden thrombophilia. Genet Med. 2011;13(1):1–16.

62. Langevitz P, Buskila D, Gladman DD, Darlington GA, Farewell VT, Lee P. HLA alleles in systemic sclerosis: association with pulmonary hypertension and outcome. Br J Rheumatol. 1992;31(9):609–13.

63. Leroyer C, Mercier B, Oger E, Chenu E, Abgrall JF, Férec C, Mottier D. Prevalence of the 20210 A allele of the prothrombin gene in venous thromboembolism patients. Thromb Haemost. 1998;80:49–51.

64. Lesca G, Plauchu H, Coulet F, Lefebvre S, Plessis G, Odent S, Rivière S, Leheup B, Goizet C, Carette MF, Cordier JF, Pinson S, Soubrier F, Calender A, Giraud S, French Rendu-Osler Network. Molecular screening of ALK1/ACVRL1 and ENG genes in hereditary hemorrhagic telangiectasia in France. Hum Mutat. 2004;23(4):289–99.

65. Loyd JE, Butler MG, Foroud TM, Conneally PM, Phillips 3rd JA, Newman JH. Genetic anticipation and abnormal gender ratio at birth in familial primary pulmonary hypertension. Am J Respir Crit Care Med. 1995;152(1):93–7.

66. Ma L, Roman-Campos D, Austin ED, Eyries M, Sampson KS, Soubrier F, Germain M, Trégouët DA, Borczuk A, Rosenzweig EB, Girerd B, Montani D, Humbert M, Loyd JE, Kass RS, Chung WK. A novel channelopathy in pulmonary arterial hypertension. N Engl J Med. 2013;369(4):351–61.

67. Ma L, Chung WK. The genetic basis of pulmonary arterial hypertension. Hum Genet. 2014;133(5):471–9.

68. Machado RD, Pauciulo MW, Thomson JR, Lane KB, Morgan NV, Wheeler L, Phillips 3rd JA, Newman J, Williams D, Galie N, Manes A, McNeil K, Yacoub M, Mikhail G, Rogers P, Corris P, Humbert M, Donnai D, Martensson G, Tranebjaerg L, Loyd JE, Trembath RC, Nichols WC. BMPR2 haploinsufficiency as the inherited molecular mechanism for primary pulmonary hypertension. Am J Hum Genet. 2001;68:92–102.

69. Machado RD, James V, Southwood M, Harrison RE, Atkinson C, Stewart S, Morrell NW, Trembath RC, Aldred MA. Investigation of second genetic hits at the BMPR2 locus as a modulator of disease progression in familial pulmonary arterial hypertension. Circulation. 2005;111(5):607–13.

70. Machado RD, Eickelberg O, Elliott CG, Geraci MW, Hanaoka M, Loyd JE, Newman JH, Phillips 3rd JA, Soubrier F, Trembath RC, Chung WK. Genetics and genomics of pulmonary arterial hypertension. J Am Coll Cardiol. 2009;54(1 Suppl):S32–42.

71. Machado RF. Sickle cell anemia-associated pulmonary arterial hypertension. J Bras Pneumol. 2007;33(5):583–91.

72. Majerus PW. Bad blood by mutation. Nature. 1994;369:14–5.

73. Mandel J, Mark E, Hales C. Pulmonary veno-occlusive disease. Am J Respir Crit Care Med. 2000;162:1964.

74. Manganelli P, Fietta P, Carotti M, Pesci A, Salaffi F. Respiratory system involvement in systemic vasculitides. Clin Exp Rheumatol. 2006;24(2 Suppl 41):S48–59.

75. Margaglione M, Brancaccio V, Giuliani N, D'Andrea G, Cappucci G, Iannaccone L, Vecchione G, Grandone E, Di Minno G. Increased risk for venous thrombosis in carriers of the prothrombin G → A20210 gene variant. Ann Intern Med. 1998;129:89–93.

76. Marinaki AM, Escuredo E, Duley JA, Simmonds HA, Amici A, Naponelli V, Magni G, Seip M, Ben-Bassat I, Harley EH, Thein SL, Rees DC. Genetic basis of hemolytic anemia caused by pyrimidine 5' nucleotidase deficiency. Blood. 2001;97(11):3327–32.

77. Martinelli I, Mannucci PM, De Stefano V, Taioli E, Rossi V, Crosti F, Paciaroni K, Leone G, Faioni EM. Different risks of thrombosis in four coagulation defects associated with inherited thrombophilia: a study of 150 families. Blood. 1998;92(7):2353–8.

78. Martinov MV, Plotnikov AG, Vitvitsky VM, Ataullakhanov FI. Deficiencies of glycolytic enzymes as a possible cause of hemolytic anemia. Biochim Biophys Acta. 2000;1474(1):75–87.

79. Matsuura S, Igarashi M, Tanizawa Y, Yamada M, Kishi F, Kajii T, Fujii H, Miwa S, Sakurai M, Nakazawa A. Human adenylate kinase deficiency associated with hemolytic anemia. A single base substitution affecting solubility and catalytic activity of the cytosolic adenylate kinase. J Biol Chem. 1989;264(17):10148–55.

80. Minucci A, Moradkhani K, Hwang MJ, Zuppi C, Giardina B, Capoluongo E. Glucose-6-phosphate dehydrogenase (G6PD) mutations database: review of the "old" and update of the new mutations. Blood Cells Mol Dis. 2012;48:154–65.

81. Montani D, Achouh L, Dorfmüller P, Le Pavec J, Sztrymf B, Tchérakian C, Rabiller A, Haque R, Sitbon O, Jaïs X, Dartevelle P, Maître S, Capron F, Musset D, Simonneau G, Humbert M. Pulmonary veno-occlusive disease: clinical, functional, radiologic, and hemodynamic characteristics and outcome of 24 cases confirmed by histology. Medicine (Baltimore). 2008;87(4):220–33.

82. Morse J, Barst R, Horn E, Cuervo N, Deng Z, Knowles J. Pulmonary hypertension in scleroderma spectrum of disease: lack of bone morphogenetic protein receptor 2 mutations. J Rheumatol. 2002;29(11):2379–81.

83. Nagaraj C, Tang B, Bálint Z, Wygrecka M, Hrzenjak A, Kwapiszewska G, Stacher E, Lindenmann J, Weir EK, Olschewski H, Olschewski A. Src tyrosine kinase is crucial for potassium channel function in human pulmonary arteries. Eur Respir J. 2013;41(1):85–95.

84. Nasim MT, Ogo T, Ahmed M, Randall R, Chowdhury HM, Snape KM, Bradshaw TY, Southgate L, Lee GJ, Jackson I, Lord GM, Gibbs JS, Wilkins MR, Ohta-Ogo K, Nakamura K, Girerd B, Coulet F, Soubrier F, Humbert M, Morrell NW, Trembath RC, Machado RD. Molecular genetic characterization of SMAD signaling molecules in pulmonary arterial hypertension. Hum Mutat. 2011;32(12):1385–9.

85. Nimmakayalu M, Major H, Sheffield V, Solomon DH, Smith RJ, Patil SR, Shchelochkov OA. Microdeletion of 17q22q23.2 encompassing TBX2 and TBX4 in a patient with congenital microcephaly, thyroid duct cyst, sensorineural hearing loss, and pulmonary hypertension. Am J Med Genet A. 2011;155A(2):418–23.

86. Olschewski A, Li Y, Tang B, Hanze J, Eul B, Bohle RM, Wilhelm J, Morty RE, Brau ME, Weir EK, Kwapiszewska G, Klepetko W, Seeger W, Olschewski H. Impact of TASK-1 in human pulmonary artery smooth muscle cells. Circ Res. 2006;98(8):1072–80.

87. Osipenko ON, Evans AM, Gurney AM. Regulation of the resting potential of rabbit pulmonary artery myocytes by a low threshold, O2-sensing potassium current. Br J Pharmacol. 1997;120(8):1461–70.

88. Pfarr N, Fischer C, Ehlken N, Becker-Grünig T, López-González V, Gorenflo M, Hager A, Hinderhofer K, Miera O, Nagel C, Schranz D, Grünig E. Hemodynamic and genetic analysis in children with idiopathic, heritable, and congenital heart disease associated pulmonary arterial hypertension. Respir Res. 2013;14:3.

89. Poort SR, Rosendaal FR, Reitsma PH, Bertina RM. A common genetic variation in the 3'-untranslated region of the prothrombin gene is associated with elevated plasma prothrombin levels and an increase in venous thrombosis. Blood. 1996;88:3698–703.

90. Porteous MEM, Burn J, Proctor SJ. Hereditary haemorrhagic telangiectasia: a clinical analysis. J Med Genet. 1992;29:527–30.

91. Rich S, Dantzker DR, Ayres SM, Bergofsky EH, Brundage BH, Detre KM, Fishman AP, Goldring RM, Groves BM, Koerner SK,

Levy PC, Reid LM, Vreim CE, Williams GW. Primary pulmonary hypertension: a national prospective study. Ann Intern Med. 1987;107:216–23.

92. Roberts KE, McElroy JJ, Wong WP, Yen E, Widlitz A, Barst RJ, Knowles JA, Morse JH. BMPR2 mutations in pulmonary arterial hypertension with congenital heart disease. Eur Respir J. 2004; 24(3):371–4.

93. Roberts KE, Kawut SM, Krowka MJ, Brown Jr RS, Trotter JF, Shah V, Peter I, Tighiouart H, Mitra N, Handorf E, Knowles JA, Zacks S, Fallon MB, Roberts KE, Kawut SM, Krowka MJ, Brown Jr RS, Trotter JF, Shah V, Peter I, Tighiouart H, Mitra N, Handorf E, Knowles JA, Zacks S, Fallon MB. Pulmonary Vascular Complications of Liver Disease Study Group. Genetic risk factors for hepatopulmonary syndrome in patients with advanced liver disease. Gastroenterology. 2010;139(1):9.e24.

94. Rodriguez-Murillo L, Subaran R, Stewart WC, Pramanik S, Marathe S, Barst RJ, Chung WK, Greenberg DA. Novel loci interacting epistatically with bone morphogenetic protein receptor 2 cause familial pulmonary arterial hypertension. J Heart Lung Transplant. 2010;29(2):174–80.

95. Rosenzweig EB, Widlitz AC, Barst RJ. Pulmonary arterial hypertension in children. Pediatr Pulmonol. 2004;38:2–22.

96. Rosenzweig EB, Morse JH, Knowles JA, Chada KK, Khan AM, Roberts KE, McElroy JJ, Juskiw NK, Mallory NC, Rich S, Diamond B, Barst RJ. Clinical implications of determining BMPR2 mutation status in a large cohort of children and adults with pulmonary arterial hypertension. J Heart Lung Transplant. 2008;27:668–74.

97. Rubin LJ. Primary pulmonary hypertension. N Engl J Med. 1997;336(2):111–7.

98. Saruhan-Direskeneli G, Hughes T, Aksu K, Keser G, Coit P, Aydin SZ, Alibaz-Oner F, Kamalı S, Inanc M, Carette S, Hoffman GS, Akar S, Onen F, Akkoc N, Khalidi NA, Koening C, Karadag O, Kiraz S, Langford CA, McAlear CA, Ozbalkan Z, Ates A, Karaaslan Y, Maksimowicz-McKinnon K, Monach PA, Ozer HT, Seyahi E, Fresko I, Cefle A, Seo P, Warrington KJ, Ozturk MA, Ytterberg SR, Cobankara V, Onat AM, Guthridge JM, James JA, Tunc E, Duzgun N, Bıcakcıgil M, Yentür SP, Merkel PA, Direskeneli H, Sawalha AH. Identification of multiple genetic susceptibility loci in Takayasu arteritis. Am J Hum Genet. 2013;93(2):298–305.

99. Saunders DN, Tindall EA, Shearer RF, Roberson J, Decker A, Wilson JA, Hayes VM. A novel SERPINA1 mutation causing serum alpha(1)-antitrypsin deficiency. PLoS One. 2012;7(12), e51762.

100. Scorza R, Caronni M, Bazzi S, Nador F, Beretta L, Antonioli R, Origgi L, Ponti A, Marchini M, Vanoli M. Post-menopause is the main risk factor for developing isolated pulmonary hypertension in systemic sclerosis. Ann N Y Acad Sci. 2002;966:238–46.

101. Selva-O'Callaghan A, Balada E, Serrano-Acedo S, Simeon Aznar CP, Ordi-Ros J. Mutations of activin-receptor-like kinase 1 (ALK-1) are not found in patients with pulmonary hypertension and underlying connective tissue disease. Clin Rheumatol. 2007;26(6):947–9.

102. Sen P, Yang Y, Navarro C, Silva I, Szafranski P, Kolodziejska KE, Dharmadhikari AV, Mostafa H, Kozakewich H, Kearney D, Cahill JB, Whitt M, Bilic M, Margraf L, Charles A, Goldblatt J, Gibson K, Lantz PE, Garvin AJ, Petty J, Kiblawi Z, Zuppan C, McConkie-Rosell A, McDonald MT, Peterson-Carmichael SL, Gaede JT, Shivanna B, Schady D, Friedlich PS, Hays SR, Palafoll IV, Siebers-Renelt U, Bohring A, Finn LS, Siebert JR, Galambos C, Nguyen L, Riley M, Chassaing N, Vigouroux A, Rocha G, Fernandes S, Brumbaugh J, Roberts K, Ho-Ming L, Lo IF, Lam S, Gerychova R, Jezova M, Valaskova I, Fellmann F, Afshar K, Giannoni E, Muhlethaler V, Liang J, Beckmann JS, Lioy J, Deshmukh H, Srinivasan L, Swarr DT, Sloman M, Shaw-Smith C, van Loon RL, Hagman C, Sznajer Y, Barrea C, Galant C, Detaille

T, Wambach JA, Cole FS, Hamvas A, Prince LS, Diderich KE, Brooks AS, Verdijk RM, Ravindranathan H, Sugo E, Mowat D, Baker ML, Langston C, Welty S, Stankiewicz P. Novel FOXF1 mutations in sporadic and familial cases of alveolar capillary dysplasia with misaligned pulmonary veins imply a role for its DNA binding domain. Hum Mutat. 2013;34(6):801–11.

103. Serrano A, Márquez A, Mackie SL, Carmona FD, Solans R, Miranda-Filloy JA, Hernández-Rodríguez J, Cid MC, Castañeda S, Morado IC, Narváez J, Blanco R, Sopeña B, García-Villanueva MJ, Monfort J, Ortego-Centeno N, Unzurrunzaga A, Marí-Alfonso B, Sánchez-Martín J, de Miguel E, Magro C, Raya E, Braun N, Latus J, Molberg O, Lie BA, Moosig F, Witte T, Morgan AW, González-Gay MA, Martin J, UK GCA Consortium Spanish GCA Consortium. Identification of the PTPN22 functional variant R620W as susceptibility genetic factor for giant cell arteritis. Ann Rheum Dis. 2013;72(11):1882–6.

104. Shintani M, Yagi H, Nakayama T, Saji T, Matsuoka R. A new nonsense mutation of SMAD8 associated with pulmonary arterial hypertension. J Med Genet. 2009;46(5):331–7.

105. Simonneau G, Gali ERL, Rubin LJ, Langleben D, Seeger W, Domenighetti G, Gibbs S, Lebrec D, Speich R, Beghetti M, Rich S, Fishman A. Clinical classification of pulmonary hypertension. J Am Coll Cardiol. 2004;43(12 Suppl S):5S–12.

106. Simsek E, Yesilyurt A, Pinarli F, Eyerci N, Ulus AT. Combined genetic mutations have remarkable effect on deep venous thrombosis and/or pulmonary embolism occurrence. Gene. 2014; 536(1):171–6.

107. Sopeña B, Pérez-Rodríguez MT, Portela D, Rivera A, Freire M, Martínez-Vázquez C. High prevalence of pulmonary hypertension in patients with hereditary hemorrhagic telangiectasia. Eur J Intern Med. 2013;24(3):e30–4.

108. Srinivasan S, Hanes MA, Dickens T, Porteous MEM, Oh SP, Hale LP, Marchuk DA. A mouse model for hereditary hemorrhagic telangiectasia (HHT) type 2. Hum Mol Genet. 2003;12:473–82.

109. Stankiewicz P, Sen P, Bhatt SS, Storer M, Xia Z, Bejjani BA, Ou Z, Wiszniewska J, Driscoll DJ, Maisenbacher MK, Bolivar J, Bauer M, Zackai EH, McDonald-McGinn D, Nowaczyk MM, Murray M, Hustead V, Mascotti K, Schultz R, Hallam L, McRae D, Nicholson AG, Newbury R, Durham-O'Donnell J, Knight G, Kini U, Shaikh TH, Martin V, Tyreman M, Simonic I, Willatt L, Paterson J, Mehta S, Rajan D, Fitzgerald T, Gribble S, Prigmore E, Patel A, Shaffer LG, Carter NP, Cheung SW, Langston C, Shaw-Smith C. Genomic and genic deletions of the FOX gene cluster on 16q24.1 and inactivating mutations of FOXF1 cause alveolar capillary dysplasia and other malformations. Am J Hum Genet. 2009;84(6):780–91.

110. Toledano K, Guralnik L, Lorber A, Ofer A, Yigla M, Rozin A, Markovits D, Braun-Moscovici Y, Balbir-Gurman A. Pulmonary arteries involvement in Takayasu's arteritis: two cases and literature review. Semin Arthritis Rheum. 2011;41(3):461–70.

111. Trembath RC, Thomson JR, Machado RD, Morgan NV, Atkinson C, Winship I, Simonneau G, Galie N, Loyd JE, Humbert M, Nichols WC, Morrell NW, Berg J, Manes A, McGaughran J, Pauciulo M, Wheeler L. Clinical and molecular genetic features of pulmonary hypertension in patients with hereditary hemorrhagic telangiectasia. N Engl J Med. 2001;345(5):325–34.

112. Valentini G, Chiarelli LR, Fortin R, Dolzan M, Galizzi A, Abraham DJ, Wang C, Bianchi P, Zanella A, Mattevi A. Structure and function of human erythrocyte pyruvate kinase. Molecular basis of nonspherocytic hemolytic anemia. J Biol Chem. 2002;277(26):23807–14.

113. Vandenbriele C, Peerlinck K, de Ravel T, Verhamme P, Vanassche T. Pulmonary arterio-venous malformations in a patient with a novel mutation in exon 10 of the ACVRL1 gene. Acta Clin Belg. 2014;69(2):139–41.

114. Vase P, Holm M, Arendrup H. Pulmonary arteriovenous fistules in hereditary haemorrhagic telangiectasia. Acta Med Scand. 1985;218:105–9.

115. West J, Fagan K, Steudel W, Fouty B, Lane K, Harral J, Hoedt-Miller M, Tada Y, Ozimek J, Tuder R, Rodman DM. Pulmonary hypertension in transgenic mice expressing a dominant-negative BMPRII gene in smooth muscle. Circ Res. 2004;94:1109–14.

116. West J, Harral J, Lane K, Deng Y, Ickes B, Crona D, Albu S, Stewart D, Fagan K. Mice expressing BMPR2R899X transgene in smooth muscle develop pulmonary vascular lesions. Am J Physiol Lung Cell Mol Physiol. 2008;295(5):L744–55.

117. Weyand CM, Hicok KC, Hunder GG, Goronzy JJ. The HLA-DRB1 locus as a genetic component in giant cell arteritis. Mapping of a disease-linked sequence motif to the antigen binding site of the HLA-DR molecule. J Clin Invest. 1992;90(6):2355–61.

118. Wieczorek S, Hellmich B, Arning L, Moosig F, Lamprecht P, Gross WL, Epplen JT. Functionally relevant variations of the interleukin-10 gene associated with antineutrophil cytoplasmic antibody-negative Churg-Strauss syndrome, but not with Wegener's granulomatosis. Arthritis Rheum. 2008;58(6):1839–48.

119. Wilcken B, Bamforth F, Li Z, Zhu H, Ritvanen A, Renlund M, Stoll C, Alembik Y, Dott B, Czeizel AE, Gelman-Kohan Z, Scarano G, Bianca S, Ettore G, Tenconi R, Bellato S, Scala I, Mutchinick OM, López MA, de Walle H, Hofstra R, Joutchenko L, Kavteladze L, Bermejo E, Martínez-Frías ML, Gallagher M, Erickson JD, Vollset SE, Mastroiacovo P, Andria G, Botto LD. Geographical and ethnic variation of the 677C-T allele of 5,10 methylenetetrahydrofolate reductase (MTHFR): findings from over 7000 newborns from 16 areas world wide. J Med Genet. 2003;40:619–25.

120. Xie G, Roshandel D, Sherva R, Monach PA, Lu EY, Kung T, Carrington K, Zhang SS, Pulit SL, Ripke S, Carette S, Dellaripa PF, Edberg JC, Hoffman GS, Khalidi N, Langford CA, Mahr AD, St Clair EW, Seo P, Specks U, Spiera RF, Stone JH, Ytterberg SR, Raychaudhuri S, de Bakker PI, Farrer LA, Amos CI, Merkel PA, Siminovitch KA. Association of granulomatosis with polyangiitis (Wegener's) with HLA-DPB1*04 and SEMA6A gene variants: evidence from genomewide analysis. Arthritis Rheum. 2013;65(9):2457–68.

121. Yeager ME, Halley GR, Golpon HA, Voelkel NF, Tuder RM. Microsatellite instability of endothelial cell growth and apoptosis genes within plexiform lesions in primary pulmonary hypertension. Circ Res. 2001;88(1):E2–11.

122. Zhao L, Chen CN, Hajji N, Oliver E, Cotroneo E, Wharton J, Wang D, Li M, McKinsey TA, Stenmark KR, Wilkins MR. Histone deacetylation inhibition in pulmonary hypertension: therapeutic potential of valproic acid and suberoylanilide hydroxamic acid. Circulation. 2012;126(4):455–67.

123. Zhu T, Martinez I, Emmerich J. Venous thromboembolism: risk factors for recurrence. Arterioscler Thromb Vasc Biol. 2009;29:298–310.

Novel Mechanisms of Disease: Network Biology and MicroRNA Signaling in Pulmonary Hypertension

Wassim H. Fares, Kusum V. Pandit, and Naftali Kaminski

Introduction

The field of network biology has been rapidly expanding in the last decade. Our understanding of the complex interactions between deoxyribonucleic acid (DNA), ribonucleic acid (RNA), proteins and drugs is much deeper than it was in the 1990's, however it is still significantly limited. We have just started to have a glimpse at this field, which is being facilitated by novel technologies and advanced computational algorithms modeling cellular interactions. The concept of static sequence of DNA to RNA to protein to functional effect now seems a naïve way to understand biology. It is rather a dynamic web of multi-way, fluid, sometimes redundant, but tightly controlled interactions between different proteins, epigenetic factors including transcription factors and microRNAs and DNA, that changes over time and under different milieus.

A microRNA is a small non-coding RNA molecule that typically contains about 18–25 nucleotides. In contrast to our traditional understanding of the role and function of RNAs, microRNAs play key roles in the regulation of gene expression both at the transcriptional and post-transcriptional levels. They are not unique to humans; microRNAs are present and functionally active in other animals, plants, and even some viruses with DNA-based genomes. MicroRNAs are among the ancient and well conserved evolutionary control mechanisms [1], although they seem to have evolved independently in animals versus plants. In contrast to plants microRNAs, animal microRNAs have more flexibility and ability to identify their target messenger RNAs (primarily on the 3'-untranslated regions of the messenger RNA) with a much smaller sequence of nucleic acids.

Although the field of classical genetics is at least a century old, the first microRNA was not characterized until the early 1990's [2] (described at the time as a 'small temporal RNA' and 'nematode idiosyncrasy' and was identified as a microRNA years later in retrospect), and the field of microRNAs did not actually boom until they were recognized as effective and independent regulatory molecules of genetics expression about 10–15 years ago. During this short period of time, almost 30,000 microRNAs have been identified, about 2000 of which have been identified so far to exist in humans [3], and they can potentially target at least ~60 % of the human protein-coding genes [1, 4]. This reflects the power, critical importance, and scope of the effect of microRNAs.

The discovery of microRNAs drastically changed our understanding of both healthy and pathologic states, which was based primarily on exons and protein-coding genes as well as protein – protein interactions. Some microRNAs are ubiquitous in different cell types or tissues, but others are tissue-specific. In contrast to the relationship between DNA and messenger RNA sequences, microRNAs are not specific to certain messenger RNAs, and messenger RNAs may also be targeted by different microRNAs [5]. It has been estimated that a single microRNA may target up to hundreds of messenger RNAs, but to a varying level of potency [6, 7]. Such diversity of microRNA/messenger RNA relationship gives rise to a huge and strong power of the microRNAs to affect a wide variety of physiologic and pathologic processes affecting multiple organ systems at different levels, and potentially escaping individual targeting repair mechanisms.

W.H. Fares, MD, MSc
Pulmonary, Critical Care and Sleep Medicine,
Yale University, School of Medicine, 300 Cedar St., TAC-441 South,
New Haven, CT 06520, USA
e-mail: wassim.fares@yale.edu

K.V. Pandit, MBBS, PhD
Division of Pulmonary, Allergy and Critical Care Medicine,
Dorothy P. and Richard P. Simmons Center for Interstitial Lung
Disease, University of Pittsburgh School of Medicine,
Pittsburgh, PA 15261, USA

Department of Medicine, University of Pittsburgh Medical Center,
Pittsburgh, PA USA

N. Kaminski, MD (✉)
Section of Pulmonary, Critical Care and Sleep Medicine,
Department of Medicine, Yale University, School of Medicine,
300 Cedar St., TAC-441 South, New Haven, CT 06520, USA
e-mail: naftali.kaminski@yale.edu

© Springer International Publishing Switzerland 2016
B.A. Maron et al. (eds.), *Pulmonary Hypertension: Basic Science to Clinical Medicine*, DOI 10.1007/978-3-319-23594-3_7

Characteristics of microRNAs

MicroRNAs are the most well studied among the class of non-coding RNAs. The other non-coding RNAs include transfer RNA (tRNA) and ribosomal RNA (rRNA), snoR-NAs, siRNAs, snRNAs, piRNAs and the long ncRNAs [8, 9]. MicroRNAs exert their effect by base-pairing with messenger RNAs obeying the standard nucleic acids base complementarity, though this base-pairing is not as perfect as other nucleic sequences pairing. The microRNA region where high affinity base pairing with the target messenger RNA is critical, though not universal, is called the seed region which is mostly located in the base pairs 2–8 of the 5' end. The shortness of the seed region, being only a few base-pairs in length, significantly increases the chances of any single microRNA to match with a large number of messenger RNAs. It is these high odds, combined with a persistent billions-of-years old evolutionary natural selection, that amplify the wide spread regulatory impact of microRNAs on such a large number of protein-coding genes [10], though at variable potency levels.

At the post-transcription level, microRNAs target messenger RNAs to selectively degrade RNAs or repress translation (e.g., by pairing with messenger RNAs and thus preventing them from being transcribed). Although microR-NAs are more known for their inhibitory or repressive effects on messenger RNAs [11], some are potentially involved in activating, stimulating, or stabilizing select protein production pathways at the transcriptional and/or translational levels [12–14].

The two other major epigenetic mechanisms that control or contribute to the regulation of the final protein products and eventual biological phenotype, in addition to microR-NAs, are DNA methylation (by DNA methyl-transferases) and histone proteins modification [15, 16]. DNA methylation involves the addition of a methyl group to the promoter region of a gene and thus silences that specific gene. Histone acetylation increases while histone de-acetylation decreases gene transcription. As stated above, they do not carry hereditary characteristics and thus their presence or absence has no direct implications regarding inheritance of genes. However, many microRNAs may actually have the ability to directly modify RNAs and thus cause the production of proteins that are not reflected by the original DNA sequences. This ability multiplies the possibilities of the diversity of produced proteins, way beyond Mendelian genetics. Biologically, microRNAs function in a similar way to post-transcriptional regulatory proteins. MicroRNA pathologies have been directly associated with certain diseases, and they are believed to play a pathologic role in some diseases [17]. MicroRNAs have been implicated in the pathogenesis of multiple diseases, including malignancies, cardiovascular, and neurologic pathologies to name a few. Their role in pulmonary vascular disease has also been explored in the last few years with multiple microRNAs being identified to play key roles in pulmonary vascular disease.

Biogenesis of MicroRNAs

In humans, most of the microRNAs are encoded within introns of coding or non-coding transcripts, a few are encoded within exons or are intergenic. Some microRNAs are located close to each other so that they are transcribed as a single unit from a common upstream promoter [18]. Though these microRNAs are polycistronic, they may undergo different post-transcriptional modifications, The canonical pathway [19] for the generation of microRNAs includes the following sequence of events (Fig. 7.1). Following transcription by RNA Polymerase II or III [20, 21], a primary microRNA transcript (pri-miRNA) is generated that is usually larger than 1 kb. This pri-miRNA contains a stem-loop structure in which the microRNA is located and single-stranded RNA segments on both 5' and 3' ends of this stem-loop. The pri-miRNA is asymmetrically processed by an RNase III endonuclease Drosha to release the precursor microRNA (pre-miRNA) that is typically about 60-70 nucleotides in length [22]. Drosha, together with its essential cofactor DGCR8 (DiGeorge Syndrome critical region-8) [23] forms the Microprocessor complex [24]. The pre-miRNA is then exported via the nuclear pore from the nucleus into the cytoplasm by a nuclear transport receptor protein called exportin-5 in the presence a GTP-binding nuclear protein of RAN-GTP. This is followed by further processing of the pre-microRNA by another RNase III enzyme, Dicer, to form a mature microRNA base-matched duplex, each of which is about 22 [18–25] nucleotides in length. For the Dicer to exert its 'dicing' or 'cutting' effect, it has to recognize a defined RNA structure, in a similar fashion to the Drosha. This RNA duplex generated by Dicer is loaded onto the Argonaute (AGO) protein to form an effector complex called RNA induced silencing complex (RISC). The guide strand or the more prevalent strand is selected on the basis of relative thermodynamic stability of the two ends of the duplex. The strand with the relatively unstable 5' terminus is preferentially selected as the guide strand. However many published studies have also demonstrated functional significance of the passenger strand (microRNA*) [25]. The better the complementarity between the microRNA and its target messenger RNA, the greater the probability of cleavage of the target transcript. If complementarity is complete, the target transcript is prevented from being translated into protein.

Fig. 7.1 The canonical pathway of microRNA processing (Reprinted by permission from Macmillan Publishers Ltd: Winter et al. [97] Nature Publishing Group)

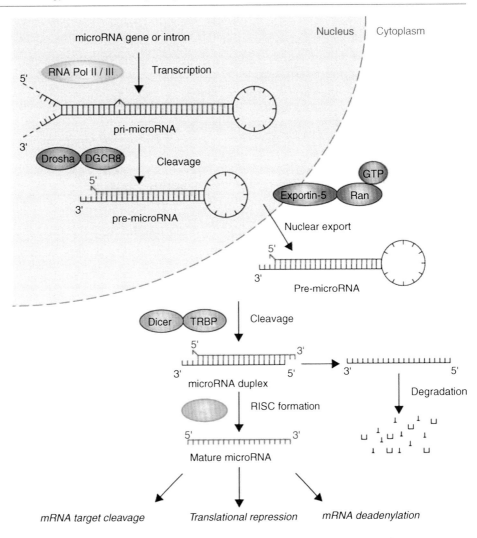

Computational Biology, Our Venue to Understand MicroRNA Network Biology

As mentioned the complexity of microRNA regulations is derived from the fact that a microRNA can target multiple mRNAs and multiple microRNAs can target a single mRNA. Thus approaches that integrate signaling from microRNAs, to mRNAs and proteins are required. However, since the microRNA field is relatively young, classification and nomenclature of microRNAs, and databases of their predicted and validated targets were required.

An online microRNA database, named miRBase, has a list of all microRNAs that are currently identified in all organisms including humans [26]. The nomenclature of microRNAs has also been standardized [26–28]. One of the more basic computational methods to identify microRNA targets and potential function includes a simple sequence analysis [29]. Such out-of-context base sequence analysis predictability has a high rate of false positive and false negative results, which makes such analyses challenging and

usually require biological validation and direct demonstration of effect on target genes.

MicroRNAs are frequently co-expressed with host genes, as well as with neighboring microRNAs [30], which highlights the networking effect and the 'team-spirit' of microRNAs, working in consortiums, rather than individually or independent of other transcription factors. The multiplicity of targets of a single microRNA [5] logarithmically increases the effect of any aberrancy in microRNAs on multiple pathways within a specific disease and potentially multiple simultaneous disease states. Efforts at creating dynamic regulatory network analysis capability and creating probabilistic modeling methods are promising [31]. Previously unknown microRNAs and new roles of known microRNAs could be predicted and identified using probabilistic modeling methods [such as the MiRNA Dynamic Regulatory Events Miner (mirDREM)] that use models to reconstruct a dynamic virtual network that explains joint regulation of microRNAs and other transcription factors of expression of protein-coding genes over a period of time [31]. Once these microRNAs and/or their roles are identified, they would then be validated/confirmed using proliferation assays for example. Transcription factors and microRNAs regulate each other, and in combination regulate protein-coding genes under different disease states [32, 33]. Computational transcription factor-microRNA networks are available for some genomes and diseases [14, 34, 35]. A wealth of data has been generated by the ENCODE project [36], however integrated analysis and experimental verification of these interactions are still ongoing.

Clinical Phenotype of Pulmonary Arterial Hypertension

As detailed in the other chapters of this book, pulmonary arterial hypertension, which is classified by the World Health Organization (WHO) as WHO group 1 pulmonary hypertension [37] is a progressive and fatal disease. The pathobiology of the pulmonary vascular disease in pulmonary arterial hypertension is diverse and not well understood [38], but it is accepted that its pathobiology is programmed in a way to tip the balance in favor of pro-inflammation, pro-coagulation particularly in-situ pro-coagulation, and pro-fibrosis. The regulatory molecules and pathways that are upstream of these pathologic end-points are not well understood or characterized. There is enough evidence now to confirm a major regulatory role of microRNAs in the pathogenesis of pulmonary vascular disease and its clinical prototype, pulmonary arterial hypertension.

Although multiple therapeutic drug families are available to treat pulmonary arterial hypertension [39], their primary effect is via vasodilatation, with only minor other contributory effects such as anti-platelets or anti-inflammatory effects. This may explain the lack of a cure for this disease at this time, and the only modest, but significant, improvement in survival of these patients over the last two decades. As our understanding of microRNAs continues to grow, the field is expected to move forward with new therapeutic pathways that will likely involve targeting microRNAs.

The challenge though, as alluded to above, is that microRNAs do not work in individual sequential pathways. They rather work in concerted efforts among 'teams' of microRNAs targeting 'teams' of genes. So typically microRNAs are down-regulated or up-regulated in global profiles [40], rather than in individual molecules or individual microRNAs. This biology network requires an eagle's view of multiple simultaneous and inter-related pathways, and the help of computational network specialists. This should not discourage scientists from going into this very exciting young field, but it has to be tackled with the right mindset. In contrast to our traditional progress in the biomedical fields over the last

century, the field of microRNAs will further progress and develop with the use of well-organized and detailed computational and biochemical quantitative models.

Pulmonary Remodeling

Though current treatments for PAH offer a survival benefit, mortality still remains high. Treatments that can effectively control cellular changes and consequent pulmonary remodeling are needed. Hypoxia, vessel injury and inflammation exacerbate the remodeling process [41]. Hyperplastic fibroblasts in the adventitial layer cause adventitial thickening. NADPH increases the reactive oxygen species in adventitia contributing to fibroblast activation. These activated fibroblasts secrete platelet-derived growth factor, endothelin-1 and serotonin causing proliferation, migration and contraction of fibroblasts and smooth muscle cells. A subset of these activated fibroblasts differentiate into myofibroblasts which are regulated by growth factors such as TGF-β [42, 43]. Myofibroblasts migrate into the medial layer increasing its thickness and deposit extracellular proteins such as collagen, fibronectin, elastin and tenascin C which in turn induces smooth muscle cell proliferation and migration within the media [41, 44, 45]. Myofibroblasts and hypertrophic smooth muscle cells considerably increase diameter of the medial layer. Hypertrophy and proliferation of endothelial cells causes intimal thickening leading to increased production of the vasoconstrictor endothelin-1 [46], and elastase which activates matrix metalloproteinases and tenascin-C further increasing smooth muscle cell proliferation. Eventually, increased proliferation of endothelial cells results in formation of plexiform lesions [47], occlusion of the lumen and diminished blood flow to distal pulmonary arteries [48].

Animal Models for PAH

Gomez-Arroyo et al. have extensively reviewed the available mouse models for pulmonary hypertension [49]. The one animal model that most closely resembles the pathobiological hallmarks of pulmonary arterial hypertension in humans is that of the combination of vascular endothelial growth factor receptor antagonist (SU5416) and chronic hypoxia [50]. SU5416 is a combined VEGF receptor 1 (Flt) and 2 (KDR) blocker. This model has been used for preclinical drug testing to determine whether the pulmonary hypertension and pulmonary vascular disease can be reversed once established. Histopathologically, the lung vascular lesions of these rats are comparable to the plexiform lesions in humans [51]. This model has also been tested in various knockout mice which has been reviewed in [52]. Since there is not an ideal mouse model for PAH yet, we cannot be certain that the results seen in pulmonary hypertension animal models can be translated to humans.

MicroRNAs in Pulmonary Hypertension

Profiling studies have identified a characteristic microRNA signature of pulmonary hypertension. Caruso et al. performed microarray analysis in rats exposed to chronic hypoxia and monocrotaline [40]. They found miR-22, miR-30 and let-7f to be downregulated while miR-322 and miR-451 were upregulated. A second study analyzed microRNA expression in pulmonary arteries of PAH patients. Amongst the upregulated microRNAs were miR-138, miR-367, miR-27b, miR-145, miR-302b and miR-450a while miR-204 was downregulated. A few microRNAs have been studied in detail to identify their roles in the pathogenesis of pulmonary hypertension. This is a non-comprehensive list of microRNAs that have been implicated in or associated with the pathogenesis of pulmonary vascular disease and has also been discussed earlier [53]. This list is expected to change rapidly as the field of microRNAs continues to exponentially grow. Here we will discuss each of these microRNAs having divided them into upregulated and downregulated microRNAs in PAH.

Upregulated microRNAs

- miR-143~145: These polycistronic microRNAs are conserved across different species, abundantly expressed in cardiac, vascular and visceral smooth muscle cells [54, 55] to maintain their contractile phenotype. MiR-145 inhibits Kruppel-like factor 5 (KLF5), thus inducing myocardin and smooth muscle cell markers such as α-smooth muscle actin, calpolin and smooth muscle myosin heavy chain [55]. MiR-143 and miR-145 are increased in human PAH and the hypoxia-induced mouse model of PH [56, 57]. PAH patients with BMPR2 mutations have increased expression of miR-145 and *in vitro* inhibition of BMPR2 induces miR-145. In vascular smooth muscle cells, TGF-β and BMP4 induce myocardin expression and nuclear transport of myocardin-related transcription factors respectively which eventually leads to increased transcription of this polycistron [58]. Inhibition of miR-145 *in vivo* prevents hypoxia-induced PH in mice [57].
- miR-210: MiR-210 is induced by hypoxia in smooth muscle cells and mouse lungs via an HIF-1-dependent pathway. It inhibits E2F3 and increases cellular resistance to apoptosis causing smooth muscle cell hyperplasia [59].

   miR-21: MiR-21 is upregulated in lungs of PAH patients and animal models of PH. In pulmonary artery smooth muscle cells, hypoxia induces miR-21 resulting a subsequent decrease in its targets PDCD4 (programmed cell death 4), SPRY2 (sprouty homolog 2) and PPARα. Inhibition of miR-21 inhibits hypoxia-induced proliferation and migration in cultured smooth muscle cells [60] and prevents and reverses hypoxia-induced PAH [61]. Using computational approaches, Parikh et al. identified miR-21 to regulate multiple pathways in PAH [62]. In pulmonary artery endothelial cells, hypoxia and BMPR2 signaling increase miR-21 expression. MiR-21 in turn downregulates BMPR2 expression forming a negative feedback loop. MiR-21 directly targets RhoB expression and Rho-kinase activity decreasing angiogenesis and vasodilatation. Inhibition of miR-21 causes the opposite effects on Rho kinase activity, exaggerating PH in animal models [62]. Decreased miR-21 in mice also activates the PDCD4/caspase-3 axis thus inducing PH. Supplementing miR-21 reduces PDCD4 and protects mice from hypoxia/SU5416-induced PH. There are a few discrepancies in the results reported for miR-21. MiR-21 is downregulated in monocrotaline-induced PH and in endothelial cells of human PAH [40, 63] but a threefold upregulation of miR-21 was observed in hypoxic human pulmonary artery smooth muscle cells, while no change was observed in rats [40, 60]. Caruso et al. demonstrated downregulation of miR-21 in rat lungs of monocrotaline-induced PH but not hypoxia-induced PH, whereas Parikh et al. demonstrated time-dependent induction of miR-21 in monocrotalin-induced PH [40, 62]. MiR-21 prevents PH in the hypoxia/SU5416 model [62, 64] but promotes it in the hypoxia alone model [61]. These contradicting results may possibly stem from the fact that miR-21 has different roles in endothelial cells and smooth muscle cells.

- miR-27a: Hypoxia induces miR-27a in pulmonary artery endothelial cells leading to increased cell proliferation and endothelin-1 expression to decrease PPARγ [65]. MiR-27a levels are increased in PPARγ knockout mice, and a PPARγ ligand, rosiglitazone attenuates hypoxia-induced miR-27a. These results suggest a negative feedback loop constituting PPARγ and miR 27a to promote PH

Downregulated microRNAs

- miR-17~92 cluster: The miR-17~92 cluster includes six mature microRNAs, miR-17, miR-18a, miR-19a, miR19b, miR-20a and miR-92a. This cluster is essential for lung development; loss of this polycistron leads to severe hypoplastic lungs in mice [66]. MiR-17~92 is downregulated in pulmonary artery smooth muscle cells from PAH patients [67] and associated with reduced expression of α-smooth muscle actin, SM22α and calpolin. Reduced cluster expression is associated with a dedifferentiated smooth muscle cell phenotype which is reversed by overexpression of the cluster. PDLIM5 (PDZ and LIM domain 5) is a direct target of this cluster. In PAH, upregulated PDLIM5 induces the TGFβ3/SMAD3 pathway contributing to PAH [67]. Transient upregulation of miR-17 in the hypoxia-induced model has been reported which was partially reversed by inhibition of miR-17 probably by inducing p21 and subsequent inhibition of proliferation of smooth muscle cells [68]. Hence in the initial stage of blood vessel remodeling, increased miR-17~92 promotes smooth muscle cell proliferation while in the later stages reduction of this cluster releases its inhibition on its target PDLIM5 to maintain the smooth muscle cell dedifferentiation. In endothelial cells, VEGF induces the miR-17~92 cluster which is required for endothelial cell proliferation and angiogenesis. A few patients with PAH have BMPR2 mutations and downregulation of BMPR2 is associated with PAH [69]. BMPR2 is a direct target of miR-17-5p and miR-20a in pulmonary artery endothelial cells. The promoter of this polycistron has a conserved STAT3 binding site. IL6 induces STA3 binding to this promoter region, thus increasing expression of miR-17~92 [70].

- miR-124: Kang et al. studied the microRNAs regulating the nuclear factor of activated T cells (NFAT) pathway which has been implicated in PAH and smooth muscle cell proliferation [71]. NFATc1, CAMTA1 and PTBP1 are direct targets of miR-124. Their inhibition results in inhibition of NFAT activity, dephosphorylation, nuclear translocation and inhibition of NFAT-dependent IL2 transcription. MiR-124 is reduced in fibroblasts isolated from PAH patients and animal models of PH [72]. MiR-124 inhibits expression of monocyte chemotactic protein-1 and polypyrimidine tract-binding protein 1 which regulate Notch1, tensin homolog/FOXO3/p21Cip1, p27Kip1 signaling to prevent hyperproliferation and migration of fibroblasts. Histone deacetylase inhibitors restore miR-124 expression and suppress fibroblast proliferation, hinting at a therapeutic role for histone deacetylase inhibitors in PAH.

- miR-204: MiR-204 is an intronic microRNA of the gene transient receptor potential melastatin 3 (TRPM3) sharing its promoter with its host gene. MiR-204 is expressed in pulmonary artery smooth muscle cells and downregulated by STAT3 [56, 73]. MiR-204 is reduced in human PAH and hypoxia-induced and monocrotaline-induced PH in rats. Endothelin-1, angiotensin –II, PDGF decrease miR-204; this microRNA reduction in turn activates the Src-STAT3-NFAT pathway by upregulating SHP2 causing smooth muscle cell proliferation and decreased apoptosis. Supplementing miR-204 reverses monocrotaline-induced PH. MiR-204 levels are negatively correlated with severity of PAH in patients and positively correlated with the levels in smooth muscle cells.

- miR-424 and 503: An intact apelin signaling pathway is essential for pulmonary vascular homeostasis. In PAH patients, reduced apelin results in increased proliferation and reduced apoptosis of endothelial cells while knockout of apelin exacerbates hypoxia-induced PH [74]. MiR-424/503 are positively regulated by apelin, and they in turn negatively regulate the fibroblast growth factor (FGF) endothelial signaling via their direct effect on FGF2 and FGF receptor-1 [75]. These microRNAs are decreased in PAH. Restoration of miR-424 and miR-503 in rat PAH models improved right ventricular function and PAH pathological molecular and antigen markers by decreasing FGF and its receptor [75].

- miR-126: Potus et al. showed decreased capillary density n peripheral skeletal muscles of PAH patients suggesting a defect in peripheral angiogenesis [76]. MiR-126, a microRNA decreased in PAH skeletal muscles and decompensated right ventricle, targets Sprouty-related EVH1 domain-containing protein 1 (SPRED-1) which is a main regulator of the VEGF/ERK pathway. Potus and colleagues also observed an increase in miR-126 and decrease in SPRED-1 in the compensated right ventricle. Supplementing miR-126 restored the angiogenic ability of PAH endothelium to normal levels in quadriceps and right ventricular endothelial cells.

This list of microRNAs is only the tip of the iceberg. A much larger number of yet unidentified microRNAs is expected to be associated or implicated in the pathobiology of pulmonary vascular disease, which includes processes such as pro-inflammation [77], pro-coagulation, pro-proliferation, intimal thickening, medial hypertrophy, and adventitial fibrosis and thickening. These involve a multitude of cells including but not limited to mononuclear cells, platelets, endothelial cell, smooth muscle cells, fibroblasts, and a wide range of cytokines and other transcription factors. These milieus and cells have direct interaction mechanisms with hypoxia [78] and flow-mediated changes. Each of these processes, molecules, milieus, and factors are likely to have their own microRNA profiles changes and networks that will collectively likely involve a much larger number of individual microRNAs. Every single biological, physiologic or pathologic process that explained any step in the pathobiology of pulmonary vascular disease likely has a microRNA regulatory mechanism that is yet to be identified. Grant et al. have summarized the studied microRNAs in the form of a regulatory network [53] (Fig. 7.2). The microRNAs depicted in this figure control pulmonary artery remodeling by targeting genes belonging to different pathways in different cell types. Thus microRNAs form complex regulatory networks by themselves, but since their expression is correlated with their target genes, they form an intertwined network involving multiple pathways. All the molecules in this network participate to maintain homeostasis. Other members of the network may rescue slight perturbations of certain molecules, however sustained excessive perturbations result in disease.

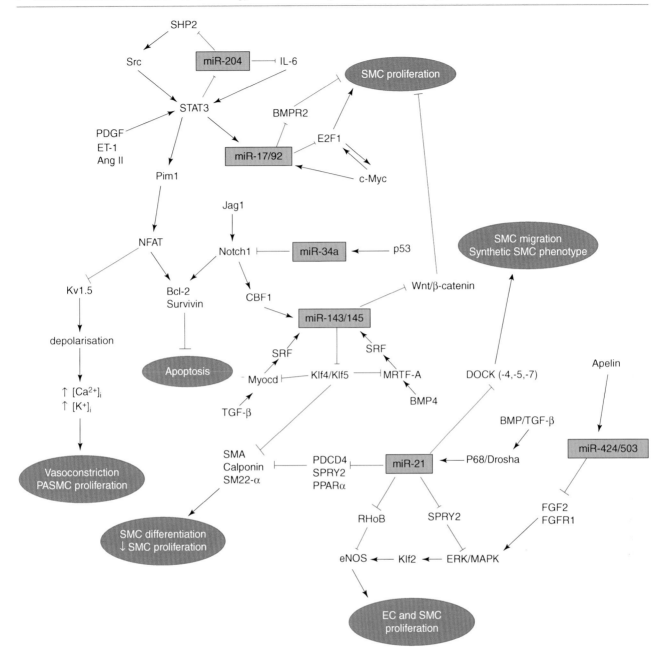

Fig. 7.2 Pathways regulated by microRNAs in pulmonary artery remodeling (Reproduced from Grant et al. [53]; Reprinted under Creative Commons Attribution (CC BY) license from Grant et al. Grant et al. [53])

Regulation of microRNAs in Pulmonary Hypertension

The most common mechanism regulating microRNAs in PAH is hypoxia. Hypoxia possibly activates certain transcription factors including hypoxia inducible factors (HIF). Mice heterozygous for HIF1α have reduced pulmonary remodeling [79]. HIF1α induces the expression of miR-210 in endothelial cells [80] and pancreatic cancer cells [81]. Hypoxia induces miR-155 by binding of HIF1α to hypoxia

responsive elements in the promoter of miR-155 [82]. HIF1α is a direct target of miR-155 thus creating a negative feedback loop.

The second process which regulates microRNA in PAH is inflammation. During inflammation, numerous cytokines, chemokines and growth factors are released which regulate microRNA expression. For example, in human airway smooth muscle cells, miR-25 is decreased following stimulation with IL-1β, TNF-α and IFN-γ [77]. However, miR-155 and miR-146 are increased by these inflammatory stimuli.

MiR-146 is induced by NF-κβ and targets TRAF6 and IRAK1 which activate NF-κβ thus forming a feedback loop [83]. Tissue damage causes NF-κβ nuclear translocation which releases IL-6. IL-6 induces miR-21 transcription in a STAT3-dependent manner [84, 85].

The third mechanism modulating microRNAs are tyrosine kinase pathways. Growth factors such as PDGF and VEGF signal through tyrosine kinase receptors which activate STAT proteins. MiR-204 and miR-17~92 are regulated by tyrosine kinase Src and STAT3 [56, 70]. The tyrosine kinase inhibitor, imatinib, which was developed for treating chronic myeloid leukemia was tested in a phase 3 trial for PAH patients [86]. Imatinib increases exercise capacity and improves hemodynamic parameters in PAH but is associated with frequent adverse effects.

MicroRNAs as Potential Biomarkers

Although microRNAs are present in the nucleus and the cytoplasm, they have also been isolated in circulation, whether in micro-vesicles, exosomes, apoptotic bodies, other types of vesicles, micro-particles, or protein- or lipid- bound [87]. It is worth noting though that the majority of circulating microRNAs seems to be carried within protein complexes [88]. The exact role and remote effect, if any, of these circulating microRNAs are yet to be fully characterized, and this characterization process will not be an easy one [89]. It is likely that microRNAs will serve as biomarkers of disease diagnosis, stratification, and/or prognosis. Establishing associations or correlations between microRNAs that are conveniently collected from the peripheral circulation, especially if they are serum or plasma that would require minimal blood sampling skills and technology would be ideal. Efficient additive combinatorial models can be improved by using microRNAs expression to weigh microRNA targets which act additively in regulating messenger RNA expression [90]. Rhodes et al. have reported reduced circulating miR-150 in peripheral blood of PAH patients and these reduced levels correlate with poor survival [91]. Another study by Schlosser et al. has reported reduced circulating miR-26a in patients with idiopathic PAH, and these miR-26a levels positively correlate with the 6-min walk distance [92].

MicroRNAs as Therapeutic Targets

The use of microRNAs as therapeutic targets did not seem possible because of the multitude of genes they regulate, their ubiquitousness, plurality, redundancy, and multiple additive targets. However microRNAs are being evaluated in clinical trials with promising results. An LNA-modified phosphorothioate oligonucleotide (SPC3649) complementary to the 5′

end of miR-122 was introduced intravenously into chimpanzees with hepatitis C [93]. The long-lasting suppression of hepatitis C viremia led to the initiation of a multicenter phase 2a clinical trial (NCT01200420) [94]. There was a dose-dependent reduction of Hepatitis C virus RNA without any viral resistance when SPC3649 was administered to patients as 5 weekly doses. These positive results have led to the initiation of a 12-week regimen clinical trial (NCT01727934) to evaluate the virologic response [95].

Another Phase I study (NCT01829971) is currently recruiting patients with primary liver cancer or liver metastasis from other cancers [96]. They will be administered the microRNA miR-34 in a liposome-formulated compound (MRX34). This study was initiated after administration of MRX34 intravenously to orthotopic mouse models of hepatocellular cancer led to increased survival. MiR-34 is a tumor suppressor that regulates p53 by targeting oncogenes such as MYC, BCL2, MET and β-catenin. However the microRNA trials in pulmonary hypertension as of date do not manipulate microRNA levels but profile them in patient samples following administration of other drugs.

Future Directions

The need for a deep understanding of the biological function of microRNAs, the extent of compensatory events in response to changes in microRNA expression, possibility of off-target effects and the lack of an ideal animal model are some of the major current obstacles for transitioning the microRNA field into a realistic therapeutic field in humans. MicroRNAs will likely play a pivotal role in further phenotyping patients with pulmonary hypertension and will likely contribute to redistributing subgroups within the WHO pulmonary hypertension classification. Temporal associations and dynamics of the microRNA-based regulatory networks are critical to understanding the roles of the microRNA profiles in different disease states. Such analyses are to be refined over time to account for not-so-highly specific interactions between the microRNAs and their targets, the variable and rapidly changing microRNA expression levels, and the effect of combinatorial microRNA binding. *In conclusion*, we should analyze profile signatures that better reflect disease states, rather than individual molecule, protein, or genetic sequence levels.

References

1. Friedman RC, Farh KK, Burge CB, Bartel DP. Most mammalian mRNAs are conserved targets of microRNAs. Genome Res. 2009;19(1):92–105.
2. Lee RC, Feinbaum RL, Ambros V. The C. elegans heterochronic gene lin-4 encodes small RNAs with antisense complementarity to lin-14. Cell. 1993;75(5):843–54.

3. Griffiths-Jones S, Grocock RJ, van Dongen S, Bateman A, Enright AJ. miRBase: microRNA sequences, targets and gene nomenclature. Nucleic Acids Res. 2006;34(Database issue):D140–4.

4. Pasquinelli AE. MicroRNAs and their targets: recognition, regulation and an emerging reciprocal relationship. Nat Rev Genet. 2012;13(4):271–82.

5. Tsang JS, Ebert MS, van Oudenaarden A. Genome-wide dissection of microRNA functions and cotargeting networks using gene set signatures. Mol Cell. 2010;38(1):140–53.

6. Baek D, Villen J, Shin C, Camargo FD, Gygi SP, Bartel DP. The impact of microRNAs on protein output. Nature. 2008;455(7209):64–71.

7. Selbach M, Schwanhausser B, Thierfelder N, Fang Z, Khanin R, Rajewsky N. Widespread changes in protein synthesis induced by microRNAs. Nature. 2008;455(7209):58–63.

8. Esteller M. Non-coding RNAs in human disease. Nat Rev Genet. 2011;12(12):861–74.

9. Ha M, Kim VN. Regulation of microRNA biogenesis. Nat Rev Mol Cell Biol. 2014;15(8):509–24.

10. Farh KK, Grimson A, Jan C, Lewis BP, Johnston WK, Lim LP, et al. The widespread impact of mammalian MicroRNAs on mRNA repression and evolution. Science. 2005;310(5755):1817–21.

11. Guo H, Ingolia NT, Weissman JS, Bartel DP. Mammalian microRNAs predominantly act to decrease target mRNA levels. Nature. 2010;466(7308):835–40.

12. Jangra RK, Yi M, Lemon SM. DDX6 (Rck/p54) is required for efficient hepatitis C virus replication but not for internal ribosome entry site-directed translation. J Virol. 2010;84(13):6810–24.

13. Vasudevan S, Tong Y, Steitz JA. Switching from repression to activation: microRNAs can up-regulate translation. Science. 2007;318(5858):1931–4.

14. Tsang J, Zhu J, van Oudenaarden A. MicroRNA-mediated feedback and feedforward loops are recurrent network motifs in mammals. Mol Cell. 2007;26(5):753–67.

15. Saco TV, Parthasarathy PT, Cho Y, Lockey RF, Kolliputi N. Role of epigenetics in pulmonary hypertension. Am J Physiol Cell Physiol. 2014;306(12):C1101–5.

16. Kim GH, Ryan JJ, Marsboom G, Archer SL. Epigenetic mechanisms of pulmonary hypertension. Pulm Circ. 2011;1(3):347–56.

17. Li M, Marin-Muller C, Bharadwaj U, Chow KH, Yao Q, Chen C. MicroRNAs: control and loss of control in human physiology and disease. World J Surg. 2009;33(4):667–84.

18. Lee Y, Jeon K, Lee JT, Kim S, Kim VN. MicroRNA maturation: stepwise processing and subcellular localization. EMBO J. 2002;21(17):4663–70.

19. Ameres SL, Zamore PD. Diversifying microRNA sequence and function. Nat Rev Mol Cell Biol. 2013;14(8):475–88.

20. Lee Y, Kim M, Han J, Yeom KH, Lee S, Baek SH, et al. MicroRNA genes are transcribed by RNA polymerase II. EMBO J. 2004;23(20):4051–60.

21. Borchert GM, Lanier W, Davidson BL. RNA polymerase III transcribes human microRNAs. Nat Struct Mol Biol. 2006;13(12):1097–101.

22. Lee Y, Ahn C, Han J, Choi H, Kim J, Yim J, et al. The nuclear RNase III Drosha initiates microRNA processing. Nature. 2003;425(6956):415–9.

23. Gregory RI, Yan KP, Amuthan G, Chendrimada T, Doratotaj B, Cooch N, et al. The Microprocessor complex mediates the genesis of microRNAs. Nature. 2004;432(7014):235–40.

24. Denli AM, Tops BB, Plasterk RH, Ketting RF, Hannon GJ. Processing of primary microRNAs by the Microprocessor complex. Nature. 2004;432(7014):231–5.

25. Chiang HR, Schoenfeld LW, Ruby JG, Auyeung VC, Spies N, Baek D, et al. Mammalian microRNAs: experimental evaluation of novel and previously annotated genes. Genes Dev. 2010;24(10):992–1009.

26. Kozomara A, Griffiths-Jones S. miRBase: annotating high confidence microRNAs using deep sequencing data. Nucleic Acids Res. 2014;42(Database issue):D68–73.

27. Ambros V, Bartel B, Bartel DP, Burge CB, Carrington JC, Chen X, et al. A uniform system for microRNA annotation. RNA. 2003;9(3):277–9.

28. Arora S, Rana R, Chhabra A, Jaiswal A, Rani V. miRNA-transcription factor interactions: a combinatorial regulation of gene expression. Mol Genet Genom MGG. 2013;288(3-4):77–87.

29. Bartel DP. MicroRNAs: target recognition and regulatory functions. Cell. 2009;136(2):215–33.

30. Baskerville S, Bartel DP. Microarray profiling of microRNAs reveals frequent coexpression with neighboring miRNAs and host genes. RNA. 2005;11(3):241–7.

31. Schulz MH, Pandit KV, Lino Cardenas CL, Ambalavanan N, Kaminski N, Bar-Joseph Z. Reconstructing dynamic microRNA-regulated interaction networks. Proc Natl Acad Sci U S A. 2013;110(39):15686–91.

32. Megraw M, Mukherjee S, Ohler U. Sustained-input switches for transcription factors and microRNAs are central building blocks of eukaryotic gene circuits. Genome Biol. 2013;14(8):R85.

33. Marson A, Levine SS, Cole MF, Frampton GM, Brambrink T, Johnstone S, et al. Connecting microRNA genes to the core transcriptional regulatory circuitry of embryonic stem cells. Cell. 2008;134(3):521–33.

34. Guo AY, Sun J, Jia P, Zhao Z. A novel microRNA and transcription factor mediated regulatory network in schizophrenia. BMC Syst Biol. 2010;4:10.

35. Delfino KR, Rodriguez-Zas SL. Transcription factor-microRNA-target gene networks associated with ovarian cancer survival and recurrence. PLoS One. 2013;8(3), e58608.

36. ENCODE Project Consortium. An integrated encyclopedia of DNA elements in the human genome. Nature. 2012;489(7414):57–74.

37. Simonneau G, Gatzoulis MA, Adatia I, Celermajer D, Denton C, Ghofrani A, et al. Updated clinical classification of pulmonary hypertension. J Am Coll Cardiol. 2013;62(25 Suppl):D34–41.

38. Tuder RM, Archer SL, Dorfmuller P, Erzurum SC, Guignabert C, Michelakis E, et al. Relevant issues in the pathology and pathobiology of pulmonary hypertension. J Am Coll Cardiol. 2013;62(25 Suppl):D4–12.

39. Galie N, Corris PA, Frost A, Girgis RE, Granton J, Jing ZC, et al. Updated treatment algorithm of pulmonary arterial hypertension. J Am Coll Cardiol. 2013;62(25 Suppl):D60–72.

40. Caruso P, MacLean MR, Khanin R, McClure J, Soon E, Southgate M, et al. Dynamic changes in lung microRNA profiles during the development of pulmonary hypertension due to chronic hypoxia and monocrotaline. Arterioscler Thromb Vasc Biol. 2010;30(4):716–23.

41. Stenmark KR, Davie N, Frid M, Gerasimovskaya E, Das M. Role of the adventitia in pulmonary vascular remodeling. Physiology (Bethesda). 2006;21:134–45.

42. Stenmark KR, Gerasimovskaya E, Nemenoff RA, Das M. Hypoxic activation of adventitial fibroblasts: role in vascular remodeling. Chest. 2002;122(6 Suppl):326S–34.

43. Jiang YL, Dai AG, Li QF, Hu RC. Transforming growth factor-beta1 induces transdifferentiation of fibroblasts into myofibroblasts in hypoxic pulmonary vascular remodeling. Acta Biochim Biophys Sin (Shanghai). 2006;38(1):29–36.

44. Chiang HY, Korshunov VA, Serour A, Shi F, Sottile J. Fibronectin is an important regulator of flow-induced vascular remodeling. Arterioscler Thromb Vasc Biol. 2009;29(7):1074–9.

45. Rabinovitch M. Pathobiology of pulmonary hypertension. Annu Rev Pathol. 2007;2:369–99.

46. Humbert M, Morrell NW, Archer SL, Stenmark KR, MacLean MR, Lang IM, et al. Cellular and molecular pathobiology of pulmonary arterial hypertension. Journal of the American College of Cardiology. 2004;43(12 Suppl S):13S–24.

47. Sakao S, Tatsumi K, Voelkel NF. Reversible or irreversible remodeling in pulmonary arterial hypertension. Am J Respir Cell Mol Biol. 2010;43(6):629–34.

48. Cool CD, Stewart JS, Werahera P, Miller GJ, Williams RL, Voelkel NF, et al. Three-dimensional reconstruction of pulmonary arteries in plexiform pulmonary hypertension using cell-specific markers. Evidence for a dynamic and heterogeneous process of pulmonary endothelial cell growth. Am J Pathol. 1999;155(2):411–9.

49. Gomez-Arroyo JG, Farkas L, Alhussaini AA, Farkas D, Kraskauskas D, Voelkel NF, et al. The monocrotaline model of pulmonary hypertension in perspective. Am J Physiol Lung Cell Mol Physiol. 2012;302(4):L363–9.

50. Ciuclan L, Bonneau O, Hussey M, Duggan N, Holmes AM, Good R, et al. A novel murine model of severe pulmonary arterial hypertension. Am J Respir Crit Care Med. 2011;184(10):1171–82.

51. Abe K, Toba M, Alzoubi A, Ito M, Fagan KA, Cool CD, et al. Formation of plexiform lesions in experimental severe pulmonary arterial hypertension. Circulation. 2010;121(25):2747–54.

52. Gomez-Arroyo J, Saleem SJ, Mizuno S, Syed AA, Bogaard HJ, Abbate A, et al. A brief overview of mouse models of pulmonary arterial hypertension: problems and prospects. Am J Physiol Lung Cell Mol Physiol. 2012;302(10):L977–91.

53. Grant JS, White K, MacLean MR, Baker AH. MicroRNAs in pulmonary arterial remodeling. Cell Mol Life Sci. 2013;70(23):4479–94.

54. Elia L, Quintavalle M, Zhang J, Contu R, Cossu L, Latronico MV, et al. The knockout of miR-143 and -145 alters smooth muscle cell maintenance and vascular homeostasis in mice: correlates with human disease. Cell Death Differ. 2009;16(12):1590–8.

55. Cheng Y, Liu X, Yang J, Lin Y, Xu DZ, Lu Q, et al. MicroRNA-145, a novel smooth muscle cell phenotypic marker and modulator, controls vascular neointimal lesion formation. Circ Res. 2009;105(2):158–66.

56. Courboulin A, Paulin R, Giguere NJ, Saksouk N, Perreault T, Meloche J, et al. Role for miR-204 in human pulmonary arterial hypertension. J Exp Med. 2011;208(3):535–48.

57. Caruso P, Dempsie Y, Stevens HC, McDonald RA, Long L, Lu R, et al. A role for miR-145 in pulmonary arterial hypertension: evidence from mouse models and patient samples. Circ Res. 2012;111(3):290–300.

58. Davis-Dusenbery BN, Chan MC, Reno KE, Weisman AS, Layne MD, Lagna G, et al. down-regulation of Kruppel-like factor-4 (KLF4) by microRNA-143/145 is critical for modulation of vascular smooth muscle cell phenotype by transforming growth factor-beta and bone morphogenetic protein 4. J Biol Chem. 2011;286(32):28097–110.

59. Gou D, Ramchandran R, Peng X, Yao L, Kang K, Sarkar J, et al. miR-210 has an antiapoptotic effect in pulmonary artery smooth muscle cells during hypoxia. Am J Physiol Lung Cell Mol Physiol. 2012;303(8):L682–91.

60. Sarkar J, Gou D, Turaka P, Viktorova E, Ramchandran R, Raj JU. MicroRNA-21 plays a role in hypoxia-mediated pulmonary artery smooth muscle cell proliferation and migration. Am J Physiol Lung Cell Mol Physiol. 2010;299(6):L861–71.

61. Yang S, Banerjee S, Freitas A, Cui H, Xie N, Abraham E, et al. miR-21 regulates chronic hypoxia-induced pulmonary vascular remodeling. Am J Physiol Lung Cell Mol Physiol. 2012;302(6):L521–9.

62. Parikh VN, Jin RC, Rabello S, Gulbahce N, White K, Hale A, et al. MicroRNA-21 integrates pathogenic signaling to control pulmonary hypertension: results of a network bioinformatics approach. Circulation. 2012;125(12):1520–32.

63. Drake KM, Zygmunt D, Mavrakis L, Harbor P, Wang L, Comhair SA, et al. Altered MicroRNA processing in heritable pulmonary arterial hypertension: an important role for Smad-8. Am J Respir Crit Care Med. 2011;184(12):1400–8.

64. White K, Dempsie Y, Caruso P, Wallace E, McDonald RA, Stevens H, et al. Endothelial apoptosis in pulmonary hypertension is controlled by a microRNA/programmed cell death 4/caspase-3 axis. Hypertension. 2014;64(1):185–94.

65. Kang BY, Park KK, Green DE, Bijli KM, Searles CD, Sutliff RL, et al. Hypoxia mediates mutual repression between microRNA-27a and PPARgamma in the pulmonary vasculature. PLoS One. 2013;8(11), e79503.

66. Ventura A, Young AG, Winslow MM, Lintault L, Meissner A, Erkeland SJ, et al. Targeted deletion reveals essential and overlapping functions of the miR-17 through 92 family of miRNA clusters. Cell. 2008;132(5):875–86.

67. Chen T, Zhou G, Zhou Q, Tang H, Ibe JC, Cheng H, et al. Loss of miR-17~92 in Smooth Muscle Cells Attenuates Experimental Pulmonary Hypertension via Induction of PDLIM5. Am J Respir Crit Care Med. 2015.

68. Pullamsetti SS, Doebele C, Fischer A, Savai R, Kojonazarov B, Dahal BK, et al. Inhibition of microRNA-17 improves lung and heart function in experimental pulmonary hypertension. Am J Respir Crit Care Med. 2012;185(4):409–19.

69. Li W, Dunmore BJ, Morrell NW. Bone morphogenetic protein type II receptor mutations causing protein misfolding in heritable pulmonary arterial hypertension. Proc Am Thorac Soc. 2010;7(6):395–8.

70. Brock M, Trenkmann M, Gay RE, Michel BA, Gay S, Fischler M, et al. Interleukin-6 modulates the expression of the bone morphogenic protein receptor type II through a novel STAT3-microRNA cluster 17/92 pathway. Circ Res. 2009;104(10):1184–91.

71. Kang K, Peng X, Zhang X, Wang Y, Zhang L, Gao L, et al. MicroRNA-124 suppresses the transactivation of nuclear factor of activated T cells by targeting multiple genes and inhibits the proliferation of pulmonary artery smooth muscle cells. J Biol Chem. 2013;288(35):25414–27.

72. Wang D, Zhang H, Li M, Frid MG, Flockton AR, McKeon BA, et al. MicroRNA-124 controls the proliferative, migratory, and inflammatory phenotype of pulmonary vascular fibroblasts. Circ Res. 2014;114(1):67–78.

73. Wang FE, Zhang C, Maminishkis A, Dong L, Zhi C, Li R, et al. MicroRNA-204/211 alters epithelial physiology. FASEB J. 2010;24(5):1552–71.

74. Chandra SM, Razavi H, Kim J, Agrawal R, Kundu RK, de Jesus PV, et al. Disruption of the apelin-APJ system worsens hypoxia-induced pulmonary hypertension. Arterioscler Thromb Vasc Biol. 2011;31(4):814–20.

75. Kim J, Kang Y, Kojima Y, Lighthouse JK, Hu X, Aldred MA, et al. An endothelial apelin-FGF link mediated by miR-424 and miR-503 is disrupted in pulmonary arterial hypertension. Nat Med. 2013;19(1):74–82.

76. Potus FPR, Breuils-Bonnet S, Tremblay E, Couture C, Michelakis ED, Provencher S, Bonnet S. Downregulation of the angiomiR-126 contributes to the failing right ventricle in pulmonary arterial hypertension. Am J Respir Crit Care Med. 2013;187:A5926.

77. Kuhn AR, Schlauch K, Lao R, Halayko AJ, Gerthoffer WT, Singer CA. MicroRNA expression in human airway smooth muscle cells: role of miR-25 in regulation of airway smooth muscle phenotype. Am J Respir Cell Mol Biol. 2010;42(4):506–13.

78. Kulshreshtha R, Ferracin M, Wojcik SE, Garzon R, Alder H, Agosto-Perez FJ, et al. A microRNA signature of hypoxia. Mol Cell Biol. 2007;27(5):1859–67.

79. Yu AY, Shimoda LA, Iyer NV, Huso DL, Sun X, McWilliams R, et al. Impaired physiological responses to chronic hypoxia in mice partially deficient for hypoxia-inducible factor 1alpha. J Clin Invest. 1999;103(5):691–6.

80. Fasanaro P, D'Alessandra Y, Di Stefano V, Melchionna R, Romani S, Pompilio G, et al. MicroRNA-210 modulates endothelial cell response to hypoxia and inhibits the receptor tyrosine kinase ligand Ephrin-A3. J Biol Chem. 2008;283(23):15878–83.

81. Huang X, Ding L, Bennewith KL, Tong RT, Welford SM, Ang KK, et al. Hypoxia-inducible mir-210 regulates normoxic gene expression involved in tumor initiation. Mol Cell. 2009;35(6):856–67.

82. Bruning U, Cerone L, Neufeld Z, Fitzpatrick SF, Cheong A, Scholz CC, et al. MicroRNA-155 promotes resolution of hypoxia-inducible factor 1alpha activity during prolonged hypoxia. Mol Cell Biol. 2011;31(19):4087–96.

83. Taganov KD, Boldin MP, Chang KJ, Baltimore D. NF-kappaB-dependent induction of microRNA miR-146, an inhibitor targeted to signaling proteins of innate immune responses. Proc Natl Acad Sci U S A. 2006;103(33):12481–6.

84. Loffler D, Brocke-Heidrich K, Pfeifer G, Stocsits C, Hackermuller J, Kretzschmar AK, et al. Interleukin-6 dependent survival of multiple myeloma cells involves the Stat3-mediated induction of microRNA-21 through a highly conserved enhancer. Blood. 2007;110(4):1330–3.

85. Niu J, Shi Y, Tan G, Yang CH, Fan M, Pfeffer LM, et al. DNA damage induces NF-kappaB-dependent microRNA-21 up-regulation and promotes breast cancer cell invasion. J Biol Chem. 2012; 287(26):21783–95.

86. Hoeper MM, Barst RJ, Bourge RC, Feldman J, Frost AE, Galie N, et al. Imatinib mesylate as add-on therapy for pulmonary arterial hypertension: results of the randomized IMPRES study. Circulation. 2013;127(10):1128–38.

87. Creemers EE, Tijsen AJ, Pinto YM. Circulating microRNAs: novel biomarkers and extracellular communicators in cardiovascular disease? Circ Res. 2012;110(3):483–95.

88. Arroyo JD, Chevillet JR, Kroh EM, Ruf IK, Pritchard CC, Gibson DF, et al. Argonaute2 complexes carry a population of circulating microRNAs independent of vesicles in human plasma. Proc Natl Acad Sci U S A. 2011;108(12):5003–8.

89. Zampetaki A, Mayr M. Analytical challenges and technical limitations in assessing circulating miRNAs. Thromb Haemost. 2012;108(4):592–8.

90. Coronnello C, Hartmaier R, Arora A, Huleihel L, Pandit KV, Bais AS, et al. Novel modeling of combinatorial miRNA targeting identifies SNP with potential role in bone density. PLoS Comput Biol. 2012;8(12), e1002830.

91. Rhodes CJ, Wharton J, Boon RA, Roexe T, Tsang H, Wojciak-Stothard B, et al. Reduced microRNA-150 is associated with poor survival in pulmonary arterial hypertension. Am J Respir Crit Care Med. 2013;187(3):294–302.

92. Schlosser K, White RJ, Stewart DJ. miR-26a linked to pulmonary hypertension by global assessment of circulating extracellular microRNAs. Am J Respir Crit Care Med. 2013;188(12):1472–5.

93. Lanford RE, Hildebrandt-Eriksen ES, Petri A, Persson R, Lindow M, Munk ME, et al. Therapeutic silencing of microRNA-122 in primates with chronic hepatitis C virus infection. Science. 2010;327(5962):198–201.

94. Santaris Pharma AS. Multiple ascending dose study of miravirsen in treatment-naïve chronic hepatitis C subjects. [Accessed 27 June 2014]. Available from: http://clinicaltrials.gov/show/NCT01200420. NLM Identifier: NCT01200420.

95. Santaris Pharma AS. Miravirsen study in null responder to pegylated interferon alpha plus ribavirin subjects with chronic hepatitis C. [Accessed 27 June 2014]. Available from: http://clinicaltrials.gov/show/NCT01727934. NLM Identifier: NCT01727934.

96. Mirna Therapeutics I. A multicenter phase I study of MRX34, MicroRNA miR-RX34 liposome injectable suspension. [Accessed 27 June 2014]. Available from: http://clinicaltrials.gov/show/NCT01829971. NLM Identifier: NCT01829971.

97. Winter J, Jung S, Keller S, Gregory RI, Diederichs S. Many roads to maturity: microRNA biogenesis pathways and their regulation. Nat Cell Biol. 2009;11(3):228–34.

Pulmonary Hypertension as a Metabolic Disease

Joshua P. Fessel and William M. Oldham

Abbreviations

2OG	2-oxoglutaric acid; α-ketoglutaric acid
ACC	Acetyl-CoA carboxylase
CPT1	Carnitine palmitoyltransferase 1
D2HG	D-2-hydroxyglutaric acid
DCA	Dichloroacetate
DON	6-diazo-5-oxo-L-norleucine; glutamine analogue
DRP1	Dynamin-related protein 1
FAO	Fatty acid oxidation
FDG	2-deoxy-2-(^{18}F)fluoro-D-glucose
FHR	Fawn hooded rat
FIS1	Mitochondrial fission protein 1
HIF	Hypoxia-inducible factor 1α
INF2	Inverted formin 2
KAT	3-ketoacyl coenzyme A thiolase
L2HG	L-2-hydroxyglutaric acid
LDH	Lactate dehydrogenase
ME	Malic enzyme
MCD	Malonyl-CoA decarboxylase
MCT	Monocrotaline
MFF	Mitochondrial fission factor
MFN	Mitofusin
MIEF1	Mitochondrial elongation factor 1, encoded by the SMCR7L gene
OPA1	Optic atrophy 1
PAB	Pulmonary artery banding
PAEC	Pulmonary artery endothelial cell
PAH	Pulmonary arterial hypertension
PASMC	Pulmonary artery smooth muscle cell
PDH	Pyruvate dehydrogenase
PDK	Pyruvate dehydrogenase kinase
PET	Positron emission tomography
PFK	Phosphofructokinase
ROS	Reactive oxygen species
RV	Right ventricle
RVEF	Right ventricular ejection fraction
SOD2	Superoxide dismutase 2
SPECT	Single photon emission computed tomography
SuH	VEGF receptor antagonist, Sugen 5416, and hypoxia
TCA	Tricarboxylic acid cycle; Krebs' cycle; citric acid cycle

J.P. Fessel, MD, PhD
Division of Allergy, Pulmonary and Critical Care Medicine,
Department of Medicine, Vanderbilt University School
of Medicine, 1161 21st Avenue South, Suite T1218 Medical
Center North, Nashville, TN, 37232, USA
e-mail: joshua.p.fessel@vanderbilt.edu

W.M. Oldham, MD, PhD (✉)
Division of Pulmonary and Critical Care Medicine,
Department of Medicine, Brigham and Women's Hospital
and Harvard Medical School, 77 Avenue Louis Pasteur, NRB 630,
Boston, MA, 02115, USA
e-mail: woldham@partners.org

Introduction

Growing evidence suggests that fundamental changes in cell metabolism are central to the pathogenesis of pulmonary arterial hypertension (PAH). The reprogramming of cellular metabolism involves all of the major carbon sources used by the pulmonary circulation and right ventricle (RV) – carbohydrates such as glucose and lactate, fatty acids, and amino acids. Metabolic reprogramming in PAH involves not only changes in the relative utilization of carbon sources, but also changes in the allocation of carbon sources to energy production *versus* macromolecule or cofactor biosynthesis. In many ways, the changes in cellular metabolism in PAH are very similar to metabolic changes that have been observed in highly proliferative cells that have undergone malignant transformation. To what extent the observed changes represent pathogenic *versus* compensatory mechanisms in PAH is an area of active investigation. In this chapter, we will address each of the major cellular metabolic pathways: glucose metabolism through glycolysis, the tricarboxylic acid (TCA)

© Springer International Publishing Switzerland 2016
B.A. Maron et al. (eds.), *Pulmonary Hypertension: Basic Science to Clinical Medicine*, DOI 10.1007/978-3-319-23594-3_8

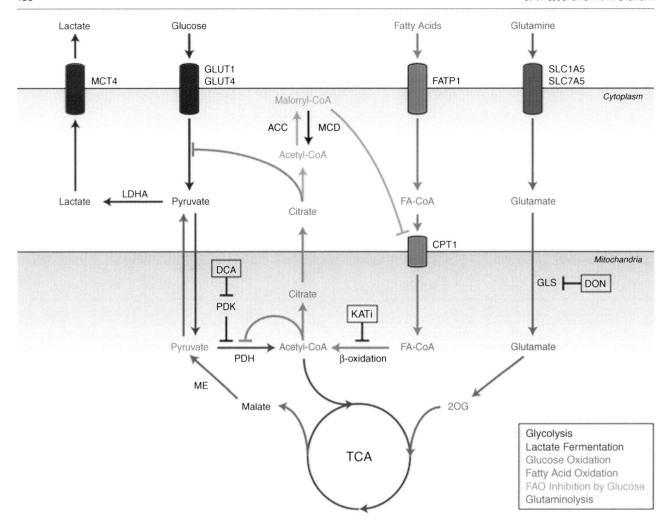

Fig. 8.1 Metabolic pathways reprogrammed in PAH. Several pathways are affected in humans with and experimental models of PAH. Increased glycolysis, lactate fermentation, and glutaminolysis are observed (*purple, pink,* and *blue*), while fatty acid oxidation (*FAO*) is decreased (*green*). Glycolysis can decrease FAO through increases in cytoplasmic malonyl-CoA inhibiting carnitine palmitoyl transferase 1 (*CPT1*) (*orange*). Levels of cytoplasmic malonyl-CoA are carefully regulated by the activities of acetyl-CoA carboxylase (*ACC*) and malonyl-CoA decarboxylase (*MCD*). FAO inhibits glycolysis as a consequence of citrate accumulation. Dichloroacetate (*DCA*) shuttles glycolytic carbon into the TCA cycle (*red*) by inhibiting pyruvate dehydrogenase kinase (*PDK*), an inhibitor of pyruvate dehydrogenase (*PDH*). The 3-ketoacyl CoA thiolase inhibitors (*KATi*), decrease FAO and relieve its inhibition of glycolysis to facilitate glucose oxidation. A glutamine analogue, 6-diazo-5-oxo-L-norleucine (*DON*) has been used in experimental models to improve RV function by inhibiting glutaminolysis

cycle, fatty acid oxidation (FAO), and oxidative phosphorylation, and how each pathway is affected in the pulmonary vasculature and right ventricle (RV) in patients with and animal models of PAH. While the metabolic changes occurring in the pulmonary vasculature and RV of patients with PAH are well described, the role of upstream signaling pathways, such as BMPRII mutations, in mediating the metabolic reprogramming is less understood. Thus, we have chosen to focus on metabolic, rather than signaling, pathways for this review.

Glycolysis, the Warburg Effect, and Hypoxia-Inducible Factor

Glycolysis, as the name implies, is the metabolic pathway by which the carbohydrate glucose is broken down into smaller carbon units that feed other metabolic pathways (Fig. 8.1).

Glycolysis is also the initial step in the conversion of glucose to usable bioenergetic fuel. Through a series of coupled enzymatic reactions, the six-carbon chain of glucose is split into two three-carbon pyruvate molecules. In the process, two molecules of ATP are consumed, but four ATP are synthesized, for a net gain of two ATP. The pyruvate molecules produced can then enter the TCA cycle (Krebs's cycle) *via* conversion to acetyl-CoA by pyruvate dehydrogenase (PDH) or they can be converted to lactate by lactate dehydrogenase (LDH). The fermentation of pyruvate to lactate oxidizes the NADH produced by glycolysis, restoring NAD^+ concentrations essential for continued glycolysis.

With the dramatic resurgence of investigations that incorporate molecular metabolism as key pieces of both theoretical and experimental design, it has become common practice to use "glycolysis" as shorthand for what is perhaps more properly described as "lactatogenic glycolysis" – glycolysis that ultimately results in the generation of lactate from the reduction of pyruvate by LDH. The terms "anaerobic glycolysis" and "aerobic glycolysis" are not especially helpful, as glycolysis is occurring regardless of oxygen availability. The intended distinction arises from the fate of pyruvate, whether it is oxidized in the TCA cycle (glucose oxidation, an aerobic process) or fermented to lactate by LDH (lactate fermentation, an anaerobic process) (Fig. 8.1). For the purposes of this discussion, the term "glycolysis" will be used in the strict sense to refer to the biochemical process of converting glucose to pyruvate.

In the early twentieth century, Otto Warburg described the phenomenon by which cells that have undergone malignant transformation change their metabolic profile to utilize lactatogenic glycolysis as the primary mode of generating ATP [1, 2]. This is a normal mode of metabolism for mammalian cells under anaerobic conditions, when oxygen deficiency is limiting oxidative metabolism of carbon subunits. However, Warburg observed this type of anaerobic metabolism in malignant transformed cells growing in oxygen concentrations that were more than sufficient to permit oxidative metabolism. He concluded that the metabolic shift from glucose oxidation to lactatogenic glycolysis for ATP production – a phenomenon commonly referred to as the Warburg effect – is a primary driver of and a required adaptation for malignant transformation.

More recently, hypoxia-inducible factor 1α (HIF) has been identified as the principal regulator of the Warburg effect in a variety of cancer cells [3]. In normal cells, as oxygen tension falls, the HIF transcription factor is stabilized, thereby activating a gene expression program leading to (1) increased glucose uptake through the expression of glucose transporters; (2) increased glycolytic flux through the expression of several glycolytic enzymes (e.g., aldolase A, phosphoglycerate kinase 1, enolase 1, triosephosphate isomerase), including the key regulators of glycolytic flux, hexokinase, phosphofructokinase L, and pyruvate kinase M [4–8]; (3) decreased oxidative phosphorylation through expression of pyruvate dehydrogenase kinases (PDK) 1–4, inhibitors of PDH [9–11]; (4) increased lactate fermentation through expression of LDHA; and (5) increased mitochondrial autophagy through expression of BNIP3 [12]. The overall goal of this gene expression program is to mitigate reactive oxygen species (ROS) generation from dysfunctional mitochondrial electron transport chains [13]. Increasing evidence suggests that abnormal HIF stabilization under normoxic conditions is responsible for the Warburg effect in malignant cells [5, 7, 9, 10, 14].

Precisely this same type of metabolic reprogramming has been observed in PAH in both the pulmonary vasculature and the RV. The earliest evidence for a shift to lactatogenic glycolysis in experimental PAH came, perhaps not surprisingly, from the chronic hypoxia rat model. With chronic hypoxia, the RV showed increased expression and activity of hexokinase, the first and rate-limiting enzyme in glycolysis, as well

as a modest increase in the expression of LDH [15]. Additional evidence of increased lactatogenic glycolysis was provided by the monocrotaline (MCT) rat model of PAH, where MCT treatment increased glycolysis and decreased FAO in cultured cardiomyocytes in a HIF-dependent manner [16]. HIF was already known to regulate glycolysis and to play some role in the pathogenesis of PAH [17–20], but this was one of the first demonstrations of a pathogenic link between glycolysis and HIF in a model of PAH.

Soon after, the observation of increased glycolysis in PAH was extended to include several different animal models of PAH as well as patients with the disease. In the Fawn hooded rat model (FHR), dysmorphic and hyperpolarized mitochondria with deficient superoxide production drove normoxic activation of HIF in pulmonary artery smooth muscle cells (PASMCs) [21]. Normoxic HIF activation was confirmed in PASMCs cultured from PAH patients. One of the implications of this study was that a glycolytic shift mediated by HIF occurs in PASMCs in PAH, but this was not directly demonstrated.

Subsequently, increased glycolytic carbon flow and lactate production were demonstrated in pulmonary artery endothelial cells (PAECs) cultured from PAH patients [22]. Positron emission tomographic imaging (PET) showed that uptake of ^{18}F-fluorodeoxyglucose (FDG) in the lungs of PAH patients was significantly increased compared to healthy controls, providing at least indirect evidence that the glycolytic reprogramming observed in vitro was also occurring in vivo in humans. As with cultured cardiomyocytes and PASMCs, the glycolytic shift in PAECs is dependent upon normoxic activation of HIF. The finding of increased glucose uptake in the lungs measured by FDG-PET has since been replicated in experimental PAH [23].

The mechanisms of normoxic HIF activation remain unclear. One hypothesis is that that epigenetic silencing of superoxide dismutase 2 (SOD2), the mitochondrial enzyme responsible for H_2O_2 generation from superoxide, leads to HIF activation through decreased cellular H_2O_2 production (or increased superoxide levels) (see below, Fig. 8.2) [24].

Similar to the pulmonary vasculature, evidence suggests that the pressure-overloaded RV has increased glycolytic flux. The MCT and pulmonary artery banding (PAB) rat models of pulmonary hypertension demonstrated increased FDG uptake and increased Glut1 expression [23, 25]. However, FDG-PET studies of the RV in patients with pulmonary hypertension have shown conflicting results [26]. Some studies have indicated that FDG uptake in the RV is increased compared to the LV in patients with pulmonary hypertension and that the uptake is proportional to disease severity [27–29], while others have not replicated these findings [30].

In contrast to the pulmonary vasculature, the role of HIF activation in mediating this metabolic change in the RV is controversial, as HIF expression has not been consistently shown to be elevated in animal models of pulmonary

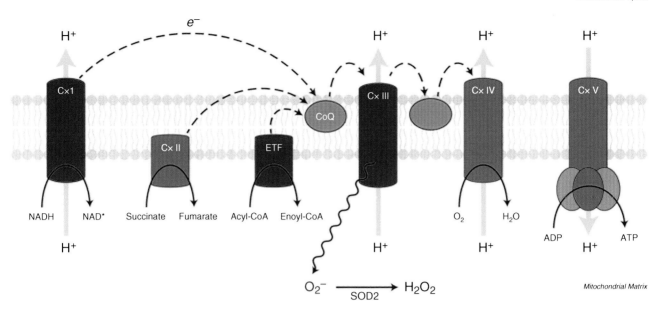

Fig. 8.2 Electron transport chain and oxidative phosphorylation. The electron transport chain transfers electrons (*e⁻, dashed lines*) from high-energy reduced carriers to molecular oxygen coupled to the generation of a proton gradient (*yellow arrows*) across the inner mitochondrial membrane. This proton gradient drives phosphorylation of ADP by ATP synthase (*Cx V*). Superoxide anion (O_2^-) can be generated by complexes I and III and by electron transferring flavoprotein dehydrogenase (*ETF*) (*red symbols*; shown only for Cx III for clarity). Dismutation of superoxide is catalyzed by superoxide dismutase 2 (*SOD2*) to form hydrogen peroxide. Epigenetic silencing of SOD2, and reduced H_2O_2 formation, has been implicated in HIF activation in the pulmonary vasculature of patients with PAH

hypertension. No change in HIF was observed in the RV of the FHR [31], while increased HIF was observed in the compensated hypertrophic RV of the MCT rat prior to RV decompensation, whereafter HIF expression was noted to decrease [25]. PDK4 is the isoform primarily responsible for the metabolic switch from glucose oxidation to lactate fermentation in the RV and it is not known to be a direct target of HIF (although PDK4 expression does increase in hypoxia in some settings [11, 32]) [23, 31]. In the FHR model, PDK4 expression is likely driven by increased FOXO1, transcription factor expression and activity, rather than HIF [31].

Tricarboxylic Acid Cycle, Glutaminolysis, and Amino Acid Metabolism

The tricarboxylic acid (TCA) cycle, also known as Krebs's cycle or the citric acid cycle, was one of the first cyclical metabolic pathways identified [33] (Fig. 8.1). The cycle is a central point of integration and regulation of carbon flow through multiple pathways within the cellular metabolic network. Regulation of carbon flow into and out of the TCA cycle is intimately linked to the balance of energy production, synthesis of biological macromolecules, cell proliferation, apoptosis, and redox homeostasis.

Classical teaching is that pyruvate generated from glycolysis is converted to acetyl-CoA by PDH, and this is the entry point into the TCA cycle. Acetyl-CoA condenses with oxaloacetate to form citrate (regenerating citrate, thus, the "citric acid cycle"), which is then converted through a series of sequential enzymatic reactions back to oxaloacetate. For each turn of the cycle, three molecules of NAD⁺ are reduced to NADH, one molecule of GTP is produced from GDP and phosphate, one molecule of ubiquinone (oxidized coenzyme Q) is reduced to ubiquinol (reduced coenzyme Q), and two molecules of CO_2 are liberated.

However, carbon flow both into and out of the TCA cycle is much more complex and dynamic than simple pyruvate entry *via* acetyl-CoA. The breakdown of amino acids and fatty acids can also contribute carbon to the TCA cycle. In general, reactions or processes that result in a net flow of carbon into the TCA cycle are termed *anaplerotic* reactions or *anaplerosis*. (Note that some sources will use this term more specifically to refer to reactions that allow carbon entry into the TCA cycle without going through acetyl-CoA as an intermediate.) The major routes for anaplerosis include (1) pyruvate directly to oxaloacetate by pyruvate carboxylase, (2) ʟ-glutamate to 2-oxoglutarate (2OG) by glutamate dehydrogenase, (3) β-oxidation of odd-chain fatty acids to succinyl-CoA as substrate for succinyl-CoA synthetase, (4) conversion of aspartate to oxaloacetate by aspartate aminotransferase, and (5) conversion of adenylosuccinate (an intermediate in purine nucleotide metabolism) to fumarate via adenylosuccinate lyase.

Reactions or processes that remove carbon from the TCA cycle to supply biosynthetic processes are termed *cataplerotic* reactions or *cataplerosis*. Carbons can exit the TCA cycle at virtually every point in the cycle to supply biosynthetic and regulatory reactions. For example, oxaloacetate and 2OG both support the synthesis of multiple amino acids. Citrate can be diverted out of the TCA cycle for the synthesis of fatty acids via ATP citrate lyase. Succinyl-CoA can be diverted from the TCA cycle to serve as the substrate for the enzymatic succinylation of lysine residues in proteins, a very recently recognized mechanism for post-translational regulation of protein structure and function [34]. Fumarate has also been shown to participate in the non-enzymatic succinylation of cysteine residues in proteins [35–38]. Clearly then, regulation of the anaplerotic/cataplerotic balance in the TCA cycle is complex, and any perturbation of this balance can have a significant impact on multiple biochemical pathways.

Glutaminolysis is one form of anaplerosis that has been linked to animal models of PAH. Glutamine is an important source of cellular energy, carbon, and nitrogen, particularly in rapidly proliferating cells [39]. Intracellular glutamine is hydrolyzed to glutamate, which is either reduced or transaminated to form 2OG (Fig. 8.1). The 2OG can be transported into the mitochondrion to enter the TCA cycle for ATP generation or reduced and carboxylated to form isocitrate for fatty acid synthesis. In the setting of impaired PDH, the increase in malate from the glutamine-fed TCA cycle is oxidized to pyruvate by malic enzyme (ME). In comparison to the PAB model, MCT rats had increased expression of glutamine transporters (SLC1A5 and SLC7A5) and increased malic enzyme induced by activation of c-Myc as a result of RV ischemia [40]. This is similar to glutaminolysis in malignancy where c-Myc expression is also increased [41]. Glutamine transporters may also be increased in the RV of patients with PAH [40].

A broader perturbation of amino acid metabolism, including increased glutamine metabolism and changes in branched chain amino acid utilization, has been shown in human PAEC expressing mutant BMPR2 *in vitro* as well as in *in vivo* measurements of transpulmonary amino acid gradients at the time of diagnostic right heart catheterization [42–44]. In contrast to c-Myc activation in the RV, normoxic activation of HIF in the pulmonary endothelium seems to be one of the key drivers of altered amino acid metabolism and altered TCA cycle carbon flux.

In addition to changes in the anaplerosis/cataplerosis balance, there is an emerging recognition of the role of novel metabolites as mediators of disease. This first came to prominence in the oncometabolism literature, with the observation that 2OG can be reduced to D-2-hydroxyglutaric acid (D2HG) in several malignancies as a result of a point mutation in the TCA cycle enzyme isocitrate dehydrogenase [45]. These mutations support oncogenesis through the inhibition of a variety of 2OG-dependent dioxygenase enzymes, such as HIF prolyl hydroxylase, histone demethylases, and TET-family 5-methylcytosine hydroxylases with a broad impact on epigenetic regulation of gene expression, collagen synthesis, and cell signaling [46, 47]. Very recently, L-2-hydroxyglutarate (L2HG) overproduction *via* reductive metabolism of 2OG has been demonstrated in response to hypoxia in PAECs and PASMCs [48]. This metabolite appears to have an important role in maintaining cellular redox homeostasis. In addition to the 2HG enantiomers, two other TCA metabolites, succinate and fumarate, also inhibit 2OG-dependent dioxygenase enzymes and may play an important role in tumorigenesis through their effect on cellular redox state [49]. Indeed, increases in succinate and other TCA metabolites have recently been shown in the lungs of PAH patients [50].

Fatty Acid Oxidation

Fatty acid oxidation is the primary metabolic fuel for the RV, and is another of the metabolic pathways affected by PAH (Fig. 8.1). In the low oxygen environment of the developing fetus, the heart relies on carbohydrate substrates that generate ATP through glucose and lactate oxidation [51]. However, shortly after birth, the heart shifts to FAO as the primary source of energy production. Fatty acids provide ~70 % of the energy for the resting heart with the balance generated from carbohydrate oxidation [52]. Importantly, the heart is flexible with regards to its energy supply; substrate availability, hormone levels (*e.g.*, insulin, epinephrine), oxygen tension, and workload regulate substrate utilization. For example, increases in serum lactate during exercise are associated with increased lactate oxidation by the heart [53]. The balance between fatty acid and glucose consumption by the heart is carefully regulated by biochemical interactions between these two metabolic pathways in the so-called "glucose-fatty acid cycle" (or "Randle cycle") initially proposed by Philip Randle and colleagues in 1963 [54, 55].

In isolated heart preparations, Randle and colleagues observed that utilization of fatty acids inhibits glucose oxidation and *vice versa*, all in the absence of hormonal regulation. Fatty acid oxidation increases mitochondrial ratios of acetyl-CoA/CoA and NADH/NAD$^+$, which inhibit PDH (Fig. 8.1). Citrate accumulates in the cytosol, inhibiting phosphofructokinase, and the resulting accumulation of glucose-6-phosphate inhibits hexokinase. Fatty acid oxidation also inhibits glucose uptake by preventing translocation of glucose transporter 4 (GLUT4) to the plasma membrane; however, the mechanism for this effect remains undetermined [55].

Inhibition of FAO by glucose oxidation in the heart is mediated through increases in cytosolic malonyl-CoA. Malonyl-CoA inhibits carnitine palmitoyltransferase 1 (CPT1), which regulates the entry and oxidation of fatty acids in the mitochondria (Fig. 8.1). Cytosolic malonyl-CoA is determined by the complex regulation of acetyl-CoA carboxylase and malonyl-CoA decarboxylase (MCD), its synthetic and degradative enzymes, respectively. Notably, FAO inhibition by glucose oxidation in the heart requires an increase in glucose uptake through GLUT4 translocation to the plasma membrane as GLUT4 transport is saturated at circulating serum glucose concentrations [55].

In addition to suppressed glucose oxidation, FHRs have suppressed FAO as demonstrated by metabolic flux analysis in a working heart model and in freshly isolated cardiac myocytes [31], although PAB animals have increased FAO assessed by similar techniques [56]. A comparison of the VEGF receptor antagonist, Sugen 5416, plus hypoxia (SuH) and PAB rats demonstrated decreased expression of PGC-1α in SuH animals that was associated with decreased expression of acyl-CoA dehydrogenases, critical enzymes for fatty acid β-oxidation, while PAB animals had increased levels of these proteins [57]. FHRs may share similar inhibition of PGC-1α-regulated metabolic pathways. The transcription of FAO metabolic enzymes is also decreased in the MCT model [58]. Impaired fatty acid uptake has been observed in pulmonary hypertension patients using single photon emission computed tomography (SPECT) of a radiolabeled fatty acid analogue [59, 60]. There is also histologic evidence of impaired fatty acid utilization in the RV of PAH patients, as evidenced by abnormal lipid accumulation and lipotoxicity within the RV cardiac myocytes of PAH patients that is not present in RV samples from patients with left ventricular failure [61].

FAO may also play an important role in the pathogenesis of PAH in the vasculature. Mice deficient for malonyl-CoA decarboxylase (MCD), the main enzyme responsible for the degradation of malonyl-CoA, are protected from hypoxic pulmonary hypertension [25]. Decreased MCD activity increases cytosolic malonyl-CoA and inhibition of CPT1, thereby decreasing FAO and increasing glucose oxidation. Interestingly, a combined genetic and metabolomic analysis of human PAH lung tissue suggested increases in FAO due to increased expression of acyl-CoA dehydrogenases and FAO intermediates [62]. Additional studies are required to characterize the role of FAO in the pathogenesis of PAH in these two tissues, RV and pulmonary vasculature, particularly in consideration of potential therapies targeted at these pathways.

Oxidative Phosphorylation, Reactive Oxygen Species, and Mitochondrial Dynamics

The net consequence of the metabolic pathways discussed above is to allow electrons to enter the electron transport system within the mitochondria (Fig. 8.2). Here, electrons are transferred from high-energy reduced carriers (such as NADH synthesized in the TCA cycle) to ubiquinone (oxi-

dized coenzyme Q). In the process, coenzyme Q is reduced to ubiquinol, and the carriers become oxidized (*e.g.*, NADH is oxidized to NAD+ by Complex I). Electrons are then transferred from ubiquinol (oxidizing it back to ubiquinone) to cytochrome *c via* Complex III. Finally, electrons are transferred from cytochrome *c* to molecular oxygen *via* Complex IV, oxidizing cytochrome *c* and converting molecular oxygen to water.

The energy from these electron transfers is coupled (for Complexes I, III, and IV) to pumping protons against their electrochemical gradient from the mitochondrial matrix into the intermembrane space. The F_1F_0 ATP synthase (sometimes referred to as Complex V) harnesses the free energy released by protons flowing back down their electrochemical gradient to power the combination of ADP and inorganic phosphate to make ATP. This is the biochemical summary of oxidative phosphorylation, a process that is stoichiometrically equivalent to a combustion reaction (compounds containing carbon and hydrogen combining with molecular oxygen to liberate CO_2, water, and energy).

Not only is this process the nexus of bioenergetics for most cell types, but oxidative phosphorylation is also intimately tied to regulation of apoptosis *via* cytochrome *c*. In addition, the mitochondrial electron transport system serves as one of the most important sources for damaging ROS. If the system works perfectly, molecular oxygen is completely reduced to water by Complex IV. However, at multiple points along the electron transport system, a single electron can be transferred to molecular oxygen, resulting in the formation of superoxide anion. Mitochondria are well equipped to deal with the constant hazard of superoxide. SOD2 (MnSOD) localizes to mitochondria and is present in concentrations that far exceed the normal concentrations of its substrate (one of the few known enzymes with this feature). SOD2 further catalyzes the already rapid dismutation of superoxide to molecular oxygen and hydrogen peroxide (Fig. 8.2). This serves to protect vulnerable lipids, proteins, and nucleic acids from oxidative damage. Indeed, SOD2 is such an important defense against baseline free radical injury that homozygous deletion of SOD2 is embryonically lethal in mice shortly after birth due to cardiomyopathy [63].

As with many other disease states, mitochondrial oxidative stress has been linked to the pathogenesis of PAH. Increased mitochondrial oxidant injury has been shown in genetic models of PAH, and driving mitochondrial free radical production enhances the development of PAH [64, 65]. Moreover, SOD2 has been shown to undergo epigenetic silencing in PAH, though the important consequence seems to be a loss of oxidative signaling from hydrogen peroxide as opposed to increased oxidant injury from superoxide. Restoring oxidative signaling by restoring SOD2 activity enhances appropriate apoptosis in the pulmonary vasculature and ameliorates the development of PAH [24].

The efficient transfer of electrons within the mitochondrial electron transport system and the proper function of antioxidant defenses require a close and tightly regulated physical relationship between the enzyme complexes and electron carriers. Disruption of the ultrastructure of mitochondria can lead directly to increased oxidant injury and an imbalance between apoptosis and proliferation. To help maintain mitochondrial ultrastructure in the face of normal and pathologic demands on bioenergetics and biosynthesis, and as a mechanism to help mitigate the effects of oxidant injury, mitochondria can combine together to form larger reticula (fusion) and can divide to form larger numbers of smaller mitochondria (fission) [66–70].

The major regulators of mitochondrial fission in mammalian cells are DRP1 (dynamin-related protein 1) and its interacting partners FIS1 (mitochondrial fission protein 1), MFF (mitochondrial fission factor), MIEF1 (mitochondrial elongation factor 1, encoded by the SMCR7L gene), and INF2 (inverted formin 2). Mitochondrial fusion is regulated by MFN1 and 2 (mitofusin 1 and 2) and by OPA1 (optic atrophy 1). The balance of fission and fusion is critical for mitochondrial quality control, mitigation of mitochondrial damage, matching of bioenergetic and biosynthetic demands to mitochondrial capacity, intracellular calcium homeostasis, and regulation of apoptosis and proliferation [66–70]. Though some general concepts have been offered, the role that fission/fusion play in regulating these processes has a large degree of situational specificity. For example, promoting mitochondrial fusion is generally seen as a way to enhance the functioning of damaged mitochondria and to be anti-apoptotic. However, in PAH, tipping the balance toward fusion by inhibition of DRP1 results in enhanced apoptosis and reduction in the hyperproliferative pheonytpe seen in PASMCs in PAH [71]. Overall, the data in PAH suggest that in the pulmonary vasculature as well as in skeletal muscle, the balance of mitochondrial dynamics is tilted to favor fission (*via* increased DRP1 expression and decreased MFN2 expression) [71–73]. Much work remains to determine which types of pulmonary hypertension are driven or modulated by changes in mitochondrial dynamics and if these processes can be effectively targeted pharmacologically *in vivo*. This topic has been recently reviewed in excellent detail [74].

Therapeutic Metabolic Reprogramming in Pulmonary Hypertension

Fortunately, several decades of biochemical exploration of these fundamental pathways of energy metabolism have provided several pharmacologic tools to interrogate the roles of these pathways in PAH disease pathogenesis. Moreover, several of these agents have shown promise in the treatment of PAH. The overarching goal of these metabolic therapies is to restore glucose oxidation in the pulmonary vasculature and improve the metabolic efficiency of the RV.

Dichloroacetate (DCA), a pharmacologic inhibitor of PDK used for many years to treat children with inborn errors of metabolism [75], has been shown in a number of experimental PAH models to ameliorate increases in RV systolic pressure and maladaptive RV remodeling and inhibit proliferation while enhancing apoptosis in the lung [21, 23, 31, 76–80]. DCA inhibits PDK, allowing PDH to shunt more pyruvate into the TCA cycle thereby increasing glucose oxidation, mitigating the adverse consequences of myocardial lactate production, and improving energetic efficiency (Fig. 8.1). DCA is generally well tolerated and has been used for the treatment of congenital lactic acidosis and a variety of malignancies. The main adverse effect is partially reversible peripheral neuropathy attributed to oxidative stress [81]. A Phase I, open label trial of DCA in PAH has been completed through the University of Alberta and Imperial College London. The primary endpoint of the study was safety and tolerability over 16 weeks of drug administration, with secondary endpoints including 6 min walk distance change, change in World Health Organization functional class for heart failure, change in pulmonary vascular resistance measured by invasive hemodynamics, changes in RV size and function by MRI, changes in serum NT-proBNP, and changes in lung and RV FDG uptake measured by PET, although complete study results are forthcoming (DCA for the treatment of pulmonary arterial hypertension; NCT01083524).

An alternative strategy of increasing glucose oxidation exploits the Randle cycle whereby inhibiting FAO, glucose oxidation is increased. Trimetazidine and ranolazine are two partial inhibitors of FAO that are available currently for clinical use in selected cardiovascular diseases [82]. These agents inhibit 3-ketoacyl coenzyme A thiolase (KAT), the last enzyme involved in fatty acid β-oxidation (Fig. 8.1). In the PAB model, KAT inhibitors increased RV glucose oxidation and ATP levels which were associated with improvements in cardiac output and exercise tolerance [56]. Trimetazidine also blocked MCT-induced mitochondrial dysfunction and ROS production [83]. Studies of the MCD null mouse suggest a beneficial effect of FAO inhibition in the pulmonary vasculature as well, likely by increasing glucose oxidation [62]. Several clinical trials are underway to assess FAO inhibitor therapy in PAH patients (NCT01839110, NCT02133352, NCT01174173, NCT01917136, NCT01953965, NCT01757808). Both DCA and KAT inhibitors activate PDH but through different mechanisms, suggesting that combined therapy with both agents may have a synergistic impact.

The glutamine antagonist, 6-diazo-5-oxo-L-norleucine (DON), decreased glutaminolysis and was associated with improvements in glucose oxidation and cardiac output in the RV working heart model as well as the MCT rat model [40]

(Fig. 8.1). Indeed, these data suggest that the increased rate of glutaminolysis is maladaptive in RV hypertrophy. The biochemical mechanisms by which glutaminolysis suppresses glucose oxidation are unclear. Unfortunately, DON likely has several targets and has demonstrated toxicity, limiting its use *in vivo*, however, novel inhibitors of glutaminolysis may find an important role as PAH therapy in the future.

Functional Consequences of Metabolic Dysregulation in the Right Ventricle

Right ventricular (RV) failure is the most common cause of death in patients with pulmonary hypertension [84]. Chronic pressure overload in patients with pulmonary hypertension leads to RV hypertrophy in an attempt to maintain cardiac output in the face of increased afterload. While partially compensatory, the adverse consequences of hypertrophy, such as ischemia [30, 85, 86], diastolic dysfunction [87], and inefficient coupling (see Chap. 17), lead to RV failure and early mortality. Indeed, clinical parameters of RV function are a major determinant of exercise capacity and prognosis in patients with RV pressure overload from any cause [88, 89]. The critical importance of RV function in the pathogenesis of pulmonary hypertension has provided strong motivation for identifying the molecular mechanisms associated with RV failure.

Interestingly, two clinical patterns of RV hypertrophy, adaptive and maladaptive, have emerged based on the rate of progression to RV failure (Table 8.1) [90]. In spite of similar RV systolic pressures and degree of hypertrophy, some patients, such as those with pulmonary arterial hypertension secondary to systemic sclerosis, progress rapidly toward RV failure [91] while others, such as those with congenital heart diseases like Eisenmenger syndrome, demonstrate prolonged periods of stability [92]. Similar effects are observed in animal models of RV pressure overload where PAB causes less RV dysfunction than either MCT or SuH treatments [23, 85].

This important distinction between adaptive and maladaptive hypertrophy provides a novel approach to thinking about the pathogenesis of RV dysfunction in PAH with the goal of understanding the molecular determinants of this pathophenotypic distinction. The association between concomitant pulmonary vascular disease and the maladaptive phenotype suggests some shared disease mechanism. Additionally, maladaptive hypertrophy has been associated histologically with RV fibrosis and capillary rarefaction, perhaps suggesting that RV ischemia may play a fundamental role in the metabolic and functional derangements in maladaptive hypertrophy [90]. Currently, the causes of RV fibrosis and decreased angiogenic gene expression are poorly understood. Moreover, while RV ischemia may lead to the

Table 8.1 Adaptive and maladaptive RV hypertrophy

	Adaptive	Maladaptive
Clinical features		
Cardiac output	Preserved, normal RVEF	Decreased, impaired RVEF
Filling pressures	Normal	Elevated
Exercise capacity	Preserved	Impaired
Patient population	Congenital heart disease	PAH, systemic sclerosis
Animal model	PAB	MCT, SuH, Chronic hypoxia
Clinical course	Stable, slow decline	Rapid progression
Anatomic features		
Hypertrophy	Concentric	Dilated
Capillary density	Preserved	Rarefied
Fibrosis	Minimal	Prominent
Ischemia	Minimal	Prominent
LV involvement	Minimal	Increased
Metabolic features		
Lactatogenic glycolysis	Mildly increased	Markedly increased
FAO	Increased	Decreased
Glutaminolysis	Unchanged	Increased

metabolic reprogramming observed, these changes in carbon utilization associated with maladaptive hypertrophy likely potentiate the "hypoxia-like" program of gene expression. The salutary consequences of increased glucose oxidation on RV function (with DCA or KAT inhibitors, for example) points to a critical role for abnormal metabolism in the pathogenesis of RV dysfunction in PAH. Identifying the molecular determinants of adaptive *versus* maladaptive RV hypertrophy may identify targets for therapeutic interventions designed to shift toward adaptive, concentric hypertrophy or break the cycle of progressive dilation, ischemia, and dysfunction. Fortunately, investigators are beginning to think about ways to model the progression of disease from compensated to decompensated RV hypertrophy and finally to RV failure [25].

Summary and Future Directions

Metabolic reprogramming is a fundamental characteristic of the pulmonary vasculature and RV of patients with PAH. The metabolic phenotype is best described by (1) increases in lactatogenic glycolysis, (2) decreased fatty acid oxidation, (3) increased glutaminolysis, and (4) inefficient oxidative phosphorylation. In a manner similar to many cancer cells, these metabolic changes may serve to facilitate the growth and proliferation of pulmonary vascular cells by blunting apoptotic signals and providing precursors for macromolecular biosynthesis. Importantly, the energetic efficiency of the RV suffers as a result of metabolic reprogramming, which has important implications for clinical outcomes like mortality and functional capacity. Fortunately, a metabolic understanding of PAH has provided novel therapeutic insights, and we anxiously await the results of clinical trials utilizing DCA and KAT inhibitors in patients with pulmonary hypertension.

Evidence for altered metabolism extends beyond the pulmonary arteries and RV to include skeletal muscle, inflammatory cells, and endothelial progenitor cells [93], offering additional evidence that pulmonary hypertension and RV failure are the most severe and consequential local manifestations of a systemic disease. As animal models of disease progression are developed and characterized and as patients are diagnosed sooner and followed longer, novel insights into the etiology and development of the PAH metabolic program will be obtained. Indeed, several of the ongoing clinical trials have a PET component where these metabolic changes can be interrogated *in vivo* in patients. Finally, the most important work left to basic and translational investigators remains to integrate the metabolic changes with the various signaling pathways and extracellular stimuli that have been implicated in studies of PAH pathogenesis.

References

1. Warburg O. On respiratory impairment in cancer cells. Science. 1956;124(3215):269–70.
2. Warburg O. On the origin of cancer cells. Science. 1956;123(3191): 309–14.
3. Semenza GL. Regulation of cancer cell metabolism by hypoxia-inducible factor 1. Semin Cancer Biol. 2009;19(1):12–6.
4. Semenza GL, Roth PH, Fang HM, Wang GL. Transcriptional regulation of genes encoding glycolytic enzymes by hypoxia-inducible factor 1. J Biol Chem. 1994;269(38):23757–63.
5. Hu CJ, Wang LY, Chodosh LA, Keith B, Simon MC. Differential roles of hypoxia-inducible factor 1alpha (HIF-1alpha) and HIF-2alpha in hypoxic gene regulation. Mol Cell Biol. 2003;23(24): 9361–74.
6. Semenza GL, Jiang BH, Leung SW, Passantino R, Concordet JP, Maire P, et al. Hypoxia response elements in the aldolase A, enolase 1, and lactate dehydrogenase A gene promoters contain essential binding sites for hypoxia-inducible factor 1. J Biol Chem. 1996; 271(51):32529–37.
7. Semenza GL. Targeting HIF-1 for cancer therapy. Nat Rev Cancer. 2003;3(10):721–32.
8. Riddle SR, Ahmad A, Ahmad S, Deeb SS, Malkki M, Schneider BK, et al. Hypoxia induces hexokinase II gene expression in human lung cell line A549. Am J Physiol Lung Cell Mol Physiol. 2000;278(2):L407–16.
9. Kim JW, Tchernyshyov I, Semenza GL, Dang CV. HIF-1-mediated expression of pyruvate dehydrogenase kinase: a metabolic switch required for cellular adaptation to hypoxia. Cell Metab. 2006;3(3): 177–85.
10. Lu CW, Lin SC, Chen KF, Lai YY, Tsai SJ. Induction of pyruvate dehydrogenase kinase-3 by hypoxia-inducible factor-1 promotes metabolic switch and drug resistance. J Biol Chem. 2008;283(42): 28106–14.
11. Takubo K, Nagamatsu G, Kobayashi CI, Nakamura-Ishizu A, Kobayashi H, Ikeda E, et al. Regulation of glycolysis by Pdk func-

12. tions as a metabolic checkpoint for cell cycle quiescence in hematopoietic stem cells. Cell Stem Cell. 2013;12(1):49–61.
12. Semenza GL. Hypoxia-inducible factors in physiology and medicine. Cell. 2012;148(3):399–408.
13. Zhang H, Bosch-Marce M, Shimoda LA, Tan YS, Baek JH, Wesley JB, et al. Mitochondrial autophagy is an HIF-1-dependent adaptive metabolic response to hypoxia. J Biol Chem. 2008;283(16):10892–903.
14. Archer SL, Gomberg-Maitland M, Maitland ML, Rich S, Garcia JG, Weir EK. Mitochondrial metabolism, redox signaling, and fusion: a mitochondria-ROS-HIF-1alpha-Kv1.5 O2-sensing pathway at the intersection of pulmonary hypertension and cancer. Am J Physiol Heart Circ Physiol. 2008;294(2):H570–8.
15. Rumsey WL, Abbott B, Bertelsen D, Mallamaci M, Hagan K, Nelson D, et al. Adaptation to hypoxia alters energy metabolism in rat heart. Am J Physiol. 1999;276(1 Pt 2):H71–80.
16. Kakinuma Y, Miyauchi T, Suzuki T, Yuki K, Murakoshi N, Goto K, et al. Enhancement of glycolysis in cardiomyocytes elevates endothelin-1 expression through the transcriptional factor hypoxia-inducible factor-1 alpha. Clin Sci. 2002;103 Suppl 48:210S–4.
17. Palmer LA, Semenza GL, Stoler MH, Johns RA. Hypoxia induces type II NOS gene expression in pulmonary artery endothelial cells via HIF-1. Am J Physiol. 1998;274(2 Pt 1):L212–9.
18. Yu AY, Frid MG, Shimoda LA, Wiener CM, Stenmark K, Semenza GL. Temporal, spatial, and oxygen-regulated expression of hypoxia-inducible factor-1 in the lung. Am J Physiol. 1998;275(4 Pt 1): L818–26.
19. Yu AY, Shimoda LA, Iyer NV, Huso DL, Sun X, McWilliams R, et al. Impaired physiological responses to chronic hypoxia in mice partially deficient for hypoxia-inducible factor 1alpha. J Clin Invest. 1999;103(5):691–6.
20. Shimoda LA, Manalo DJ, Sham JS, Semenza GL, Sylvester JT. Partial HIF-1alpha deficiency impairs pulmonary arterial myocyte electrophysiological responses to hypoxia. Am J Physiol Lung Cell Mol Physiol. 2001;281(1):L202–8.
21. Bonnet S, Michelakis ED, Porter CJ, Andrade-Navarro MA, Thebaud B, Bonnet S, et al. An abnormal mitochondrial-hypoxia inducible factor-1alpha-Kv channel pathway disrupts oxygen sensing and triggers pulmonary arterial hypertension in fawn hooded rats: similarities to human pulmonary arterial hypertension. Circulation. 2006;113(22):2630–41.
22. Xu W, Koeck T, Lara AR, Neumann D, DiFilippo FP, Koo M, et al. Alterations of cellular bioenergetics in pulmonary artery endothelial cells. Proc Natl Acad Sci U S A. 2007;104(4):1342–7.
23. Piao L, Fang YH, Cadete VJ, Wietholt C, Urboniene D, Toth PT, et al. The inhibition of pyruvate dehydrogenase kinase improves impaired cardiac function and electrical remodeling in two models of right ventricular hypertrophy: resuscitating the hibernating right ventricle. J Mol Med (Berl). 2010;88(1):47–60.
24. Archer SL, Marsboom G, Kim GH, Zhang HJ, Toth PT, Svensson EC, et al. Epigenetic attenuation of mitochondrial superoxide dismutase 2 in pulmonary arterial hypertension: a basis for excessive cell proliferation and a new therapeutic target. Circulation. 2010;121(24):2661–71.
25. Sutendra G, Dromparis P, Paulin R, Zervopoulos S, Haromy A, Nagendran J, et al. A metabolic remodeling in right ventricular hypertrophy is associated with decreased angiogenesis and a transition from a compensated to a decompensated state in pulmonary hypertension. J Mol Med (Berl). 2013;91(11):1315–27.
26. van de Veerdonk MC, Marcus JT, Bogaard HJ, Vonk Noordegraaf A. State of the art: advanced imaging of the right ventricle and pulmonary circulation in humans (2013 Grover Conference series). Pulm Circ. 2014;4(2):158–68.
27. Can MM, Kaymaz C, Tanboga IH, Tokgoz HC, Canpolat N, Turkyilmaz E, et al. Increased right ventricular glucose metabolism in patients with pulmonary arterial hypertension. Clin Nucl Med. 2011;36(9):743–8.

28. Fang W, Zhao L, Xiong CM, Ni XH, He ZX, He JG, et al. Comparison of 18 F-FDG uptake by right ventricular myocardium in idiopathic pulmonary arterial hypertension and pulmonary arterial hypertension associated with congenital heart disease. Pulm Circ. 2012;2(3):365–72.

29. Kluge R, Barthel H, Pankau H, Seese A, Schauer J, Wirtz H, et al. Different mechanisms for changes in glucose uptake of the right and left ventricular myocardium in pulmonary hypertension. J Nucl Med. 2005;46(1):25–31.

30. Wong YY, Ruiter G, Lubberink M, Raijmakers PG, Knaapen P, Marcus JT, et al. Right ventricular failure in idiopathic pulmonary arterial hypertension is associated with inefficient myocardial oxygen utilization. Circ Heart Fail. 2011;4(6):700–6.

31. Piao L, Sidhu VK, Fang YH, Ryan JJ, Parikh KS, Hong Z, et al. FOXO1-mediated upregulation of pyruvate dehydrogenase kinase-4 (PDK4) decreases glucose oxidation and impairs right ventricular function in pulmonary hypertension: therapeutic benefits of dichloroacetate. J Mol Med (Berl). 2013;91(3):333–46.

32. Lee JH, Kim EJ, Kim DK, Lee JM, Park SB, Lee IK, et al. Hypoxia induces PDK4 gene expression through induction of the orphan nuclear receptor ERRgamma. PLoS One. 2012;7(9):e46324.

33. Krebs HA, Johnson WA. Metabolism of ketonic acids in animal tissues. Biochem J. 1937;31(4):645–60.

34. Zhang Z, Tan M, Xie Z, Dai L, Chen Y, Zhao Y. Identification of lysine succinylation as a new post-translational modification. Nat Chem Biol. 2011;7(1):58–63.

35. Alderson NL, Wang Y, Blatnik M, Frizzell N, Walla MD, Lyons TJ, et al. S-(2-Succinyl)cysteine: a novel chemical modification of tissue proteins by a Krebs cycle intermediate. Arch Biochem Biophys. 2006;450(1):1–8.

36. Nagai R, Brock JW, Blatnik M, Baatz JE, Bethard J, Walla MD, et al. Succination of protein thiols during adipocyte maturation: a biomarker of mitochondrial stress. J Biol Chem. 2007;282(47):34219–28.

37. Blatnik M, Frizzell N, Thorpe SR, Baynes JW. Inactivation of glyceraldehyde-3-phosphate dehydrogenase by fumarate in diabetes: formation of S-(2-succinyl)cysteine, a novel chemical modification of protein and possible biomarker of mitochondrial stress. Diabetes. 2008;57(1):41–9.

38. Blatnik M, Thorpe SR, Baynes JW. Succination of proteins by fumarate: mechanism of inactivation of glyceraldehyde-3-phosphate dehydrogenase in diabetes. Ann N Y Acad Sci. 2008;1126:272–5.

39. Lunt SY, Vander Heiden MG. Aerobic glycolysis: meeting the metabolic requirements of cell proliferation. Annu Rev Cell Dev Biol. 2011;27:441–64.

40. Piao L, Fang YH, Parikh K, Ryan JJ, Toth PT, Archer SL. Cardiac glutaminolysis: a maladaptive cancer metabolism pathway in the right ventricle in pulmonary hypertension. J Mol Med (Berl). 2013;91(10):1185–97.

41. Anso E, Mullen AR, Felsher DW, Mates JM, Deberardinis RJ, Chandel NS. Metabolic changes in cancer cells upon suppression of MYC. Cancer Metab. 2013;1(1):7.

42. Fessel JP, Hamid R, Wittmann BM, Robinson LJ, Blackwell T, Tada Y, et al. Metabolomic analysis of bone morphogenetic protein receptor type 2 mutations in human pulmonary endothelium reveals widespread metabolic reprogramming. Pulm Circ. 2012;2(2):201–13.

43. Fessel JP, Shah AT, Egnatchik R, Skala MC, Young JD, Kang CJ, et al. Increased glutamine metabolism is a key feature of the metabolic reprogramming in BMPR2 mutant pulmonary endothelium. Am J Respir Crit Care Med. 2013;187(American Thoracic Society International Conference Abstracts):A1743.

44. Fessel JP, Fares WH, Brittain EL, Hemnes AR, Austin ED, Monahan KJ, et al. Targeted in vivo metabolomics reveals multiple functional abnormalities in the lung vasculature of pulmonary hypertension patients. Am J Respir Crit Care Med. 2014;189(American Thoracic Society International Conference Abstracts):A6637.

45. Ward PS, Patel J, Wise DR, Abdel-Wahab O, Bennett BD, Coller HA, et al. The common feature of leukemia-associated IDH1 and IDH2 mutations is a neomorphic enzyme activity converting alpha-ketoglutarate to 2-hydroxyglutarate. Cancer Cell. 2010;17(3):225–34. Epub 2010/02/23. eng.

46. Xu W, Yang H, Liu Y, Yang Y, Wang P, Kim SH, et al. Oncometabolite 2-hydroxyglutarate is a competitive inhibitor of alpha-ketoglutarate-dependent dioxygenases. Cancer Cell. 2011;19(1):17–30.

47. Cairns RA, Mak TW. Oncogenic isocitrate dehydrogenase mutations: mechanisms, models, and clinical opportunities. Cancer Discov. 2013;3(7):730–41.

48. Oldham WM, Clish CB, Yang Y, Loscalzo J. Hypoxia-Mediated Increases in l-2-hydroxyglutarate Coordinate the Metabolic Response to Reductive Stress. Cell Metab. 2015;22(2):291–303.

49. Cardaci S, Ciriolo MR. TCA cycle defects and cancer: when metabolism tunes redox state. Int J Cell Biol. 2012;2012:161837.

50. Zhao Y, Peng J, Lu C, Hsin M, Mura M, Wu L, et al. Metabolomic heterogeneity of pulmonary arterial hypertension. PLoS One. 2014;9(2):e88727.

51. Rajabi M, Kassiotis C, Razeghi P, Taegtmeyer H. Return to the fetal gene program protects the stressed heart: a strong hypothesis. Heart Fail Rev. 2007;12(3–4):331–43.

52. Neely JR, Morgan HE. Relationship between carbohydrate and lipid metabolism and the energy balance of heart muscle. Annu Rev Physiol. 1974;36:413–59.

53. Bergman BC, Tsvetkova T, Lowes B, Wolfel EE. Myocardial glucose and lactate metabolism during rest and atrial pacing in humans. J Physiol. 2009;587(Pt 9):2087–99.

54. Randle PJ, Garland PB, Hales CN, Newsholme EA. The glucose fatty-acid cycle. Its role in insulin sensitivity and the metabolic disturbances of diabetes mellitus. Lancet. 1963;1(7285):785–9.

55. Hue L, Taegtmeyer H. The Randle cycle revisited: a new head for an old hat. Am J Physiol Endocrinol Metab. 2009;297(3):E578–91.

56. Fang YH, Piao L, Hong Z, Toth PT, Marsboom G, Bache-Wiig P, et al. Therapeutic inhibition of fatty acid oxidation in right ventricular hypertrophy: exploiting Randle's cycle. J Mol Med (Berl). 2012;90(1):31–43.

57. Gomez-Arroyo J, Santos-Martinez LE, Aranda A, Pulido T, Beltran M, Munoz-Castellanos L, et al. Differences in right ventricular remodeling secondary to pressure overload in patients with pulmonary hypertension. Am J Respir Crit Care Med. 2014;189(5):603–6.

58. Buermans HP, Redout EM, Schiel AE, Musters RJ, Zuidwijk M, Eijk PP, et al. Microarray analysis reveals pivotal divergent mRNA expression profiles early in the development of either compensated ventricular hypertrophy or heart failure. Physiol Genomics. 2005;21(3):314–23.

59. Nagaya N, Goto Y, Satoh T, Uematsu M, Hamada S, Kuribayashi S, et al. Impaired regional fatty acid uptake and systolic dysfunction in hypertrophied right ventricle. J Nucl Med. 1998;39(10):1676–80.

60. Kim Y, Goto H, Kobayashi K, Sawada Y, Miyake Y, Fujiwara G, et al. Detection of impaired fatty acid metabolism in right ventricular hypertrophy: assessment by I-123 beta-methyl iodophenyl pentadecanoic acid (BMIPP) myocardial single-photon emission computed tomography. Ann Nucl Med. 1997;11(3):207–12.

61. Hemnes AR, Brittain EL, Trammell AW, Fessel JP, Austin ED, Penner N, et al. Evidence for right ventricular lipotoxicity in heritable pulmonary arterial hypertension. Am J Respir Crit Care Med. 2014;189(3):325–34.

62. Sutendra G, Bonnet S, Rochefort G, Haromy A, Folmes KD, Lopaschuk GD, et al. Fatty acid oxidation and malonyl-CoA decarboxylase in the vascular remodeling of pulmonary hypertension. Sci Transl Med. 2010;2(44):44ra58.

63. Li Y, Huang TT, Carlson EJ, Melov S, Ursell PC, Olson JL, et al. Dilated cardiomyopathy and neonatal lethality in mutant mice lack-

ing manganese superoxide dismutase. Nat Genet. 1995;11(4): 376–81.

64. Fessel JP, Flynn CR, Robinson LJ, Penner NL, Gladson S, Kang CJ, et al. Hyperoxia synergizes with mutant bone morphogenic protein receptor 2 to cause metabolic stress, oxidant injury, and pulmonary hypertension. Am J Respir Cell Mol Biol. 2013;49(5):778–87.

65. Lane KL, Talati M, Austin E, Hemnes AR, Johnson JA, Fessel JP, et al. Oxidative injury is a common consequence of BMPR2 mutations. Pulm Circ. 2011;1(1):72–83.

66. Braschi E, McBride HM. Mitochondria and the culture of the Borg: understanding the integration of mitochondrial function within the reticulum, the cell, and the organism. Bioessays. 2010;32(11): 958–66.

67. Friedman JR, Nunnari J. Mitochondrial form and function. Nature. 2014;505(7483):335–43.

68. Hoppins S, Nunnari J. The molecular mechanism of mitochondrial fusion. Biochim Biophys Acta. 2009;1793(1):20–6.

69. Lackner LL, Nunnari JM. The molecular mechanism and cellular functions of mitochondrial division. Biochim Biophys Acta. 2009;1792(12):1138–44.

70. Shutt TE, McBride HM. Staying cool in difficult times: mitochondrial dynamics, quality control and the stress response. Biochim Biophys Acta. 2013;1833(2):417–24.

71. Marsboom G, Toth PT, Ryan JJ, Hong Z, Wu X, Fang YH, et al. Dynamin-related protein 1-mediated mitochondrial mitotic fission permits hyperproliferation of vascular smooth muscle cells and offers a novel therapeutic target in pulmonary hypertension. Circ Res. 2012;110(11):1484–97.

72. Ryan JJ, Marsboom G, Fang YH, Toth PT, Morrow E, Luo N, et al. PGC1alpha-mediated mitofusin-2 deficiency in female rats and humans with pulmonary arterial hypertension. Am J Respir Crit Care Med. 2013;187(8):865–78.

73. Batt J, Ahmed SS, Correa J, Bain A, Granton J. Skeletal muscle dysfunction in idiopathic pulmonary arterial hypertension. Am J Respir Cell Mol Biol. 2014;50(1):74–86.

74. Archer SL. Mitochondrial dynamics–mitochondrial fission and fusion in human diseases. N Engl J Med. 2013;369(23):2236–51.

75. Saudubray JM, Sedel F, Walter JH. Clinical approach to treatable inborn metabolic diseases: an introduction. J Inherit Metab Dis. 2006;29(2–3):261–74.

76. Bonnet S, Archer SL, Allalunis-Turner J, Haromy A, Beaulieu C, Thompson R, et al. A mitochondria-K+ channel axis is suppressed in cancer and its normalization promotes apoptosis and inhibits cancer growth. Cancer Cell. 2007;11(1):37–51.

77. Archer SL, Fang YH, Ryan JJ, Piao L. Metabolism and bioenergetics in the right ventricle and pulmonary vasculature in pulmonary hypertension. Pulm Circ. 2013;3(1):144–52.

78. Michelakis ED, McMurtry MS, Wu XC, Dyck JR, Moudgil R, Hopkins TA, et al. Dichloroacetate, a metabolic modulator, prevents and reverses chronic hypoxic pulmonary hypertension in rats: role of increased expression and activity of voltage-gated potassium channels. Circulation. 2002;105(2):244–50.

79. McMurtry MS, Bonnet S, Wu X, Dyck JR, Haromy A, Hashimoto K, et al. Dichloroacetate prevents and reverses pulmonary hypertension by inducing pulmonary artery smooth muscle cell apoptosis. Circ Res. 2004;95(8):830–40.

80. Guignabert C, Tu L, Izikki M, Dewachter L, Zadigue P, Humbert M, et al. Dichloroacetate treatment partially regresses established pulmonary hypertension in mice with SM22alpha-targeted overexpression of the serotonin transporter. FASEB J. 2009;23(12):4135–47.

81. Kankotia S, Stacpoole PW. Dichloroacetate and cancer: new home for an orphan drug? Biochim Biophys Acta. 2014;1846(2):617–29.

82. Fragasso G, Spoladore R, Cuko A, Palloshi A. Modulation of fatty acids oxidation in heart failure by selective pharmacological inhibition of 3-ketoacyl coenzyme-A thiolase. Curr Clin Pharmacol. 2007;2(3):190–6.

83. Guarnieri C, Muscari C. Beneficial effects of trimetazidine on mitochondrial function and superoxide production in the cardiac muscle. Cardiovasc Drugs Ther. 1990;4 Suppl 4:814–5.

84. Tonelli AR, Arelli V, Minai OA, Newman J, Bair N, Heresi GA, et al. Causes and circumstances of death in pulmonary arterial hypertension. Am J Respir Crit Care Med. 2013;188(3):365–9.

85. Bogaard HJ, Natarajan R, Henderson SC, Long CS, Kraskauskas D, Smithson L, et al. Chronic pulmonary artery pressure elevation is insufficient to explain right heart failure. Circulation. 2009;120(20): 1951–60.

86. Ruiter G, Ying Wong Y, de Man FS, Louis Handoko M, Jaspers RT, Postmus PE, et al. Right ventricular oxygen supply parameters are decreased in human and experimental pulmonary hypertension. J Heart Lung Transplant. 2013;32(2):231–40.

87. Chen EP, Craig DM, Bittner HB, Davis RD, Van Trigt P. Pharmacological strategies for improving diastolic dysfunction in the setting of chronic pulmonary hypertension. Circulation. 1998;97(16):1606–12.

88. Sztrymf B, Souza R, Bertoletti L, Jais X, Sitbon O, Price LC, et al. Prognostic factors of acute heart failure in patients with pulmonary arterial hypertension. Eur Respir J. 2010;35(6):1286–93.

89. Brickner ME, Hillis LD, Lange RA. Congenital heart disease in adults. First of two parts. N Engl J Med. 2000;342(4):256–63.

90. Ryan JJ, Archer SL. The right ventricle in pulmonary arterial hypertension: disorders of metabolism, angiogenesis and adrenergic signaling in right ventricular failure. Circ Res. 2014;115(1):176–88.

91. Kawut SM, Taichman DB, Archer-Chicko CL, Palevsky HI, Kimmel SE. Hemodynamics and survival in patients with pulmonary arterial hypertension related to systemic sclerosis. Chest. 2003;123(2):344–50.

92. Hopkins WE, Ochoa LL, Richardson GW, Trulock EP. Comparison of the hemodynamics and survival of adults with severe primary pulmonary hypertension or Eisenmenger syndrome. J Heart Lung Transplant. 1996;15(1 Pt 1):100–5.

93. Sutendra G, Michelakis ED. The metabolic basis of pulmonary arterial hypertension. Cell Metab. 2014;19(4):558–73.

Renin-Angiotensin-Aldosterone and Other Neurohumoral Factors in the Pathogenesis of Pulmonary Hypertension

9

Bradley A. Maron, Thomas E. Stephens, and Jane A. Leopold

Introduction

Pulmonary arterial hypertension (PAH) is characterized by intimal hypertrophy, fibrosis, and plexogenic remodeling of distal pulmonary arterioles. These changes increase pulmonary vascular resistance, and, consequently, disrupt normal right ventricular (RV)-pulmonary arterial performance to promote right heart failure [1]. The contribution of circulating, endogenously synthesized vasoactive hormones and/or neurohumoral factors to RV-pulmonary vascular dysfunction in PAH is increasingly recognized. Findings from basic science, translational, and clinical reports identify catecholamines, angiotensin(s), the mineralocorticoid hormone aldosterone, and selected estrogen/androgen sex hormone derivatives in the development of pulmonary vascular remodeling, RV dysfunction, and as markers of PAH prevalence [2, 3]. In this chapter, we will review current concepts relating to the effects of these factors to RV and pulmonary arterial function in the context of the pulmonary hypertension clinical phenotype.

The significance of these effectors to the pathobiology of PAH, however, is complex and extends beyond extrapolating their role(s) from left-sided to right-sided heart disease. The intrinsic properties of RV cardiomyocytes and pulmonary vascular cells are principally distinctive compared to left ventricular (LV) cardiomyocytes and vascular cells from systemic circulatory beds, respectively. For example, substantial heterogeneity between pulmonary and systemic vascular cells is observed in response to hypoxia, while the adrenergic-dependent inotropic potential of RV and LV cardiomyocytes is dissimilar [3]. These observations illustrate that hormonal regulation of systemic blood vessels does not necessarily predict pulmonary vascular function. Thus, the fact that many biological factors under discussion here may be elevated in systemic vascular compartments in PAH does not refute the assertion that RV/pulmonary vascular remodeling occurs in this disease in the absence of substantial LV or systemic vascular disease.

Cardiopulmonary Targets of the Autonomic Nervous System

The cardiopulmonary system is a key target of each branch of the autonomic nervous system. Endogenous catecholamines, which include norepinephrine, epinephrine, and dopamine, are synthesized in sympathetic nerve endings from the uptake and sequential hydroxylation of the essential amino acid phenylalanine. In turn, adrenergic receptors (ARs) are well represented in RV cardiomyocytes and pulmonary blood vessels. Stimulation of the AR subtype α_1 by (nor)epinephrine induces vasoconstriction and blood vessel thickening. Interestingly, α_1 expression levels are virtually equal in pulmonary vascular compared to resistance arteriole tissue, and receptor density is substantially greater than is observed in conduit blood vessels, such as aorta (Table 9.1) [4]. Likewise, the primary dopamine-selective receptor in

B.A. Maron, MD (✉)
Division of Cardiovascular Medicine, Department of Medicine, Brigham and Women's Hospital and Harvard Medical School, 77 Ave. Louis Pasteur, New Research Building (NRB), Room 0630-N, Boston, MA, 02115, USA

Department of Cardiology, Veterans Affairs Boston Healthcare System, Boston, MA, 02115, USA
e-mail: bmaron@partners.org

T.E. Stephens, BA
Division of Cardiovascular Medicine, Department of Medicine, Brigham and Women's Hospital and Harvard Medical School, 77 Ave. Louis Pasteur, New Research Building (NRB), Room 0654, Boston, MA, 02115, USA

J.A. Leopold, MD
Division of Cardiovascular Medicine, Department of Medicine, Brigham and Women's Hospital and Harvard Medical School, 77 Ave. Louis Pasteur, New Research Building (NRB), Room 0630-K, Boston, MA, 02115, USA

Table 9.1 Total α_1-adrenergic receptor (AR) density in the human vasculature

Vessel type	Artery	Mean α_1-AR density (fmol/mg protein)
Arteries		
Central	Aorta	9.8 ± 1.8
Small somatic	Mammary	6.0 ± 1.3
Splanchnic	Mesenteric	13 ± 6.1
	Splenic	28 ± 7.7
	Hepatic	28 ± 5.9
Renal	Renal	23 ± 5.9
Pulmonary	**Pulmonary artery**	**24 ± 5.2**
Coronary	Epicardial coronary	2.1 ± 0.67
Veins		
Central	Vena cava	16 ± 2.8
Small somatic	Saphenous	10 ± 1.2
Renal	Renal vein	18 ± 5.8
Pulmonary	**Pulmonary vein**	**18 ± 4.6**

Reproduced with permission from Rudner et al. [4]

cardiovascular tissue, D_1, is constitutively expressed in RV cardiomyocytes at similar levels reported for LV cardiomyocytes [5].

The neural innervation of the lung ultrastructure is complex and involves a network of efferent, sensory, and neurohumoral pathways. Amine Precursor Uptake and Decarboxylation (APUD) cell clusters, which express catecholamine synthesis potential, are also distributed throughout the pulmonary vascular bed [5]. Whereas APUD-regulated catecholamine control of epithelial smooth muscle cell function is linked to the development of airway disease, such as asthma, the influence of these cells to the pathogenesis of pulmonary vascular disease is less well defined. Nevertheless, pulmonary vascular/lung nerve stimulation is associated with frequency-dependent increases in pulmonary artery perfusion pressure [6], while surgical or chemical denervation of proximal pulmonary arterioles influences pulmonary artery and RV systolic pressure directly in experiment pulmonary hypertension *in vivo* [7]. In one single center study of 13 PAH patients, changes from baseline at 3 months following pulmonary artery denervation were noted for mean pulmonary artery pressure (mPAP) (55 ± 5 vs. 36 ± 5 mmHg, p<0.01), 6-min walk distance (6-MWD) (324 ± 21 vs. 491 ± 38 m, p<0.01), and Tei index (e.g., assessment of RV systolic function) (0.7 ± 0.04 vs. 0.5 ± 0.04, p<0.01) [8], providing preliminary data to support future investigations assessing the validity of this strategy for use in clinical practice.

Despite these collective observations, studies quantifying neurohumoral activation in PAH patients report variable conclusions. Plasma venous norepinephrine levels correlated inversely in PAH (N=60) with cardiac output (r=−0.29, p<0.05) in one study [9], which is a finding supported by other data demonstrating an association between circulating norepinephrine levels (N=21) and pulmonary artery pressure (r=0.66, P<0.01), cardiac index (r=−0.56, P<0.01), and pulmonary vascular resistance (r=0.69, P<0.001) [10]. Sympathetic over-activation in PAH is supported further by work from Velez-Rosa and colleagues [11], who analyzed muscle sympathetic nerve activity (MSNA) in 17 PAH patients. They observed that MSNA, which measures electrical activity of the peroneal nerve fascicle using tungsten microelectrodes to assess muscle-directed sympathetic nerve trafficking, was increased by 33 % (P<0.01) in PAH patients compared with controls. A significant, inverse relationship between MSNA and exercise capacity, assessed by New York Heart Association functional class, was also observed.

Adrenergic Signaling and PAH

The G-protein coupled AR subtypes β_1 and β_2, are expressed constitutively in human pulmonary artery endothelial cells (PAECs) in a 1:3 distribution [6]. Stimulation of β_1 and β_2 receptors, in turn, is linked to endothelium-dependent regulation of pulmonary vascular tone. For example, extra-lobar pulmonary arteries dissected from mice and treated with isoproterenol (10^{-9}–10^{-5} mol/L), the selective β_2-AR agonist procaterol (0.1 μM), but not the β_3 agonist CL316243, demonstrated a significant pulmonary vascular relaxation response. In turn, this effect was attenuated by inhibition of endothelial nitric oxide synthase (eNOS) with L-NG-Nitroarginine Methyl Ester (L-NAME) (300 μM) or selective pharmacological antagonism of the β_1- or β_2- AR, and was abolished fully in transgenic mice lacking eNOS [12].

Perturbation to the redox balance of RV cardiomyocytes and pulmonary vascular cells is also implicated in abnormal β-AR-nitric oxide (NO•) signal transduction. In cultured pulmonary artery endothelial cells, peroxynitrite ($ONOO^-$) oxidizes eNOS to decrease bioavailable levels of NO•, which disrupts pulmonary vascular tone and promotes adverse remodeling. Increases in RV cardiomyocyte $ONOO^-$ levels assessed with anti-nitrotyrosine immunohistochemistry are observed in pulmonary hypertensive rats and are associated with RV dysfunction and decreased cardiac output *in vivo* [13]. In turn, pertussis toxin restores β-AR signaling in pulmonary artery smooth muscle cells [14], suggesting that Gi uncoupling induced by ONOO- may be an important mechanism by which β-AR-NO• signaling is disrupted under conditions of increased pulmonary vascular oxidant stress, as has been reported in various forms of pulmonary vascular disease.

In contrast to the beneficial effects of β-AR signal transduction on RV and pulmonary vascular function, α-AR stimulation is linked to *adverse* pulmonary arterial remodeling and the development of pulmonary hypertension. For example, stimulation of α_1-AR in PASMCs and adventitial fibroblasts by norepinephrine promotes a maladaptive pulmonary vascular hypertrophy induced by hypoxia in pulmonary hypertensive mice [15]. In turn, transgenic mice deficient in epinephrine and norepinephrine synthesis or α_1-AR expression appear protected from luminal occlusion and intimal thickening under the same conditions [15]. The determinates of pathogenic α_1-AR stimulation are largely unknown, but may involve cross-talk between α- and β-AR signaling, particularly with respect to α_1-AR-dependent regulation of β-AR chloride (Cl$^-$) conductance, which has been shown to inhibit β-AR signal transduction targets [16].

Adrenergic Signaling in PAH: The Right Ventricle

Pharmacological modification of catecholamine signal transduction through β-, α-, and D-receptor antagonism or antagonism is a *bona fide* treatment strategy for patients with various stages of heart failure due to left ventricular dysfunction. Despite the routine use of these therapies for this purpose, the differential effect of manipulating catecholamine function on RV performance in patients with left-sided or right-sided heart failure is not well established. Furthermore, the extent to which changes in adrenergic receptor expression or activity *promotes* RV dysfunction under conditions of increased RV afterload, such as in pulmonary hypertension, is incompletely characterized.

Piao and colleagues recently addressed these areas of uncertainty by characterizing changes to the β-AR- and D$_1$-signaling profiles in various models of experimental RV dysfunction *in vivo* [17]. They observed a greater decrease in RV cardiomyocyte α_1- and β_1-AR protein/mRNA expression levels in the hypertrophied RV under conditions of chronic inflammatory pulmonary vascular injury compared to acute pulmonary occlusion through pulmonary artery banding. These data are in concert with earlier studies demonstrating that compared to control hearts or patients with biventricular heart failure, β_1-AR expression levels are decreased in the RV of PAH patients with isolated right heart failure [18, 19]. The authors assert that this finding distinguishes, in part, adaptive from maladaptive RV hypertrophic remodeling, respectively, as pulmonary hypertension was common to both experimental models. In that study, intracellular cAMP production was attenuated and activity of G protein–coupled receptor kinase-2 (GRK2), which is implicated in adrenergic receptor down regulation in LV cardiomyocytes, was increased in the maladaptive RV hypertrophied hearts. Collectively, these findings were in support of additional findings indicating RV cardiomyocyte β_1-AR desensitization in PAH and the potential superiority of inotropic agents that maintain adenylyl cyclase coupling

under these conditions, including dobutamine to preserve contractility in the failing RV.

These and similar observations from others [20] suggest that strategies to modulate RV hypertrophy directly may offset abnormal adrenergic signaling patterns in PAH. Several investigators have explored this to observe that pharmacological inhibition of α_1-/β_1-/β_2-signaling improves RV structure and performance in experimental PAH without differentially affecting pulmonary vascular function *in vivo*. Bogaard and colleagues [21] reported that although no significant change was noted in pulmonary arterioles of Sugen-5416/hypoxia-PAH rats treated with carvedilol, drug treatment promoted RV reverse remodeling and improved tricuspid plane annular excursion (TAPSE), and increased cardiac output. This effect was associated with decreased RV thickness and intramyocardial fibrosis burden, as well as alterations to the molecular signature of the hypertrophied RV vis-á-vis cardiomyocyte fetal gene activation, including decreased α-myosin heavy chain gene and increased fetal β-myosin heavy chain expression levels. Similar findings are observed for the selective β_1-AR antagonist bisoprolol, which decreased RV thickness and improved ventricular elastance in one study of monocrotaline-PAH [22], while the beneficial effects of selected other AR antagonists on RV function is also reported under alternative experimental conditions such as high altitude and hypobaric hypoxia [23].

Translating AR Axis Interventions to PAH Clinically

Reconciling the favorable effects of β-AR stimulation in RV or pulmonary vascular tissue (e.g., increased NO• bioactivity) under normal conditions with benefits linked to β-AR *antagonism* in experimental PAH is an important area of active investigation. It is interesting to note that AR signal transduction regulates interleukin 6 (IL-6) and vascular endothelial growth factor (VEGF) [24], which are both involved in pulmonary endothelial injury and recapitulation of PAH experimentally. It is also possible that dysregulated catecholamine-AR signaling in PAH is a consequence of pathogenic changes to intermediaries downstream of AR activation. For example, the β_1-AR target sarcoplasmic reticulum Ca^{2+}-ATPase 2a (SERCA2a), which regulates intracellular Ca^{2+} content in vascular smooth muscle cells, is down regulated in PASMCs and pulmonary arterioles in monocrotaline-PAH [25], while gene transfer via intratracheal delivery of aerosolized adeno-associated virus serotype 1 (AAV1) carrying SERCA2a reverses pulmonary endothelial dysfunction, decreases PAP, vascular remodeling, and RV hypertrophy significantly in PAH *in vivo* [25].

It is possible that the functional consequences of β-AR signaling on pulmonary vascular function vary in the intact *versus* injured pulmonary endothelium. Overall, the balance of available data points to dysregulated adrenergic signaling in pulmonary vascular and RV tissue in PAH, although the identification of factors responsible for mediating a transition from healthy to maladaptive AR signaling in PAH remain incompletely characterized. Along these lines, consensus is pending regarding the risk-reward balance of AR-modulating pharmacotherapeutics clinically. While attempts to replicate in PAH/RV dysfunction patients the (substantial) benefits of AR antagonists observed in left heart disease, this strategy has been evaluated empirically only in small observational studies limited largely to patients with selected forms of pulmonary vascular disease (e.g., portopulmonary hypertension) and in whom treatment was with early generation drugs (propranolol or atenolol) at high doses [26]. Some PAH experts maintain reservations regarding the safety profile of AR antagonists [27], particularly owing to the association of this drug class with diminished functional capacity due to chronotropic/RV inotropic insufficiency in patients with (exercise-induced) pulmonary vascular disease, while recently published expert consensus guidelines referenced insufficient clinical data to outline formal recommendations for their use in practice [28]. To bridge this knowledge gap, several randomized, prospective clinical trials have been announced assessing the effect of AR antagonists, including carvedilol, on outcome in PAH (NCT00964678; NCT01723371; NCT01586156; NCT0225394 at clinicaltrials.gov) (Table 9.2), while further efforts are also required to clarify optimal AR agonist therapy in the critically ill PAH patient with severely impaired cardiac output.

Aldosterone as a PAH Disease Modifier

Elevated levels of aldosterone in lung has been demonstrated in monocrotaline- and Sugen-5416/hypoxia-PAH in rats and the porcine pulmonary vein banding model of PAH [29]. In patients with PAH pulmonary arterial aldosterone levels are increased by 4.9-fold compared with controls [30]. In that study, aldosterone levels correlated inversely with cardiac output and positively with key measures of pulmonary vascular remodeling, including pulmonary vascular resistance and transpulmonary gradient. Adrenal stimulation by renin-angiotensin axis upregulation is likely to be the chief source of aldosterone production in PAH; however, the possibility that pulmonary vascular tissue functions as an extra-adrenal source of aldosterone production has been reported. Endocrine functionality was suggested originally five decades ago by several groups based on observations demonstrating that isolated synthesis of angiotensin I occurs in lung tissue [31]. In support of this are data demonstrating a transpulmonary increase in plasma levels of the aldosterone secretagogues angiotensin II [32] and the endothelin-1 precursor Big endothelin-1 [33] in patients with selected forms of pulmonary hypertension. Whether autonomous aldosterone synthesis in lung or pulmonary vascular tissue occurs or is relevant to PAH pathobiology in patients *per se*, requires further investigations [34].

It is noteworthy that key proteins required for *de novo* aldosterone synthesis, including steroidogenic acute regulatory protein (StAR), CYP11B1 (11-beta-hydroxylase), and CYP11B2 (aldosterone synthase) are constitutively expressed or inducible in cardiomyocytes, PASMCs, and/or PAECs by factors associated with pulmonary vascular injury [35, 36]. Treatment of human PAECs with ET-1 at levels similar to those observed in PAH patients induces association of the steroidogenic transcription factors steroidogenic factor-1 (SF-1) and PGC-1α to the CYP11B2 promoter, which increases pulmonary endothelial CYP11B2 expression and aldosterone levels by twofold *in vitro* (Fig. 9.1) [37]. Furthermore, pharmacological antagonism of the mineralocorticoid receptor with spironolactone attenuates angiotensin-II-mediated PASMC hypertrophy [35], providing some evidence in support of functionally active aldosterone biosynthesized in pulmonary vascular tissue.

The Vasculopathy of Hyperaldosteronism

Elevated levels of aldosterone promote a vasculopathy in systemic blood vessels that overlaps, in part, with the histopathophenotype of PAH. In patients with primary hyperaldosteronism (i.e., unstimulated adrenal aldosterone synthesis), for example, VSMC proliferation, increased arterial stiffness, and vascular fibrosis define the remodeling pattern of resistance blood vessels [38].

Aldosterone-induced reactive oxygen species generation is one mechanism proposed to account for adverse pulmonary vascular remodeling and pulmonary hypertension. Pathophysiologically relevant levels of aldosterone (10^{-9}–10^{-7} mol/l) have been shown to increase NADPH oxidase type-4 (NOX4)-derived hydrogen peroxide generation in cultured human PAECs that oxidatively modifies the endothelin-B (ET_B) receptor at cysteines in position 402, 403, and 405 (Cys402/403/405). As a consequence of Cys402/403/405 oxidation, ET_B signal transduction, and, thus, ET_B-dependent NO• synthesis is impaired, which is associated with the development of pulmonary vascular fibrosis in monocrotaline- and Sugen-5416/hypoxia-PAH (Fig. 9.2) [37].

Aldosterone is also a mitogenic trigger in pulmonary vascular cells and RV cardiomyocytes [39]. Treatment of PASMCs harvested from idiopathic PAH patients with aldosterone (10^{-7} mol/l) stimulates cellular proliferation and mitosis [40], in part, through upregulation of mitogen activated protein kinase (MAPK). This effect is exacerbated by co-incubation of aldosterone with bone morphogenic pro-

Table 9.2 Registered clinical trials investigating the effect of therapies that influence neurohumoral and/or hormonal signaling on outcome in pulmonary arterial hypertension (PAH)

Study name	Identifier/duration	Treatment	Inclusion criteria	Endpoint	Primary secondary
Beta-blockers for the treatment of PAH in children	NCT01723371 6 mo End date: 9/2014	Carvedilol	Age: ≥8 and ≤17.5 yr mPAP >25 mmHg PCWP <15 mmHg PVR >3 Wood units Clinically stable (3 mo)	Adverse event incidence	Δ 6MWD, VO$_2$ Δ TAPSE Δ RVEF
Beta-blockers in PAH	NCT01246037 6 mo End date: 4/2014	Bisoprolol	Age: ≥18 yr Stable iPAH WHO Class II/III	ΔRVEF by CMR Safety measures	RV diastolic function Sympathetic activity levels
PAH treatment with carvedilol for heart failure (PAHTCH)	NCT01586156 6 months End date: 7/2018	Carvedilol	Age: 18–65 yr PAH WHO Class I-III	ΔHIF/NO/ AR recovery ΔRV function	
Pilot study of the safety and efficacy of carvedilol in PAH	NCT00964678 6 mo End date: 5/2014	Carvedilol	Age: ≥18 yr WHO Group 1 PH NHYA Class II/III mPAP >25 mmHg 6MWD >100 m	ΔRVEF by CMR	ΔRVESV Δ6MWD ΔTAPSE
Spironolactone for PAH	NCT01712620 6 mo End date: 11/2015	Spironolactone	Age: ≥18 yr WHO Group 1 PH Stable therapy (4 wk) mPAP >25 mmHg PCWP <15 mmHg PVR >3.0 Wood units NYHA Class I-III	Δ6MWD Clinical worsening	ΔVO$_2$ ΔRV function Inflammation biomarkers Drug safety
Effects of spironolactone on collagen metabolism in patients with PAH	NCT01468571 16 wk End date: 12/2015	Spironolactone	Age: ≥18 yr Body weight >40 kg WHO Group 1 PH Stable therapy (4 wk)	ΔFibrosis markers	Adverse events Δ6MWD ΔFunctional class Clinical worsening
Modulating effects of lisinopril on sildenafil activity in PAH (MELISSA)	NCT01181284 32 wk End date: 7/2011	Lisinopril added to sildenafil	Age: 18–75 yr WHO Group I PAH PVR >3 Wood units PCWP ≤16 6MWD 150–575 m PDE-Vi (3 mo)	ACE-I tolerability	ΔN-BNP levels ΔGas exchange measures Δ6MWD
Combined ambrisentan plus spironolactone in patients with pulmonary arterial hypertension (CAPS-PAH)	NCT0225394 6 mo End date: 6/2017	Spironolactone added to ambrisentan	Age: 16–75 yr WHO Group I PAH PVR >3 Wood units PCWP ≤16 6MWD 150–575 m Ambrisentan/PDE-Vi (3 mo)	Combined: (a) 6-MWD (b) pVO$_2$	Fibrosis markers RV function QOL
Hormonal, metabolic, and signaling interactions in PAH	NCT01884051 5 yr End date: 9/2017	ACE-2 Metformin		Sex hormone metabolite levels Δ6MWD Glucose metabolism	Hemodynamics PET scan results

NCT national clinical trial (clinicaltrials.gov), *mPAP* mean pulmonary artery pressure, *PVR* pulmonary vascular resistance, *PCWP* pulmonary capillary wedge pressure, *6MWD* 6-min walk distance, *VO2* peak volume of oxygen consumption, *TAPSE* tricuspid annual plane excursion, *RVEF* right ventricular ejection fraction, *iPAH* idiopathic pulmonary arterial hypertension, *WHO* World Health Organization, *CMR* cardiac magnetic resonance, *PH* pulmonary hypertension, *NYHA* New York Heart Association, *PDE-Vi* phosphodiesterase-type 5 inhibitor, *ACE-I* angiotensin converting enzyme inhibitor, *N-BNP* N-terminal brain natriuretic peptide, *PET* positron emission tomography, *QOL* quality of life, *mo* month, *wk* week, *yr* year. Reproduced with permission from Maron et al. [82]

teins (BMP)-2 and BMP-7, which are factors implicated in the proliferative and vasoconstrictive pathophenotype of PAH, and, thus, identifies hormonal regulation of PAH-associated proteins as a potential mechanistic underpinning of adverse pulmonary vascular remodeling. Findings from our laboratory [41] (Abstract) are in concert with this principle by suggesting that aldosterone also upregulates the protein kinase mammalian target of rapamycin (mTOR), which is known to stimulate apoptosis-resistance and dysregulated cell growth patterns in PASMCs in iPAH patients [42].

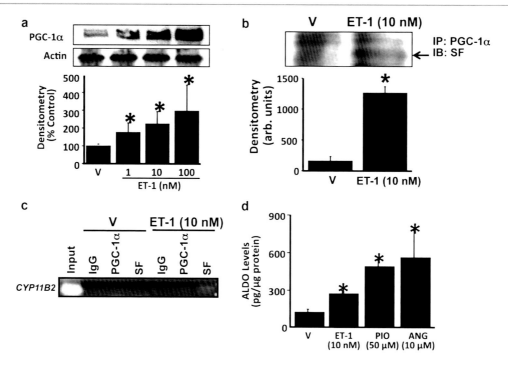

Fig. 9.1 Endothelin-1 (*ET-1*) stimulates PGC-1α-dependent association of steroidogenesis factor (*SF*) with *CYP11B2* to increase aldosterone levels. (**a**) The effect of ET-1 on PGC-1α expression was assessed by Western analysis (n = 4). (**b**) Co-immunoprecipitation experiments demonstrated that incubation of human pulmonary artery endothelial cells with ET-1 (10 nM) for 24 h induced the association of PGC-1α with steroidogenesis factor-1 (*SF*) (n = 3). (**c**) Chromatin immunoprecipitation (n = 3) of cell lysates using antibodies to PGC-1α, SF, and immunoglobulin-G (*IgG*) as a negative control was followed by PCR amplification of the proximal region of the *CYP11B2* (aldosterone synthase) promoter region containing the gonadotrope-specific element. (**d**) The functional effect of PGC-1α stimulation on aldosterone production was assessed in cells treated with the selective PGC-1α agonist pioglitazone (50 μM) for 24 h (n = 4), or with ET-1 (10 nM) or angiotensin II (*ANG*) (10 μM) for 24 h as positive controls. *p < 0.05 vs. V. *PGC-1α* PPAR-γ co-activator-1α; *arb. units* arbitrary units, *IP* immunoprecipitation, *IB* immunoblot (Data are presented as mean ± S.E.M. Representative blots are shown. *Reproduced with permission from* Maron et al. [37])

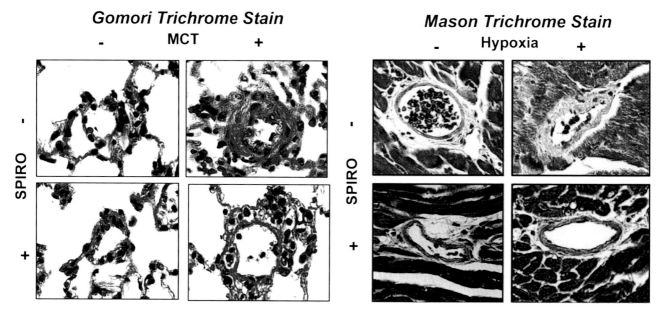

Fig. 9.2 Pharmacological inhibition of aldosterone with spironolactone abrogates maladaptive cardiovascular fibrosis in experimental pulmonary arterial hypertension (PAH) *in vivo*. (**a**) Pulmonary arterioles harvested from controls or rats with monocrotaline-PAH treated with vehicle or spironolactone in the drinking water (25 mg/kg/d) was subjected to Gomori trichrome staining to assess differences in pulmonary vascular collagen deposition (N = 4–6 rats/condition) (*Adapted with permission from* Maron et al. [37]). (**b**) Mice exposed to normoxia or hypoxia were treated with vehicle or spironolactone (15 mg/kg/d) and right ventricular sections were stained with mason trichrome for collagen assessment (N = 8–10 mice/condition) (*Adapted with permission from* Preston et al. [39])

Fig. 9.3 Crossroads of estradiol metabolism in PAH. Activities of 2-hydroxylation, 16alpha-hydroxylation, and 17beta-HSD pathways may determine the overall biological effects of estradiol in PAH. *COMT* Catechol-O-methyltransferase, *HSD* hydroxysteroid dehydrogenase (*Reproduced with permission from* Austin et al. [46])

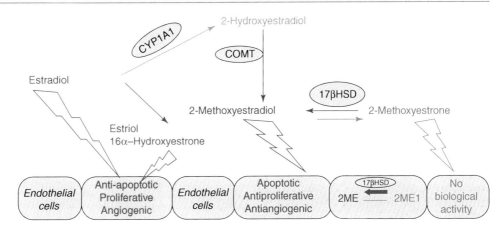

The Fibrosis Pathophenotype of PAH and Aldosterone

Pulmonary vascular and RV fibrosis is a critical component of the cardiopulmonary remodeling pattern in PAH and, when present, is an end-stage finding associated with increased mortality [43]. Activation of transforming growth factor-β (TGF-β) signaling by aldosterone promotes collagen deposition in pulmonary vascular, cardiovascular, and various non-vascular tissue beds [44]. Likewise, TGF-β is a master regulator of lung and pulmonary vascular fibrosis, and is implicated in the development of pulmonary hypertension in PAH patients [45]. Aldosterone increases levels of the profibrotic CCN (acronym for Connective tissue growth factor [CTGF], Cysteine rich protein, Nephroblastoma) protein and TGF-β target CTGF, in specific, to upregulate collagen deposition and the matrix remodeling proteins MMP-2 and MMP-9 in cultured human PAECs (Fig. 9.3). In turn, these changes are associated with fibrillar collagen deposition in pulmonary arterioles and frank RV replacement fibrosis in PAH *in vivo* (Fig. 9.2) [37, 39]. Aldosterone may also exert these pathogenic effects on cardiopulmonary tissue through alternative fibrotic signaling pathways involving mineralocorticoid receptor stimulation, including activation of reactive oxygen species generating enzymes, NF-κB, and VCAM-1 [47, 48], among others.

Aldosterone Inhibition: A Novel Pharmacotherapeutic Target in PAH

The potential therapeutic role of aldosterone antagonism has been evaluated extensively in experimental animal models of PAH *in vivo*. Work from our laboratory demonstrated that in MCT-PAH rats, spironolactone (25 mg/kg/d) treatment administered using a disease prevention model increased pulmonary artery acceleration time (14.1 ± 1.2 versus 22.3 ± 2.2 ms, $P < 0.005$, n=6) and decreased

pulmonary artery systolic pressure (89.3 ± 5.2 versus 69.5 ± 5.4 mmHg, $P < 0.01$, n=6), RV free-wall thickness (1.07 ± 0.05 versus 0.86 ± 0.03 mm, $P < 0.03$, n=6) and RV weight (0.43 ± 0.07 versus 0.35 ± 0.04 RV weight/LV septum weight, $P = 0.22$, n=5) compared to vehicle-treated rats. These hemodynamic changes were directionally similar to findings observed in SU-Hypox-PAH rats treated with the selective mineralocorticoid receptor antagonist eplerenone (0.4 mg/g chow) at a time point following evidence of pulmonary vascular injury. In a disease prevention drug treatment protocol, eplerenone decreased pulmonary hypertension severity in SU-Hypox-PAH and improved cardiac index (72.6 ± 41.5 vs. 119 ± 40.1 ml/min/g, $P = 0.1$, N=5–6) and indexed pulmonary vascular resistance (46.2 ± 12.9 vs. 15.4 ± 3.6 mmHg/min/[g/ml], $P < 0.05$, n=5–6) compared to SU-Hypox-PAH rats treated with vehicle control. Preston and colleagues also demonstrated that daily treatment with spironolactone (40 mg/kg/d) initiated at the time of chronic hypoxia exposure decreased the number of musclarized pulmonary arterioles to improve right ventricular systolic pressure and mice significantly [37, 39].

Despite these observations plus long-standing availability of mineralocorticoid therapies, well-established safety profile of this drug class, and proven benefits of aldosterone inhibition in other forms of cardiovascular disease, the efficacy of this pharmacotherapy in PAH is limited to case reports or small observational studies series [49].

Owing to data identifying aldosterone-induced oxidation of the ET_B receptor as a potential treatment target to improve pulmonary vascular function PAH, we performed a retrospective analysis of the Pulmonary Arterial Hypertension, Randomized Double-Blind, Placebo-Controlled, Multicenter, Efficacy Study 1 (ARIES-1) and Study 2 (ARIES-2) trial [50] to test the hypothesis that coupling therapies that inhibit endothelin type-A (ET_A) receptor-mediated pulmonary vasoconstriction with spironolactone to improve ET_B signaling is a useful strategy to treat PAH [30].

We observed that among the entire study cohort, 15 % (mean dose 31.2 mg/d) of patients reported spironolactone use. From 67 patients randomized to receive ambrisentan (10 mg/d), concurrent spironolactone use was identified in 10 patients. Compared to ambrisentan alone (N = 57), therapy with ambrisentan plus spironolactone improved change from baseline at 12 weeks in 6-MWD (mean ± SE, +38.2 ± 8.1 vs. +74.2 ± 27.4 m, p = 0.11), decreased plasma brain natriuretic peptide levels by 1.7-fold (P = 0.08), and improved in functional class (P = 0.08). Furthermore, whereas progressive illness, PAH-associated hospitalizations or death occurred as an end-point for 5.3 % of patients treated with ambrisentan alone, no patients in the ambrisentan + spironolactone group achieved any of these end-points. These findings provide preliminary data in support of a recently announced multi-center, prospective, randomized clinical trial testing the effect of spironolactone (50 mg/d) vs. placebo on cardiopulmonary fitness (combined primary end-point of change from baseline in peak volume of oxygen consumption [VO_2] and 6-min walk distance) in ambrisentan-treated patients (NCT 02253394). In this regard, a number of other prospective clinical trials have been proposed to test the effects of mineralocorticoid receptor antagonism on outcome in PAH (NCT01468571; NCT01712620) (Table 9.2).

The Renin-Angiotensin System (RAS) in PAH

Lung tissue has long been recognized as a rich source of angiotensin converting enzyme (ACE), although RAS inhibition in the treatment of PAH is controversial. Findings from small clinical trials performed in the era prior to the availability of PAH-specific therapy linked systemic hypotension to ACE-inhibitor (ACE-I) use despite noted improvements to cardiopulmonary hemodynamics and RV structure [51]. However, a resurgence of interest in RAS as a modifiable contributor to PAH in patients has emerged in tandem with improved understanding of angiotensin vascular biology [52] and contemporary strategies for early PAH diagnosis in advance of systemic hypotension [53].

Seminal observations reported over 2 decades ago determined that ACE-I attenuated hypoxic pulmonary vasoconstriction and the attendant pathological changes to RV function by decreasing levels of angiotensin II directly rather than altering levels of angiotensin-II-associated vasoactive factors, such as via bradykinin metabolism [54]. In pulmonary hypertensive mice exposed to chronic hypoxia, increased anti-angiotensin II immunohistochemical staining is evident in the pulmonary blood vessel wall despite a decrease in levels in whole lung, and ACE-I decreases PASMC proliferation and concentric thickening of pulmonary arterioles [55]. It has been proposed that angiotensin II promotes adverse pulmonary vascular remodeling, in part, by upregulating hypoxia

inducible factor-1α (HIF-1α), increasing vascular reactive oxygen species formation [56], and inducing cell cycle arrest through a mechanism involving activation of the G1 phase cyclin-dependent kinase p27 (Kip1), which is an inhibitor of G1 phase cyclin-dependent kinase [56].

Recently, de Man and colleagues [57] noted that both PASMCs and PAECs from PAH patients express increased levels of ACE and the angiotensin-II receptor type 1 (AT1R), which mediates angiotensin-II-dependent pulmonary vasoconstriction. The functional importance of AT1R to PAH was confirmed by experiments demonstrating that the selective AT1R inhibitor losartan delayed progression of pulmonary hypertension and improved RV-pulmonary arterial coupling in monocrotaline-PAH rats *in vivo*. In light of earlier observations suggesting potential harm by ACE-I in PAH, the authors postulate that selective AT-1R antagonists may be more appropriate than ACE-I in this patient population owing to a comparatively lower risk of systemic hypotension.

Additional Angiotensin Peptides and PAH Pathobiology

The true complexity of RAS signaling is increasingly evident through the identification of vasoactive angiotensin I derivatives: angiotensin- (1–9) and angiotensin- (1–7), and angiotensin-(1–5), as well as the angiotensin-(1–7) receptor, Mas [58]. In contrast to classical angiotensin-II-AT-1 signaling, upregulation of angiotensin-(1–7) exerts anti-hypertrophic, anti-fibrotic, and vasodilatory effects on LV cardiomyocytes and systemic blood vessels, leading to speculation that ACE-2, which converts angiotensin-I to angiotensin-(1–7), may represent a potential therapeutic target in PAH. Lung and RV tissue express increased ACE-2 levels in experimental PAH [59] and administration of recombinant human ACE-2 to mice with pulmonary artery banding-PAH decreases RV hypertrophy, RV end-diastolic pressure and RV diastolic time [60]. While these effects do not appear contingent on changes to RV fibrosis content, ACE-2 treatment normalizes expression of connexin 37, which regulates myocardial contractility. Targeting ACE-2/Mas in the pulmonary vasculature has also been demonstrated to decrease arteriole muscularization and pulmonary hypertension severity in monocrotlaine-PAH [61, 62], although little data are currently available with respect to the relevance of this signaling pathway, other angiotensin derivatives, or renin *per se* to patients with PAH.

Sex Hormones and PAH: Unraveling the Estrogen Paradox

Among the earliest epidemiologic trends described in PAH was a disparity in disease prevalence favoring women to men, ultimately determined via registry analyses to be ~2.0–2.5:1, with females accounting for up to 70 % of incident cases [63]. Despite this, however, there are compelling large-scale population science data indicating that PAH is more severe and associated with a less favorable prognosis in men compared to women [64]. For example, a recent meta-analysis of baseline hemodynamics from 11 randomized clinical trials (N = 1,211) demonstrated that compared to women, cardiac index was lower by −0.14 L/min/m^2 (95 % confidence interval [CI] −0.23–0.04, p = 0.01) and PVR was higher by 1.23 Wood units (95 % CI, 0.18–2.27, p = 0.02) in men [65]. The hormonal profile of women relative to men, particularly with respect to estrogen, estrogen derivatives, and androgens, has therefore served as the chief biological focus of efforts that aim to account for these collective differences. The juxtaposition of increased PAH prevalence *and* probability of survival in women is often referred to as the "estrogen paradox." [46]

Estrogen Metabolism and PAH

The possibility that sex differences in PAH pathobiology is linked to estrogen metabolism has been studied previously. Data from Affymetrix® dChip array analyses of lymphocytes isolated from patients with PAH occurring due to an inactivating mutation in the gene encoding for BMPR-2, which is the most well-studied monogenetic pulmonary vascular disease, indicated important differences in estrogen metabolites [66]. Findings from this seminal work identified that expression levels of the estrogen-metabolizing enzyme CYP1B1 were ~10-fold lower in BMPR-2-PAH patients compared to controls, while no differences were observed between female and male PAH patients. Subsequent observations from a nested case-control study associated the CYP1B1 Asn453Ser genotype with overproduction of 16α-hydroxyoestrone that is a potent stimulator of estrogen receptor-dependent proliferation in PASMCs [67].

White and colleagues subsequently determined that CYP1B1 and 16α-hydroxyoestrone levels are increased in remodeled pulmonary arterioles from mice with hypoxia- and Sugen-5416/hypoxia-PAH, as well as PAH patients. In genetically engineered CYP1B1$^{-/-}$ mice exposed to hypoxia, as well as hypoxia- or Sugen-5416/hypoxia-PAH mice treated with the CYP1B1 inhibitor 2,3′,4,5′-tetramethoxystilbene (TMS), pulmonary vascular remodeling, RV hypertrophy, and cardiopulmonary hemodynamics were improved significantly compared to wild type or untreated animals [68]. Dexfenfluramine-induced upregulation of tryptophan hydroxylase, which is the rate-limiting enzyme in the synthesis of serotonin also promotes CYP1B1-mediated PASMC proliferation in pulmonary hypertensive mice [69], and, thus, it is interesting to speculate that CYP1B1 upregulation by serotonin may provide mechanistic insights regarding the link between dexfenfluramine use and annorexigen-PAH.

In contrast to 16α-hydroxyoestrone, the non-estrogenic metabolites of estrogen, 2-methoxyestradiol (2-ME) and 2-hydroxyestrogen (2-OHE), appear to exert anti-inflammatory and anti-fibrotic properties in pulmonary vascular cells and cardiomyocytes from monocrotaline-PAH rats (Fig. 9.3) [70]. Although this effect is hypothesized to involve 2-ME-induced suppression of epidermal growth factor (EGF)-dependent growth and migration of vascular endothelial cells [71], the precise mechanism(s) underpinning the effect of these estrogen derivatives on pulmonary vascular function, the generalizability of these findings to other pulmonary vascular diseases, or the larger question of estrogen receptor involvement in PAH disease trajectory is unresolved.

Androgens and PAH

Dehydroepiandrosterone (DHEA) and the DHEA 3β-sulphate ester (DHEA-S) are vasoactive intermediates of the androgen biosynthesis pathway, and are the most abundant circulating hormones in humans [72]. The synthesis of DHEA requires the mitochondrial cholesterol side-chain cleavage enzyme (CYP11A1) that converts cholesterol to pregnenolone, and 17-α-hydroxylase and 17, 20 lyase (CYP17) that synthesizes DHEA from pregnenolone in the endoplasmic reticulum [72]. In vascular cells and cardiomyocytes DHEA is associated with a diverse range of biological effects including inhibition of Akt/Glycogen-synthase-kinase-3β and Src/STAT3 signaling that regulates proliferation and apoptosis in pulmonary vascular cells, respectively [73], and promotes soluble guanylyl cyclase-dependent pulmonary arterial relaxation through PKG-1α dimerization [74]. On the other hand, DHEA is a noncompetitive inhibitor of the anti-oxidant enzyme glucose-6-phosphate dehydrogenase, which, in turn, is linked to increased reactive oxygen species generation that is detrimental to vascular endothelial and smooth muscle cells, among other cell lines relevant to pulmonary vascular disease [75, 76]. This association notwithstanding, the observation that DHEA regulates large conductance Ca^{2+}-activated channels and voltage-gated K$^+$ channels that mediate cellular contractile status in PASMCs due to hypoxia prompted further investigations to determine if DHEA is therapeutically relevant in PAH [77].

The administration of DHEA prevents pulmonary vascular remodeling, RV dysfunction and pulmonary hypertension in rats exposed to chronic hypoxia, while acute drug administration is a potent stimulator of pulmonary vasodilation [78]. It is hypothesized that perturbation to the redox status of vascular cells toward oxidation by DHEA is sufficient to stimulate repolarization of Ca^{2+}-activated channels and voltage-gated K$^+$ channels that ultimately improves pulmonary vascular tone [79]. Alternatively, DHEA is also linked to improved cardiopulmonary performance via diminished activity of the anti-apoptotic kinase RhoA/Rho kinase (ROCK) [80] in the pulmonary vasculature, as well as decreased reactive oxygen species accumulation in RV cardiomyocytes in various hypoxic models of PAH. Evidence in support of a therapeutic benefit by DHEA in patients, however, is limited at this time to a single small pilot study indicating some clinical benefit in selected chronic obstructive pulmonary disease patients [81].

Conclusions

Evidence from numerous lines of research implicates neurohumoral and hormonal involvement in the pathobiology of pulmonary vascular disease. In particular, sound mechanistic data are available associating β/α-adrenergic receptor stimulation, angiotensin II aldosterone, estrogen metabolite 16α-hydroxyoestrone and the androgen derivative DHEA to the development of cornerstone pulmonary vascular and RV histopathophenotypic changes observed in experimental models of PAH and in PAH patients. Enhanced insight into the potential therapeutic benefits of targeting these factors in PAH is anticipated through the completion of several ongoing clinical trials.

References

1. Forfia PR, Fisher MR, Mathai SC, Housten-Harris T, Hemnes AR, Borlaug BA, et al. Tricuspid annular displacement predicts survival in pulmonary hypertension. Am J Respir Crit Care Med. 2006; 174(9):1034–41.
2. Mehra MR, Park MH, Landzberg MJ, Lala A, Waxman AB. Right heart failure: toward a common language. J Heart Lung Transplant. 2014;33(2):123–6.
3. Wang GY, McCloskey DT, Turcato S, Swigart PM, Simpson PC, Baker AJ. Contrasting inotropic responses to alpha1-adrenergic receptor stimulation in left versus right ventricular myocardium. Am J Physiol Heart Circ Physiol. 2006;291(4):H2013–7.
4. Rudner XL, Berkowitz DE, Booth JV, Funk BL, Cozart KL, D'Amico EB, et al. Subtype specific regulation of human vascular alpha(1)-adrenergic receptors by vessel bed and age. Circulation. 1999;100(23):2336–43.
5. Cavallotti C, Mancone M, Bruzzone P, Sabbatini M, Mignini F. Dopamine receptor subtypes in the native human heart. Heart Vessels. 2010;25(5):432–7.
6. Barnes PJ, Liu SF. Regulation of pulmonary vascular tone. Pharmacol Rev. 1995;47(1):87–131.
7. Chen SL, Zhang YJ, Zhou L, Xie DJ, Zhang FF, Jia HB, et al. Percutaneous pulmonary artery denervation completely abolishes experimental pulmonary arterial hypertension in vivo. EuroIntervention. 2013;9(2):269–76.
8. Chen SL, Zhang FF, Xu J, Xie DJ, Zhou L, Nguyen T, et al. Pulmonary artery denervation to treat pulmonary arterial hypertension: the single-center, prospective, first-in-man PADN-1 study (first-in-man pulmonary artery denervation for treatment of pulmonary artery hypertension). J Am Coll Cardiol. 2013;62(12):1092–100.
9. Nagaya N, Nishikimi T, Uematsu M, Satoh T, Kyotani S, Sakamaki F, et al. Plasma brain natriuretic peptide as a prognostic indicator in patients with primary pulmonary hypertension. Circulation. 2000;102(8):865–70.
10. Nootens M, Kaufmann E, Rector T, Toher C, Judd D, Francis GS, et al. Neurohormonal activation in patients with right ventricular failure from pulmonary hypertension: relation to hemodynamic variables and endothelin levels. J Am Coll Cardiol. 1995;26(7): 1581–5.
11. Velez-Roa S, Ciarka A, Najem B, Vachiery JL, Naeije R, van de Borne P. Increased sympathetic nerve activity in pulmonary artery hypertension. Circulation. 2004;110(10):1308–12.
12. Leblais V, Delannoy E, Fresquet F, Begueret H, Bellance N, Banquet S, et al. beta-adrenergic relaxation in pulmonary arteries: preservation of the endothelial nitric oxide-dependent beta2 component in pulmonary hypertension. Cardiovasc Res. 2008;77(1): 202 10.
13. Kim GH, Ryan JJ, Archer SL. The role of redox signaling in epigenetics and cardiovascular disease. Antioxid Redox Signal. 2013;18(15):1920–36.
14. Chakraborti S, Roy S, Chowdhury A, Mandal A, Chakraborti T. Role of PKCalpha-p38 MAPK-Gialpha axis in peroxynitrite-mediated inhibition of beta-adrenergic response in pulmonary artery smooth muscle cells. Cell Signal. 2013;25(2):512–26.
15. Faber JE, Szymeczek CL, Salvi SS, Zhang H. Enhanced alpha1-adrenergic trophic activity in pulmonary artery of hypoxic pulmonary hypertensive rats. Am J Physiol Heart Circ Physiol. 2006; 291(5):H2272–81.
16. Hool LC, Oleksa LM, Harvey RD. Role of G proteins in alpha1-adrenergic inhibition of the beta-adrenergically activated chloride current in cardiac myocytes. Mol Pharmacol. 1997;51(5):853–60.
17. Piao L, Fang YH, Parikh KS, Ryan JJ, D'Souza KM, Theccanat T, et al. GRK2-mediated inhibition of adrenergic and dopaminergic signaling in right ventricular hypertrophy: therapeutic implications in pulmonary hypertension. Circulation. 2012;126(24):2859–69.
18. Bristow MR, Minobe W, Rasmussen R, Larrabee P, Skerl L, Klein JW, et al. Beta-adrenergic neuroeffector abnormalities in the failing human heart are produced by local rather than systemic mechanisms. J Clin Invest. 1992;89(3):803–15.
19. Ungerer M, Bohm M, Elce JS, Erdmann E, Lohse MJ. Altered expression of beta-adrenergic receptor kinase and beta 1-adrenergic receptors in the failing human heart. Circulation. 1993;87(2): 454–63.
20. Leineweber K, Brandt K, Wludyka B, Beilfuss A, Ponicke K, Heinroth-Hoffmann I, et al. Ventricular hypertrophy plus neurohumoral activation is necessary to alter the cardiac beta-adrenoceptor system in experimental heart failure. Circ Res. 2002;91(11):1056–62.
21. Bogaard HJ, Natarajan R, Mizuno S, Abbate A, Chang PJ, Chau VQ, et al. Adrenergic receptor blockade reverses right heart remodeling and dysfunction in pulmonary hypertensive rats. Am J Respir Crit Care Med. 2010;182(5):652–60.
22. de Man FS, Handoko ML, van Ballegoij JJ, Schalij I, Bogaards SJ, Postmus PE, et al. Bisoprolol delays progression towards right heart failure in experimental pulmonary hypertension. Circ Heart Fail. 2012;5(1):97–105.
23. Voelkel NF, McMurtry IF, Reeves JT. Chronic propranolol treatment blunts right ventricular hypertrophy in rats at high altitude. J Appl Physiol Respir Environ Exerc Physiol. 1980;48(3):473–8.
24. Madden KS, Szpunar MJ, Brown EB. beta-Adrenergic receptors (beta-AR) regulate VEGF and IL-6 production by divergent pathways in high beta-AR-expressing breast cancer cell lines. Breast Cancer Res Treat. 2012;130(3):747–58.
25. Hadri L, Kratlian RG, Benard L, Maron BA, Dorfmuller P, Ladage D, et al. Therapeutic efficacy of AAV1.SERCA2a in monocrotaline-induced pulmonary arterial hypertension. Circulation. 2013;128(5): 512–23.
26. Provencher S, Herve P, Jais X, Lebrec D, Humbert M, Simonneau G, et al. Deleterious effects of beta-blockers on exercise capacity

and hemodynamics in patients with portopulmonary hypertension. Gastroenterology. 2006;130(1):120–6.

27. Peacock A, Ross K. Pulmonary hypertension: a contraindication to the use of {beta}-adrenoceptor blocking agents. Thorax. 2010; 65(5):454–5.

28. Gomberg-Maitland M, Bull TM, Saggar R, Barst RJ, Elgazayerly A, Fleming TR, et al. New trial designs and potential therapies for pulmonary artery hypertension. J Am Coll Cardiol. 2013;62(25 Suppl):D82–91.

29. Aguero J, Ishikawa K, Hadri L, Santos-Gallego C, Fish K, Hammoudi N, et al. Characterization of right ventricular remodeling and failure in a chronic pulmonary hypertension model. Am J Physiol Heart Circ Physiol. 2014;307(8):H1204–15.

30. Maron BA, Opotowsky AR, Landzberg MJ, Loscalzo J, Waxman AB, Leopold JA. Plasma aldosterone levels are elevated in patients with pulmonary arterial hypertension in the absence of left ventricular heart failure: a pilot study. Eur J Heart Fail. 2013;15(3):277–83.

31. Heinemann HO, Ryan JW, Ryan US. Is the lung a para-endocrine organ? Am J Med. 1977;63(4):595–603.

32. Wenz M, Steinau R, Gerlach H, Lange M, Kaczmarczyk G. Inhaled nitric oxide does not change transpulmonary angiotensin II formation in patients with acute respiratory distress syndrome. Chest. 1997;112(2):478–83.

33. Wilkens H, Bauer M, Forestier N, Konig J, Eichler A, Schneider S, et al. Influence of inhaled iloprost on transpulmonary gradient of big endothelin in patients with pulmonary hypertension. Circulation. 2003;107(11):1509–13.

34. Peacock AJ, Matthews A. Transpulmonary angiotensin II formation and pulmonary haemodynamics in stable hypoxic lung disease: the effect of captopril. Respir Med. 1992;86(1):21–6.

35. Takeda Y, Miyamori I, Yoneda T, Hatakeyama H, Inaba S, Furukawa K, et al. Regulation of aldosterone synthase in human vascular endothelial cells by angiotensin II and adrenocorticotropin. J Clin Endocrinol Metab. 1996;81(8):2797–800.

36. Young MJ, Clyne CD, Cole TJ, Funder JW. Cardiac steroidogenesis in the normal and failing heart. J Clin Endocrinol Metab. 2001; 86(11):5121–6.

37. Maron BA, Zhang YY, White K, Chan SY, Handy DE, Mahoney CE, et al. Aldosterone inactivates the endothelin-B receptor via a cysteinyl thiol redox switch to decrease pulmonary endothelial nitric oxide levels and modulate pulmonary arterial hypertension. Circulation. 2012;126(8):963–74.

38. Farquharson CA, Struthers AD. Aldosterone induces acute endothelial dysfunction in vivo in humans: evidence for an aldosterone-induced vasculopathy. Clin Sci (Lond). 2002;103(4):425–31.

39. Preston IR, Sagliani KD, Warburton RR, Hill NS, Fanburg BL, Jaffe IZ. Mineralocorticoid receptor antagonism attenuates experimental pulmonary hypertension. Am J Physiol Lung Cell Mol Physiol. 2012;304(10):L678–88.

40. Yamanaka R, Otsuka F, Nakamura K, Yamashita M, Otani H, Takeda M, et al. Involvement of the bone morphogenetic protein system in endothelin- and aldosterone-induced cell proliferation of pulmonary arterial smooth muscle cells isolated from human patients with pulmonary arterial hypertension. Hypertens Res. 2010;33(5):435–45.

41. Aghamohammedzadeh R, Heagerty A, Loscalzo J, Maron BA, Leopold JA, editors. Raptor activation by aldoseterone promotes apoptosis resistance in pulmonary artery smooth muscle cells to modulate adverse pulmonary vascular remodeling in pulmonary arterial hypertension (abstract). 2013 Federation of American Societies for Experimental Biology National Meeting. Boston; 2013.

42. Goncharov DA, Kudryashova TV, Ziai H, Ihida-Stansbury K, DeLisser H, Krymskaya VP, et al. Mammalian target of rapamycin complex 2 (mTORC2) coordinates pulmonary artery smooth muscle cell metabolism, proliferation, and survival in pulmonary arterial hypertension. Circulation. 2014;129(8):864–74.

43. Carlsen J, Hasseriis Andersen K, Boesgaard S, Iversen M, Steinbruchel D, Bogelund Andersen C. Pulmonary arterial lesions in explanted lungs after transplantation correlate with severity of pulmonary hypertension in chronic obstructive pulmonary disease. J Heart Lung Transplant. 2013;32(3):347–54.

44. Weber KT, Sun Y, Bhattacharya SK, Ahokas RA, Gerling IC. Myofibroblast-mediated mechanisms of pathological remodelling of the heart. Nat Rev Cardiol. 2013;10(1):15–26.

45. Graham BB, Chabon J, Gebreab L, Poole J, Debella E, Davis L, et al. Transforming growth factor-beta signaling promotes pulmonary hypertension caused by Schistosoma mansoni. Circulation. 2013;128(12):1354–64.

46. Austin ED, Lahm T, West J, Tofovic SP, Johansen AK, Maclean MR, et al. Gender, sex hormones and pulmonary hypertension. Pulm Circ. 2013;3(2):294–314.

47. Brown NJ. Contribution of aldosterone to cardiovascular and renal inflammation and fibrosis. Nat Rev Nephrol. 2013;9(8):459–69.

48. Caprio M, Newfell BG, la Sala A, Baur W, Fabbri A, Rosano G, et al. Functional mineralocorticoid receptors in human vascular endothelial cells regulate intercellular adhesion molecule-1 expression and promote leukocyte adhesion. Circ Res. 2008;102(11):1359–67.

49. Kokubu T, Kazatani Y, Hamada M, Matsuzaki K, Ito T, Nishimura K, et al. Is captopril effective in primary pulmonary hypertension? Jpn Circ J. 1982;46(10):1095–7.

50. Maron BA, Waxman AB, Opotowsky AR, Gillies H, Blair C, Aghamohammadzadeh R, et al. Effectiveness of spironolactone plus ambrisentan for treatment of pulmonary arterial hypertension (from the [ARIES] study 1 and 2 trials). Am J Cardiol. 2013;112(5):720–5.

51. Bertoli L, Fusco M, Lo Cicero S, Micallef E, Busnardo I. Influence of ACE inhibition on pulmonary haemodynamics and function in patients in whom beta-blockers are contraindicated. Postgrad Med J. 1986;62 Suppl 1:47–51.

52. Bader M. ACE2, angiotensin-(1–7), and Mas: the other side of the coin. Pflugers Arch. 2013;465(1):79–85.

53. Hoeper MM, Bogaard HJ, Condliffe R, Frantz R, Khanna D, Kurzyna M, et al. Definitions and diagnosis of pulmonary hypertension. J Am Coll Cardiol. 2013;62 Suppl):D42–50.

54. Morrell NW, Morris KG, Stenmark KR. Role of angiotensin-converting enzyme and angiotensin II in development of hypoxic pulmonary hypertension. Am J Physiol. 1995;269(4 Pt 2):H1186–94.

55. Morrell NW, Atochina EN, Morris KG, Danilov SM, Stenmark KR. Angiotensin converting enzyme expression is increased in small pulmonary arteries of rats with hypoxia-induced pulmonary hypertension. J Clin Invest. 1995;96(4):1823–33.

56. Wolf G. Role of reactive oxygen species in angiotensin II-mediated renal growth, differentiation, and apoptosis. Antioxid Redox Signal. 2005;7(9–10):1337–45.

57. de Man FS, Tu L, Handoko ML, Rain S, Ruiter G, Francois C, et al. Dysregulated renin-angiotensin-aldosterone system contributes to pulmonary arterial hypertension. Am J Respir Crit Care Med. 2012;186(8):780–9.

58. Zhang R, Wu Y, Zhao M, Liu C, Zhou L, Shen S, et al. Role of HIF-1alpha in the regulation ACE and ACE2 expression in hypoxic human pulmonary artery smooth muscle cells. Am J Physiol Lung Cell Mol Physiol. 2009;297(4):L631–40.

59. Johnson JA, West J, Maynard KB, Hemnes AR. ACE2 improves right ventricular function in a pressure overload model. PLoS One. 2011;6(6):e20828.

60. Yamazato Y, Ferreira AJ, Hong KH, Sriramula S, Francis J, Yamazato M, et al. Prevention of pulmonary hypertension by Angiotensin-converting enzyme 2 gene transfer. Hypertension. 2009;54(2):365–71.

61. Ferreira AJ, Shenoy V, Yamazato Y, Sriramula S, Francis J, Yuan L, et al. Evidence for angiotensin-converting enzyme 2 as a therapeutic target for the prevention of pulmonary hypertension. Am J Respir Crit Care Med. 2009;179(11):1048–54.

62. Ling Y, Johnson MK, Kiely DG, Condliffe R, Elliot CA, Gibbs JS, et al. Changing demographics, epidemiology, and survival of incident pulmonary arterial hypertension: results from the pulmonary hypertension registry of the United Kingdom and Ireland. Am J Respir Crit Care Med. 2012;186(8):790–6.

63. Humbert M, Sitbon O, Chaouat A, Bertocchi M, Habib G, Gressin V, et al. Survival in patients with idiopathic, familial, and anorexigen-associated pulmonary arterial hypertension in the modern management era. Circulation. 2012;122(2):156–63.

64. Benza RL, Miller DP, Gomberg-Maitland M, Frantz RP, Foreman AJ, Coffey CS, et al. Predicting survival in pulmonary arterial hypertension: insights from the Registry to Evaluate Early and Long-Term Pulmonary Arterial Hypertension Disease Management (REVEAL). Circulation. 2012;122(2):164–72.

65. Ventetuolo CE, Praestgaard A, Palevsky HI, Klinger JR, Halpern SD, Kawut SM. Sex and haemodynamics in pulmonary arterial hypertension. Eur Respir J. 2014;43(2):523–30.

66. West J, Cogan J, Geraci M, Robinson L, Newman J, Phillips JA, et al. Gene expression in BMPR2 mutation carriers with and without evidence of pulmonary arterial hypertension suggests pathways relevant to disease penetrance. BMC Med Genomics. 2008;1:45.

67. Austin ED, Cogan JD, West JD, Hedges LK, Hamid R, Dawson EP, et al. Alterations in oestrogen metabolism: implications for higher penetrance of familial pulmonary arterial hypertension in females. Eur Respir J. 2009;34(5):1093–9.

68. White K, Johansen AK, Nilsen M, Ciuclan L, Wallace E, Paton L, et al. Activity of the estrogen-metabolizing enzyme cytochrome P450 1B1 influences the development of pulmonary arterial hypertension. Circulation. 2012;126(9):1087–98.

69. Shang W, Konidari I, Schomberg DW. 2-Methoxyestradiol, an endogenous estradiol metabolite, differentially inhibits granulosa and endothelial cell mitosis: a potential follicular antiangiogenic regulator. Biol Reprod. 2001;65(2):622–7.

70. Dempsie Y, MacRitchie NA, White K, Morecroft I, Wright AF, Nilsen M, et al. Dexfenfluramine and the oestrogen-metabolizing enzyme CYP1B1 in the development of pulmonary arterial hypertension. Cardiovasc Res. 2013;99(1):24–34.

71. Tofovic SP, Zhang X, Zhu H, Jackson EK, Rafikova O, Petrusevska G. 2-Ethoxyestradiol is antimitogenic and attenuates monocrotaline-induced pulmonary hypertension and vascular remodeling. Vascul Pharmacol. 2008;48(4–6):174–83.

72. Auchus RJ. Overview of dehydroepiandrosterone biosynthesis. Semin Reprod Med. 2004;22(4):281–8.

73. Paulin R, Meloche J, Jacob MH, Bisserier M, Courboulin A, Bonnet S. Dehydroepiandrosterone inhibits the Src/STAT3 constitutive activation in pulmonary arterial hypertension. Am J Physiol Heart Circ Physiol. 2011;301(5):H1798–809.

74. Oka M, Karoor V, Homma N, Nagaoka T, Sakao E, Golembeski SM, et al. Dehydroepiandrosterone upregulates soluble guanylate cyclase and inhibits hypoxic pulmonary hypertension. Cardiovasc Res. 2007;74(3):377–87.

75. Leopold JA, Dam A, Maron BA, Scribner AW, Liao R, Handy DE, et al. Aldosterone impairs vascular reactivity by decreasing glucose-6-phosphate dehydrogenase activity. Nat Med. 2007;13(2):189–97.

76. Leopold JA, Loscalzo J. Cyclic strain modulates resistance to oxidant stress by increasing G6PDH expression in smooth muscle cells. Am J Physiol Heart Circ Physiol. 2000;279(5):H2477–85.

77. Bonnet S, Dumas-de-La-Roque E, Begueret H, Marthan R, Fayon M, Dos Santos P, et al. Dehydroepiandrosterone (DHEA) prevents and reverses chronic hypoxic pulmonary hypertension. Proc Natl Acad Sci U S A. 2003;100(16):9488–93.

78. Archer SL, Weir EK, Reeve HL, Michelakis E. Molecular identification of O2 sensors and O2-sensitive potassium channels in the pulmonary circulation. Adv Exp Med Biol. 2000;475:219–40.

79. Liu Y, Suzuki YJ, Day RM, Fanburg BL. Rho kinase-induced nuclear translocation of ERK1/ERK2 in smooth muscle cell mitogenesis caused by serotonin. Circ Res. 2004;95(6):579–86.

80. Dumas de La Roque E, Savineau JP, Metivier AC, Billes MA, Kraemer JP, Doutreleau S, et al. Dehydroepiandrosterone (DHEA) improves pulmonary hypertension in chronic obstructive pulmonary disease (COPD): a pilot study. Ann Endocrinol (Paris). 2012;73(1):20–5.

81. Alzoubi A, Toba M, Abe K, O'Neill KD, Rocic P, Fagan KA, et al. Dehydroepiandrosterone restores right ventricular structure and function in rats with severe pulmonary arterial hypertension. Am J Physiol Heart Circ Physiol. 2013;304(12):H1708–18.

82. Maron BA, Leopold JA. Emerging concepts in the molecular basis of pulmonary arterial hypertension: Part II: Neurohumoral signaling contributes to the pulmonary vascular and right ventricular pathophenotype of pulmonary arterial hypertension. Circulation 2015;131(23):2079–91.

Part III

Translational and Clinical Principles of Pulmonary Vascular Disease and Right Ventricular Dysfunction

Animal Models of Pulmonary Hypertension

Jose Gomez-Arroyo, Ivana Nikolic, and Paul B. Yu

Introduction

Animal models have been an essential tool for understanding pulmonary vascular disease, and for the development of usable therapies. Classic physiologic experiments such as those performed by von Euler and Liljestrand describing the paradoxical (vasoconstrictive) effect of hypoxia in the lung circulation of cats in 1946 [1], and subsequent efforts in large and small animals have helped to establish principles of pulmonary vascular physiology. More recently, the deployment of molecular biological tools and the use of genetically modified organisms in models designed to recapitulate different aspects of pulmonary vascular disease have helped to frame traditional concepts of pulmonary vascular physiology within contemporary concepts of cellular biology such as signaling, inflammation, and metabolism [2]. Human pulmonary vascular disease represents a heterogeneous spectrum of phenotypes and underlying etiologies. As in many diseases, there is no single animal model of pulmonary hypertension that entirely recapitulates a given human pulmonary hypertension phenotype in its entirety [3–6]. Here we review several of the most influential and widely used models of pulmonary arterial hypertension. We cover some of the practical as well as scientific advantages and disadvantages of each and ways in which these models are complementary in representing the phenotypic spectrum of clinical disease. This discussion will focus on models that have been designed to recapitulate aspects of PAH typically associated with World Health Organization Group I PAH, which includes disease that is idiopathic, heritable, or associated with toxin

exposure, connective tissue disease, liver disease, human immunodeficiency virus (HIV) infection, congenital heart disease, or schistosomiasis [7]. The classic models entail various combinations of exposure to hypoxia, toxin-mediated injury to the pulmonary vasculature, as well as the creation of systemic to pulmonary shunts. Newer models have utilized the blockade of vascular endothelial growth factor signaling. Finally, we discuss efforts to model schistosomiasis or HIV-infection associated PAH, most recently in non-human primates.

Monocrotaline-Injury Model

Along with chronic hypoxia, the pyrrolizidine alkaloid monocrotaline (MCT) has long been utilized to induce pulmonary hypertension [2]. When administered to rats, MCT induces reproducible pulmonary arterial hypertension and arteriolar remodeling as part of a syndrome that may sporadically express other features such as pulmonary fibrosis, hepatic venoclussive disease, myocarditis and acute lung injury [3]. Although the MCT model has been extensively characterized in the past 40 years, the precise molecular and cellular effects by which monocrotaline induces PAH remain elusive, but several mechanisms have been proposed. After being metabolized to its active form in the rat liver, MCT is metabolized to dehydro-monocrotaline, a.k.a., monocrotaline pyrrole (MCTP), a moderately reactive alkylating agent which appears to induce endothelial apoptosis [8, 9]. MCTP can induce endothelial cell damage by mechanisms that include disruption of intracellular membrane trafficking [10], deregulation of nitric oxide signaling [11] and dysregulation of bone morphogenetic protein receptor II (BMPRII) expression and downstream SMAD signaling [12], affecting a receptor and signaling axis implicated in the majority of heritable forms of PAH. Paradoxically, while MCT potently induces endothelial cell damage, the model is characterized mainly by smooth muscle cell proliferation and therefore vessel media thickening (Fig. 10.1) [3]. This paradox might be explained by the

J. Gomez-Arroyo, MD, PhD
Department of Anesthesiology and Critical Care Medicine,
Johns Hopkins University, Baltimore, MD, 21287, USA

I. Nikolic, MD • P.B. Yu, MD, PhD (✉)
Division of Cardiovascular Medicine, Department of Medicine,
Harvard Medical School, Brigham and Women's Hospital,
75 Francis Street, Boston, MA, 02115, USA
e-mail: pbyu@partners.org

© Springer International Publishing Switzerland 2016
B.A. Maron et al. (eds.), *Pulmonary Hypertension: Basic Science to Clinical Medicine*, DOI 10.1007/978-3-319-23594-3_10

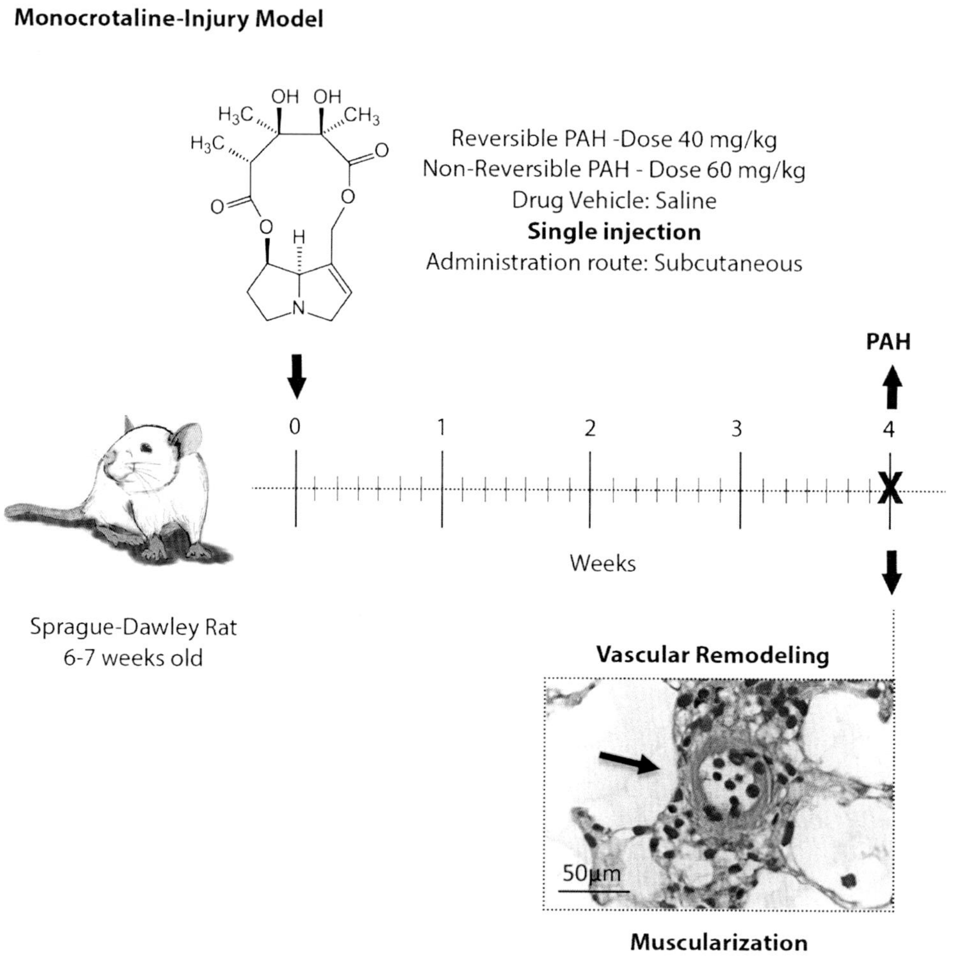

Fig. 10.1 Pulmonary arterial hypertension time-course and type of vascular remodeling pattern secondary to exposure to the monocrotraline pyrrole. A single subcutaneous injection of monocrotaline at a dose of 60 mg/kg causes non-reversible PAH associated with vascular remodeling mainly characterized by media muscularization. *Black arrow* shows time of injection. *X* marks time of tissue harvesting. Chemical structure of monocrotaline was obtained from Wikimedia Commons (Public domain) (Micrograph from lung vessel was modified with permission from Gomez-Arroyo et al. [3])

Monocrotaline-Injury Model

Reversible PAH -Dose 40 mg/kg
Non-Reversible PAH - Dose 60 mg/kg
Drug Vehicle: Saline
Single injection
Administration route: Subcutaneous

Sprague-Dawley Rat
6-7 weeks old

PAH

Weeks

Vascular Remodeling

50 μm

Muscularization

disruption of normally homeostatic effects of an intact intima upon the underlying media, abnormal paracrine effects between the injured endothelium and vascular smooth muscle cell layer, or direct toxic effects of MCTP on the media that are otherwise not yet elucidated [9, 13]. It is also notable that the development of pulmonary hypertension occurs with delayed kinetics following a single exposure to MCT: PAH typically occurs 3–4 weeks after MCT challenge, yet MCT and MCTP are metabolized rapidly and cleared from the circulation [14]. The phenotype may result from delayed effects of endothelial injury versus persistent effects of MCT that has accumulated in erythrocytes, where it conserves its capability to interact with lung tissue.

The MCT model offers great advantages against other models of PAH such as cost, accessibility, and reproducibility. The response to MCT is very dose sensitive, such that an injection of 40 mg/kg of MCT will yield modest PAH, whereas a single dose of 60 mg/kg will produce more severe PAH at 3 weeks, and significant mortality after 4–5 weeks [15]. Importantly, MCT induces PAH without the need for other exposures such as hypoxia, which requires the housing of animals in a nitrogen dilution chamber that might not readily available and, in turn, can be

costly to acquire and maintain. In addition, because chronic hypoxia is not required, the model can be readily characterized in a longitudinal fashion, allowing researchers to study the impact of mild to severely increased pulmonary afterload upon the development of right ventricular hypertrophy by a variety of invasive and non-invasive means [16, 17] as well as the impact upon exercise adaptation [18], for example. Similar to tissues obtained from human PAH, tissues from MCT-induced PAH exhibit exaggerated TGF-β signaling and pro-fibrotic transcriptional activity, and suppressed expression of BMPR2 and downstream BMP signaling activity [19]. Based on this molecular signature, as well as histology, the MCT model has been suggested to be particularly helpful for highlighting the contributions of fibrosis, inflammation, and lung injury in pulmonary vascular disease [3], a notion that is supported by the observation that numerous experimental and approved therapies with potential anti-fibrotic and anti-inflammatory effects have demonstrated efficacy in the MCT model [19–24]. Because MCT pro-toxin requires metabolism by the liver the generate an active metabolite, and because MCT can also cause hepatic inflammation and hepatotoxicity, experimental design in this model must account for the potential effects

Fig. 10.2 Pulmonary arterial hypertension time-course and type of vascular secondary to exposure to SU5416/Hypoxia. A single subcutaneous injection of SU5416 at a dose of 20 mg/kg in combination with chronic hypoxia (10 %) exposure causes severe, irreversible PAH at 4 weeks, characterized by angioobliteration and muscularization. *Black arrow* shows time of injection. *X* marks time of tissue harvesting. Chemical structure of SU5416 was obtained from Wikimedia Commons (Public domain) (Micrograph from lung vessel was modified with permission from Gomez-Arroyo et al. [3])

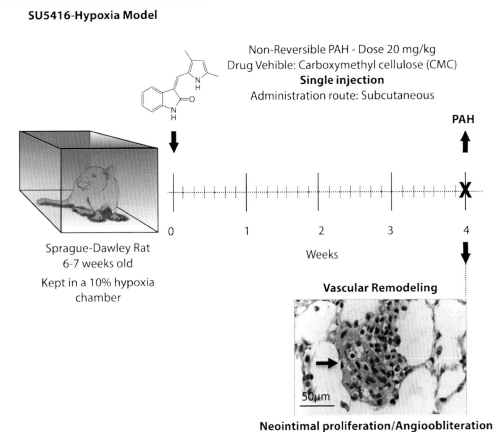

SU5416-Hypoxia Model

Non-Reversible PAH - Dose 20 mg/kg
Drug Vehible: Carboxymethyl cellulose (CMC)
Single injection
Administration route: Subcutaneous

PAH

Sprague-Dawley Rat
6-7 weeks old
Kept in a 10% hypoxia
chamber

Weeks

Vascular Remodeling

50µm

Neointimal proliferation/Angioobliteration

of MCT on the metabolism and pharmacokinetics of experimental drugs, and conversely, exogenous agents or experimental conditions which alter the function of hepatic cytochrome P450 monooxygenases may modulate the availability and pulmonary vascular toxicity of MCTP [13]. MCT may exert direct toxicity on the heart or other organs by impacting the microcirculation of those organs, with potentially confounding effects that make it difficult to isolate the effects of pressure-overload on the right ventricle versus direct toxic effects on the right ventricle, for example. The activity of MCT is generally believed to be a species-specific phenomenon in the rat. In earlier studies, administration to mice of as much as 600 mg/kg of MCT, tenfold greater than those required to elicit pulmonary vascular remodeling in the rat, was observed to generate pneumotoxicity without significant pulmonary vascular remodeling or right ventricular hypertrophy [25], a finding attributed to the lack of cytochrome P450 monooxygenases in mice required to convert MCT to MCTP. However, in more recent studies, similarly high doses of MCT, or direct administration of MCTP have been reported to generate successful models of PAH in standard mouse backgrounds, as well as genetically modified mice [26–28]. While the use of MCT/MCTP in mice would provide significant new opportunities for investigation, further investigation may be needed to standardize MCT or MCTP regimens and their consequent phenotypes in this species.

SUGEN 5416-based Models

SUGEN 5416 (SU5416), 1,3-Dihydro-3-[(3,5-dimethyl-1H-pyrrol-2-yl)methylene]-2H-indol-2-one also known as semaxinib, (Fig. 10.2) is a potent ATP-competitive inhibitor of VEGF receptor kinases 1 and 2 [29], which was originally developed for use as an adjuvant anti-angiogenic agent in the treatment of cancer by the former SUGEN company in the late 1990s [30]. At the same time, it was observed that VEGF and VEGFR2 mRNA and protein are overexpressed in the obstructive and plexiform lesions of human and rodent pulmonary arterial hypertension, the histology of which were suggested to resemble a process of disordered angiogenesis [31–33]. SU5416 was initially administered to rats to test the hypothesis that VEGF is required for the maintenance of airways, and was found to induce alveolar septal cell apoptosis, emphysema, as well as pruning of the distal pulmonary vasculature [34]. When the same group tried to combine the effect of VEGF receptor blockade with chronic hypoxia in order to worsen emphysema, they observed, surprisingly, that rats exposed to SU5416-hypoxia developed severe vascular remodeling (Fig. 10.2) and non-reversible PAH associated with severe right ventricular dysfunction, right ventricular failure and death when left untreated [35]. In contrast to hypoxia alone and MCT-induced models, this model resulted in neointimal and plexiform lesions populated by proliferating endothelial cells, and was thus one of the first animal models to recapitulate these pathognomonic features of human pulmonary vascular disease [36]. The fact that chronic hypoxia in combination with an anti-angiogenic VEGFR2 inhibitor would cause PAH might seem counterintuitive, given the angiogenic activity and overexpression of VEGF signaling molecules observed at sites of remodeling [37]. Since treatment with a pan-caspase inhibitor prevented the development of angio-obliterative pulmonary hypertension after SU5416-hypoxia exposure [35], a mechanism invoking endothelial cell apoptosis as a triggering event was postulated [38]. Subsequently, *in-vitro* studies have bolstered the concept that proliferation of apoptosis-resistant endothelial cells contributes to PAH in the SU5416-hypoxia model [39], providing additional evidence for the "cancer paradigm" as a model for understanding the pathophysiology of PAH as a proliferative disorder [38, 40].

The SU5416-hypoxia model has permitted the introduction of contemporary scientific concepts to understanding further the factors regulating PAH pathobiology, such as the contributions of pulmonary endothelial cell mitochondrial fragmentation [41], endothelial apelin-fibroblast growth factor signaling dysregulation [42], and dysregulation of multiple miRNA species [43]. This model has helped to elucidate the requirement for copper [44] and thyroid (T4) hormone [45] for the development of angioproliferative lesions. Recently, SU5416-hypoxia was used to demonstrate the role of Forkhead box O (FoxO) transcription factor 1 in the regulation of cell cycle control and bone morphogenic protein receptor type 2 (BMPR2) signaling in experimental PAH [46].

Two key advantages that the SU5416-hypoxia model has provided to the field of PAH-research are that (i) this model does not require genetic manipulation, underscoring the critical role of VEGF in adult lung biology, and (ii) that severe pulmonary vascular remodeling occur even in the absence of chronic hypoxia [47]. Not too long after the first report of SU5416-hypoxia-induced PAH was published, attempts to generate alternative models of PAH prompted researchers to combine SU5416 with other insults or "hits" [47]. Several of these modifications have resulted in seminal contributions to field, in particular, the athymic-SU5416 rat model of PAH. Taraseviciene-Stewart, Nicolls, Voelkel and collaborators demonstrated that administration of a single dose of SU5416 to athymic nude rats lacking T cells resulted in severe angio-obliterative PAH and RV dysfunction even in the absence of chronic hypoxia [48]. This model yielded an early opportunity to evaluate the role of chronic inflammation and immune dysregulation in a histologically faithful model of PAH, providing evidence for the role of regulatory T cells [49] and macrophage-derived proinflammatory mediators [50] in the pathogenesis of PAH [51].

The SU5416-hypoxia model has also been studied extensively to evaluate the pathobiology of chronic right ventricular (RV) dysfunction secondary to PAH. The RV in the SU5416-hypoxia rat model responds to pulmonary hypertension with robust hypertrophy, followed by dysfunction and systolic failure [52]. Based on data derived from this model, it has been proposed that maladaptive/dysfunctional RV hypertrophy is characterized by capillary rarefaction [53], myocardial ischemia [54], cardiomyocyte apoptosis and fibrosis [55, 56], and significant metabolic remodeling and mitochondrial dysfunction [57]. These molecular and cellular changes are associated with decreased cardiac output, marked RV dilatation and decreased exercise capacity. Importantly, the administration of SU5416 by itself does not induce capillary rarefaction in the right ventricle, despite its potential effects on the myocardial microcirculation, whereas pure pressure overload by pulmonary arterial banding elicits pathophysiologic effects similar to that seen with SU5416-hypoxia, supporting the relevance of the SU5416-hypoxia model in studying RV pathophysiology.

Like any other experimental model of disease, there are several limitations that should be considered when utilizing SU5416-hypoxia for study in PAH. For example, neither chronic hypoxia nor VEGF blockade has been implicated directly in human PAH. Based on the dysregulation of VEGF signaling activity in affected tissues, however, a potential role of imbalance between angiogenic and anti-angiogenic activity has been posited [37]. In contrast to the effects of SU5416, administration of imatinib, a small molecule multi-kinase inhibitor targeting an overlapping set of tyrosine kinase growth factor receptors including VEGFR and PDGFR, has been proposed as a therapy for limiting the progression of PAH [58]. Multi-kinase inhibitors such as nilotinib and dasatinib with overlapping effects on PDGFR and Src were found to ameliorate experimental PAH more potently than imatinib [59]. Yet nilotinib has been associated with peripheral arterial occlusive disease in man [60, 61], and more vexingly, dasatinib has been associated with incident PAH in previously unaffected patients receiving these drugs for cancer therapy [62]. The relationship of VEGF/VEGFR signaling to the many other signaling axes targeted by these small molecules, and their pathogenetic roles remains incompletely defined. While SU5416 has clearly highlighted the importance of VEGF and VEGFR signaling as a possible trigger for PAH, it is not known if environmental factors might engender similar effects upon this signaling axis to contribute to the development of PAH in man. Other smaller, but non-trivial considerations accompany the use of this animal model are cost and equipment. Requiring rats, inhibitor compound, and access to chronic hypoxia facilities, the cost of generating the SU5416-hypoxia model is significantly greater than that of monocrotaline. Moreover, akin to MCT, there appears to be some species specificity for SU5416-hypoxia, which requires the use of rats for induction of the PAH histopathophenotype. Some researchers have reported a similar phenotype when the SU5416-hypoxia model is employed in mice [63], affording the opportunity to explore a potentially robust PAH model in genetically modified mice. However, several factors should be considered when using SU5416-hypoxia in mice: (1) the degree of vascular remodeling is not the same as that of rats, lacking neo-intimal remodeling [64], (2) the disease in mice is reversible upon return to normoxia [63] and (3) severe RV failure has not been documented [4].

Strain-Specific and Genetically-Modified Models of PAH

The Fawn-hooded rat (FHR) strain has been known to be exquisitely sensitive to the development of PAH and pulmonary vascular remodeling in response to mild or moderate hypoxia in comparison to other rat strains [65, 66], and develops spontaneous PAH at 20 weeks of age, culminating in mortality at 60 weeks of age [67]. The sensitivity of FHR to hypoxia has been attributed to mitochondrial abnormalities, particularly in the pulmonary artery smooth muscle, preceding the development of PAH and persisting in culture. A relative deficiency in mitochondrial reactive oxygen species production appears to cause aberrant activation of hypoxia inducible factor (HIF-1α), which in turn inhibits the expression of oxygen sensing, voltage-gated potassium channels such as Kv1.5, leading to a disruption of normal oxygen sensing to mimic chronic hypoxia [67]. A number of oxygen-sensitive candidate genes potentially affected by the known rearrangement of chromosome 1 in FHR have been suggested to contribute the molecular mechanism of the PAH phenotype. This model has been particularly useful in highlighting potential contributions of mitochondrial and metabolic function to the pathogenesis of PAH, as well as therapeutic interventions acting upon these pathways.

A recent transgenic mouse model has tested a longstanding and controversial hypothesis that inflammation and immune dysregulation contribute to the pathogenesis of PAH [68]. Patients with idiopathic or familial PAH have been observed to express increased circulating levels of IL-1β, IL-6, IL-8, IL-10, and TNF-α, with levels of IL-6, IL-8, and IL-10 being associated with increased mortality [69, 70]. The fact that IL-6 is also elevated in other inflammatory diseases associated with PAH including systemic lupus erythematosus suggested a particularly important role of this cytokine [71]. Steiner and colleagues showed that a transgenic mouse expressing IL-6 under the control of the Clara

cell promoter in the lung did not develop pulmonary hypertension spontaneously, but developed severe PAH (with an average RVSP of 60 mmHg) and right ventricular hypertrophy following exposure to chronic hypoxia [72]. In fact the vascular remodeling seen in this context, which included neointimal remodeling, had some features that were reminiscent of human plexiform lesions, including overexpression of VEGF, as well as of pro-survival proteins such as survivin and Bcl-2. It is not known if these mice will spontaneously regress upon return to normoxia, or under other experimental therapies. Given the potential relevance to human PAH associated with immune dysregulation, whether or not this model might be responsive to therapeutic modulation of inflammation is an important subject of further investigation.

Heterozygous loss-of-function mutations in BMPR2, expressing the bone morphogenetic protein type II receptor (BMPRII) are known to occur in 75–80 % of patients with familial or heritable forms of PAH, 10–25 % of patients with sporadic idiopathic PAH [73–78], with a reduced penetrance of approximately 20 %. Testing whether or not this mutation might be sufficient to engender PAH in animal models has been a long-term pursuit in the field. West and colleagues showed in 2004 that overexpression of a dominant negative BMPRII transgene in the smooth muscle of mice led to increased muscularization of pulmonary arterioles, and increased right ventricular systolic pressures at Denver altitude [79]. While expression at high levels of a dominant negative BMPRII transgene suppressed BMP signaling and led to pulmonary vascular disease, it was acknowledged that this model might not necessarily recapitulate the functionally haploinsufficient state found in most mutation-positive humans [76, 77]. In 2005, Beppu and colleagues found that a Bmpr2 heterozygous knock-out mouse developed minimally increased right ventricular systolic pressures under normoxia or hypoxia, and with very modest changes in alveolar capillary structure [80]. These haploinsufficient mice developed more significant pulmonary hypertension and medial hypertrophy of distal vessels following intratracheal gene transfer of 5-lipoxygenase, suggesting that inflammation might unmask a latent phenotype in these animals. Since BMPR2-null mice are arrested in early development [81], conditional gene targeting of Bmpr2 in mice [82] combined with endothelial-specific recombination via an endothelial (Alk1 promoter driven) Cre recombinase was required to test the effects of postnatal, tissue specific ablation [83]. These endothelial targeted conditional Bmpr2-null mice were reported to have spontaneous PAH, albeit with variable penetrance, accompanied by increased distal pulmonary arteriolar muscularization and mild right ventricular hypertrophy. This phenotype of endothelial targeted conditional Bmpr2-null mice, despite being sporadic and generally mild, has been revisited in the context of therapy by other groups. Attenuation of leukocyte recruitment and extravasation by the inhibition of chemokine receptors CXCR1 and 2 was sufficient to normalize pulmonary hypertension in this model [84]. In a study by Spiekerkoetter and colleagues, pulmonary hypertension was exacerbated in this model by chronic hypoxia, and the resulting PAH and right ventricular hypertrophy was normalized by administration of FK506, based on a mechanism of enhanced BMP signaling via the inhibition of BMP type I receptor regulatory molecule FKBP12 [85]. The studies using endothelial ablation of *Bmpr2* in conditional knockout mice importantly demonstrated that complete ablation of BMPRII from the vascular endothelium was by itself insufficient to generate consistently severe PAH or remodeling by itself, yet could be additive with other insults. These studies leave open the role of BMPRII loss-of-function in other vascular tissues (e.g., smooth muscle) or tissue compartments, and other potential environmental insults that might contribute.

Systemic-to-Pulmonary Shunting, Pneumonectomy, Overflow and Banding Models

It has been long been recognized that left-to-right sided shunts, such as those associated with congenital heart disease, or systemic veno-venous shunts, such as those associated with porto-pulmonary syndrome, can be associated with PAH. Eisenmenger syndrome, a condition that commonly results from unrepaired post-tricuspid congenital cardiac defects – such as ventriculo-septal defects or patent ductus arteriosus – has challenged many researchers to evaluate the role of flow-induced shear stress in the development of vascular remodeling [38].

Models of over-circulation-induced PAH have been described in the rat by means of an aorto-caval shunt [86], or alternatively, by a single injection of monocrotaline after the removal of a lung lobe (pneumonectomy) by White and colleagues [87]. This combination results not only in the development of pulmonary hypertension but also the development of neointimal proliferative lesions, a feature not seen with MCT treatment alone.

Because of size restrictions, most of the animal models of flow-induced pulmonary hypertension have been performed in medium to large size animals such as miniature swine, piglets and domesticated pigs. Rondelet, Naeije and collaborators demonstrated that anastomosis of the left subclavian artery to the pulmonary arterial trunk in piglets resulted in pulmonary arterial hypertension and lung vascular remodeling characterized mainly by vessel muscularization [88]. Interestingly, this model exhibits other features associated with human PAH such as increased levels of circulating vascular endothelial growth factor and plasma endothelin-1 level, decreased expression of BMPRII and endothelin-1 receptors [89] and has even been associated with right ventricular failure [90]. The development of right ventricular failure in this model contrasts with observations from Eisenmenger syndrome cohort studies, in which signs or symptoms of heart failure are not observed until late in disease. The piglet shunt model develops severe RV dysfunction in the setting of relatively mild pulmonary hypertension, leading some to speculate whether or not RV dysfunction might be a more direct consequence of decreased expression of angiogenic factors angiopoietin-2 and VEGF, and the increased expression of pro-inflammatory cytokines interleukin (IL)-1α, IL-1β, and tumour necrosis factor-α (TNF-α) that are observed in the RV tissues of these animals [89, 90].

Recently a model of PAH was described using Yorkshire pigs subjected to repeated distal pulmonary arterial embolization with dextran beads and selective coiling of proximal pulmonary arteries with silk suture material [91]. This procedure elicited acute and sustained increases in pulmonary arterial pressures, with the development of pulmonary vascular remodeling, accompanied by decreased right ventricular function and right ventricular hypertrophy. In order to model post-capillary pulmonary hypertension, pulmonary vein banding has also been applied in the pig model, leading to robust increases in pulmonary arterial pressures and pulmonary vascular resistance, accompanied by distal pulmonary arterial remodeling, and RV dysfunction [92]. While pulmonary hypertension was a consistent finding in this model, a subsequent analysis of the natural history of pigs subjected to pulmonary vein banding revealed subsets which developed right ventricular failure, and those which remain compensated [93], suggesting that this model could be used to help understand factors which dictate the variable natural history of PH in man.

Thus, swine-based models of PH have been advantageous particularly for the study of shunt-based, overflow-mediated, or obstructive forms of pulmonary vascular disease. The high cost of maintaining these larger animals, and the paucity of commercially available reagents for performing genetic and protein analysis on porcine tissues are major limitations, however. A key advantage of swine based models, however, is the ability to perform survival surgery, critical for studying mechanical interventions such as shunt closure or right ventricular assist devices. Larger animals such as miniature and domesticated swine, by virtue of the human-like proportions of their cardiopulmonary system, permit sophisticated and detailed invasive measurements of hemodynamics, and imaging techniques for assessing myocardial function by approaches similar if not identical to those deployed in human disease [91–93].

Models of Schistosomiasis-Associated PAH

PAH associated with schistosomiasis infection (Sch-PAH) is among the most prevalent causes of PAH worldwide. PAH occurs almost exclusively in patients with chronic hepatosplenic *Schistosomiasis mansoni* infection, yet not all chronically infected individuals develop PAH, and the factors determining penetrance are not well elucidated [7, 94]. It is thought that infection of lung tissues with *Schistosoma* eggs elicits a powerful host immune response leading to granuloma formation and obliterative remodeling in pulmonary arteries [95]. Treatment of the underlying infection in affected individuals does not generally reverse PAH, but may arrest progression. The broad worldwide impact of Sch-PAH and the limited understanding of underlying pathophysiology has motivated the development of suitable animal models.

Crosby and colleagues observed pulmonary remodeling in a mouse model of schistosomiasis generated by transcutaneous infection of mice with *S. mansoni* cercariae [96]. Despite exhibiting significant pulmonary vascular remodeling, including medial hypertrophy of small pulmonary arteries and plexiform-like lesions, and a Th2 as well as Th1 inflammatory signature reminiscent of human Sch-PAH, these mice did not develop pulmonary hypertension or right ventricular hypertrophy after 12 weeks of infection. Similar results were by Kolosionek at al., using a similar model of transcutaneous infection, and attributed the lack of PAH to the patchy extent of involvement in mouse lungs under these conditions [97]. The lack of PAH or RVH was surprising given that plexiform lesions generally signify severe pulmonary vascular remodeling, and are recapitulated by few animal models, particularly mice. Graham and colleagues found similarly that transcutaneous infection with cercariae, or intravenous injection of viable eggs, thought to mimic embolization of eggs to the lung via shunts that develop in chronically infected animals, were unable to induce PAH. However, the combination of these two treatments in sequence, eliciting pre-sensitization, infection, and embolization, resulted in modest PAH, possibly due to more widespread lung involvement, but without RVH [98]. Sequential pre-sensitization and intravenous injection also elicited a Th2 inflammatory response with IL-13 being implicated as a key effector. Independent of the mode of infection, the duration of infection may be critical, however, as subsequent studies by Crosby and colleagues extending observation to 25 weeks following inoculation have revealed pulmonary arterial hypertension and RVH, both of which were attenuated by treatment with Praziquantel, likely by decreasing the local production of Th2 inflammatory cytokines [99]. These studies suggest that neither hepatic infection nor lung embolization alone are sufficient for the development of PAH as a complication of Schistosoma infection, but an additional "hit" of pre-sensitization, as well sustained infection may be required. It is unclear if the penetrance of PAH in these models is due to the presence or absence of portal hypertension, as has been postulated in human Sch-PAH, or due to some other factor that would be dependent on the repeated cycles of infection and chronicity seen in human disease.

Despite their limitations, these initial animal studies have identified a number of potentially important mediators of Sch-PAH, with therapeutic implications. The contribution of Th2 cytokines has been demonstrated by several groups, and particularly the role of IL-13 has been confirmed by gain- and loss-of-function studies in mice [98, 99]. Importantly, IL-13 has been shown to upregulate TGF-β1 signaling, and requires TGF-β signaling pathway function for its profibrotic effects [100]. Consistent with a possible role of IL-13-mediated activation of TGF-β, the phosphorylation of the downstream effect Smad2 is upregulated in pulmonary granulomas of schistosomiasis infected mice [98]. In fact, concurrent therapy of mice challenged with intraperitoneal cercariae and intravenous *S. mansoni* eggs with a pan-TGF-β neutralizing antibody resulted in improved RVSP and pulmonary vascular remodeling [101].

Models of Human Immunodeficiency Virus-Associated Pulmonary Arterial Hypertension

HIV-associated PAH represents a cause of PAH that likely poses a larger global healthcare burden than all other causes of Group I PAH apart from schistosomiasis. PAH can be present as part of the HIV-Associated Non-AIDS conditions [102] and indeed, the presence of PAH is an independent predictor of mortality in this group of patients [103, 104]. Generating a suitable animal model to reproduce such a complex condition like HIV-associated PAH involves several challenges, however. A major obstacle is that HIV cannot infect non-human primates other than chimpanzees, an endangered species. Moreover, chimpanzees do not develop AIDS reliably after viral inoculation [105], making this species inefficient as an experimental model. In the late 1980s, a simian immunodeficiency virus (SIV) was isolated from rhesus macaques (*macaca mulatta*) [106–108], which infects macaques with high levels of replication [109]. SIV-infected macaques develop an AIDS-like condition which mimics human disease including CD4+ T cell depletion, weight loss, thymic and lymphoid atrophy, and susceptibility to opportunistic infections [110]. More recently, it was shown that these animals develop pulmonary vascular remodeling [111] associated with moderate pulmonary arterial hypertension [112]. The degree of vascular remodeling in this model may be multifactorial, as rhesus macaques treated with morphine as a "second hit" develop severe pulmonary vascular remodeling including plexiform lesions [113]. It has been postulated that morphine could lead to increased oxidative stress-mediated endothelial cell apoptosis and that proliferation of endothelial cells may result from exposure to viral proteins [113, 114], however the exact mechanism whereby HIV/SIV contributes to pulmonary vascular remodeling remains unresolved.

This complex animal model offers several advantages not only for gaining insights into HIV-related pulmonary arterial hypertension, but into mechanisms of PAH in general. Unlike other experimental models, non-human primates infected with SIV develop PAH without requiring any genetic or pharmacological manipulation, which limits off-target effects that may confound other models [3]. SIV-associated PAH in non-human primates represents the only robust model of PAH in which the inciting factor is essentially identical to the cause in man. Furthermore, since the animals used in this preclinical model are outbred, the individualized responses of each primate to SIV infection affords the opportunity to characterize factors contributing to the penetrance of the phenotype, including the degree to which individual animals develop PAH or RV failure. Lastly, this model allows for a standardized timing of infection, serial sampling and tissue recovery, offering the opportunity to dissect pathogenetic factors early in the course of disease in a human-like model. This is in contrast to less-specific end-stage phenomena that are typically seen in clinical human studies of PAH. Some of the advantages of the SIV-infected macaque model also represent limitations, however. The heterogeneous responses to infection and intervention may require larger and more expensive cohorts in order to demonstrate statistically significant findings during experimentation, and the underlying host factors contributing to variable penetrance may be challenging to ascertain even with next generation sequencing methodologies. The SIV-infection related PAH model in macques may be prohibitively expensive for most labs, as the approximate price for housing a SIV-infected cohort of 12 macaques may approach $250,000 USD for 1 year, not including the cost of any interventions or analysis. Expense notwithstanding, SIV-associated PAH in macaques is potentially the most authentic model of any etiology of human PAH and affords a tremendous opportunity to unravel the early pathogenetic events in a primate model.

Conclusions

Currently available small animal and large animal models offer a host of complementary advantages and disadvantages for the investigation of mechanism and therapeutic intervention in PAH. Larger animal models generally offer greater histopathologic and pathophysiologic similarity to human PAH disease, but require a significantly greater financial and technical investment. Inbred strains of mice and rats offer significant advantages in cost and scalability, but individually may lack critical aspects of the disease phenotype. Reliance on a single rodent model could potentially generate artifactual findings, particularly in the mouse, and should be supported by mechanistically distinct models preferably in another species such as the rat. A key challenge for the study of pathophysiology relevant to human disease remains generating PAH in

animals that results from similar precipitating factors known to trigger PAH in man. A common motif throughout most models of PAH is that a single physiologic challenge or insult is generally insufficient to generate substantial PAH, pulmonary vascular remodeling and right ventricular hypertrophy/failure, whereas a combination of two distinct insults can potently elicit these findings. Recent modifications to existing models have improved their reproducibility, or their ability to capture distinct facets of the PAH phenotypic spectrum, even in mouse and rat species, suggesting that further potential yet exists to optimize these models further. Despite their limitations, numerous pathophysiologic and translatable insights have been obtained from studying PAH in currently available models. The advent of novel technologies to permit genome editing and humanization of large genetic loci within rodents and larger species is anticipated to facilitate more authentic and relevant PAH models in the near future.

References

1. von Euler US, Liljestrand G. Observations on the pulmonary arterial blood pressure in the cat. Acta Physiol Scand. 1946;12:301–20.
2. Stenmark KR, Meyrick B, Galie N, Mooi WJ, McMurtry IF. Animal models of pulmonary arterial hypertension: the hope for etiological discovery and pharmacological cure. Am J Physiol Lung Cell Mol Physiol. 2009;297:L1013–32.
3. Gomez-Arroyo JG, Farkas L, Alhussaini AA, Farkas D, Kraskauskas D, Voelkel NF, Bogaard HJ. The monocrotaline model of pulmonary hypertension in perspective. Am J Physiol Lung Cell Mol Physiol. 2012;302:L363–9.
4. Gomez-Arroyo J, Saleem SJ, Mizuno S, Syed AA, Bogaard HJ, Abbate A, Taraseviciene-Stewart L, Sung Y, Kraskauskas D, Farkas D, Conrad DH, Nicolls MR, Voelkel NF. A brief overview of mouse models of pulmonary arterial hypertension: problems and prospects. Am J Physiol Lung Cell Mol Physiol. 2012;302: L977–91.
5. Voelkel NF, Tuder RM. Hypoxia-induced pulmonary vascular remodeling: a model for what human disease? J Clin Invest. 2000;106:733–8.
6. Ryan J, Bloch K, Archer SL. Rodent models of pulmonary hypertension: harmonisation with the world health organisation's categorisation of human PH. Int J Clin Pract Suppl. 2011;(172): 15–34.
7. Simonneau G, Gatzoulis MA, Adatia I, Celermajer D, Denton C, Ghofrani A, Gomez Sanchez MA, Krishna Kumar R, Landzberg M, Machado RF, Olschewski H, Robbins IM, Souza R. Updated clinical classification of pulmonary hypertension. J Am Coll Cardiol. 2013;62:D34–41.
8. Thomas HC, Lame MW, Dunston SK, Segall HJ, Wilson DW. Monocrotaline pyrrole induces apoptosis in pulmonary artery endothelial cells. Toxicol Appl Pharmacol. 1998;151:236–44.
9. Reindel JF, Roth RA. The effects of monocrotaline pyrrole on cultured bovine pulmonary artery endothelial and smooth muscle cells. Am J Pathol. 1991;138:707–19.
10. Sehgal PB, Mukhopadhyay S. Dysfunctional intracellular trafficking in the pathobiology of pulmonary arterial hypertension. Am J Respir Cell Mol Biol. 2007;37:31–7.

11. Huang J, Wolk JH, Gewitz MH, Mathew R. Progressive endothelial cell damage in an inflammatory model of pulmonary hypertension. Exp Lung Res. 2010;36:57–66.

12. Ramos M, Lame MW, Segall HJ, Wilson DW. Monocrotaline pyrrole induces Smad nuclear accumulation and altered signaling expression in human pulmonary arterial endothelial cells. Vascul Pharmacol. 2007;46:439–48.

13. Roth RA, Reindel JF. Lung vascular injury from monocrotaline pyrrole, a putative hepatic metabolite. Adv Exp Med Biol. 1991;283:477–87.

14. Estep JE, Lame MW, Morin D, Jones AD, Wilson DW, Segall HJ. [14C]monocrotaline kinetics and metabolism in the rat. Drug Metab Dispos. 1991;19:135–9.

15. Ruiter G, de Man FS, Schalij I, Sairras S, Grunberg K, Westerhof N, van der Laarse WJ, Vonk-Noordegraaf A. Reversibility of the monocrotaline pulmonary hypertension rat model. Eur Respir J. 2013;42:553–6.

16. Hessel MH, Steendijk P, den Adel B, Schutte CI, van der Laarse A. Characterization of right ventricular function after monocrotaline-induced pulmonary hypertension in the intact rat. Am J Physiol Heart Circ Physiol. 2006;291:H2424–30.

17. Urboniene D, Haber I, Fang YH, Thenappan T, Archer SL. Validation of high-resolution echocardiography and magnetic resonance imaging vs. high-fidelity catheterization in experimental pulmonary hypertension. Am J Physiol Lung Cell Mol Physiol. 2010;299:L401–12.

18. Handoko ML, de Man FS, Happe CM, Schalij I, Musters RJ, Westerhof N, Postmus PE, Paulus WJ, van der Laarse WJ, Vonk-Noordegraaf A. Opposite effects of training in rats with stable and progressive pulmonary hypertension. Circulation. 2009;120:42–9.

19. Long L, Crosby A, Yang X, Southwood M, Upton PD, Kim DK, Morrell NW. Altered bone morphogenetic protein and transforming growth factor-beta signaling in rat models of pulmonary hypertension: potential for activin receptor-like kinase-5 inhibition in prevention and progression of disease. Circulation. 2009;119:566–76.

20. Zaiman AL, Podowski M, Medicherla S, Gordy K, Xu F, Zhen L, Shimoda LA, Neptune E, Higgins L, Murphy A, Chakravarty S, Protter A, Sehgal PB, Champion HC, Tuder RM. Role of the TGF-beta/Alk5 signaling pathway in monocrotaline-induced pulmonary hypertension. Am J Respir Crit Care Med. 2008;177:896–905.

21. Thomas M, Docx C, Holmes AM, Beach S, Duggan N, England K, Leblanc C, Lebret C, Schindler F, Raza F, Walker C, Crosby A, Davies RJ, Morrell NW, Budd DC. Activin-like kinase 5 (ALK5) mediates abnormal proliferation of vascular smooth muscle cells from patients with familial pulmonary arterial hypertension and is involved in the progression of experimental pulmonary arterial hypertension induced by monocrotaline. Am J Pathol. 2009;174:380–9.

22. Prie S, Leung TK, Cernacek P, Ryan JW, Dupuis J. The orally active ET(A) receptor antagonist (+)-(S)-2-(4,6-dimethoxy-pyrimidin-2-yloxy)-3-methoxy-3,3-diphenyl-propionic acid (LU 135252) prevents the development of pulmonary hypertension and endothelial metabolic dysfunction in monocrotaline-treated rats. J Pharmacol Exp Ther. 1997;282:1312–8.

23. Hill NS, Warburton RR, Pietras L, Klinger JR. Nonspecific endothelin-receptor antagonist blunts monocrotaline-induced pulmonary hypertension in rats. J Appl Physiol (1985). 1997;83:1209–15.

24. Czer GT, Marsh J, Konopka R, Moser KM. Low-dose PGI2 prevents monocrotaline-induced thromboxane production and lung injury. J Appl Physiol (1985). 1986;60:464–71.

25. Molteni A, Ward WF, Ts'ao CH, Solliday NH. Monocrotaline pneumotoxicity in mice. Virchows Arch B Cell Pathol Incl Mol Pathol. 1989;57:149–55.

26. Aliotta JM, Pereira M, Amaral A, Sorokina A, Igbinoba Z, Hasslinger A, El-Bizri R, Rounds SI, Quesenberry PJ, Klinger JR. Induction of pulmonary hypertensive changes by extracellular vesicles from monocrotaline-treated mice. Cardiovasc Res. 2013;100:354–62.

27. Qiao L, Nishimura T, Shi L, Sessions D, Thrasher A, Trudell JR, Berry GJ, Pearl RG, Kao PN. Endothelial fate mapping in mice with pulmonary hypertension. Circulation. 2014;129:692–703.

28. Guignabert C, Izikki M, Tu LI, Li Z, Zadigue P, Barlier-Mur AM, Hanoun N, Rodman D, Hamon M, Adnot S, Eddahibi S. Transgenic mice overexpressing the 5-hydroxytryptamine transporter gene in smooth muscle develop pulmonary hypertension. Circ Res. 2006;98:1323–30.

29. Itokawa T, Nokihara H, Nishioka Y, Sone S, Iwamoto Y, Yamada Y, Cherrington J, McMahon G, Shibuya M, Kuwano M, Ono M. Antiangiogenic effect by SU5416 is partly attributable to inhibition of Flt-1 receptor signaling. Mol Cancer Ther. 2002;1:295–302.

30. Fong TA, Shawver LK, Sun L, Tang C, App H, Powell TJ, Kim YH, Schreck R, Wang X, Risau W, Ullrich A, Hirth KP, McMahon G. SU5416 is a potent and selective inhibitor of the vascular endothelial growth factor receptor (Flk-1/KDR) that inhibits tyrosine kinase catalysis, tumor vascularization, and growth of multiple tumor types. Cancer Res. 1999;59:99–106.

31. Cool CD, Stewart JS, Werahera P, Miller GJ, Williams RL, Voelkel NF, Tuder RM. Three-dimensional reconstruction of pulmonary arteries in plexiform pulmonary hypertension using cell-specific markers. Evidence for a dynamic and heterogeneous process of pulmonary endothelial cell growth. Am J Pathol. 1999;155:411–9.

32. Tuder RM, Groves B, Badesch DB, Voelkel NF. Exuberant endothelial cell growth and elements of inflammation are present in plexiform lesions of pulmonary hypertension. Am J Pathol. 1994;144:275–85.

33. Tuder RM, Chacon M, Alger L, Wang J, Taraseviciene-Stewart L, Kasahara Y, Cool CD, Bishop AE, Geraci M, Semenza GL, Yacoub M, Polak JM, Voelkel NF. Expression of angiogenesis-related molecules in plexiform lesions in severe pulmonary hypertension: evidence for a process of disordered angiogenesis. J Pathol. 2001;195:367–74.

34. Kasahara Y, Tuder RM, Taraseviciene-Stewart L, Le Cras TD, Abman S, Hirth PK, Waltenberger J, Voelkel NF. Inhibition of VEGF receptors causes lung cell apoptosis and emphysema. J Clin Invest. 2000;106:1311–9.

35. Taraseviciene-Stewart L, Kasahara Y, Alger L, Hirth P, Mc Mahon G, Waltenberger J, Voelkel NF, Tuder RM. Inhibition of the VEGF receptor 2 combined with chronic hypoxia causes cell death-dependent pulmonary endothelial cell proliferation and severe pulmonary hypertension. FASEB J. 2001;15:427–38.

36. Abe K, Toba M, Alzoubi A, Ito M, Fagan KA, Cool CD, Voelkel NF, McMurtry IF, Oka M. Formation of plexiform lesions in experimental severe pulmonary arterial hypertension. Circulation. 2010;121:2747–54.

37. Voelkel NF, Gomez-Arroyo J. The role of vascular endothelial growth factor in pulmonary arterial hypertension. The angiogenesis paradox. Am J Respir Cell Mol Biol. 2014;51:474–84.

38. Voelkel NF, Gomez-Arroyo J, Abbate A, Bogaard HJ, Nicolls MR. Pathobiology of pulmonary arterial hypertension and right ventricular failure. Eur Respir J. 2012;40:1555–65.

39. Sakao S, Taraseviciene-Stewart L, Lee JD, Wood K, Cool CD, Voelkel NF. Initial apoptosis is followed by increased proliferation of apoptosis-resistant endothelial cells. FASEB J. 2005;19:1178–80.

40. Rai PR, Cool CD, King JA, Stevens T, Burns N, Winn RA, Kasper M, Voelkel NF. The cancer paradigm of severe pulmonary arterial hypertension. Am J Respir Crit Care Med. 2008;178:558–64.

41. Ryan JJ, Marsboom G, Fang YH, Toth PT, Morrow E, Luo N, Piao L, Hong Z, Ericson K, Zhang HJ, Han M, Haney CR, Chen CT, Sharp WW, Archer SL. PGC1alpha-mediated mitofusin-2 deficiency in female rats and humans with pulmonary arterial hypertension. Am J Respir Crit Care Med. 2013;187:865–78.

42. Kim J, Kang Y, Kojima Y, Lighthouse JK, Hu X, Aldred MA, McLean DL, Park H, Comhair SA, Greif DM, Erzurum SC, Chun HJ. An endothelial apelin-FGF link mediated by miR-424 and miR-503 is disrupted in pulmonary arterial hypertension. Nat Med. 2013;19:74–82.

43. Bertero T, Lu Y, Annis S, Hale A, Bhat B, Saggar R, Wallace WD, Ross DJ, Vargas SO, Graham BB, Kumar R, Black SM, Fratz S, Fineman JR, West JD, Haley KJ, Waxman AB, Chau BN, Cottrill KA, Chan SY. Systems-level regulation of microRNA networks by miR-130/301 promotes pulmonary hypertension. J Clin Invest. 2014;124:3514–28.

44. Bogaard HJ, Mizuno S, Guignabert C, Al Hussaini AA, Farkas D, Ruiter G, Kraskauskas D, Fadel E, Allegood JC, Humbert M, Vonk Noordegraaf A, Spiegel S, Farkas L, Voelkel NF. Copper dependence of angioproliferation in pulmonary arterial hypertension in rats and humans. Am J Respir Cell Mol Biol. 2012;46:582–91.

45. Al Husseini A, Bagnato G, Farkas L, Gomez-Arroyo J, Farkas D, Mizuno S, Kraskauskas D, Abbate A, Van Tassel B, Voelkel NF, Bogaard HJ. Thyroid hormone is highly permissive in angioproliferative pulmonary hypertension in rats. Eur Respir J. 2013;41:104–14.

46. Savai R, Al-Tamari HM, Sedding D, Kojonazarov B, Muecke C, Teske R, Capecchi MR, Weissmann N, Grimminger F, Seeger W, Schermuly RT, Pullamsetti SS. Pro-proliferative and inflammatory signaling converge on FoxO1 transcription factor in pulmonary hypertension. Nat Med. 2014;20:1289–300.

47. Nicolls MR, Mizuno S, Taraseviciene-Stewart L, Farkas L, Drake JI, Al Husseini A, Gomez-Arroyo JG, Voelkel NF, Bogaard HJ. New models of pulmonary hypertension based on VEGF receptor blockade-induced endothelial cell apoptosis. Pulm Circ. 2012;2:434–42.

48. Taraseviciene-Stewart L, Nicolls MR, Kraskauskas D, Scerbavicius R, Burns N, Cool C, Wood K, Parr JE, Boackle SA, Voelkel NF. Absence of T cells confers increased pulmonary arterial hypertension and vascular remodeling. Am J Respir Crit Care Med. 2007;175:1280–9.

49. Tamosiuniene R, Tian W, Dhillon G, Wang L, Sung YK, Gera L, Patterson AJ, Agrawal R, Rabinovitch M, Ambler K, Long CS, Voelkel NF, Nicolls MR. Regulatory T cells limit vascular endothelial injury and prevent pulmonary hypertension. Circ Res. 2011;109:867–79.

50. Tian W, Jiang X, Tamosiuniene R, Sung YK, Qian J, Dhillon G, Gera L, Farkas L, Rabinovitch M, Zamanian RT, Inayathullah M, Fridlib M, Rajadas J, Peters-Golden M, Voelkel NF, Nicolls MR. Blocking macrophage leukotriene b4 prevents endothelial injury and reverses pulmonary hypertension. Sci Transl Med. 2013;5:200ra117.

51. Rabinovitch M, Guignabert C, Humbert M, Nicolls MR. Inflammation and immunity in the pathogenesis of pulmonary arterial hypertension. Circ Res. 2014;115:165–75.

52. Oka M, Homma N, Taraseviciene-Stewart L, Morris KG, Kraskauskas D, Burns N, Voelkel NF, McMurtry IF. Rho kinase-mediated vasoconstriction is important in severe occlusive pulmonary arterial hypertension in rats. Circ Res. 2007;100:923–9.

53. Bogaard HJ, Natarajan R, Henderson SC, Long CS, Kraskauskas D, Smithson L, Ockaili R, McCord JM, Voelkel NF. Chronic pulmonary artery pressure elevation is insufficient to explain right heart failure. Circulation. 2009;120:1951–60.

54. Gomez A, Bialostozky D, Zajarias A, Santos E, Palomar A, Martinez ML, Sandoval J. Right ventricular ischemia in patients with primary pulmonary hypertension. J Am Coll Cardiol. 2001;38:1137–42.

55. Bogaard HJ, Natarajan R, Mizuno S, Abbate A, Chang PJ, Chau VQ, Hoke NN, Kraskauskas D, Kasper M, Salloum FN, Voelkel NF. Adrenergic receptor blockade reverses right heart remodeling and dysfunction in pulmonary hypertensive rats. Am J Respir Crit Care Med. 2010;182:652–60.

56. Lang M, Kojonazarov B, Tian X, Kalymbetov A, Weissmann N, Grimminger F, Kretschmer A, Stasch JP, Seeger W, Ghofrani HA, Schermuly RT. The soluble guanylate cyclase stimulator riociguat ameliorates pulmonary hypertension induced by hypoxia and SU5416 in rats. PLoS One. 2012;7:e43433.

57. Gomez-Arroyo J, Mizuno S, Szczepanek K, Van Tassell B, Natarajan R, dos Remedios CG, Drake JI, Farkas L, Kraskauskas D, Wijesinghe DS, Chalfant CE, Bigbee J, Abbate A, Lesnefsky EJ, Bogaard HJ, Voelkel NF. Metabolic gene remodeling and mitochondrial dysfunction in failing right ventricular hypertrophy secondary to pulmonary arterial hypertension. Circ Heart Fail. 2013;6:136–44.

58. Ghofrani HA, Seeger W, Grimminger F. Imatinib for the treatment of pulmonary arterial hypertension. N Engl J Med. 2005; 353:1412–3.

59. Pullamsetti SS, Berghausen EM, Dabral S, Tretyn A, Butrous E, Savai R, Butrous G, Dahal BK, Brandes RP, Ghofrani HA, Weissmann N, Grimminger F, Seeger W, Rosenkranz S, Schermuly RT. Role of Src tyrosine kinases in experimental pulmonary hypertension. Arterioscler Thromb Vasc Biol. 2012;32:1354–65.

60. Aichberger KJ, Herndlhofer S, Schernthaner GH, Schillinger M, Mitterbauer-Hohendanner G, Sillaber C, Valent P. Progressive peripheral arterial occlusive disease and other vascular events during nilotinib therapy in CML. Am J Hematol. 2011;86:533–9.

61. Valent P, Hadzijusufovic E, Schernthaner G, Wolf D, Rea D, le Coutre P. Vascular safety issues in CML patients treated with BCR/ABL1 kinase inhibitors. Blood. 2015;125(6):901–6.

62. Montani D, Bergot E, Gunther S, Savale L, Bergeron A, Bourdin A, Bouvaist H, Canuet M, Pison C, Macro M, Poubeau P, Girerd B, Natali D, Guignabert C, Perros F, O'Callaghan DS, Jais X, Tubert-Bitter P, Zalcman G, Sitbon O, Simonneau G, Humbert M. Pulmonary arterial hypertension in patients treated by dasatinib. Circulation. 2012;125:2128–37.

63. Ciuclan L, Bonneau O, Hussey M, Duggan N, Holmes AM, Good R, Stringer R, Jones P, Morrell NW, Jarai G, Walker C, Westwick J, Thomas M. A novel murine model of severe pulmonary arterial hypertension. Am J Respir Crit Care Med. 2011;184:1171–82.

64. Vitali SH, Hansmann G, Rose C, Fernandez-Gonzalez A, Scheid A, Mitsialis SA, Kourembanas S. The Sugen 5416hypoxia mouse model of pulmonary hypertension revisited: long-term follow-up. Pulm Circ. 2014;4(4):619–29.

65. Sato K, Webb S, Tucker A, Rabinovitch M, O'Brien RF, McMurtry IF, Stelzner TJ. Factors influencing the idiopathic development of pulmonary hypertension in the fawn hooded rat. Am Rev Respir Dis. 1992;145:793–7.

66. Nagaoka T, Muramatsu M, Sato K, McMurtry I, Oka M, Fukuchi Y. Mild hypoxia causes severe pulmonary hypertension in fawn-hooded but not in Tester Moriyama rats. Respir Physiol. 2001; 127:53–60.

67. Bonnet S, Michelakis ED, Porter CJ, Andrade-Navarro MA, Thebaud B, Haromy A, Harry G, Moudgil R, McMurtry MS, Weir EK, Archer SL. An abnormal mitochondrial-hypoxia inducible factor-1alpha-Kv channel pathway disrupts oxygen sensing and triggers pulmonary arterial hypertension in fawn hooded rats: similarities to human pulmonary arterial hypertension. Circulation. 2006;113:2630–41.

68. Nicolls MR, Taraseviciene-Stewart L, Rai PR, Badesch DB, Voelkel NF. Autoimmunity and pulmonary hypertension: a perspective. Eur Respir J. 2005;26:1110–8.

69. Humbert M, Monti G, Brenot F, Sitbon O, Portier A, Grangeot-Keros L, Duroux P, Galanaud P, Simonneau G, Emilie D. Increased interleukin-1 and interleukin-6 serum concentrations in severe primary pulmonary hypertension. Am J Respir Crit Care Med. 1995;151:1628–31.

70. Soon E, Holmes AM, Treacy CM, Doughty NJ, Southgate L, Machado RD, Trembath RC, Jennings S, Barker L, Nicklin P,

Walker C, Budd DC, Pepke-Zaba J, Morrell NW. Elevated levels of inflammatory cytokines predict survival in idiopathic and familial pulmonary arterial hypertension. Circulation. 2010;122:920–7.

71. Yoshio T, Masuyama JI, Kohda N, Hirata D, Sato H, Iwamoto M, Mimori A, Takeda A, Minota S, Kano S. Association of interleukin 6 release from endothelial cells and pulmonary hypertension in SLE. J Rheumatol. 1997;24:489–95.

72. Steiner MK, Syrkina OL, Kolliputi N, Mark EJ, Hales CA, Waxman AB. Interleukin-6 overexpression induces pulmonary hypertension. Circ Res. 2009;104:236–44, 228p following 244.

73. Deng Z, Morse JH, Slager SL, Cuervo N, Moore KJ, Venetos G, Kalachikov S, Cayanis E, Fischer SG, Barst RJ, Hodge SE, Knowles JA. Familial primary pulmonary hypertension (gene PPH1) is caused by mutations in the bone morphogenetic protein receptor-II gene. Am J Hum Genet. 2000;67:737–44.

74. International PPHC, Lane KB, Machado RD, Pauciulo MW, Thomson JR, Phillips 3rd JA, Loyd JE, Nichols WC, Trembath RC. Heterozygous germline mutations in BMPR2, encoding a TGF-beta receptor, cause familial primary pulmonary hypertension. Nat Genet. 2000;26:81–4.

75. Aldred MA, Vijayakrishnan J, James V, Soubrier F, Gomez-Sanchez MA, Martensson G, Galie N, Manes A, Corris P, Simonneau G, Humbert M, Morrell NW, Trembath RC. BMPR2 gene rearrangements account for a significant proportion of mutations in familial and idiopathic pulmonary arterial hypertension. Hum Mutat. 2006;27:212–3.

76. Machado RD, Aldred MA, James V, Harrison RE, Patel B, Schwalbe EC, Gruenig E, Janssen B, Koehler R, Seeger W, Eickelberg O, Olschewski H, Elliott CG, Glissmeyer E, Carlquist J, Kim M, Torbicki A, Fijalkowska A, Szewczyk G, Parma J, Abramowicz MJ, Galie N, Morisaki H, Kyotani S, Nakanishi N, Morisaki T, Humbert M, Simonneau G, Sitbon O, Soubrier F, Coulet F, Morrell NW, Trembath RC. Mutations of the TGF-beta type II receptor BMPR2 in pulmonary arterial hypertension. Hum Mutat. 2006;27:121–32.

77. Machado RD, Pauciulo MW, Thomson JR, Lane KB, Morgan NV, Wheeler L, Phillips 3rd JA, Newman J, Williams D, Galie N, Manes A, McNeil K, Yacoub M, Mikhail G, Rogers P, Corris P, Humbert M, Donnai D, Martensson G, Tranebjaerg L, Loyd JE, Trembath RC, Nichols WC. BMPR2 haploinsufficiency as the inherited molecular mechanism for primary pulmonary hypertension. Am J Hum Genet. 2001;68:92–102.

78. Thomson J, Machado R, Pauciulo M, Morgan N, Yacoub M, Corris P, McNeil K, Loyd J, Nichols W, Trembath R. Familial and sporadic primary pulmonary hypertension is caused by BMPR2 gene mutations resulting in haploinsufficiency of the bone morphogenetic protein type II receptor. J Heart Lung Transplant. 2001;20:149.

79. West J, Fagan K, Steudel W, Fouty B, Lane K, Harral J, Hoedt-Miller M, Tada Y, Ozimek J, Tuder R, Rodman DM. Pulmonary hypertension in transgenic mice expressing a dominant-negative BMPRII gene in smooth muscle. Circ Res. 2004;94:1109–14.

80. Beppu H, Ichinose F, Kawai N, Jones RC, Yu PB, Zapol WM, Miyazono K, Li E, Bloch KD. BMPR-II heterozygous mice have mild pulmonary hypertension and an impaired pulmonary vascular remodeling response to prolonged hypoxia. Am J Physiol Lung Cell Mol Physiol. 2004;287:L1241–7.

81. Beppu H, Kawabata M, Hamamoto T, Chytil A, Minowa O, Noda T, Miyazono K. BMP type II receptor is required for gastrulation and early development of mouse embryos. Dev Biol. 2000;221:249–58.

82. Yu PB, Beppu H, Kawai N, Li E, Bloch KD. Bone morphogenetic protein (BMP) type II receptor deletion reveals BMP ligand-specific gain of signaling in pulmonary artery smooth muscle cells. J Biol Chem. 2005;280:24443–50.

83. Hong KH, Lee YJ, Lee E, Park SO, Han C, Beppu H, Li E, Raizada MK, Bloch KD, Oh SP. Genetic ablation of the BMPR2 gene in pulmonary endothelium is sufficient to predispose to pulmonary arterial hypertension. Circulation. 2008;118:722–30.

84. Burton VJ, Holmes AM, Ciuclan LI, Robinson A, Roger JS, Jarai G, Pearce AC, Budd DC. Attenuation of leukocyte recruitment via CXCR1/2 inhibition stops the progression of PAH in mice with genetic ablation of endothelial BMPR-II. Blood. 2011;118:4750–8.

85. Spiekerkoetter E, Tian X, Cai J, Hopper RK, Sudheendra D, Li CG, El-Bizri N, Sawada H, Haghighat R, Chan R, Haghighat L, de Jesus PV, Wang L, Reddy S, Zhao M, Bernstein D, Solow-Cordero DE, Beachy PA, Wandless TJ, Ten Dijke P, Rabinovitch M. FK506 activates BMPR2, rescues endothelial dysfunction, and reverses pulmonary hypertension. J Clin Invest. 2013;123:3600–13.

86. van Albada ME, Berger RM, Niggebrugge M, van Veghel R, Cromme-Dijkhuis AH, Schoemaker RG. Prostacyclin therapy increases right ventricular capillarisation in a model for flow-associated pulmonary hypertension. Eur J Pharmacol. 2006;549:107–16.

87. White RJ, Meoli DF, Swarthout RF, Kallop DY, Galaria II, Harvey JL, Miller CM, Blaxall BC, Hall CM, Pierce RA, Cool CD, Taubman MB. Plexiform-like lesions and increased tissue factor expression in a rat model of severe pulmonary arterial hypertension. Am J Physiol Lung Cell Mol Physiol. 2007;293:L583–90.

88. Rondelet B, Kerbaul F, Motte S, van Beneden R, Remmelink M, Brimioulle S, McEntee K, Wauthy P, Salmon I, Ketelslegers JM, Naeije R. Bosentan for the prevention of overcirculation-induced experimental pulmonary arterial hypertension. Circulation. 2003;107:1329–35.

89. Rondelet B, Kerbaul F, Van Beneden R, Motte S, Fesler P, Hubloue I, Remmelink M, Brimioulle S, Salmon I, Ketelslegers JM, Naeije R. Signaling molecules in overcirculation-induced pulmonary hypertension in piglets: effects of sildenafil therapy. Circulation. 2004;110:2220–5.

90. Rondelet B, Dewachter C, Kerbaul F, Kang X, Fesler P, Brimioulle S, Naeije R, Dewachter L. Prolonged overcirculation-induced pulmonary arterial hypertension as a cause of right ventricular failure. Eur Heart J. 2012;33:1017–26.

91. Aguero J, Ishikawa K, Fish KM, Hammoudi N, Hadri L, Garcia-Alvarez A, Ibanez B, Fuster V, Hajjar RJ, Leopold JA. Combination proximal pulmonary artery coiling and distal embolization induces chronic elevations in pulmonary artery pressure in Swine. PLoS One. 2015;10:e0124526.

92. Pereda D, Garcia-Alvarez A, Sanchez-Quintana D, Nuno M, Fernandez-Friera L, Fernandez-Jimenez R, Garcia-Ruiz JM, Sandoval E, Aguero J, Castella M, Hajjar RJ, Fuster V, Ibanez B. Swine model of chronic postcapillary pulmonary hypertension with right ventricular remodeling: long-term characterization by cardiac catheterization, magnetic resonance, and pathology. J Cardiovasc Transl Res. 2014;7:494–506.

93. Aguero J, Ishikawa K, Hadri L, Santos-Gallego C, Fish K, Hammoudi N, Chaanine A, Torquato S, Naim C, Ibanez B, Pereda D, Garcia-Alvarez A, Fuster V, Sengupta PP, Leopold JA, Hajjar RJ. Characterization of right ventricular remodeling and failure in a chronic pulmonary hypertension model. Am J Physiol Heart Circ Physiol. 2014;307:H1204–15.

94. Graham BB, Bandeira AP, Morrell NW, Butrous G, Tuder RM. Schistosomiasis-associated pulmonary hypertension: pulmonary vascular disease: the global perspective. Chest. 2010;137:20S–9.

95. Kolosionek E, Crosby A, Harhay MO, Morrell N, Butrous G. Pulmonary vascular disease associated with schistosomiasis. Expert Rev Anti Infect Ther. 2010;8:1467–73.

96. Crosby A, Jones FM, Southwood M, Stewart S, Schermuly R, Butrous G, Dunne DW, Morrell NW. Pulmonary vascular remodeling correlates with lung eggs and cytokines in murine schistosomiasis. Am J Respir Crit Care Med. 2010;181:279–88.

97. Kolosionek E, King J, Rollinson D, Schermuly RT, Grimminger F, Graham BB, Morrell N, Butrous G. Schistosomiasis causes remodeling of pulmonary vessels in the lung in a heterogeneous localized manner: detailed study. Pulm Circ. 2013;3:356–62.

98. Graham BB, Mentink-Kane MM, El-Haddad H, Purnell S, Zhang L, Zaiman A, Redente EF, Riches DW, Hassoun PM, Bandeira A, Champion HC, Butrous G, Wynn TA, Tuder RM. Schistosomiasis-induced experimental pulmonary hypertension: role of interleukin-13 signaling. Am J Pathol. 2010;177:1549–61.

99. Crosby A, Jones FM, Kolosionek E, Southwood M, Purvis I, Soon E, Butrous G, Dunne DE, Morrell NW. Praziquantel reverses pulmonary hypertension and vascular remodeling in murine schistosomiasis. Am J Respir Crit Care Med. 2011;184:467–73.

100. Lee CG, Homer RJ, Zhu Z, Lanone S, Wang X, Koteliansky V, Shipley JM, Gotwals P, Noble P, Chen Q, Senior RM, Elias JA. Interleukin-13 induces tissue fibrosis by selectively stimulating and activating transforming growth factor beta(1). J Exp Med. 2001;194:809–21.

101. Graham BB, Chabon J, Gebreab L, Poole J, Debella E, Davis L, Tanaka T, Sanders L, Dropcho N, Bandeira A, Vandivier RW, Champion HC, Butrous G, Wang XJ, Wynn TA, Tuder RM. Transforming growth factor-beta signaling promotes pulmonary hypertension caused by Schistosoma mansoni. Circulation. 2013;128:1354–64.

102. Mehta NJ, Khan IA, Mehta RN, Sepkowitz DA. HIV-related pulmonary hypertension: analytic review of 131 cases. Chest. 2000;118:1133–41.

103. Degano B, Guillaume M, Savale L, Montani D, Jais X, Yaici A, Le Pavec J, Humbert M, Simonneau G, Sitbon O. HIV-associated pulmonary arterial hypertension: survival and prognostic factors in the modern therapeutic era. AIDS. 2010;24:67–75.

104. Opravil M, Pechere M, Speich R, Joller-Jemelka HI, Jenni R, Russi EW, Hirschel B, Luthy R. HIV-associated primary pulmonary hypertension. A case control study. Swiss HIV Cohort Study. Am J Respir Crit Care Med. 1997;155:990–5.

105. Alter HJ, Eichberg JW, Masur H, Saxinger WC, Gallo R, Macher AM, Lane HC, Fauci AS. Transmission of HTLV-III infection from human plasma to chimpanzees: an animal model for AIDS. Science. 1984;226:549–52.

106. Daniel MD, Letvin NL, King NW, Kannagi M, Sehgal PK, Hunt RD, Kanki PJ, Essex M, Desrosiers RC. Isolation of T-cell tropic HTLV-III-like retrovirus from macaques. Science. 1985;228:1201–4.

107. Benveniste RE, Morton WR, Clark EA, Tsai CC, Ochs HD, Ward JM, Kuller L, Knott WB, Hill RW, Gale MJ, et al. Inoculation of baboons and macaques with simian immunodeficiency virus/Mne, a primate lentivirus closely related to human immunodeficiency virus type 2. J Virol. 1988;62:2091–101.

108. O'Connor DH, Mothe BR, Weinfurter JT, Fuenger S, Rehrauer WM, Jing P, Rudersdorf RR, Liebl ME, Krebs K, Vasquez J, Dodds E, Loffredo J, Martin S, McDermott AB, Allen TM, Wang C, Doxiadis GG, Montefiori DC, Hughes A, Burton DR, Allison DB, Wolinsky SM, Bontrop R, Picker LJ, Watkins DI. Major histocompatibility complex class I alleles associated with slow simian immunodeficiency virus disease progression bind epitopes recognized by dominant acute-phase cytotoxic-T-lymphocyte responses. J Virol. 2003;77:9029–40.

109. Hahn BH, Shaw GM, De Cock KM, Sharp PM. AIDS as a zoonosis: scientific and public health implications. Science. 2000;287:607–14.

110. Baskin GB, Martin LN, Rangan SR, Gormus BJ, Murphey-Corb M, Wolf RH, Soike KF. Transmissible lymphoma and simian acquired immunodeficiency syndrome in rhesus monkeys. J Natl Cancer Inst. 1986;77:127–39.

111. George MP, Brower A, Kling H, Shipley T, Kristoff J, Reinhart TA, Murphey-Corb M, Gladwin MT, Champion HC, Morris A, Norris KA. Pulmonary vascular lesions are common in SIV- and SHIV-env-infected macaques. AIDS Res Hum Retroviruses. 2011;27:103–11.

112. George MP, Champion HC, Simon M, Guyach S, Tarantelli R, Kling HM, Brower A, Janssen C, Murphy J, Carney JP, Morris A, Gladwin MT, Norris KA. Physiologic changes in a nonhuman primate model of HIV-associated pulmonary arterial hypertension. Am J Respir Cell Mol Biol. 2013;48:374–81.

113. Spikes L, Dalvi P, Tawfik O, Gu H, Voelkel NF, Cheney P, O'Brien-Ladner A, Dhillon NK. Enhanced pulmonary arteriopathy in simian immunodeficiency virus-infected macaques exposed to morphine. Am J Respir Crit Care Med. 2012;185:1235–43.

114. Marecki JC, Cool CD, Parr JE, Beckey VE, Luciw PA, Tarantal AF, Carville A, Shannon RP, Cota-Gomez A, Tuder RM, Voelkel NF, Flores SC. HIV-1 Nef is associated with complex pulmonary vascular lesions in SHIV-nef-infected macaques. Am J Respir Crit Care Med. 2006;174:437–45.

The Cardiopulmonary Hemodynamic Evaluation of Pulmonary Hypertension

11

Yonatan Buber and Alexander R. Opotowsky

Introduction

Pulmonary hypertension (PHT), elevated pulmonary artery pressure, is a clinical finding that can be caused by diverse pathophysiological and hemodynamic causes related to a wide array of clinical conditions. In recognition of the various contributors to its development, PHT is currently categorized into five clinical groups with specific characteristics [1–6]. These distinctions are largely, although not entirely, based on hemodynamic data. In addition to addressing the pathophysiologic basis for each sub-type of PHT, this classification also aims to guide the treating clinician in diagnosis, risk stratification, and therapy of PHT.

The term PHT refers simply to elevated pulmonary artery pressure. Normal mean pulmonary artery pressure (mPAP) at rest is ~14±3 mmHg, with an upper limit of normal ~20 mmHg [7, 8]. Although the presence of PHT may be initially suspected using noninvasive studies such as echocardiography, PHT is defined as a mean pulmonary artery pressure (mPAP) >25 mmHg at rest assessed by right heart catheterization (RHC) [9–11]. The prevalence of each subgroup of PHT is not well defined, but left heart disease (World Health Organization Group 2) is the most common cause, likely followed by lung disease (World Health Organization Group 3) [12].

As noted above, definitive diagnosis requires invasive hemodynamic assessment with cardiac catheterization. In addition to establishing the diagnosis of PHT, hemodynamic evaluation provides data on pathophysiology, disease severity and prognosis. Catheterization also provides objective data on therapeutic response for patients with known PHT.

Many tests play an important role in the diagnosis and assessment of PHT, including the electrocardiogram, laboratory testing, nuclear imaging, cardiopulmonary CT angiography, and cardiovascular magnetic resonance. There are also important hemodynamic concepts and relationships, such as ventriculo-arterial coupling that are not commonly addressed in clinical evaluation [13]. In this chapter, we focus on the current clinical hemodynamic evaluation of PHT, which depends predominantly on 3 tests: physical examination, transthoracic echocardiography and invasive catheterization. We discuss cardinal indices for each modality and provide clinical context for interpretation.

Physical Examination for Hemodynamic Evaluation of Pulmonary Hypertension

The general examination can direct attention to systemic causes of PHT but our focus will be on its role in providing indirect and direct insight into the current hemodynamics of PHT. Pallor may suggest severe anemia causing high pulmonary blood flow, which itself can result in PHT. The pattern of breathing is usually normal, but may be helpful in suggesting one or another cause (e.g., Cheyne-Stokes respirations in severe left heart failure, pursed lip breathing with chronic obstructive lung disease). Lung sounds are normal with pulmonary arterial hypertension; 'wet' crackles suggest elevated left ventricular end diastolic pressure, while 'dry' inspiratory crackles may point towards interstitial lung disease [14]. Hepatomegaly, elevated jugular venous pressure, peripheral edema, ascites and cool extremities are consistent with congestion and low output right heart failure, indicating more advanced disease.

Elevated jugular venous pressure can be seen in any type of PHT, whether due to left heart disease or elevated pulmonary vascular resistance (PVR). Sustained elevation of the jugular

Y. Buber, MD
Department of Cardiology, Boston Children's Hospital and Brigham and Women's Hospital, Harvard Medical School, Boston, MA, USA

Heart Institute, Sheba Medical Center, Tel Aviv University Faculty of Medicine, Ramat Gan, Israel

Sackler Faculty of Medicine, Tel Aviv University, Tel Aviv, Israel

A.R. Opotowsky, MD, MPH, MMSc (✉)
Department of Cardiology, Boston Children's Hospital, Brigham and Women's Hospital and Harvard Medical School, 300 Longwood Avenue, Boston, MA 02115, USA
e-mail: sasha@tch.harvard.edu

© Springer International Publishing Switzerland 2016
B.A. Maron et al. (eds.), *Pulmonary Hypertension: Basic Science to Clinical Medicine*, DOI 10.1007/978-3-319-23594-3_11

venous pressure in response to external pressure applied to the abdomen (abdominojugular or hepatojugular reflux) is more specific for elevated left heart filling pressure but can also be seen in other settings. Abdominojugular reflux is provoked by applying consistent pressure over the right upper abdominal quadrant for at least 10 s. A sustained rise >3 cm in the venous pressure for at least 10–15 s is abnormal. The patient should refrain from holding his or her breath or performing a Valsalva maneuver (see below). Abdominojugular reflux is useful in predicting heart failure and a pulmonary arterial wedge pressure >15 mmHg [15], though its specificity for left heart failure in patients referred for evaluation of PHT is unknown.

Blood pressure response to the Valsalva maneuver is a sensitive and specific indicator of elevated left heart filling pressure [16]. The Valsalva maneuver is performed with the blood pressure cuff inflated ~10–15 mmHg above the systolic blood pressure. While the clinician is auscultating over the brachial artery, the semi recumbent patient is asked to perform a forced expiratory effort against a closed glottis casing increased intrathoracic pressure. A normal response consists of four phases:

Phase 1: there is a rise in the systolic blood pressure at the onset of Valsalva with audible Korotkoff sounds which usually last ~2–4 heart beats.

Phase 2: with continued Valsalva there is reduced venous return to the left heart with a decrease in stroke volume and pulse pressure and a decline in systolic blood pressure (observed by the disappearance of Korotkoff sounds); there is also reflex tachycardia.

Phase 3: after Valsalva release there is a sudden drop in the systolic blood pressure due to the decrease in the intrathoracic pressure.

Phase 4: after a delay, there increased systolic blood pressure ("overshoot" relative to baseline systolic pressure) accompanied by reflex decrease in heart rate due to an increase in the venous return, with re-appearance of Korotkoff sounds.

Two distinct abnormal blood pressure responses to the Valsalva maneuver can be recognized by sphygmomanometer: a sustained or square-wave response and absence of the phase 4 overshoot. The absent overshoot pattern may suggest decreased systolic function; the square-wave response indicates elevated left-heart filling pressure for any reason [17]. The Valsalva response can be quantified using the pulse amplitude ratio, though this is only possible with invasive monitoring or specialized technology (arterial applanation tonometry) which is not widely available. This ratio compares the minimum pulse pressure at the end of the strain phase with the maximum pulse pressure at the onset of the strain phase; a higher ratio is consistent with a square-wave response. Note that the response of heart rate to each phase of Valsalva is opposite to that seen for blood pressure (i.e., when blood pressure rises, heart rate decreases).

The cardiac examination includes palpation of the chest for heaves and thrills, as well as to define the size and character of the point of maximal impulse. The right ventricle (RV) is anteriorly positioned, directly behind the sternum and chest wall; a palpable 'right ventricular' heave or lift may be present when the RV is enlarged. This is best appreciated using the heel of the hand placed at the inferior left lower sternal border or with the finger tips just below the xiphoid process during normal inspiration. Auscultation may include a loud pulmonary component of the second heart sound (P2), a holosystolic murmur of tricuspid regurgitation, a decrescendo diastolic murmur of pulmonary regurgitation or a right-sided S3 gallop. Tricuspid regurgitation in the setting of markedly elevated RV systolic pressure and an enlarged RV may produce a laterally positioned high-pitched murmur reminiscent of mitral regurgitation. Augmentation of the murmur with inspiration differentiates the right-sided tricuspid from left-sided mitral regurgitant murmur.

Echocardiographic Hemodynamic Evaluation of Pulmonary Hypertension

Transthoracic echocardiography (TTE) is an integral part of both the initial workup and follow up in PHT regardless of etiology. It is also frequently used for screening patients at high risk of PHT, including patients with certain connective tissue disorders such as scleroderma, HIV or a family history of PHT. Combined with quantitative hemodynamic calculations (summarized in Table 11.1 and discussed in this section), TTE can provide clinically useful approximations of pulmonary vascular and right ventricle (RV) hemodynamics. Many important variables do not require calculations, including assessment of size and function of the RV and left ventricle (LV) as well as right and left atrial size [18].

Systolic Pulmonary Artery Pressure

Systolic pulmonary artery pressure (sPAP) is equal to RV systolic pressure in the absence of pulmonary valve stenosis or another cause of RV outflow tract or PA obstruction. RV systolic pressure, and therefore sPAP, can be estimated by addition of right atrial (RA) pressure (RAP) to the pressure gradient between the right chambers. The maximal systolic pressure gradient between the RV and RA can be estimated using the simplified modified Bernoulli equation:

$$\Delta P = 4\,v^2$$

where v is peak tricuspid regurgitant flow velocity (Fig. 11.1). Although widely accepted as a screening test, this method is only moderately accurate. While initial reports of TTE estimates of sPAP as compared with RHC suggested a correlation coefficient >0.9, larger subsequent research studies and reviews of clinical TTEs have reported a less robust association, with

Table 11.1 Variables used for echocardiographic hemodynamic evaluation

Variable	Criteria used
Elevated mean right atrial pressure/central venous pressure	Inferior vena cava dimension >2.1 cm and inferior vena cava inspiratory collapse < 50 % Prominent diastolic flow in the superior vena cava, hepatic veins or jugular veins Bulging of the atrial septum towards the left atrium
Systolic PA pressure	4 × (peak tricuspid valve regurgitation jet velocity)^2 + estimated right atrial pressure
Diastolic PA pressure	4 × (end diastolic pulmonic valve jet velocity)^2 + estimated right atrial pressure
	4 × (tricuspid valve regurgitation jet velocity at the time of pulmonary valve opening)^2 + right atrial pressure
Mean PA pressure	4 × (peak pulmonic valve regurgitation jet velocity)^2 + estimated right atrial pressure
	Mean tricuspid valve regurgitant pressure gradient + estimated right atrial pressure
	0.61 × PA systolic pressure + 2 mmHg
Pulmonary vascular resistance	$PVR = \dfrac{PASP}{RVOT\,VTI} + 3 \; if \; notch \; present$
Measures of right ventricular function	Myocardial perfusion index (Tei index): $\dfrac{ICT+IRV}{systolic\ ejection\ time}$
	Tricuspid annular plane systolic excursion (TAPSE): longitudinal distance traveled of lateral tricuspid annulus in apical 4-chamber view towards apex during systole
	Right ventricular fractional area change (RV-FAC): $\dfrac{end\text{-}diastolic\ area - end\text{-}systolic\ area \times 100}{end\text{-}diastolic\ area}$

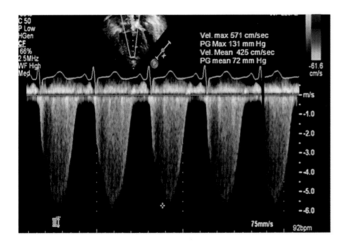

Fig. 11.1 Estimation of the systolic pulmonary arterial pressure (sPAP) using the simplified modified Bernoulli equation ($\Delta P = 4v^2$). Shown is the spectral continuous-wave Doppler signal of the tricuspid regurgitation corresponding to the right ventricular–right atrial pressure gradient. sPAP can be estimated using the sum of the estimated right atrial pressure and the peak RV-RA pressure gradient. In this example, SPAP is estimated at 131 (= 4 × 5.71^2) + central venous pressure, or 146 mmHg, if RAP is estimated at 15 mmHg, indicating severe pulmonary hypertension. The mean pulmonary arterial pressure can be calculated in a similar fashion using the mean systolic gradient based on TR velocity: 72 mmHg + assumed RAP of 15 mmHg = 87 mmHg

r ~ 0.7. Mean difference between TTE and RHC ranges from 3 to 40 mmHg, and sPAP may be underestimated by at least 20 mmHg in >30 % of patients; overestimation also occurs [19–22]. Causes of sPAP underestimation by TTE include inaccurate estimation of RAP (see below) and incomplete tricuspid regurgitation envelopes or incorrect determination of peak velocity. The probe incident angle must be meticulously

aligned with the tricuspid regurgitant jet to avoid underestimation. Respiratory variation adds additional (true) variability in sPAP. It is thus recommended that this velocity be measured in multiple views and the maximal velocity jet should be used for the calculation, especially when high sensitivity for PHT is the goal, such as when TTE is being used as a screening test. Fewer than 80 % of patients have a dependable TR envelope, however, and even patients with severe PHT may have little or no TR. Poor regurgitant signals can be enhanced with the use of contrast, either proprietary products or an agitated mix of air-blood-saline. In general, it is preferable to provide an accurate range of possible sPAP values based on expected variance rather than a single integer estimate that encourages unrealistic expectation of precision. An additional shortcoming of TTE for sPAP estimation is specific to patients with severe tricuspid regurgitation; since RAP increases during systole as the result of high volume TR, this technique may underestimate sPAP.

Despite technical limitations and only moderate correlation with invasive measurements, this approach to sPAP estimation is clinically useful and remains by far the most commonly applied TTE variable to evaluate right heart hemodynamics. There is certainly a role for using this measure in *screening* for suspected PHT and or in patients at high risk for PHT, as long as there is a fundamental understanding of the limitations inherent to the technique [23]. It must be highlighted that TTE sPAP estimates cannot diagnose PHT and this approach should never be used as a rationale to treat patients with selective pulmonary vasodilator medications or to monitor the efficacy of that therapy.

Various cut-offs have been proposed to screen for PHT. European guidelines for the diagnosis and treatment of PHT propose that PHT is "likely" if tricuspid regurgitation jet velocity is >3.4 m/s (or estimated sPAP is >50 mmHg) and "possible" when the velocity is between 2.9 and 3.4 m/s (or estimated sPAP is 37–50 mmHg), with or without additional echocardiographic signs suggestive of PHT, or when the velocity is ≤2.8 m/s (or sPAP is ≤36 mmHg) with additional variables suggestive of PHT [9]. This last point cannot be overemphasized adequately. TTE evaluation of PHT should neither start nor finish with sPAP estimation. Other guideline documents are less specific, suggesting that in the absence of other potential etiologies of PHT (e.g., left heart disease or advanced lung disease), an estimated RV systolic pressure >40 mmHg generally warrants further evaluation in the patient with unexplained dyspnea [10, 11].

Systolic PAP (in the absence of RV outflow obstruction) equals the pressure difference (gradient) between RA and RV during systole as estimated above plus the RAP. In the absence of obstruction, central venous pressure (CVP), RAP and RV end diastolic pressure (EDP) are essentially the same, and can be estimated, albeit with modest accuracy, by measuring size, flow patterns and the respiratory variation of the inferior vena cava (IVC) [20]. With normal RAP, systolic flow predominates. As right heart filling pressure increases, this pattern is blunted and the relation between systolic and diastolic flows may equalize or even reverse. Negative intrathoracic pressure, induced by a sniff or during normal respiration, causes flow from the abdominal IVC into the intrathoracic venous system causing "collapse" of the intrahepatic IVC. This collapse is blunted with elevated venous pressure, though it should be noted that without measurement of the shift in intrathoracic pressure the extent of expected collapse is difficult to predict. It has been proposed that IVC diameter <2.1 cm and collapse greater than 50 % on inspiration suggests normal RAP (0–5 mmHg). The presence of either greater diameter or lesser collapse (but not both) suggest mildly elevated RAP (~5–10 mmHg); diameter >2.1 cm with <50 % collapse suggests RAP>10 mmHg [24]. The precision of the cut-offs belies the modest clinical accuracy of these estimates [25]. This constitutes an important source of error when estimating PA pressure, and it is reasonable to instead use the estimate of right atrial pressure based on jugular venous findings on physical examination. The IVC can be enlarged for other reasons, such as with positive pressure ventilation and in highly trained athletes. Additional TTE markers of elevated RAP include: presence of prominent diastolic flow in the superior vena cava, hepatic veins or jugular veins); bulging of the intraatrial septum towards the left atrium; dilation of the coronary sinus; pericardial effusion; and tricuspid E/e' ratio >6 of the tricuspid inflow Doppler/ tricuspid annular tissue Doppler evaluation. Regardless of the method used for the evaluation of the RA pressure, jugular venous pressure estimates of experienced clinicians generally better estimate RA pressure than any TTE variable or combination of variables.

Mean Pulmonary Artery Pressure

Mean pulmonary arterial pressure (mPAP) can also be estimated with TTE. One advantage to estimating mPAP rather than sPAP is that PHT is defined based on mPAP. Possibly the simplest method of calculating the mean pulmonary arterial pressure (mPAP) is:

$$mPAP = 0.61 \times PA\ systolic\ pressure + 2\ mmHg\ [26].$$

For obvious reasons, this has little advantage to estimating sPAP and has the same limitations. While sPAP and mPAP are strongly correlated ($r^2 \sim 0.95$) this relationship varies with high stroke volume, and may be problematic in patients with high pulmonary stroke volume those with severe anemia or intracardiac left-to-right shunt. Considering the limitations mentioned above of evaluation of the sPAP using the tricuspid regurgitation velocity jet, alternative methods have been developed in an aim to provide a more accurate assessment of the mPAP.

Method 1: Use of the Pulmonary Valve Regurgitation Jet

The pulmonary regurgitation Doppler velocity pattern is characterized by a rapid rise immediately after the closure of the pulmonary valve and a gradual deceleration until the end of diastole. The pulmonary regurgitation velocity corresponds to the diastolic pressure gradient between the PA and RV through diastole (i.e., both the velocity and gradient decline). The peak pulmonary regurgitation velocity at the start of diastole reflects the pressure gradient between the PA and RV the start of diastole. Application of the modified simplified Bernoulli equation to peak pulmonary regurgitation velocity (Fig. 11.2) with the addition of estimated RAP provides a reasonable estimate of mPAP [27]. Pulmonary regurgitation envelopes are often incomplete or absent, however, precluding this approach in many patients. Further, since the mPAP is lower than the sPAP, an inaccurate RAP estimate has a proportionally greater impact on mPAP estimates. Thus, while this method can be useful qualitatively to confirm sPAP estimates or when the TR envelope is of poor quality, it is not generally as robust or as commonly used.

Method 2: RV-RA Mean Systolic Gradient

The mean RV-RA systolic gradient can be derived from the Doppler profile of the tricuspid regurgitation (Fig. 11.1). The sum of this estimate and estimated RAP correlates with RHC mPAP [28]. This method depends on the presence a pristine complete tricuspid regurgitation Doppler envelope; in that situation, it has the advantage of 'averaging the error' of measurement over systole compared with a quadratic function a single velocity.

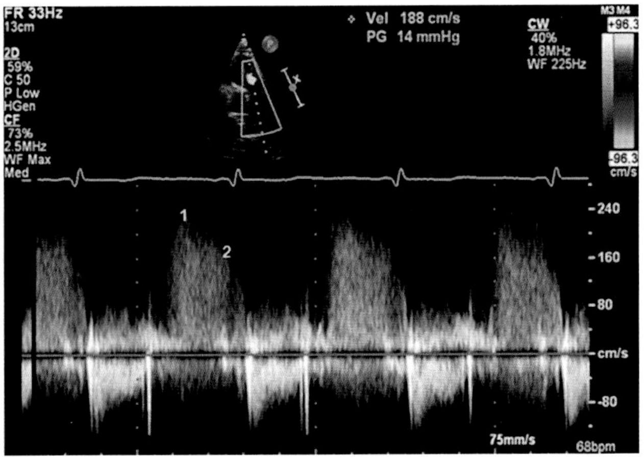

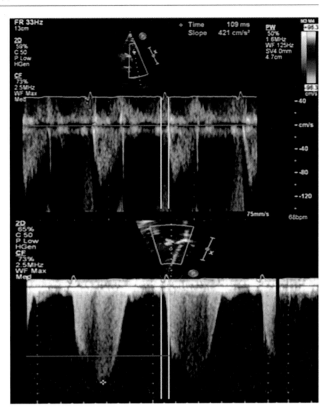

Fig. 11.2 Doppler echocardiographic estimation of mean pulmonary artery pressure (mPAP) and diastolic PA pressure by continuous-wave Doppler signal of pulmonary regurgitation. *Point 1* marks the maximal pulmonary regurgitation velocity at the beginning of diastole. Mean PA pressure correlates with 4 * (early PR velocity)^2 + estimated RAP, in this example 21 mmHg + RAP. *Point 2* marks the diastolic PR velocity at the onset of atrial contraction. PA diastolic pressure is estimated by 4 *(end PR velocity ~ 1.6 m/s)^2 + estimated RAP. In this example, PA diastolic pressure is ~10 mmHg + RAP. Note that the point selected in this case is actually not truly at end diastole but rather before the A wave. Depending on how RAP is estimated and the magnitude of the A wave pressure augmentation (which can be large in a patient with good atrial function and a stiff RV), there can be marked variation in the correct RAP estimate for this calculation. Also notable is the presence of respiratory variation

Method 3: Calculation from the Systolic and the Diastolic Pressures

The third method consists of estimating the PA systolic and diastolic pressures (see below) and calculating mPAP value using a standard equation:

$$mPAP = \frac{(2 \times dPAP + sPAP)}{3}$$

Where dPAP denotes diastolic PA pressure.

Diastolic Pulmonary Artery Pressure

Two noninvasive echocardiographic methods can be utilized to evaluate the diastolic pulmonary artery pressure (dPAP): the first consists of evaluation of the end-diastolic PA-RV gradient and the second consists of assessment of the RV pressure at the time of pulmonary valve opening. Of course, these events are essentially simultaneous and both correspond to end diastole.

Method 1: Use of End-Diastolic PA-RV Gradient

The end diastolic PA-RV pressure gradient can be estimated by applying the modified simplified Bernoulli equation to the end-diastolic pulmonary regurgitation velocity (Fig. 11.2). Adding the RAP to this calculation

Fig. 11.3 Diastolic PA pressure may be estimated by the Doppler velocity of tricuspid regurgitation at the time of pulmonary valve opening. Transpulmonary flow (*top*) and tricuspid regurgitant flow (*bottom*). It is apparent that very small errors in measurement of timing (whether by measurement or changes in heart rate) may result in important error. *Yellow lines*: time between Q wave and pulmonary valve opening. *Blue line*: TR velocity at the time of pulmonary valve opening

estimates dPAP; in research settings this correlates well with invasive dPAP measurements in select patients [29, 30]. As with tricuspid regurgitation, inadequate pulmonary regurgitant Doppler signals can be enhanced with the use of contrast or air-blood-saline mixture. The limitations described for mPAP Method 1 estimation apply here as well.

Method 2: RV Pressure Assessment at the Time of the Pulmonary Valve Opening

RV end diastolic pressure equals PA pressure at the moment of pulmonary valve opening. Given that the gradient between the RV and RA can be estimated by the velocity of the tricuspid valve regurgitant jet, applying the simplified Bernoulli at the time of pulmonary valve opening and adding the RAP to this value allows an estimation of dPAP [31]. The tricuspid valve regurgitant velocity Doppler sign needs to be aligned with the time from the QRS complex to the onset of pulmonary flow on the regurgitation velocity envelope (Fig. 11.3). While this method requires more effort and practice to allow reproducible demarcation of timing, it does correlated reasonably well with invasively measured dPAP in the research setting [31, 32].

Pulmonary Vascular Resistance

As will be further elaborated in the section discussing the invasive hemodynamic study, pulmonary vascular resistance (PVR) is a critical variable in understanding PHT physiology and appropriate management. PVR cannot be directly measured by TTE or RHC, and rather is estimated as a function of transpulmonary gradient and pulmonary blood flow.

Several methods have been proposed to estimate PVR with TTE. The first such technique consists of determining the ratio between the tricuspid regurgitation velocity and the velocity time integral of flow across the pulmonary annulus/RV outflow tract [33]. This ratio corresponds, with important exceptions, to the ratio of transpulmonary gradient to the cardiac output at the pulmonary bed used to estimate PVR by RHC. An equation was proposed to estimate PVR (in Wood units):

$$PVR = 10 \times \frac{TTFV}{RVOTVTI} + 0.16$$

In the initial report, TTFV to RVOT VTI ratio < 0.2 predicted PVR < 2 WU with 70 % sensitivity and 94 % specificity [33]. In a study of patients with cirrhosis, a ratio > 0.12 had 100 % sensitivity and negative predictive value for the detection of PVR > 1.5 WU; all patients with ratios < 0.12 could safely proceed to liver transplantation without the need for invasive hemodynamic assessment to exclude portopulmonary hypertension [34]. This method has several notable limitations. First, it does not account for the quadratic relationship between TTFV and pressure, and therefore markedly underestimates high PVR. Second, TTFV estimates of PA pressure do not reflect transpulmonary gradient (mPAP-PAWP). The accuracy of this method and others like it is unclear in patients with very high PAWP. Finally, the ratio does not have an intuitive interpretation and the equation to estimate true PVR (multiplying by 10 and then adding a small constant) is also not intuitive.

A modification of this approach was developed empirically and involved a ratio of estimated PA pressure to velocity time integral of flow across the pulmonary valve [35]:

$$PVR = \frac{PASP}{RVOT\,VTI} + 3 \ \ if \ \ notch \ \ present$$

Of note, there a constant of +3 is added if there is notching of the RVOT Doppler envelope (see below). This equation is slightly more accurate than the original approach and is easier to apply in clinical practice [36].

There are several other techniques listed below. While all are reasonable, they require additional calculation and are less useful in a busy clinical practice.

A third method consists of measuring the ratio between sPAP and velocity time integral at the RVOT corrected for heart rate [37]. Compared with the tricuspid regurgitation velocity and the velocity time integral index, this ratio takes into account RAP and heart rate. When evaluated in a population with PHT and high PVR versus invasive measurement of PVR, it was found that a cutoff value of 0.076 had 86 % sensitivity and 82 % specificity in determining indexed PVR > 15 resistance units.

A fourth technique consists of measuring the pre-ejection period (the time between the onset of tricuspid regurgitation and the onset of pulmonary systolic flow), the time interval between the onset of ejection and the time of peak flow velocity, or AcT), and total systolic time (the sum of the pre-ejection period and pulmonary ejection time) [38].

A final method is to estimate each component of PVR (mPAP, PAWP, pulmonary flow) using a set of different validated equations and then calculate PVR. This is appealing, and might be expected to provide more accurate estimates. Given the inaccuracy of TTE PAWP and pulmonary flow estimates, however, the resulting data are disappointing. Because of the labor involved and lack of incremental benefit, this method is of limited clinical relevance.

Ancillary Findings: Status of Right and Left Heart Chambers

Severe PHT causes RV and RA dilatation, RV dysfunction, abnormal ventricular septal motion, coronary sinus dilation and pericardial effusion [39]. Many of these findings are apparent only with severe disease, and may not reflect good variables for PHT screening; abnormal septal motion is an exception. Furthermore, right heart findings are not perfectly correlated to the severity of pulmonary vascular disease and are a function of multiple factors such as disease etiology, speed of disease progression, presence of tricuspid regurgitation, co-existing right coronary disease, other associated cardiac and vascular morbidities, and, presumably, genetic predisposition. Many of these findings may improve after initiation of pulmonary vasodilator therapy, and routine echocardiographic follow up is also indicated to monitor the effects of such treatment [9–11]. These data taken in conjunction with change in patient symptom burden and 6 min walk distance constitute the core variables used to assess adequacy of medical therapy for pulmonary arterial hypertension.

Right Atrial Dimensions
RA dimensions, including diameter and area, measured in the four chamber apical view should be measured. RA area >20 cm^2 is considered abnormal and area >27 cm^2 portends poor prognosis among patients with pulmonary arterial hypertension [40].

Right Ventricular Indexes
It is well recognized that the RV is more challenging to assess with TTE than the LV because of its heavier trabecula-

tions, and complicated geometry with the presence of an infundibulum. The initial physiologic response of the RV to pressure overload often includes dilatation. The apical four chamber view provides the most comprehensive view of the ventricle, though no single view is adequate (Fig. 11.4). A dilated RV often assumes a more globular shape, compared to the usual triangular appearance in the apical view. The ratio between the diastolic inflow diameters and areas of the RV and the LV correlates with the degree of RV dilatation: an area ratio ranging from 0.6–1 typically indicates mild RV dilation, while severe RV dilation is associated with a ratio > 1 [41]. Despite various attempts to quantify RV size, however, this remains a notable weakness of TTE evaluation of PHT.

Estimation of RV function may be accomplished via several methods. Percentage RV fractional area change (FAC),

defined as [(end-diastolic area − end-systolic area)/end-diastolic area] × 100, is a measure of RV systolic function that has been shown to correlate with RV ejection fraction (EF) by magnetic resonance imaging (MRI) [42, 43]. RV FAC is an independent predictor of heart failure, sudden death, stroke, and/or mortality in patients after pulmonary embolism [44] and myocardial infarction [45, 46]. FAC is obtained by tracing the RV endocardium in systole and diastole from the annulus to the apex along the free wall (below the trabeculations), and then back to the annulus along the ventricular septum. The lower reference value for normal RV FAC is ~35 % [24]. Complex RV geometry, however, limits the accuracy of any 2D technique. 3 dimensional TTE is promising, but not yet widely available. Assessment of the RV myocardial performance index, also known as the Tei index, is an alternative, non-geometric approach. This index is defined as the ratio of the isovolumic contraction time plus isovolumic relaxation time to systolic ejection time [47]. With progressive ventricular dysfunction, ejection constitutes a shorter portion of this time period. In pediatric idiopathic PHT, RV performance index is closely related with invasive mPAP and that it can be used to monitor mPAP after initiation of medical therapy [48]. A smaller study conducted in patients with connective tissue disease demonstrated that a myocardial performance index > 0.36 combined with sPAP ≥ 35 mmHg may improve TTE accuracy in predicting PHT. The Tei index has also been shown to have important prognostic implications: in a series of 53 PHT patients, an elevated Tei index was associated with an increased risk of clinical events and death [49]. One important caveat to use of this method in monitoring to response to therapy may be its relative independence to changes in afterload [50]. The Tei index is less commonly used in clinical practice, perhaps because of its lack of direct correspondence to any single physiologic parameter and unintuitive interpretation.

RV contraction has a predominantly longitudinal component (as opposed to torsion of the LV), and simply measuring the distance travelled by the tricuspid annulus during contraction provides a reasonable estimate of RV function [9]. This measurement is termed tricuspid annular plane systolic excursion (TAPSE) and is usually measured by M-mode echocardiography of the lateral tricuspid annulus (though it can be estimated from 2D images) (Fig. 11.5). Normal TAPSE is > 1.6–1.7 cm (though most normal people have TAPSE > 2–2.2 cm) and is reduced with RV dysfunction [51]. Low TAPSE (< 1.8 cm in one study) predicts increased risk of death in pulmonary arterial hypertension [52]. RV function also predicts outcome in patients with left heart failure. Important limitations to this method include its angle and load dependency, its focus on a single dimension of right ventricular motion and the fact that the tricuspid annular motion may be affected by overall heart motion [53].

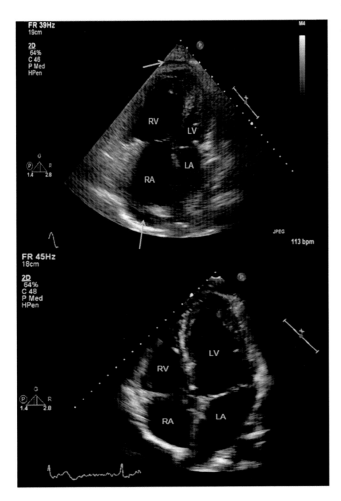

Fig. 11.4 Apical 4 chamber views of a normal size right ventricle and right atrium (*top*) and of a markedly enlarged right ventricle and right atrium in a patient with pulmonary arterial hypertension. Note the round shape assumed by the right ventricle in the bottom image as compared to the normal, crescent shape right ventricle in the top image. Also noted is the presence of a small pericardial effusion (*arrows*). *RV* right ventricle, *RA* right atrium, *LV* left ventricle, *LA* left atrium

Fig. 11.5 (**a**, **b**) Measurement of the tricuspid annular plane systolic excursion (TAPSE) by M-mode echocardiography. (**a**) Low TAPSE is reduced in the setting of pulmonary arterial hypertension related to systemic sclerosis. (**b**) A patient with chronic thromboembolic pulmonary hypertension but preserved RV function (TAPSE ~ 2.4 cm). Increasing brightness and contrast on M-Mode images can help define TAPSE

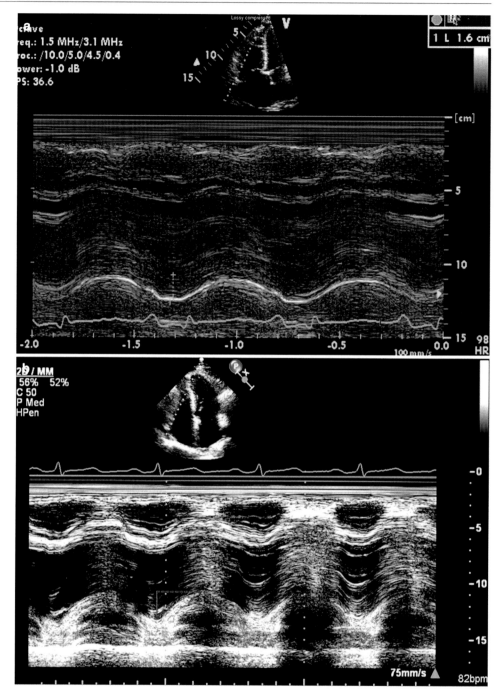

Morphology of the Pulmonary Flow Velocity Curve

The "domelike" morphology (parabolic curve) of Doppler pulmonary flow velocity in individuals with normal pulmonary pressure and resistance assumes a more "triangular" shape skewed towards late systole in patients with PHT (Fig. 11.6). Peak velocity appears during early ejection compared with mid-ejection in normal people. In some cases there is flow deceleration in mid systole followed by a second late-ejection increase in velocity, resulting in the appearance of mid-systolic notching [54, 55]. The pulmonary flow acceleration time (defined as the time interval from the onset of forward flow in the pulmonary artery to the peak velocity) is inversely related to sPAP, mPAP and PVR [56, 57]. Both notching and short acceleration time correspond to true late ejection flow deceleration secondary to reflected pressure waves; therefore, they are present in patients with elevated PVR and non-compliant pulmonary arteries but not in patients with PHT due to left heart disease.

Fig. 11.6 The pattern of systolic (ejection) flow across the pulmonary valve in a patient without (**a**) and with (**b**) pulmonary arterial hypertension. Acceleration time, the time between onset of flow and peak velocity, is normal (>100 ms) in the top example and there is a normal parabolic flow envelope. Three distinctive features of pulmonary arterial hypertension with elevated pulmonary vascular resistance are depicted on the bottom image: a more triangular shape of systolic flow skewed towards the end of systole, notching of the systolic flow (*orange arrow*) and short acceleration time of <80 milliseconds (*red lines*)

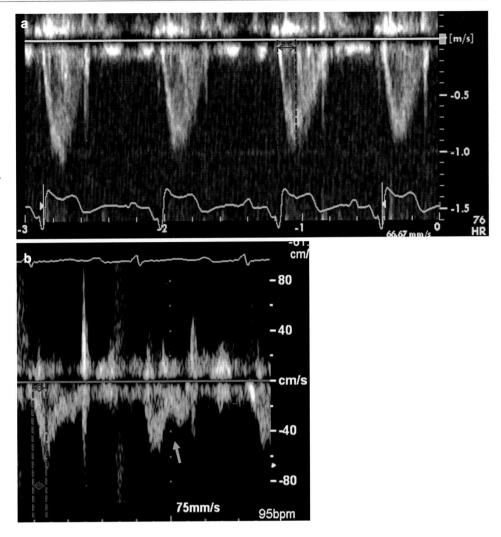

Impact on the Left Heart and Cardiac Output

By altering RV size and geometry PHT may cause compression of the left heart chambers, resulting in impaired LV filling (preload limitation) and reduced cardiac output [39, 58, 59]. LV compression can be quantified using the eccentricity index, the ratio of anterior-inferior to septal-lateral short axis dimensions of the left ventricle, both in diastole and in systole [60]. Eccentricity index is assessed on the two-dimensional short-axis view of the LV (Fig. 11.7). Late systolic septal flattening (systolic eccentricity index >1) is a sensitive marker of elevated RV impedance, largely as the result of prolonged RV contraction [61]. The consequently abnormal LV filling can be assessed by the evaluating the Doppler appearance of the mitral inflow, with E < A velocities (Grade I "diastolic dysfunction") [39]. Compression of the LV cavity with limited ventricular diastolic filling is associated with worse prognosis in patients with PHT [62].

Additional Findings Associated with PHT

Coronary sinus dilation suggests elevated RAP in the absence of alternative explanation (e.g., left superior vena cava draining to the coronary sinus). The presence of a pericardial effusion (Fig. 11.4) has similar pathophysiology and has important prognostic implications [63]. Such pericardial effusions are rarely hemodynamically important in patients with severe pulmonary arterial hypertension; pericardiocentesis is contraindicated as it often has catastrophic consequences related to changes in RV geometry. This recommendation does not apply to patients with other forms of PHT or mild PAH with alternative causes for pericardial effusion. Right-to-left shunting through a patent foramen ovale can be present at rest or with exercise. This causes hypoxemia unresponsive to O_2 supplementation. The diagnosis can be confirmed by intravenous injection of agitated saline or proprietary contrast material can make this diagnosis and may explain hypoxemia observed in a subset of patients with PHT.

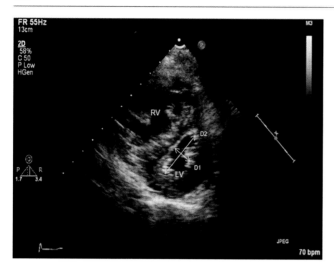

Fig. 11.7 Measurement of the eccentricity index. Normally, D2/D1 ratio approximates 1 throughout the cardiac cycle. In this example of a patient with pulmonary arterial hypertension, the ratio markedly >1 in this late systolic frame. Of note, less prominent end diastolic ventricular septal flattening is often present among patients with elevated PA impedance in the absence of any volume loading of the right ventricle. *RV* right ventricle, *LV* left ventricle

Invasive Hemodynamic Assessment of PHT

Preparation of the Patient for Cardiac Catheterization

Patients are usually asked to fast for at least 4–6 h prior to catheterization, though this is not absolutely necessary if administration of sedative agents is not planned. A peripheral intravenous line should be placed if sedation will be administered or if the patient is considered to be at elevated risk for adverse events. Most chronic medications should be continued as prescribed, including pulmonary vasodilators. It is reasonable to hold a diuretic dose on the morning of a catheterization in stable patients. There is variability in the approach to oral anticoagulant use. While continuing anticoagulants is associated with increased bleeding risk, the absolute risk of serious bleeding from venous catheterization is low even with therapeutic anticoagulation. We generally continue warfarin without change in regimen, and proceed with RHC as long as INR is <3. The INR should not be supratherapeutic, however, as this increases risk with no benefit. The risk-benefit calculus will vary depending on the indication for anticoagulation. For example, uninterrupted anticoagulation is strongly merited in the presence of a mechanical mitral valve but is less important if the indication is primary prevention of stroke in the setting atrial fibrillation. The approach to newer anticoagulants must be similarly approached, though in general holding doses prior is reasonable for most patients, with the duration depending on the specific pharmacokinetics of the drug, and will undoubtedly

evolve as more experience is accrued with these agents. The timing for discontinuation of dabigatran prior to the catheterization procedure varies by kidney function and bleeding risk; for patients with glomerular filtration rate >60 ml/min and a low bleeding risk it is reasonable to hold the medication for 24 h prior to the procedure. This time frame is also recommended for patients at low bleeding risk treated with rivaroxaban and apixaban, regardless of their kidney function. Aspirin or other oral antiplatelet agents can usually be continued without interruption, though those on dual antiplatelet therapy are at increased risk for bleeding. Given a small risk for lactic acidosis, patients taking metformin and scheduled for an elective procedure during which intravenous iodinated contrast material may be administered should hold this medication the morning of the procedure and restart after renal function is confirmed to be stable for at least 48 h after the procedure if contrast is used [64]. Other considerations include allergies, especially to heparin or latex which may require use of different techniques and equipment.

We believe that conscious sedation (e.g., intravenous benzodiazepines or opiates) prior to or during the catheterization procedure should not be routine but rather should be considered on an individual basis. While providers vary in their use of sedation, in the absence of severe anxiety diagnostic RHC is usually tolerated without subjective distress. Conversely, although some prior studies have raised the concern that administrating systemic sedation to patients with PAH may be associated with adverse outcomes [65], the risk is likely small in hemodynamically stable patients unless liver or kidney function is impaired. An additional downside to sedation is that patients must be monitored for a more extended period after the procedure if sedation is administered; this is inconvenient for patients and requires additional resources. Another reason for avoiding systemic sedation is the potential effect on the patient's hemodynamic profile during catheterization. There are two potential mechanisms: first, administration may result in systemic hypotension [66] leading to unrepresentative (low relative to the unsedated state) readings of certain variables, such as LV end diastolic pressure; second, benzodiazepines have a variable negative inotropic effect with resulting worsening RV function, an effect that has been shown in patients with pre-existing LV diastolic dysfunction [67]. These effects are usually not clinically apparent or relevant but the lack of benefit from routine sedation makes the potential for even minor or rare adverse effects unacceptable. Indirect effects via respiratory inhibition with subsequent hypercapnia can also affect hemodynamic values.

If mechanical ventilation is clinically indicated, the potential associated hemodynamic effects must be considered. There is often an increase in RV afterload and decline in RV contractility, along with a number of other effects. With the use of positive end expiratory pressure (PEEP), positive intrathoracic pressure is variably transmitted to the central circulation, thus affecting right-sided pressures (especially during forced inspiration) [68–70]. The extent to which PEEP affects right-sided pressures is unpredictable and depends on various variables: baseline filling pressure, compliance of the chest wall, lung and of cardiac chamber compliance, and intravascular/cardiac volume status. There is no universal adjustment to account for the effect of PEEP on the PAWP, but PEEP < 10 cm H_2O does not importantly affect PAWP [70]. For values above that, one suggested correction is that PAWP rises ~2–3 cm for every 5 cm H_2O increment in PEEP [71]. To avoid unnecessary uncertainty, PEEP should be maintained as low as clinically reasonable.

A second alteration to be considered is an inaccurately elevated PAWP reading due to unexpected lung zone position of the catheter tip. In the upright position, lung zone 3 is located at the base of the lung, where alveolar pressure is lower than both pulmonary arterial and pulmonary venous pressure; position of the catheter tip in zone 3 allows pressure transmission directly from the left atrium to the wedged catheter tip. Under normal conditions, lung zone 3 is where the PAWP accurately reflects left atrial pressure [70]. With mechanical ventilation, the catheter tip is less likely to be located in zone 3, since alveolar pressure is increased and zone 3 accounts for a smaller portion of the lung. Use of PEEP and hypovolemia exacerbate this. Demonstrating that the catheter tip is below the level of the left atrium suggests zone 3 location [72]. Note that when the patient is supine, one cannot confirm position with AP imaging, since zone 3 is posterior to, not inferior/caudal to, the left atrium. It is reasonable to obtain hemodynamic measurements in various pulmonary segments, preferably in both the right and left lungs, to support the assertion that any single measurement is representative of underlying hemodynamics.

Percutaneous Access Sites and Catheter Choice

All roads lead to Rome and all systemic veins lead to the heart; therefore, any systemic vein could be used for venous access. Considerations as to optimal access sites include size of the vein, ease of vascular access, directness of course from access site to right heart, and requirements for monitoring after sheath removal.

The most common access sites used in catheterization for hemodynamic assessment of PHT are the femoral vein and the right internal jugular vein (IJ). The right IJ is preferred unless there is planned concomitant femoral arterial access or specific procedures (e.g., probing for PFO) are expected. Access via the left internal jugular vein or left subclavian vein does not provide as direct a catheter course, but is reasonable when right IJ access is not a good option (e,g., thrombosis). Proximal arm veins can also be used for

venous access. This is commonly the favored approach when radial arterial access is used for a simultaneous left heart catheterization, but it limits catheter size and manipulation. Several groups have reported on their experience with the IJ access technique in large groups of patients; when performed by experienced personnel, IJ access is quick (<15 min) and associated with a very low complication rate (1–1.7 %); hemostasis can be rapidly achieved and patients (in the absence of sedation) can be discharged directly following the procedure in most cases [73, 74].To facilitate both cannulation success and speed, 2D ultrasound guidance may be used to locate the IJ and adjacent carotid artery. Ultrasound guidance is especially encouraged when technical difficulties are suspected (i.e. patients with short or thick neck) or when difficulties are encountered at the time of the procedure. Potential complications with IJ access are uncommon and include pulmonary hemorrhage, pneumothorax, carotid puncture, sinus bradycardia (vasovagal, usually transient and responsive to fluid; rarely requiring atropine administration) and complete heart block (especially in setting of pre-existing left bundle branch block). When considering catheter advancement to the pulmonary artery, one should keep in mind that IJ access will usually lead the catheter to the right PA, whereas femoral access will more commonly lead to catheter position in the left PA. When femoral venous catheterization is performed, patients are usually observed in the supine position for at least 2 h following removal of the sheath to ensure adequate venous hemostasis prior to ambulation. In the setting of active anticoagulation or a larger sheath, observation may be extended. Vascular closure devices, such as the Perclose ProGlide Suture-Mediated Closure System (Abbot Vascular, USA) can decrease bleeding time and access site complications. Sheath size is typically required to be 5 French or larger when using closure devices, and other contraindications should be checked with the manufacturer prior to usage. In the authors opinion, the internal jugular approach is preferable when no other interventions are planned, as it allows easier catheter manipulation through the right ventricular outflow tract and into the pulmonary arteries and, barring complications, the patient can be discharged home soon after sheath removal.

When deciding upon access site in a given patient, historical data regarding prior venous and arterial access and potential obstructions, compressions, complex anatomical courses and prior procedural complications should be obtained. Patients with kidney disease on hemodialysis, congenital heart disease, pacemakers, or indwelling chronic venous access for other reasons (e.g., intravenous prostanoids) are more likely to have had multiple prior procedures and vascular injury or thrombosis. Imaging of the vascular bed may be established by various modalities including ultrasound, computed tomography and magnetic resonance angiography.

The quality of hemodynamic data depends on an array of variables. First, the quality of tracings depends on the frequency response of the fluid filled catheter system. Frequency response is directly proportional to the size of the lumen and inversely related to length of tubing. Thus, optimal tracings are obtained with catheters with large lumens and minimal excess tubing.

Of note, the external diameter of the catheter is not always indicative of lumen size. A large catheter with multiple ports (e.g., 8 F catheter with RA, thermodilution and PA ports) will often have slower frequency response than a smaller single port catheter (e.g., 6 F single lumen catheter). Frequency response is generally <12 Hz [75]. Selection of catheter balances the risk associated with larger access sheath (albeit a very small risk), benefits of additional ports or technologies (e.g., ability to perform thermodilution cardiac output estimates) and quality of hemodynamic tracings.

Catheters with end holes are necessary to measure occlusion (wedge) pressures and for sampling pressures within small chambers or when discerning pressure gradients over short distances. While catheters with side holes are preferable to measure intra-cardiac pressures to prevent erroneous readings due to damping effect resulting from obstruction of the catheter tip by cardiac tissue this is a modest concern and issues are recognizable (blunted waveforms) and can be addressed with catheter repositioning. Generally only in the context of congenital heart disease are side-ports truly needed for this reason.

A "Swan-Ganz" catheter is commonly used for measuring right-heart pressures when thermodilution is considered for evaluation of the cardiac output (see below). In addition to the balloon at the tip for flotation, it consists of an end-hole port, a side-hole port 30 cm from the catheter tip, and a thermistor for measurement of cardiac output by the thermodilution method. Other balloon flotation catheters include: the Berman catheter, which includes multiple side-holes near the tip and no end hole or thermistor and is used mainly for angiography; catheters with an RV side port to allow a pacing via a temporary pacemaker wire; and the balloon-wedge catheter, which contains an end-hole similar to the Swan-Ganz catheter but no thermistor for cardiac output measurement or additional infusion or pressure monitoring ports [70].

It is not infrequent that coronary anatomy also must be visualized during catheterization to assess PHT. The reasons for this may be numerous: evaluation of the coronary anatomy as part of surgical planning, evaluation for a coronary fistula to the right sided chambers as a possible source of left to right shunt, evaluation of atherosclerotic coronary artery disease as a possible reason for impaired LV function or elevated filling pressure, and evaluation of the anatomic relations between the coronary arteries and the pulmonary arteries for specific procedures (e.g., percutaneous prosthetic pulmonary valve implantation). This is not part of the hemodynamic evaluation of PHT and will not be further detailed. There is debate on the additive value of left heart catheterization to the hemodynamic evaluation of PHT. PAWP and LV end diastolic pressure usually differ by a small amount though sometimes may vary by >5 mmHg [76, 77]. Use of strict cut-offs for diagnosis (e.g., PAWP > 15 mmHg) highlights the possible importance of this difference. While some have used this to suggest that LVEDP should be measured directly, PAWP may be a better indicator of pulmonary venous pressure through the entire cardiac cycle in most situations including for patients with mitral valve disease. However, the issue is probably less the measurements and more the false assertion that any single dichotomous cut-off reflects true physiology and diagnosis. Direct measurement of LVEDP is indicated in a small subset of patients but should not be used in routine evaluation of PHT both because of limited additive data in the context of real additional risk, patient inconvenience, and resource use.

Equipment Selection and Specialized Techniques for Hemodynamic Catheterization

Table mounted fluid-filled pressure transducers are currently used by most catheterization laboratories. The pressure wave is transmitted through the fluid-filled catheter to a membrane in the transducer; this alters membrane configuration via oscillatory waves, resulting in a change in electrical resistance. The electrical signal is transmitted to a computer, which in turn converts the signal to temporal pressure data and provides a graphic representation of the pressure over time. These transducers usually arrive precalibrated but the accuracy of this calibration must be confirmed prior to the procedure. It is important to establish a standardized physiologic reference point for subsequent pressure measurements ("zeroing") before measurements are made. Based on experimental data, the patient's midchest is often used, as this site approximates the location of the right atrium. Significant pressure changes and erroneous readings can be caused by improper transducer location and misidentification of the zero point; a transducer placed above the true zero position will lead to falsely low measured pressure reading, while a transducer placed below the true zero position will result in a falsely high pressure measurements. Of note, pressure gradients are not affected by such error. Although widely accepted, the practice of transducer placement at the mid-chest level has been repeatedly challenged as it has been shown to result in systematic overestimation of the intracardiac pressures due to hydrostatic effects, thus producing physiologically significant error in the measurement of diastolic intracardiac pressure [78–80]. A more accurate yet time consuming method consists of aligning the external fluid-filled transducer with the uppermost blood level in the chamber in which pressure is to be measured (as assessed by fluoroscopy or echocardiography), a method that highlights the fact that the only factor that contributes to measured hydrostatic pressure with a fluid-filled catheter system is the position of the transducer with respect to the uppermost fluid level in the container or chamber in which pressure is being measured [80].

Dissipation of the energy inside the pressure measuring system is called damping. Optimal damping is achieved by use of a short, wide-bore, non-compliant catheter system that is directly connected to the transducer with use of a low-density liquid from which all air bubbles have been removed [81]. Over-damping results in loss of high-frequency events, causing underestimation of the systolic pressure and overestimation of the diastolic pressure, while under-damping (sometimes called "ringing") results in narrow, sharp upstrokes of the pressure waves. Additional important potential sources of error include catheter whip artifacts (motion of the tip of the catheter within the measured chamber) and catheter tip obstruction within small vessels or valvular orifices occurring because of the size of the catheter itself. When pressure is measured head-on (not an issue in routine RHC), there can also be error related to kinetic force related to blood flow. Formation of small thrombi in catheters can cause changes in pressure contour, especially in catheters with small internal diameters. Thus, we encourage the practice of rebalancing the zero baseline during pressure evaluation at each chamber or vessel and intermittent catheter flushing with saline or heparinized saline in order to avoid this.

Pressure can be directly measured by using a small transducer (micromanometer) mounted at the tip of a catheter, thus avoiding the limitations of a fluid-filled system [82]. Frequency response is much better than with fluid filled systems and this detailed data can be used to understand pulsatile components of flow and generate impedance spectra. Micromanometer catheters are expensive and not routinely used during clinical RHC, but rather they form the basis of the pressure wire used for measurement of intracoronary pressures and are used for research studies.

In patients with a markedly enlarged right heart right atrium or severe tricuspid valve regurgitation, pulmonary valve regurgitation or abnormal right ventricular outflow tract anatomy (such as present in certain congenital heart diseases such as physiologically corrected transposition of the great arteries or tetralogy of Fallot), manipulation of the catheter from the RV to the main PA may pose a technical challenge. To reiterate, choice of venous access site plays a large role in ease of catheter positioning. In difficult situations, several methods can be used to facilitate the advancement of the catheter towards and through the RV to the PA:

- Instead of attempting to advance the catheter in a direct fashion from the RA to the RV and out to the PA, the catheter is directed towards the lateral wall of the right atrium and with the balloon inflated, it is gently pushed against its wall. This will loop the catheter in the atrium, with its tip directed downwards towards the tricuspid valve. This loop provides mechanical support and this may allow transit in the setting of a large atrium or tricuspid valve regurgitation. Once the catheter has been advanced into the RV, the tip is directed up towards the PA.
- The relatively soft shaft of an end-hole catheter makes it more challenging to torque. In that circumstance, a stiff wire with soft tip guide wire can be advanced through the tip of the catheter and maneuvered into the pulmonary artery. The wire is then advanced until its body is well past the orifice. Even a relatively stiff catheter will usually follow a guide wire when the stiff portion of the wire is positioned well distal to the proximal PA. An alternative, and often preferable, technique is to deflect the tip of the catheter toward, or even into, the orifice with an active deflector wire or a stiff, static deflector wire after manually curving the wire (typically with a single curve, but occasionally requiring a double "S" shaped curve) and then the catheter is advanced into the PA off the wire. Once it has been demonstrated that the tip of the catheter is directed precisely toward or into the PA with a deflector wire, the catheter is advanced off the deflector wire and into and through the vessel.
- If the above methods fail, a different catheter should be considered. Several catheter options exist, and the choice is operator dependent. The most commonly used catheters include Judkins right, Bentson, multi-purpose and, occasionally, cobra catheters which provide a 1:1 torque and are pre-formed in a manner that can facilitate crossing both the tricuspid valve and the RV outflow tract. The same wire maneuvers described above can be applied to these catheters. Given their relatively small size, however, once positioned in the PA, they should be exchanged over a wire for a balloon tipped end hole catheter to allow more accurate pressure measurement.

Pressure Measurements and Cardiac Output Determination

Once the pulmonary arterial catheter has been placed in the desired positions, measurements of saturations and pressures from the various chambers can be obtained. A hemodynamic study should be an interactive and dynamic procedure; each measurement obtained adds a piece to the puzzle until a final picture is obtained. Data needs to be constantly re-interpreted and measurements should be repeated if a single value does not align with the emerging picture. Based on the sum of the findings, further testing and interventions are considered; these can include nitric oxide or other vasodilator administration to assess pulmonary vaso-reactivity (see below), oxygen supplementation, diuretic or nitroglycerin for isolated elevated left heart filling pressures or balloon occlusion of a patent shunt lesion.

For non-ventilated patients, hemodynamic pressure measurements should reflect the time of most neutral intrathoracic pressure, usually at end expiration. Mean pressures should not be considered an adequate substitute to end expiratory pressures. Very rarely, in the cases of severe labored breathing, estimation of intrathoracic pressure using esophageal manometry may be of value [83]. End-expiratory maneuvers (extended slow expiration without Valsalva or Mueller) are useful in select patients to provide an extended period of neutral intrathoracic pressure.

Reference pressure values for the various chambers and vessels are provided in **Table** 11.2. There are notable variations in "normal" based on patient position, size, clinical state, and sex. It should be noted that there is often a gap between truly normal values and values felt to reflect clinically relevant pathophysiology. For example, normal PAWP is 12 mmHg or lower, but values ≤15 mmHg are usually not considered sufficient for a diagnosis of left heart failure. Likewise, mPAP is normally <20 mmHg but a value ≥25 mmHg is required for a diagnosis of PHTN

The normal right atrial (RA) pressure is 0–5 mmHg; the height of the "a" wave typically exceeds the 'v' wave (Fig. 11.8). Possible reasons for encountering elevated RA "v" waves are tricuspid regurgitation and a non-compliant RV. A non-compliant RV causes accentuation of the "a" wave in the setting of normal RA contractility. Constrictive

Table 11.2 Normal invasive hemodynamic data [121, 122]

	Average	Range	
Pressures			
Right atrium			
a wave	6	3–6	mmHg
v wave	5	1–4	mmHg
Mean	3	1–5	mmHg
Right ventricle			
Systolic	25	20–30	mmHg
End-diastolic	4	2–7	mmHg
Pulmonary artery			
Systolic	25	16–30	mmHg
Diastolic	9	4–13	mmHg
Mean	15	9–18	mmHg
Pulmonary capillary wedge			
Mean	9	5–12	mmHg
Left atrium			
a wave	10	4–14	mmHg
v wave	12	6–16	mmHg
Mean	8	6–11	mmHg
Left ventricle			
Peak systolic	120	90–140	mmHg
End-diastolic	8	6–12	mmHg
Vascular resistances			
Systemic vascular resistance	1100–1400	700–1600	Dynes*sec/cm-5
Total pulmonary resistance	200	100–300	Dynes*sec/cm-5
Pulmonary vascular resistance	70	20–180	Dynes*sec/cm-5
Blood Flow			
Stroke volume	90	50–150	mL/beat
Cardiac output	5.8	3.6–8	L/min
Cardiac index	3.3	2.2–5	L/min/m^2

These data reflect general guidelines for adults when supine at rest. It is critical to consider the clinical context, which often diverges importantly from ideal conditions, in interpretation such as sedation, anxiety, position, body size and gender

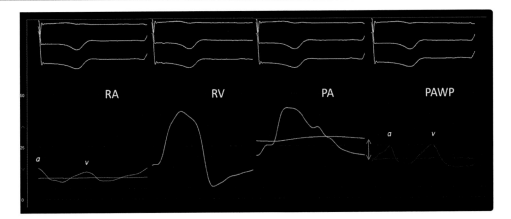

Fig. 11.8 Signal averaged hemodynamic tracings in a patient with pulmonary hypertension due to elevated left heart filling pressure. From left to right are tracings fro the right atrium, right ventricle, pulmonary artery and pulmonary artery wedge position. The *blue double ended arrow* designates the transpulmonary gradient, the difference between mean PAP and mean PAWP. In this case the transpulmonary gradient is <10 mmHg (normal). Right atrial and pulmonary artery wedge tracings are similar with subtle differences. First, the a and v waves occur earlier in the right atrium, since it is measuring the right atrial pressure changes simultaneously while the pulmonary artery wedge position requires transmission of pressure through the pulmonary vasculature. Second, *a* wave pressure is usually higher than the pressure of the *v* wave in the right atrium while *v* wave pressure is generally higher in the left atrium/pulmonary artery wedge pressure. In the normal circulation, left atrial/pulmonary artery wedge pressure is higher than right atrial pressure. *RA* right atrium, *RV* right ventricle, *PA* pulmonary artery, *PAWP* pulmonary artery wedge pressure

pericarditis and tamponade may cause equalization of the "a" and the "v" waves.

Elevated RA pressure implies more clinically severe disease or other causes of volume overload. Elevated RA pressure, along with low cardiac index (CI) and elevated mean PA pressures have been incorporated in a formula to predict prognosis in a National Institutes of Health (NIH) registry study, published in 1991 [84]. Despite the fact that this study was conducted in an era when no US Food and Drug Administration-approved therapies for PAH were available, the adverse prognosis associated with elevated RA pressure persists [85]. Thus, markedly elevated RA pressure (>15 or >20 mmHg) is highlighted as a poor prognostic sign in patients with PHT [86, 87].

The normal RV systolic pressure is 20–30 mmHg, and the normal RV end-diastolic pressure is 0–8 mmHg. PHT causes RV hypertrophy with elevated filling pressures; it can also cause progressive tricuspid regurgitation, and RV diastolic and systolic dysfunction [88, 89]. Since these pathophysiological change may take place in a staged manner, the hemodynamics (and hence the pressure tracings) may vary depending on the disease stage; in the setting of preserved RV contractility the peak rate of RV pressure rise may be increased by up to 10 times the normal value [90]. Occasionally, prominent "a" waves (large pressure augmentation with atrial contraction) will be present on the RV waveforms at this disease state, indicating decreased compliance of the RV: the compliant RV is able to normally "accommodate" the contraction of the RA without a substantial rise in pressure, and this finding suggests RV non-compliance. With severe or chronic PHT, RV systolic dysfunction results

in depressed upstroke and delayed relaxation on pressure tracings.

The driving pressure of the flow across the pulmonary circulation is referred to as the transpulmonary pressure gradient (TPG), and is the calculated result of subtracting the pulmonary venous pressure, estimated by PAWP, from the mean PA pressure:

$$TPG = \left[\begin{array}{l} \text{mean PA pressure} \\ - \text{pulmonary artery wedge pressure} \left(PAWP \right) \end{array} \right].$$

The pulmonary circulation presents low resistance to flow compared with the systemic circulation. The normal PA systolic pressure is 20–30 mmHg, and the normal diastolic pressure is 4–12 mmHg. RV and PA systolic pressure should be approximately equal; a systolic pressure drop between the RV and the PA suggests pulmonary valve stenosis or subpulmonary muscular obstruction; a gradient in the distal pulmonary circulation may be caused by pulmonary artery (main or branch) stenosis or obstruction. This is uncommon but has important treatment implications and constitutes another reason for measuring PA pressure bilaterally.

As mentioned above, the definition of PHT is mPAP >25 mmHg at rest. Pulmonary arterial hypertension (PAH) refers to PHT with elevated pulmonary vascular resistance (PVR) >3 Wood units and normal left heart filling pressure (PAWP ≤ 15 mmHg). TPG calculation (shown above) is major determinant in differentiating precapillary from postcapillary PHT. TPG >12 mmHg suggests some degree of "precapillary" PHT (whether due to active vasoconstriction, arteriolar remodeling or another process). As detailed below, however, the same hemodynamic pattern is seen in pulmonary venoocclusive disease. In the setting of high PAWP, the diastolic PA pressure to PAWP pressure gradient can also be used to identify the presence of a degree of pulmonary vascular disease not entirely related to elevated left heart filling pressures. A gradient >5–7 mmHg is abnormal (Fig. 11.8) [91]. The clinical importance of this finding in patients left heart disease remains to be defined [92, 93], but in theory this may identify a subset of patients who could respond to directed pulmonary vasodilator medical therapy.

Pulmonary wedge angiography can be performed to confirm wedge placement by hand injection of a small amount (2–5 mL) of contrast material distal to a 'wedged' pulmonary artery catheter to opacify the distal pulmonary vasculature (Fig. 11.9). The balloon is deflated, allowing contrast to flow through the pulmonary vasculature, thus outlining the pulmonary venous drainage. Obtaining a sample of wedge blood with oxygen saturation greater than 90 % from the catheter tip strongly supports the achievement of good wedge position, though such samples are not always easy to obtain from a wedged catheter and the procedure carries some risk of damage to the pulmonary vasculature [70]. Wedge angiography is also informative in providing a measure of the physical appearance of the branch pulmonary arteries and perfusion, the presence of pulmonary arteriovenous malformations, and possible evidence of macroscopic pulmonary venous obstruction. The operator should be aware that high pulmonary arterial pressure creates difficulty in obtaining a true "wedge". It

can be difficult to completely obstruct antegrade flow in the setting of elevated PA pressure, and even a small amount of systolic forward flow can cause inaccurately high PAWP estimates relative to the left atrial pressure [94, 95]. It is often helpful to deflate the balloon by ~0.5–1 mL; this results in forward movement of the balloon into a smaller branch vessel with a more secure seal. An additional option is to deliver a small soft tipped 0.018 in. guide wire out of the catheter tip and advance it further into the PA. The soft tips of these wires limit vessel wall injury, and are platinum covered in order to provide enhanced visibility. Different operators use different wires based on personal experience and level of comfort. Most choose soft-tipped wires with 1:1 torque, such as Flex T wire©, BMW wire©, or Whisper wire©. Once the wire reaches the desired position, the catheter can be slowly advanced over it. It is not uncommon for this "tracking" to be challenging, especially when attempted in tortuous vessels; however, one should not give in to the temptation to use a stiffer wire given the much higher risk of vessel wall injury. The use of double-balloon insufflation in the wedge position to secure catheter position is controversial, as it may also lead to vessel wall injury or balloon rupture; it can be useful but should only be used in specific situations by experienced operators. These issues are important in the patient with large left-sided v waves, when PAWP tracing can be similar to the PA tracing with subtle clues to differentiate them (Fig. 11.10).

While the terms wedge pressure, occlusion pressure and capillary pressure tend to be used interchangeably, there are technical differences between them. In clinical practice, the

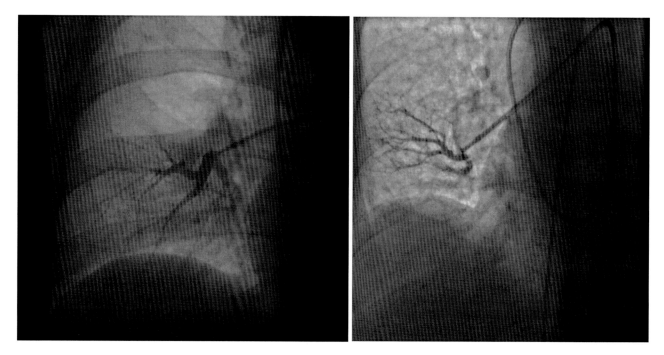

Fig. 11.9 Injection of contrast material through the end-hole port with fluoroscopic confirmation of wedge positioning, with no contrast-free forward flow

Fig. 11.10 Hemodynamic tracings from pulmonary artery (*green*) and pulmonary artery wedge (*red*) positions in a patient with large v waves in the context of left heart non-compliance. If care is not taken, the wedge tracing morphology can appear similar to the pulmonary artery morphology. Since only one of the two tracings is usually displayed at time, this can cause confusion and possibly lead to an adverse event if wedge position is not identified and therefore maintained for an extended period. A key difference is that, the peak of the v wave occurs after the peak of pulmonary artery systolic pressure, and well after the electrocardiographic T wave (highlighted in *yellow* for the 3rd contraction)

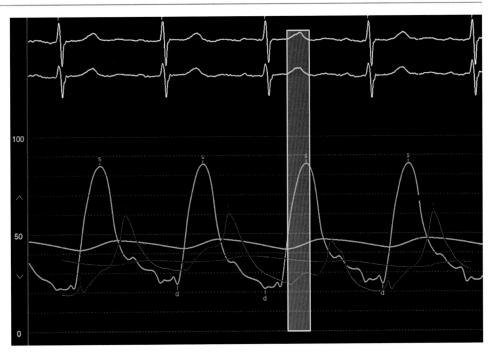

distinction is rarely relevant. Pulmonary capillary wedge pressure refers to occlusion of a small branch pulmonary artery with an end hole catheter without a balloon tip, while "pulmonary artery occlusion pressure" is a more accurate term for what is usually referred to clinically as wedge pressure. Wedge pressure is slightly higher than occlusion pressure, a fact related to continued flow through distal veins via collateral vessels when only a small branch artery is occluded. Because wedge and occlusion pressures prevent flow through the capillaries and small venules, these techniques underestimate true capillary pressure [96]. While this error is usually clinically unimportant, it is importantly misleading in the small subset of patients with pulmonary venoocclusive disease (normal PAWP despite markedly elevated pulmonary capillary pressure, and thus have a hemodynamic picture indistinguishable from PAH). Also of note, a massively dilated right heart can compress the left ventricle and impair filling, resulting in elevated left sided filling pressures. Such an increase in PAWP must be discriminated from the more common reason of elevation of PAWP, i.e. left-sided lesions or systolic or diastolic dysfunction. In theory, the shape of change in pressure with time after occlusion of the pulmonary artery with a balloon tipped catheter can help define true capillary pressure [97], but this is difficult to apply in clinical practice.

Cardiac Output Measurements

The determination of cardiac output (CO) is essential for the diagnostic work-up and follow-up in patients with PHT. The two most commonly used methods for this evaluation are the Fick method and the thermodilution method. When reviewing the results of a right heart study, one should acknowledge the fact that no completely accurate clinical method of measuring CO in all patients exists, yet a value can be estimated on the basis of various assumptions. For comparison among patients, cardiac output should be indexed to the patient's body surface area and expressed as cardiac index (CI).

Fick Method

The Fick principle 'assumes' that the rate at which oxygen is consumed is a function of the rate of blood flow times the rate of oxygen pick-up by the red blood cells [98, 99]. The basic assumption made in this principle is that the same number of red blood cells that enter the lungs must leave them if no intracardiac shunt is present. Hence, the rate of flow of the red blood cells as they pass through the lung can be determined if the numbers of oxygen molecules that are attached to the red blood cells entering the lung, the number of oxygen molecules that are attached to the red blood cells leaving the lung, and the number of oxygen molecules consumed during travel through the lung are known. This can be expressed as the follows:

$$\text{Cardiac output}\left(\text{liter / minute}\right) = \frac{\text{oxygen consumption}\left(\text{ml / min}\right)}{\Delta A - V O_2 \times 1.36 \times \text{Hemoglobin}\left(\text{mg / dL}\right) \times 10}$$

Where ΔA-V O_2 is the arterial-venous oxygen saturation difference and the constant 1.36 is the oxygen-carrying capacity of hemoglobin (expressed in mL O_2/g Hgb).

By reviewing the equation above, it can be appreciated that the important variables to be recorded at the hemodynamic study are A-V O_2 content difference and oxygen consumption. The A-V O_2 content difference is measured by simultaneously obtaining systemic arterial and mixed venous blood samples and analyzing the percent oxygen saturation. Ideally, the arterial blood sample should be obtained from the pulmonary veins; however, in the absence of a right-to-left intracardiac shunt, the femoral or central aortic artery oxygen content provide very close approximations. The PA is the most reliable site for obtaining mixed venous blood. In other sites, such as either vena cava, right atrium, or right ventricle, there may be significant variation in blood oxygen content within the chamber. Potential errors at the time of A-V O_2 difference determination are usually mainly due to improper collection of the mixed venous or arterial blood samples. Ideally, these blood samples should be collected close to simultaneously in a steady state environment. Further, the location of sampling should maximize the likelihood of obtaining representative mixed samples, limiting the impact of streaming. In addition, care should be taken to ensure that the mixed venous sample is not sampled from the wedge position due to catheter migration, as this will falsely elevate the oxygen saturation.

The other important measurement in Fick's method is the oxygen uptake (also referred to as consumption). At steady state, oxygen consumption is the rate at which oxygen is taken up by the blood from the lungs and should ideally be measured directly in the catheterization laboratory. Cardiac output using the Fick principle can be calculated using either the "direct" or the "indirect" methods. Direct Fick refers to measuring every component required to apply the Fick principle: mixed venous and systemic arterial oxygen content (usually very closely estimated by [Hgb] and oxygen saturation] and total body oxygen consumption. The most common variable which is not measured, and rather assumed, is O_2 consumption. Often, however, systemic arterial saturation is estimated (albeit not assumed) by non-invasive pulse oximetry. Oxygen consumption should be measured or cardiac output should also be estimated using a dilution technique to confirm accuracy; isolated indirect Fick estimates should be avoided for reasons detailed below.

Available commercial systems typically use a fitting gas exchange mask or mouthpiece that collects and measures the oxygen content of expired air. Measurement of oxygen uptake may prolong the duration of the study, though only in catheterization laboratories which do not regularly perform this measurement. It requires a cooperative or ventilated patient, a steady state environment, and trained personnel. Unfortunately, most catheterization laboratories choose to forgo this precise and rigorous technique and rather use an estimated (often referred to as "assumed") value for oxygen uptake based on the patient's age, sex and body surface area. Many labs use an estimate of 125 mL/min/m² of body surface area for all patients (approach of Dehmer); others use this estimate for most patients and 110 mL/ min/m² for elderly patients. There are alternative approaches (LaFarge, Bergstra) to estimate VO₂ using age, heart rate and sex, but these are less frequently used in adult clinical practice. Body surface area can be estimated by a number of different equations. As is the case for many other "assumed" values in medical calculations, differences among patients who undergo right heart studies would likely make these estimates inaccurate [100–102]. Depending on the predictive equation used, cardiac output estimates are inaccurate (relative to direct Fick) by >25 % in at least 1 of 6 patients. The error is >10 % in well over half of patients [103]. The degree of error is especially striking in obese patients, but none of the clinically used formulas provide adequately reliable estimates for patients of any body mass index.

The Fick method is often favored in patients with low cardiac output rather than the thermodilution method (discussed below). Because the Fick equation requires a steady state of O_2 consumption and delivery, changes in output are not captured in real time. Also, ventilation of subjects with inspiratory O_2 fractions larger than 60 % require consideration of the contribution dissolved arterial O_2 or this can cause inaccurate estimates [102].

Thermodilution Method

In this method, CO is calculated by using an equation that considers the temperature and specific gravity of an injected solution and the temperature and specific gravity of the blood along with this solution volume. The thermodilution procedure requires injection of a bolus of liquid (usually normal saline) into the proximal port of the catheter. The change in temperature in the sample is measured by a thermistor mounted in the distal end of the catheter. The change in temperature versus time is then graphically displayed, and a calibration factor is used. The cardiac output is inversely related to the area under a thermodilution curve, shown as a function of temperature versus time, with a smaller area under the curve indicative of a higher cardiac output. Temperature fluctuation in the circuit can affect accuracy however, and the use of two thermistors can significantly improve the accuracy of this technique [104, 105]. The thermodilution method has several advantages. Perhaps its greatest advantage is the rapid display of results with computerized methods, and other advantages are the lack of need for withdrawal of arterial blood since it is less affected by recirculation than other indicator methods. Thermodilution cannot be used in the presence of intracardiac shunting. Many hold that thermodilution can be inaccurate in patients with severe tricuspid regurgitation, extremes of cardiac output or an irregular rhythm. Hoeper *et al.* compared the Fick and the thermodilution methods for evaluation of CO in patients with severe PHT, and reported that the accuracy of thermodilution was similar to the Fick method over a broad range of CO values (1.7–7.8 L/min). Importantly, the agreement between the two methods was not affected by the severity of tricuspid regurgitation [106]. Hillis *et al.* also reported good agreement between the Fick and the indicator dilution methods (combination of thermodilution and indocyanine green dye) in patients without PHT with broad range of CO values (difference of <10 % and <20 % in 67 % and 91 %, respectively, of the 808 patients studied) [107].

As can be predicted from the Fick principle, CO can be roughly assessed by the mixed venous oxygen saturation. Assuming normal hemoglobin concentration and normal arterial oxygen saturation, low mixed venous oxygen saturations indicate low cardiac output. Understanding the principles allows one to avoid misinterpretation of situations where low mixed venous saturation may be present with normal cardiac output (e.g., arterial hypoxemia, severe anemia, situations with high oxygen consumption such as exercise). While low cardiac output or index is a universal marker of adverse outcomes, decreased venous saturation itself may be a strong predictor of poor outcome in pulmonary arterial hypertension patients [108, 109], though some investigators failed to observe this prognostic implication in other cohorts [84].

Finally, CO can also be estimated by angiographic estimation of stroke volume. This can be calculated by tracing the LV end-diastolic and end-systolic images. Stroke volume is the amount of blood ejected with each beat. Calibration of the images with grids or ventricular phantoms is often necessary to obtain accurate ventricular volumes. Angiographic approaches are rarely used, and are not depended upon as a primary method to estimate CO. The main technical drawback of this method is the inherent inaccuracy of calibrating angiographic volumes. Such large contrast volume loads can also cause adverse clinical events in patients with important PHT. In cases of valvular regurgitation or atrial fibrillation, angiographic cardiac output does not accurately measure true systemic outputs.

Pulmonary Vascular Resistance

PVR is calculated as:

$$PVR = \frac{(Mean\ PA\ pressure - PAWP)}{Cardiac\ output\ (CO)} = \frac{(TPG)}{CO}$$

Multiplying the resistance thus calculated (Wood units: mmHg/L/min) by 80 converts to the resistance unit of dynes*sec/cm^5; normal supine resting PVR is <200 dynes*sec/cm^5 (or 2.5 Woods units). PVR can be indexed to the patient's body size (PVRI=PVR × BSA). This is necessary in children given the marked differences in body size, but also has some advantage in adults. Using PVR instead of PVRI may result in important underestimation of the prevalence of PHT in patients with markedly elevated body mass index. [110] Also, PVRI may be a better marker of adverse outcome after cardiac transplant than unindexed PVR [111]. Elevated PVR is considered to mainly reflect pathological changes in the pulmonary vascular bed and the functional status of pulmonary vascular endothelium and smooth muscle cells; however, it is also related to blood viscosity and to changes in perivascular alveolar and pleural pressure [96, 112–114]. Normal PVRI increases with age. The upper limit for PVRI in normal subjects increases from about 2.8 WU*m^2 (6–10 yrs) to 3.2 WU*m^2 (32–45 yrs) to 4.6 WU*m^2 (60–83 yrs) [112, 113].

Direct Measurement of Left Heart Pressure

Evaluation of left sided pressures requires arterial access unless a known patent inter-atrial communication that can be safely crossed exists and only left atrial and pulmonary venous pressures need to be directly assessed. This requirement has to be appreciated in advance, especially in patients who are taking anticoagulants and in those with known difficult access sites. Possible conditions in which direct evaluation of the left sided pressures may be required include one or more of the following:

– Uncertainty about a direct correlation between the PAWP and the left atrial pressure/LV end-diastolic pressure, such as in patients with suspected pulmonary vein obstruction or cor triatriatum.
– Clinical or imaging-based suspicion of restrictive/constrictive physiology, requiring concomitant measurement of RV and LV pressures.
– Left-sided valvular disease that is suspected to contribute to the overall hemodynamic picture, requiring direct evaluation of the pressure gradient across the involved valve(s).
– Known or suspected coronary artery disease requiring direct visualization of the coronary bed.

Provocative Maneuvers in the Cardiac Catheterization Lab

Vasoreactivity Testing

Pulmonary vasoreactivity testing is typically performed during the second stage of the invasive hemodynamic study after all the basic data has been collected. The main historical purpose of acute pulmonary vasoreactivity testing is to identify a small subpopulation of patients who can benefit from treatment with calcium channel blocker agents (CCBs). Until the 1990s, these were the only clinically used agents available for treating PAH. The usefulness of testing and benefit from long term CCB therapy was demonstrated predominantly in patients with idiopathic PAH. In patients with PAH due to other etiologies such as heritable PAH, connective tissue disease, and HIV, the usefulness of acute vasoreactivity tests and long-term treatment with CCBs is less clear.

Acute vasoreactivity testing should be performed with short-acting agents that have little or no systemic effects. The agent most commonly used in acute testing is nitric oxide (NO), while inhaled epoprostenol or intra-venous epoprostenol or adenosine can also be used as alternatives (with the caveat that intravenous administration may cause systemic vasodilation). Simply administering a high concentration of inhaled oxygen is not sufficient, though can be helpful in determining if supplemental oxygen is likely to have a notable clinical benefit. The most widely used definition of "a positive" acute response is both reduction of mean PA pressure by ≥ 10 mmHg *and* resulting absolute mPAP ≤ 40 mmHg with increased or unchanged cardiac output [9–11]. Using these criteria, about 10 % of the patients with idiopathic pulmonary arterial hypertension are considered "responsive". Acute responders are likely to show a sustained response to long-term treatment with high doses of CCBs; responders have excellent prognosis, with up to 95 % survival at 5 years [115, 116]. The value of performing a vasoreactivity testing and the usefulness of long term CCB treatment are less clear in patients with PHT associated with congenital heart disease, PAH associated with scleroderma or other associated PAH, as acute response as defined above is exceptionally rare.

In addition to assisting in patient management, the results of vasodilator testing have also been shown to have important prognostic implications, as the extent of acute response correlates with prognosis. However, the usefulness of this incremental prognostic information is unclear in caring for the patient and some clinicians do not perform vasodilator therapy on patients other than the subset eligible for possible treatment with CCB.

Exercise Testing and Fluid Administration

Not uncommonly, basic hemodynamic studies in individuals with PHT reveal borderline elevated left sided filling pressures, which can become truly elevated in states of vigorous myocardial contraction or of high volume load, Typically, these patients also have evidence of diastolic dysfunction by echocardiography (see above), further raising the concern for elevated left sided filling pressures contributing to the their symptoms. When the level of suspicion is sufficient, this option should be fully explored during the catheterization procedure, as elevated left sided filling pressures could be potentially amenable to medical therapy.

In attempting to relate the patient's symptoms to the physiologic and hemodynamic state, provocation of elevated left sided filling pressures should be attempted by performing maneuvers that will closely imitate the physiologic conditions that cause enhanced myocardial contraction and volume overload. The two commonly used methods for this purpose are exercise and a fluid challenge. Common cath lab exercise protocols include supine cycle ergometry (often starting at a 20-W workload and increasing by 10-W increments in 3-min stages to maximum tolerated levels) and outstretched arm adduction lifting of weights (if femoral access had been obtained with repetition frequency gradually increased to fatigue) [117]. Elevation of PAWP >25 mmHg is commonly used to define a positive response. Because intrathoracic pressure swings are enhanced with the increased work of breathing during exercise, pressures should be measured as the mean of inspiration and expiration. When possible, values should be confirmed with the left ventricular end diastolic pressure. Fluid challenge protocols vary between laboratories, the most common consisting of a bolus infusion of 10–15 mL/kg of isotonic saline. Similar definitions and considerations for positive response and simultaneous left ventricular end diastolic pressure measurement exist for fluid challenges [118]. However, the response to fluid is not equivalent to that seen with exercise; with sufficient volume IV fluid will increase filling pressures even normal people. Exercise is more sensitive, specific, and physiologic than administration of intravenous fluid [119].

Special Considerations: Hemodynamic Measurement in the Setting of Congenital Heart Disease

The invasive hemodynamic study is an integral part of the standard evaluation and follow up of patients with various types of congenital heart disease (CHD). The spectrum of CHD is wide, and it is beyond the scope of this chapter to discuss the various anatomies or the distinctive hemodynamic features accompanying each type of lesion. However, several important considerations should be mentioned with regards to the invasive hemodynamic studies in patients suspected or known to have CHD, as they differ from those in patients with assumed normal cardiac anatomy:

A. Vascular Access Site
In general, the same considerations discussed above regarding femoral and IJ access apply for patients with CHD. However,

the presence of certain lesions may recommend a particular access site and not another. One common example is the presence of an atrial septal defect or a patent foramen ovale, in which femoral access is preferred. Catheters introduced through the IJ veins are typically oriented towards the tricuspid valve and into the RV (i.e., anterior-inferior direction), whereas in order to engage the atrial septum the catheter should be aimed in the posterior-superior direction. Similar considerations exist for a membranous or outlet-type ventricular septal defect, whereas in apical muscular-type ventricular septal defect the jugular approach is preferred for the converse reason. Occluded venous access sites are common in CHD patients. Access through uncommon sites, such as the hepatic vein, may be necessary. This type of access should be performed by trained, operators. Briefly, a needle (typically Chiba needle) is passed under ultrasound guidance between the mid and anterior axillary line, near the costal margin between the diaphragm and the inferior liver edge. The needle is advanced posteriorly and cephalated toward the intrahepatic IVC or just below the IVC-RA junction, to within a few centimeters of the right border of the spine. When contrast injection confirms entry into a large central hepatic vein, a sheath and dilator are advanced over a guide wire to the atrium. At the end of the procedure, a catheter (usually one French size smaller than the entry catheter) is exchanged, and this sheath is withdrawn, with hand injection of contrast until the tip of the sheath is seen to be out of the vessel and within the liver parenchymal tract. This tract is then occluded using coils, vascular plug, or Gelfoam.

B. Choice of Gas to Fill Balloons

Balloon catheters use in CHD patients: whereas in the non CHD patients the floating balloons of end hole, side hole (Berman catheter) or Swan-Ganz catheters are filled with regular room air, in patients with known or suspected intracardiac or vascular shunts, CO_2 filling is preferred. CO_2 is approximately 20 times more soluble than oxygen in blood, reducing the likelihood of a catastrophic outcome in the setting of balloon rupture and embolization of the contents in the setting of shunting.

C. Locating an Intracardiac or Great Vessel Shunt

All patients with PHT should be evaluated for presence of an intracardiac or great vessel shunt. These shunts can be either the cause of the disease (i.e., Eisenmenger syndrome), the result of the disease (i.e., opening of a patent foramen ovale in the face of elevated right sided filling pressures) or merely an unrelated bystander (i.e. small restrictive ventricular septal defect) [120]. In order to locate and determine the magnitude of the shunt, the oxygen saturation of blood should be measured at multiple levels of the heart and great vessels (often termed an "oximetry run" or "shunt run"). This allows

evaluation of a significant "step-up" or "step-down" in the saturations, indicating the presence of a shunt. For a complete oximetry run, blood should be sampled at the inferior vena cava, RA (to avoid sampling of low saturated blood entering the RA from the coronary sinus, sampling should be obtained with the catheter directed towards the lateral RA wall), high superior vena cava, low superior vena cava, RV inflow, RV outflow, main pulmonary artery, left ventricle, ascending aorta and descending aorta. The LA and the pulmonary veins can be easily accessed in the presence of an atrial septal defect or a patent foramen ovale (via femoral vein access). Special maneuvers, such as trans-septal puncture, are needed to enter the LA in the absence of these communications in order to determine the pulmonary venous saturation in the presence of a right to left shunt at the pulmonary venous level (such as in patients with total or partial pulmonary anomalous venous connection). Samples should be obtained in quick succession to minimize the effect of normal temporal variation in oxygen uptake, cardiac output and loading conditions, and, therefore, variation in oxygen saturations. A significant step-up is considered present if the increase to the PA is $\geq 6-7\%$ from the atrial level or mean absolute difference $\geq 5\%$ at the ventricular levels.

Quantification of shunt magnitude. Shunt quantification is expressed usually by a ratio of the pulmonary blood flow ("Qp") to systemic blood flow ("Qs").

Qp is inversely proportional to the difference between pulmonary venous saturation and pulmonary arterial saturation). Qs is inversely proportional to the difference between systemic arterial saturation and mixed venous saturation.

When Qp is greater than Qs (Qp/Qs >1), this indicates a left-to-right shunt. Qp/Qs between 1.0 and 1.5 indicates a "small" left-to-right shunt, and a Qp/Qs >2.0 indicates a larger left to-right shunt, though context remains critical. Conversely, Qs>Qp (Qp/QS<1) indicates a predominantly right-to left shunt. Fig. 11.11 shows an example of the hemodynamic findings in a patient with PHT and an atrial septal defect.

Certain considerations regarding the oximetry run in patients with congenital heart disease should be recognized:

1. Shunt detection is enhanced in the presence of low systemic venous saturation.
2. High systemic flow may diminish arterio-venous oxygen saturation difference across the systemic bed, leading to higher mixed venous oxygen saturation which may falsely emphasize the degree of left-to-right shunt.

Calculation of the Pulmonary Vascular Resistance

Whereas in patients without CHD systemic blood flow (Qs) approximates pulmonary blood flows (Qp) closely, this is not true for many patients with CHD. Thus, when calculating the PVR in this patient population, when using the formula

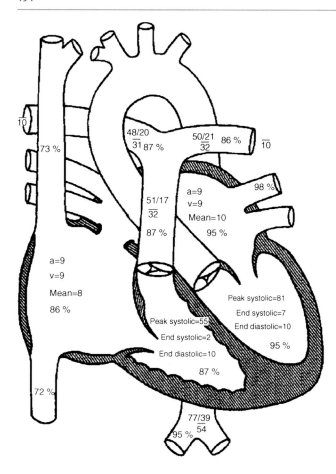

Fig. 11.11 Example of a cardiac diagram with hemodynamic data of a patient with a secundum atrial septal defect and pulmonary hypertension. Notice the "step up" in the saturations between the vena cava and the pulmonary artery, as well as the elevated pulmonary arterial pressures

$$PVR = \frac{\left(\text{Mean PA pressure} - \text{PAWP}\right)}{\text{Cardiac output}\left(\text{CO}\right)}$$

The pulmonary blood flow, or

$$\frac{O_2 \text{ consumption}}{\left(\text{PV sat} - \text{PA sat}\right) \times \left(\left[\text{Hgb}\right]\right) \times \left(1.36 \times 10\right)}$$

should be used for the denominator.

Conclusions

Hemodynamic evaluation in patients with suspected or known pulmonary hypertension does not start with catheterization. Rather, a large part of the history and physical examination aim to define the likely hemodynamic underpinning of the patients symptoms. Transthoracic echocardiography has assumed a major role in the hemodynamic evaluation of pulmonary hypertension. The focus is often too narrowly on the systolic pulmonary artery pressure estimate, but echocardiography can provide extensive

information on the full array of hemodynamic variables. Catheterization remains a requisite part of definitive diagnosis and understanding of pulmonary hypertension hemodynamics. A comprehensive understanding of the techniques and pitfalls of each of these approaches is required to ensure that hemodynamic data obtained are valid, representative and accurate.

References

1. Simonneau G, Robbins IM, Beghetti M, Channick RN, Delcroix M, Denton CP, Elliott CG, Gaine SP, Gladwin MT, Jing ZC, Krowka MJ, Langleben D, Nakanishi N, Souza R. Updated clinical classification of pulmonary hypertension. J Am Coll Cardiol. 2009;54:S43–54.
2. Hachulla E, Gressin V, Guillevin L, Carpentier P, Diot E, Sibilia J, Kahan A, Cabane J, Frances C, Launay D, Mouthon L, Allanore Y, Tiev KP, Clerson P, de Groote P, Humbert M. Early detection of pulmonary arterial hypertension in systemic sclerosis: a French nationwide prospective multicenter study. Arthritis Rheum. 2005;52:3792–800.
3. Humbert M, Sitbon O, Chaouat A, Bertocchi M, Habib G, Gressin V, Yaici A, Weitzenblum E, Cordier JF, Chabot F, Dromer C, Pison C, Reynaud-Gaubert M, Haloun A, Laurent M, Hachulla E, Simonneau G. Pulmonary arterial hypertension in France: results from a national registry. Am J Respir Crit Care Med. 2006;173:1023–30.
4. Peacock AJ, Murphy NF, McMurray JJ, Caballero L, Stewart S. An epidemiological study of pulmonary arterial hypertension. Eur Respir J. 2007;30:104–9.
5. Duffels MG, Engelfriet PM, Berger RM, van Loon RL, Hoendermis E, Vriend JW, van der Velde ET, Bresser P, Mulder BJ. Pulmonary arterial hypertension in congenital heart disease: an epidemiologic perspective from a Dutch registry. Int J Cardiol. 2007;120:198–204.
6. Condliffe R, Kiely DG, Gibbs JS, Corris PA, Peacock AJ, Jenkins DP, Hodgkins D, Goldsmith K, Hughes RJ, Sheares K, Tsui SS, Armstrong IJ, Torpy C, Crackett R, Carlin CM, Das C, Coghlan JG, Pepke-Zaba J. Improved outcomes in medically and surgically treated chronic thromboembolic pulmonary hypertension. Am J Respir Crit Care Med. 2008;177:1122–7.
7. Kovacs G, Berghold A, Scheidl S, Olschewski H. Pulmonary arterial pressure during rest and exercise in healthy subjects: a systematic review. Eur Respir J. 2009;34:888–94.
8. Badesch DB, Champion HC, Sanchez MA, Hoeper MM, Loyd JE, Manes A, McGoon M, Naeije R, Olschewski H, Oudiz RJ, Torbicki A. Diagnosis and assessment of pulmonary arterial hypertension. J Am Coll Cardiol. 2009;54:S55–66.
9. Galie N, Hoeper MM, Humbert M, Torbicki A, Vachiery JL, Barbera JA, Beghetti M, Corris P, Gaine S, Gibbs JS, Gomez-Sanchez MA, Jondeau G, Klepetko W, Opitz C, Peacock A, Rubin L, Zellweger M, Simonneau G. Guidelines for the diagnosis and treatment of pulmonary hypertension: the Task Force for the Diagnosis and Treatment of Pulmonary Hypertension of the European Society of Cardiology (ESC) and the European Respiratory Society (ERS), endorsed by the International Society of Heart and Lung Transplantation (ISHLT). Eur Heart J. 2009;30:2493–537.
10. McLaughlin VV, Archer SL, Badesch DB, Barst RJ, Farber HW, Lindner JR, Mathier MA, McGoon MD, Park MH, Rosenson RS, Rubin LJ, Tapson VF, Varga J. ACCF/AHA 2009 expert consensus

document on pulmonary hypertension a report of the American College of Cardiology Foundation Task Force on Expert Consensus Documents and the American Heart Association developed in collaboration with the American College of Chest Physicians; American Thoracic Society, Inc.; and the Pulmonary Hypertension Association. J Am Coll Cardiol. 2009;53:1573–619.

11. Hoeper MM, Bogaard HJ, Condliffe R, Frantz R, Khanna D, Kurzyna M, Langleben D, Manes A, Satoh T, Torres F, Wilkins MR, Badesch DB. Definitions and diagnosis of pulmonary hypertension. J Am Coll Cardiol. 2013;62:D42–50.

12. Gabbay E, Yeow W, Playford D. Pulmonary arterial hypertension (PAH) is an uncommon cause of pulmonary hypertension (PH) in an unselected population: the Armadale echocardiography study. Am J Resp Crit Care Med. 2007;A713.

13. Champion HC, Michelakis ED, Hassoun PM. Comprehensive invasive and noninvasive approach to the right ventricle-pulmonary circulation unit: state of the art and clinical and research implications. Circulation. 2009;120:992–1007.

14. McGee SR. Evidence-based physical diagnosis. Philadelphia: Elsevier/Saunders; 2012.

15. Wiese J. The abdominojugular reflux sign. Am J Med. 2000;109:59–61.

16. Opotowsky AR, Ojeda J, Rogers F, Arkles J, Liu T, Forfia PR. Blood pressure response to the valsalva maneuver. A simple bedside test to determine the hemodynamic basis of pulmonary hypertension. J Am Coll Cardiol. 2010;56:1352–3.

17. Felker GM, Cuculich PS, Gheorghiade M. The Valsalva maneuver: a bedside "biomarker" for heart failure. Am J Med. 2006;119:117–22.

18. Opotowsky AR, Ojeda J, Rogers F, Prasanna V, Clair M, Moko L, Vaidya A, Afilalo J, Forfia PR. A simple echocardiographic prediction rule for hemodynamics in pulmonary hypertension. Circ Cardiovasc Imaging. 2012;5:765–75.

19. McGoon M, Gutterman D, Steen V, Barst R, McCrory DC, Fortin TA, Loyd JE. Screening, early detection, and diagnosis of pulmonary arterial hypertension: ACCP evidence-based clinical practice guidelines. Chest. 2004;126:14S–34.

20. Rich JD, Shah SJ, Swamy RS, Kamp A, Rich S. Inaccuracy of Doppler echocardiographic estimates of pulmonary artery pressures in patients with pulmonary hypertension: implications for clinical practice. Chest. 2011;139:988–93.

21. Giardini A. Limitations inherent to the simplified Bernoulli equation explain the inaccuracy of Doppler echocardiographic estimates of pulmonary artery pressures in patients with pulmonary hypertension. Chest. 2011;140:270; author reply 270–271.

22. Fisher MR, Criner GJ, Fishman AP, Hassoun PM, Minai OA, Scharf SM, Fessler HE. Estimating pulmonary artery pressures by echocardiography in patients with emphysema. Eur Respir J. 2007;30:914–21.

23. Fisher MR, Forfia PR, Chamera E, Housten-Harris T, Champion HC, Girgis RE, Corretti MC, Hassoun PM. Accuracy of Doppler echocardiography in the hemodynamic assessment of pulmonary hypertension. Am J Respir Crit Care Med. 2009;179:615–21.

24. Rudski LG, Lai WW, Afilalo J, Hua L, Handschumacher MD, Chandrasekaran K, Solomon SD, Louie EK, Schiller NB. Guidelines for the echocardiographic assessment of the right heart in adults: a report from the American Society of Echocardiography endorsed by the European Association of Echocardiography, a registered branch of the European Society of Cardiology, and the Canadian Society of Echocardiography. J Am Soc Echocardiogr. 2010;23:685–713; quiz 786–688.

25. Brennan JM, Blair JE, Goonewardena S, Ronan A, Shah D, Vasaiwala S, Kirkpatrick JN, Spencer KT. Reappraisal of the use of inferior vena cava for estimating right atrial pressure. J Am Soc Echocardiogr. 2007;20:857–61.

26. Abbas AE, Fortuin FD, Schiller NB, Appleton CP, Moreno CA, Lester SJ. Echocardiographic determination of mean pulmonary artery pressure. Am J Cardiol. 2003;92:1373–6.

27. Aduen JF, Castello R, Lozano MM, Hepler GN, Keller CA, Alvarez F, Safford RE, Crook JE, Heckman MG, Burger CD. An alternative echocardiographic method to estimate mean pulmonary artery pressure: diagnostic and clinical implications. J Am Soc Echocardiogr. 2009;22:814–9.

28. Lee RT, Lord CP, Plappert T, Sutton MS. Prospective Doppler echocardiographic evaluation of pulmonary artery diastolic pressure in the medical intensive care unit. Am J Cardiol. 1989;64:1366–70.

29. Ge Z, Zhang Y, Ji X, Fan D, Duran CM. Pulmonary artery diastolic pressure: a simultaneous Doppler echocardiography and catheterization study. Clin Cardiol. 1992;15:818–24.

30. Stephen B, Dalal P, Berger M, Schweitzer P, Hecht S. Noninvasive estimation of pulmonary artery diastolic pressure in patients with tricuspid regurgitation by Doppler echocardiography. Chest. 1999;116:73–7.

31. Selimovic N, Rundqvist B, Bergh CH, Andersson B, Petersson S, Johansson L, Bech-Hanssen O. Assessment of pulmonary vascular resistance by Doppler echocardiography in patients with pulmonary arterial hypertension. J Heart Lung Transplant. 2007;26:927–34.

32. Abbas AE, Fortuin FD, Schiller NB, Appleton CP, Moreno CA, Lester SJ. A simple method for noninvasive estimation of pulmonary vascular resistance. J Am Coll Cardiol. 2003;41:1021–7.

33. Farzaneh-Far R, McKeown BH, Dang D, Roberts J, Schiller NB, Foster E. Accuracy of Doppler-estimated pulmonary vascular resistance in patients before liver transplantation. Am J Cardiol. 2008;101:259–62.

34. Haddad F, Zamanian R, Beraud AS, Schnittger I, Feinstein J, Peterson T, Yang P, Doyle R, Rosenthal D. A novel non-invasive method of estimating pulmonary vascular resistance in patients with pulmonary arterial hypertension. J Am Soc Echocardiogr. 2009;22:523–9.

35. Opotowsky AR, Clair M, Afilalo J, Landzberg MJ, Waxman AB, Moko L, Maron BA, Vaidya A, Forfia PR. A simple echocardiographic method to estimate pulmonary vascular resistance. Am J Cardiol. 2013;112:873–82.

36. Opotowsky AR, Santos M, Maron BA, Afilalo J, Waxman AB, Landzberg MJ, Forfia PR. Towards widespread noninvasive assessment of pulmonary vascular resistance in clinical practice. J Am Soc Echocardiogr. 2014;27:108–9.

37. Scapellato F, Temporelli PL, Eleuteri E, Corra U, Imparato A, Giannuzzi P. Accurate noninvasive estimation of pulmonary vascular resistance by Doppler echocardiography in patients with chronic failure heart failure. J Am Coll Cardiol. 2001;37:1813–9.

38. Bossone E, Duong-Wagner TH, Paciocco G, Oral H, Ricciardi M, Bach DS, Rubenfire M, Armstrong WF. Echocardiographic features of primary pulmonary hypertension. J Am Soc Echocardiogr. 1999;12:655–62.

39. Bustamante-Labarta M, Perrone S, De La Fuente RL, Stutzbach P, De La Hoz RP, Torino A, Favaloro R. Right atrial size and tricuspid regurgitation severity predict mortality or transplantation in primary pulmonary hypertension. J Am Soc Echocardiogr. 2002;15:1160–4.

40. Jardin F, Dubourg O, Bourdarias JP. Echocardiographic pattern of acute cor pulmonale. Chest. 1997;111:209–17.

41. Lai WW, Gauvreau K, Rivera ES, Saleeb S, Powell AJ, Geva T. Accuracy of guideline recommendations for two-dimensional quantification of the right ventricle by echocardiography. Int J Cardiovasc Imaging. 2008;24:691–8.

42. Anavekar NS, Gerson D, Skali H, Kwong RY, Yucel EK, Solomon SD. Two-dimensional assessment of right ventricular function: an

echocardiographic-MRI correlative study. Echocardiography. 2007;24:452–6.

43. Nass N, McConnell MV, Goldhaber SZ, Chyu S, Solomon SD. Recovery of regional right ventricular function after thrombolysis for pulmonary embolism. Am J Cardiol. 1999;83:804–6, A810.

44. Zornoff LA, Skali H, Pfeffer MA, St John Sutton M, Rouleau JL, Lamas GA, Plappert T, Rouleau JR, Moye LA, Lewis SJ, Braunwald E, Solomon SD. Right ventricular dysfunction and risk of heart failure and mortality after myocardial infarction. J Am Coll Cardiol. 2002;39:1450–5.

45. Anavekar NS, Skali H, Bourgoun M, Ghali JK, Kober L, Maggioni AP, McMurray JJ, Velazquez E, Califf R, Pfeffer MA, Solomon SD. Usefulness of right ventricular fractional area change to predict death, heart failure, and stroke following myocardial infarction (from the VALIANT ECHO Study). Am J Cardiol. 2008;101:607–12.

46. Tei C, Dujardin KS, Hodge DO, Bailey KR, McGoon MD, Tajik AJ, Seward SB. Doppler echocardiographic index for assessment of global right ventricular function. J Am Soc Echocardiogr. 1996;9:838–47.

47. Dyer KL, Pauliks LB, Das B, Shandas R, Ivy D, Shaffer EM, Valdes-Cruz LM. Use of myocardial performance index in pediatric patients with idiopathic pulmonary arterial hypertension. J Am Soc Echocardiogr. 2006;19:21–7.

48. Yeo TC, Dujardin KS, Tei C, Mahoney DW, McGoon MD, Seward JB. Value of a Doppler-derived index combining systolic and diastolic time intervals in predicting outcome in primary pulmonary hypertension. Am J Cardiol. 1998;81:1157–61.

49. Eidem BW, O'Leary PW, Tei C, Seward JB. Usefulness of the myocardial performance index for assessing right ventricular function in congenital heart disease. Am J Cardiol. 2000;86:654–8.

50. Ueti OM, Camargo EE, Ueti Ade A, de Lima-Filho EC, Nogueira EA. Assessment of right ventricular function with Doppler echocardiographic indices derived from tricuspid annular motion: comparison with radionuclide angiography. Heart. 2002;88:244–8.

51. Forfia PR, Fisher MR, Mathai SC, Housten-Harris T, Hemnes AR, Borlaug BA, Chamera E, Corretti MC, Champion HC, Abraham TP, Girgis RE, Hassoun PM. Tricuspid annular displacement predicts survival in pulmonary hypertension. Am J Respir Crit Care Med. 2006;174:1034–41.

52. Badano LP, Ginghina C, Easaw J, Muraru D, Grillo MT, Lancellotti P, Pinamonti B, Coghlan G, Marra MP, Popescu BA, De Vita S. Right ventricle in pulmonary arterial hypertension: haemodynamics, structural changes, imaging, and proposal of a study protocol aimed to assess remodelling and treatment effects. Eur J Echocardiogr. 2010;11:27–37.

53. Naeije R, Torbicki A. More on the noninvasive diagnosis of pulmonary hypertension: Doppler echocardiography revisited. Eur Respir J. 1995;8:1445–9.

54. Kitabatake A, Inoue M, Asao M, Masuyama T, Tanouchi J, Morita T, Mishima M, Uematsu M, Shimazu T, Hori M, Abe H. Noninvasive evaluation of pulmonary hypertension by a pulsed Doppler technique. Circulation. 1983;68:302–9.

55. Arkles JS, Opotowsky AR, Ojeda J, Rogers F, Liu T, Prassana V, Marzec L, Palevsky HI, Ferrari VA, Forfia PR. Shape of the right ventricular Doppler envelope predicts hemodynamics and right heart function in pulmonary hypertension. Am J Respir Crit Care Med. 2011;183:268–76.

56. Dabestani A, Mahan G, Gardin JM, Takenaka K, Burn C, Allfie A, Henry WL. Evaluation of pulmonary artery pressure and resistance by pulsed Doppler echocardiography. Am J Cardiol. 1987;59:662–8.

57. Burgess MI, Bright-Thomas RJ, Ray SG. Echocardiographic evaluation of right ventricular function. Eur J Echocardiogr. 2002;3:252–62.

58. Haddad F, Hunt SA, Rosenthal DN, Murphy DJ. Right ventricular function in cardiovascular disease, part I: anatomy, physiology, aging, and functional assessment of the right ventricle. Circulation. 2008;117:1436–48.

59. Ryan T, Petrovic O, Dillon JC, Feigenbaum H, Conley MJ, Armstrong WF. An echocardiographic index for separation of right ventricular volume and pressure overload. J Am Coll Cardiol. 1985;5:918–27.

60. Raymond RJ, Hinderliter AL, Willis PW, Ralph D, Caldwell EJ, Williams W, Ettinger NA, Hill NS, Summer WR, de Boisblanc B, Schwartz T, Koch G, Clayton LM, Jobsis MM, Crow JW, Long W. Echocardiographic predictors of adverse outcomes in primary pulmonary hypertension. J Am Coll Cardiol. 2002;39:1214–9.

61. Marcus JT, Gan CT, Zwanenburg JJ, Boonstra A, Allaart CP, Gotte MJ, Vonk-Noordegraaf A. Interventricular mechanical asynchrony in pulmonary arterial hypertension: left-to-right delay in peak shortening is related to right ventricular overload and left ventricular underfilling. J Am Coll Cardiol. 2008;51:750–7.

62. Hinderliter AL, Willis PW, Long W, Clarke WR, Ralph D, Caldwell EJ, Williams W, Ettinger NA, Hill NS, Summer WR, de Biosblanc B, Koch G, Li S, Clayton LM, Jobsis MM, Crow JW. Frequency and prognostic significance of pericardial effusion in primary pulmonary hypertension. PPH Study Group. Primary pulmonary hypertension. Am J Cardiol. 1999;84:481–4, A410.

63. Heupler Jr FA. Guidelines for performing angiography in patients taking metformin. Members of the Laboratory Performance Standards Committee of the Society for Cardiac Angiography and Interventions. Cathet Cardiovasc Diagn. 1998;43:121–3.

64. Cote P, Campeau L, Bourassa MG. Therapeutic implications of diazepam in patients with elevated left ventricular filling pressure. Am Heart J. 1976;91:747–51.

65. Francis GS, Cohn JN. The autonomic nervous system in congestive heart failure. Annu Rev Med. 1986;37:235–47.

66. Groeneveld AB, Berendsen RR, Schneider AJ, Pneumatikos IA, Stokkel LA, Thijs LG. Effect of the mechanical ventilatory cycle on thermodilution right ventricular volumes and cardiac output. J Appl Physiol (1985). 2000;89:89–96.

67. Couture P, Denault AY, Shi Y, Deschamps A, Cossette M, Pellerin M, Tardif JC. Effects of anesthetic induction in patients with diastolic dysfunction. Can J Anaesth. 2009;56:357–65.

68. Biondi JW, Schulman DS, Soufer R, Matthay RA, Hines RL, Kay HR, Barash PG. The effect of incremental positive end-expiratory pressure on right ventricular hemodynamics and ejection fraction. Anesth Analg. 1988;67:144–51.

69. Theres H, Binkau J, Laule M, Heinze R, Hundertmark J, Blobner M, Erhardt W, Baumann G, Stangl K. Phase-related changes in right ventricular cardiac output under volume-controlled mechanical ventilation with positive end-expiratory pressure. Crit Care Med. 1999;27:953–8.

70. Ragosta M. Normal waveforms, artifacts, and pitfalls. In: Textbook of clinical hemodynamics. Philadelphia: Saunders/Elsevier; 2008.

71. Summerhill EM, Baram M. Principles of pulmonary artery catheterization in the critically ill. Lung. 2005;183:209–19.

72. Dehmer GJ, Firth BG, Hillis LD. Oxygen consumption in adult patients during cardiac catheterization. Clin Cardiol. 1982;5:436–40.

73. Ranu H, Smith K, Nimako K, Sheth A, Madden BP. A retrospective review to evaluate the safety of right heart catheterization via the internal jugular vein in the assessment of pulmonary hypertension. Clin Cardiol. 2010;33:303–6.

74. Hemnes AR, Forfia PR, Champion HC. Assessment of pulmonary vasculature and right heart by invasive haemodynamics and echocardiography. Int J Clin Pract Suppl. 2009;162:4–19.

75. Rutten AJ, Nancarrow C, Ilsley AH, Runciman WB. An assessment of six different pulmonary artery catheters. Crit Care Med. 1987;15:250–5.

76. Oliveira RK, Ferreira EV, Ramos RP, Messina CM, Kapins CE, Silva CM, Ota-Arakaki JS. Usefulness of pulmonary capillary wedge pressure as a correlate of left ventricular filling pressures in pulmonary arterial hypertension. J Heart Lung Transplant. 2014;33:157–62.

77. Ryan JJ, Rich JD, Thiruvoipati T, Swamy R, Kim GH, Rich S. Current practice for determining pulmonary capillary wedge pressure predisposes to serious errors in the classification of patients with pulmonary hypertension. Am Heart J. 2012;163:589–94.

78. Sabbah HN, Anbe DT, Stein PD. Negative intraventricular diastolic pressure in patients with mitral stenosis: evidence of left ventricular diastolic suction. Am J Cardiol. 1980;45:562–6.

79. Paulus WJ, Vantrimpont PJ, Rousseau MF. Diastolic function of the nonfilling human left ventricle. J Am Coll Cardiol. 1992;20:1524–32.

80. Courtois M, Fattal PG, Kovacs Jr SJ, Tiefenbrunn AJ, Ludbrook PA. Anatomically and physiologically based reference level for measurement of intracardiac pressures. Circulation. 1995;92:1994–2000.

81. Baim DS, Grossman W. Grossman's cardiac catheterization, angiography, and intervention. Philadelphia: Lippincott Williams & Wilkins; 2006.

82. Falsetti HL, Mates RE, Carroll RJ, Gupta RL, Bell AC. Analysis and correction of pressure wave distortion in fluid-filled catheter systems. Circulation. 1974;49:165–72.

83. Irvin CG, Sampson M, Engel L, Grassino AE. Effect of breathing pattern on esophageal pressure gradients in humans. J Appl Physiol Respir Environ Exerc Physiol. 1984;57:168–75.

84. D'Alonzo GE, Barst RJ, Ayres SM, Bergofsky EH, Brundage BH, Detre KM, Fishman AP, Goldring RM, Groves BM, Kernis JT, et al. Survival in patients with primary pulmonary hypertension. Results from a national prospective registry. Ann Intern Med. 1991;115:343–9.

85. Thenappan T, Shah SJ, Rich S, Tian L, Archer SL, Gomberg-Maitland M. Survival in pulmonary arterial hypertension: a reappraisal of the NIH risk stratification equation. Eur Respir J. 2010;35:1079–87.

86. Dias CA, Assad RS, Caneo LF, Abduch MC, Aiello VD, Dias AR, Marcial MB, Oliveira SA. Reversible pulmonary trunk banding. II. An experimental model for rapid pulmonary ventricular hypertrophy. J Thorac Cardiovasc Surg. 2002;124:999–1006.

87. Chen EP, Craig DM, Bittner HB, Davis RD, Van Trigt P. Pharmacological strategies for improving diastolic dysfunction in the setting of chronic pulmonary hypertension. Circulation. 1998;97:1606–12.

88. Stein PD, Sabbah HN, Anbe DT, Marzilli M. Performance of the failing and nonfailing right ventricle of patients with pulmonary hypertension. Am J Cardiol. 1979;44:1050–5.

89. Chemla D, Castelain V, Herve P, Lecarpentier Y, Brimioulle S. Haemodynamic evaluation of pulmonary hypertension. Eur Respir J. 2002;20:1314–31.

90. Fishman AP, Fisher AB. The respiratory system. Bethesda: American Physiological Society, Distributed by Williams & Wilkins; 1985.

91. Naeije R, Vachiery JL, Yerly P, Vanderpool R. The transpulmonary pressure gradient for the diagnosis of pulmonary vascular disease. Eur Respir J. 2013;41:217–23.

92. Tedford RJ, Beaty CA, Mathai SC, Kolb TM, Damico R, Hassoun PM, Leary PJ, Kass DA, Shah AS. Prognostic value of the pre-transplant diastolic pulmonary artery pressure-to-pulmonary capillary wedge pressure gradient in cardiac transplant recipients with pulmonary hypertension. J Heart Lung Transplant. 2014;33:289–97.

93. Tampakakis E, Leary PJ, Selby VN, De Marco T, Cappola TP, Felker GM, Russell SD, Kasper EK, Tedford RJ. The diastolic pulmonary gradient does not predict survival in patients with pulmonary hypertension due to left heart disease. JACC Heart Fail. 2015;3:9–16.

94. Zidulka A, Hakim TS. Wedge pressure in large vs. small pulmonary arteries to detect pulmonary venoconstriction. J Appl Physiol (1985). 1985;59:1329–32.

95. Hellems HK, Haynes FW, Dexter L. Pulmonary capillary pressure in man. J Appl Physiol. 1949;2:24–9.

96. Kafi SA, Melot C, Vachiery JL, Brimioulle S, Naeije R. Partitioning of pulmonary vascular resistance in primary pulmonary hypertension. J Am Coll Cardiol. 1998;31:1372–6.

97. Teboul JL, Andrivet P, Ansquer M, Besbes M, Rekik N, Lemaire F, Brun-Buisson C. Bedside evaluation of the resistance of large and medium pulmonary veins in various lung diseases. J Appl Physiol (1985). 1992;72:998–1003.

98. Cournand A, Riley RL, Breed ES, Baldwin ED, Richards DW, Lester MS, Jones M. Measurement of cardiac output in man using the technique of catheterization of the right auricle or ventricle. J Clin Invest. 1945;24:106–16.

99. Stead EA, Warren JV, Merrill AJ, Brannon ES. The cardiac output in male subjects as measured by the technique of right atrial catheterization. Normal values with observations on the effect of anxiety and tilting. J Clin Invest. 1945;24:326–31.

100. Kendrick AH, West J, Papouchado M, Rozkovec A. Direct Fick cardiac output: are assumed values of oxygen consumption acceptable? Eur Heart J. 1988;9:337–42.

101. Fakler U, Pauli C, Hennig M, Sebening W, Hess J. Assumed oxygen consumption frequently results in large errors in the determination of cardiac output. J Thorac Cardiovasc Surg. 2005;130:272–6.

102. Ultman JS, Bursztein S. Analysis of error in the determination of respiratory gas exchange at varying FIO2. J Appl Physiol Respir Environ Exerc Physiol. 1981;50:210–6.

103. Narang N, Thibodeau JT, Levine BD, Gore MO, Ayers CR, Lange RA, Cigarroa JE, Turer AT, de Lemos JA, McGuire DK. Inaccuracy of estimated resting oxygen uptake in the clinical setting. Circulation. 2014;129:203–10.

104. Moise SF, Sinclair CJ, Scott DH. Pulmonary artery blood temperature and the measurement of cardiac output by thermodilution. Anaesthesia. 2002;57:562–6.

105. Lehmann KG, Platt MS. Improved accuracy and precision of thermodilution cardiac output measurement using a dual thermistor catheter system. J Am Coll Cardiol. 1999;33:883–91.

106. Hoeper MM, Maier R, Tongers J, Niedermeyer J, Hohlfeld JM, Hamm M, Fabel H. Determination of cardiac output by the Fick method, thermodilution, and acetylene rebreathing in pulmonary hypertension. Am J Respir Crit Care Med. 1999;160:535–41.

107. Hillis LD, Firth BG, Winniford MD. Analysis of factors affecting the variability of Fick versus indicator dilution measurements of cardiac output. Am J Cardiol. 1985;56:764–8.

108. Rich S, Dantzker DR, Ayres SM, Bergofsky EH, Brundage BH, Detre KM, Fishman AP, Goldring RM, Groves BM, Koerner SK, et al. Primary pulmonary hypertension. A national prospective study. Ann Intern Med. 1987;107:216–23.

109. Sandoval J, Bauerle O, Palomar A, Gomez A, Martinez-Guerra ML, Beltran M, Guerrero ML. Survival in primary pulmonary hypertension. Validation of a prognostic equation. Circulation. 1994;89:1733–44.

110. McGregor M, Sniderman A. On pulmonary vascular resistance: the need for more precise definition. Am J Cardiol. 1985;55:217–21.

111. Addonizio LJ, Gersony WM, Robbins RC, Drusin RE, Smith CR, Reison DS, Reemtsma K, Rose EA. Elevated pulmonary vascular resistance and cardiac transplantation. Circulation. 1987;76:V52–5.

112. Tartulier M, Bourret M, Deyrieux F. Pulmonary arterial pressures in normal subjects. Effects of age and muscular exercise. Bull Physiopathol Respir (Nancy). 1972;8:1295–321.

113. Ehrsam RE, Perruchoud A, Oberholzer M, Burkart F, Herzog H. Influence of age on pulmonary haemodynamics at rest and during supine exercise. Clin Sci (Lond). 1983;65:653–60.

114. Weir EK, Reeves JT. Pulmonary hypertension. Mount Kisco: Futura Pub. Co.; 1984.

115. Sitbon O, Humbert M, Jais X, Ioos V, Hamid AM, Provencher S, Garcia G, Parent F, Herve P, Simonneau G. Long-term response to calcium channel blockers in idiopathic pulmonary arterial hypertension. Circulation. 2005;111:3105–11.

116. Barst RJ, Langleben D, Frost A, Horn EM, Oudiz R, Shapiro S, McLaughlin V, Hill N, Tapson VF, Robbins IM, Zwicke D, Duncan B, Dixon RA, Frumkin LR. Sitaxsentan therapy for pulmonary arterial hypertension. Am J Respir Crit Care Med. 2004;169:441–7.

117. Borlaug BA, Nishimura RA, Sorajja P, Lam CS, Redfield MM. Exercise hemodynamics enhance diagnosis of early heart failure with preserved ejection fraction. Circ Heart Fail. 2010;3:588–95.

118. Fujimoto N, Borlaug BA, Lewis GD, Hastings JL, Shafer KM, Bhella PS, Carrick-Ranson G, Levine BD. Hemodynamic responses to rapid saline loading: the impact of age, sex, and heart failure. Circulation. 2013;127:55–62.

119. Andersen MJ, Olson TP, Melenovsky V, Kane GC, Borlaug BA. Differential hemodynamic effects of exercise and volume expansion in people with and without heart failure. Circ Heart Fail. 2015;8:41–8.

120. Opotowsky AR. Clinical evaluation and management of pulmonary hypertension in the adult with congenital heart disease. Circulation. 2015;131:200–10.

121. Lentner C. Geigy scientific tables: heart and circulation. West Caldwell: CIBA-GEIGY Corporation; 1990.

122. Davidson CJ, Bonow R. Cardiac catheterization. In: Braunwald's heart disease: a textbook. Philadelphia: Elsevier Saunders; 2012. p. 383–405.

Geeshath Jayasekera and Andrew J. Peacock

The definite haemodynamic diagnosis of pulmonary hypertension (PH) requires right heart catheterization (RHC) and direct measurements of right ventricular, pulmonary artery and pulmonary capillary wedge pressures and cardiac output. As this is an invasive test with risk and cost implications diagnostic algorithms have been devised that combines clinical assessment, non-imaging cardio-respiratory assessment and non-invasive imaging in patients suspected of having pulmonary hypertension. The initial aim is to establish a tentative diagnosis of pulmonary hypertension, to assess its severity and to identify the underlying etiology. Diagnosis must then be confirmed by RHC. Subsequently non-invasive imaging techniques may be used to monitor disease progression as well as response to treatment in patients with pulmonary hypertension as an alternative to repeat invasive right heart catheterization. In the future these imaging techniques may also help us to understand the cellular and molecular mechanisms responsible for the pathophysiology of pulmonary hypertension in both the pulmonary circulation and the right ventricle (RV).

Echocardiography

Morphological Assessment of the Right Heart and Pulmonary Circulation

Two-dimensional echocardiography using a subcostal/apical 4-chamber view has been used to obtain various variables in the assessment of right ventricle morphology in patients with pulmonary hypertension. In two studies the right ventricular

end diastolic dimension alone and the right ventricular end diastolic dimension indexed to body surface area correlated well with mean pulmonary artery pressure (mPAP) [1, 2] (Fig. 12.1).

Volume calculations of the right ventricle are essential for quantification of RV systolic function. Due to the partly retrosternal location of the right ventricle and the heavily trabeculated RV border, imaging of the right ventricle by conventional echocardiography is challenging. However using complex biplane and multi-slice methods to evaluate RV geometry did not improve the accuracy of the results compared to simple mono-plane area length method [3, 4]. Measurements of RV free wall thickness and RV mass are less practical due to the trabeculations of the RV endocardial surface and the complex RV shape.

To differentiate RV dilation secondary to RV pressure overload from RV dilatation due to increased preload, systolic and diastolic positioning of the inter-ventricular septum (IVS) may be used (Fig. 12.2). Increased RV preload resulted in predominantly end-diastolic leftward IVS displacement while in pure pressure overload this was maximum at end systole [5]. Ryan et al. used a left ventricular eccentricity

G. Jayasekera, MBChB, MRCP
Scottish Pulmonary Vascular Unit, Golden Jubilee National Hospital, Glasgow, UK

A.J. Peacock, MPhil, MD (✉)
Scottish Pulmonary Vascular Unit, Regional Heart and Lung Centre, Golden Jubilee National Hospital, Agamemnon Street, Glasgow G12 8DY, UK
e-mail: apeacock@udcf.gla.ac.uk

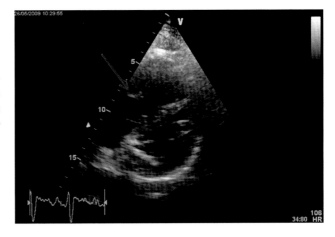

Fig. 12.1 2D echocardiogram – Short axis view of a patient with idiopathic pulmonary arterial hypertension showing RV dilatation (*red arrow*)

© Springer International Publishing Switzerland 2016
B.A. Maron et al. (eds.), *Pulmonary Hypertension: Basic Science to Clinical Medicine*, DOI 10.1007/978-3-319-23594-3_12

index, defined as the ratio of the length of two perpendicular minor axis diameters, which were obtained at end systole and end diastole. One of these diameters bisected and was perpendicular to the inter-ventricular septum. In normal subjects in the study the index was 1.0, while in RV volume overload the index was significantly increased at end diastole, and approximately 1.0 at end systole. In the group of patients with RV pressure overload the index was greater than 1.0 in both end systole and end diastole [6].

Haemodynamic Assessment of the Right Heart and the Pulmonary Circulation

Bernoulli equation (pressure gradient $= 4 V^2$ mmHg) is used to calculate the pressure gradient driving blood through a cardiac orifice (Fig. 12.3). Tricuspid valve regurgitant jet

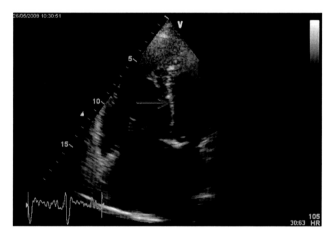

Fig. 12.2 2D echocardiogram – Apical chamber view of patient with idiopathic pulmonary arterial hypertension. There is inter-ventricular septal bowing (*arrow*) and marked dilatation of right sided chambers

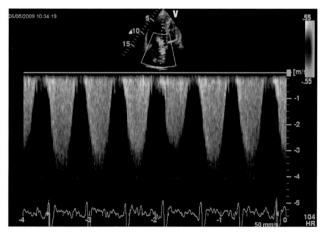

Fig. 12.3 Continuous wave Doppler mapping of the tricuspid regurgitant jet. A tricuspid regurgitant velocity of 4 m/s^2 is demonstrated. Using the Bernoulli equation (pressure gradient $= 4 V^2$ mmHg) a TRPG of 64 mmHg could be derived

velocity from the apical 4-chamber view is usually used to calculate tricuspid regurgitant pressure gradient (TRPG) (V = peak tricuspid regurgitant velocity at end diastole). The calculation of systolic pulmonary arterial pressure (sPAP) uses the equation, sPAP = TRPG + Right Atrial Pressure (RAP). This calculation is based on the assumption that there is no right ventricular outflow tract stenosis allowing the right ventricular systolic pressure to be equivalent to sPAP. Although not routinely used in the diagnosis and follow up of pulmonary hypertension echocardiography derived diastolic pulmonary artery pressure (dPAP) and mean pulmonary pressure (mPAP) may be useful when tricuspid regurgitant jets cannot be used. In a study by Lei et al. the peak diastolic and end diastolic pulmonary artery to right ventricular pressure gradients derived by Doppler flow profiles correlated well with measurements at right heart catheterization. A correlation was also observed between pulmonary artery diastolic pressure and Doppler derived end diastolic pressure gradient [7].

Right atrial pressure measurement is required to calculate sPAP from tricuspid and pulmonary regurgitant jets. In an early study by Nakao et al., they suggested that inferior vena cava (IVC) diameter of more than 1 cm and area of more than 2.0 cm^2 measured by echocardiography at the left lateral position to have sensitivities of 84 % and 73 % and specificities of 95 % and 100 % for the diagnosis of raised right atrial pressure (8 mmHg) respectively [8]. Kircher et al. analysed the respiratory motion of the IVC by two-dimensional echocardiography. They measured the inspiratory and expiratory IVC diameters and suggested the use of percentage collapse (Caval Index) as a predictor of Right atrial pressure (Caval index < 50 % indicate RA pressure ≥ 10 mmHg) [9].

Echocardiography Definition of Pulmonary Hypertension

Pulmonary hypertension is defined as mPAP exceeding 25 mmHg at rest during right heart catheterization. Various attempts have been made to define non-invasive diagnostic criteria of pulmonary hypertension based on echocardiographic findings thus studies have concentrated on defining normal echocardiogram derived pulmonary artery pressures. In a study of 53 healthy people TRPG ranged from 12.6 to 29.3 mmHg. The study authors concluded that TRPG of 30 mmHg should be considered the upper limit of normal [10]. In an analysis of the Massachusetts General Hospital echocardiographic database, 3790 echocardiographically normal subjects had a measured sPAP documented. The estimated upper 95 % limit for sPAP was 37.2 mmHg (RAP = 10 mmHg). A sPAP >40 mmHg was found in 6 % of those >50 years old and 5 % of those with a BMI >30 kg/m^2 [11]. The alternative approach has been to estimate mPAP based on pulmonary artery pressures measured by echocardiography. Syyed et al. identified a relationship between sPAP from echocardiography and mPAP from right heart catheterization. They identified a linear relationship (sPAP = 1.5 mPAP + 0.46) which was maintained following changes in posture and activity [12].

Pulsatile Pulmonary Haemodynamics

Kitabatke et al. used a Doppler technique to study the flow velocity patterns of the right ventricular outflow tract. They identified characteristic abnormalities of the pulmonary valve motion in pulmonary hypertension including rapid opening slope in systole and mid-systolic semi-closure of the pulmonary valve. In patients with pulmonary hypertension the flow velocity pattern demonstrated a rapid acceleration reaching a peak level sooner than the normal cohort. Mid systolic notching due to a secondary slower rise during deceleration was also observed in some of the patients. They observed that the time to peak flow (AcT) and the ratio AcT/RVET (Right ventricular ejection time) decreased with rising mPAP [13]. However AcT was shown to be longer in patients with low cardiac index [14] and high pulmonary blood flow in congenital cardiac diseases [15] and shorter in patients with high body surface area [16] and proximal pulmonary emboli [17].

Prognostic Staging and Follow Up

There are specific echocardiographic findings that are important in terms of prognosis in patients with pulmonary hypertension. In a study by Raymond et al. the abnormal echocardiographic findings of presence of pericardial effusion, right atrial enlargement and septal displacement during diastole reflected the severity of right heart failure and predicted adverse events in patients with severe pulmonary hypertension [18]. Tei et al. introduced a Doppler derived index (Tei index or Myocardial performance index) that combined elements of systolic and diastolic function for the assessment of global right ventricular function. The index is calculated using tissue Doppler recordings and is defined as (A-B)/B where A is the time interval between the end and onset of the trans-tricuspid flow and B is the right ventricular ejection time. The A interval includes the isovolumetric contraction time (IVCT), isovolumetric relaxation time (IVRT) and the ejection time, thus the Tei index can also be expressed by the formula (IVCT + IVRT)/RVET. The Tei index was a strong predictor of clinical status and survival and was relatively unaffected by heart rate, right ventricular pressure, right ventricular dilatation or tricuspid regurgitation [19]. Vogel et al. examined the effect of acute changes in loading conditions and contractile functions on the Tei index. In a study of Yorkshire pigs the relationship between dP/dt_{max} and the Tei index was inconsistent post Dobutamine infusion. The index was significantly affected by acute changes in afterload and preload [20].

In contrast to the left ventricle, which shortens relatively symmetrically in the transverse and longitudinal planes, the right ventricle contraction is predominantly on a longitudinal plane. Thus the displacement of the tricuspid annulus towards the RV apex at systole is correlated with the RV ejection fraction. This measure, known as TAPSE (Tricuspid annular plane systolic excursion) have been found to be highly reproducible and practical [21, 22]. In a prospective observational study by Forfia et al. a TAPSE of less than 1.8 cm was associated with greater RV systolic dysfunction, right heart remodelling and RV/LV disproportion. A high TAPSE (1.8 cm or more) also predicted survival with a 1 and 2-year survival rates of 94 % and 88 % compared to 60 % and 50 % in the low TAPSE group [23]. In a later study in 59 idiopathic pulmonary arterial hypertension (IPAH) patients, the group with TAPSE ≤ 15 mm and a left ventricular eccentricity index ≥1.7 had the highest adverse event rate. Higher TAPSE and a lack of TR predicted a favourable prognosis [24]. An important point to consider is that TAPSE could be pseudonormalised in significant volume loading as seen in left to right shunting or severe functional TR.

A novel measurement, pulmonary vascular capacitance (PVCAP), was assessed as a predictor of morality in patients with pulmonary arterial hypertension (PAH) in a recent study. PVCAP was defined as stroke volume/pulmonary artery pulse pressure and is measured by two-dimensional and Doppler echocardiography. Patients in the highest PVCAP quartile had a 39 % mortality against 7 % in the lowest quartile [25].

Differential Diagnosis

Echocardiography may also aid in identifying the cause of pulmonary hypertension including left heart disease, congenital cardiac diseases and valvular pathology. It may also help in identifying alternative causes of right ventricular dilatation including right ventricular arrythmogenic dysplasia and right ventricular infarction.

New Developments in Echocardiography

RV measurements by 2-dimensional echocardiography are difficult due to its complex shape. 3-dimensional echocardiography (3D Echo) has been used frequently in the volumetry of the left ventricle and Grapsa et al. compared RV volume and mass data obtained by 3D echo against cardiac

MR imaging (Fig. 12.4). They measured RV end diastolic and end systolic volumes, stroke volume and RV mass and compared these findings with CMR. Although CMR showed less inter-observer variability for some measures, RV volume and mass were similar for CMR and 3D echo in PAH patients [26]. In a study comparing 2-D echo to 3D echo, an index of RV contractility corrected for preload (dP/dt/EDV) and right ventricular end-diastolic volume (RVEDV) was measured. The 2D Echo derived contractility index did not correlate with disease severity while 3D echo derived values were potential markers of disease severity [27]. Comparing the two imaging modalities de Bello and colleagues showed that 3D echo derived RV diastolic and systolic volumes as well as ejection fraction to have a higher discriminating power compared to the 2D derived variables [28].

More recently 3-D speckle tracking which has been used extensively in left ventricular functional assessment, has been used to assess patients with pulmonary hypertension. Myocardial strain is defined as the relative lengthening or shortening of a myocardial segment expressed as a percentage of its initial length. The PH population had reduced right ventricular strain and dysynchronous ventricles. Although area strain, longitudinal strain, circumferential strain and radial strain were all reduced in patients with PH, area strain correlated best with RVEF and was the only predictor of mortality [29] (Fig. 12.5).

In patients with dilated right ventricles 3D echocardiography has the disadvantage of suboptimal images, and the resulting exclusion of the RV free wall from the imaging has lead to inaccurate volumes. As an alternative to this, Bhave et al. suggested using a "knowledge based reconstruction" method for 3D modelling of the RV endocardium from 2D images. This involved acquiring 2D images localised in 3 dimensional space by a magnetic field generator located under the patient and a magnetic field sensor, then using a reconstruction algorithm to construct a 3D model. This is based on identifying specific landmarks and a reconstructing algorithm using these landmarks to fit sub regions of the right ventricle to hearts in a database of patients with similar pathology. These provided valuable and accurate RV volumes, which compared with CMR, but larger studies are required to determine the practicality of this approach [30].

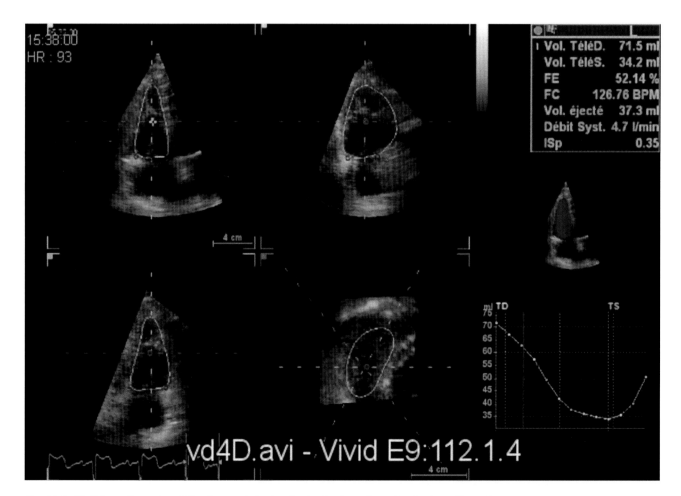

Fig. 12.4 3D Echocardiography – RV volume and ejection fraction by three-dimensional echocardiography

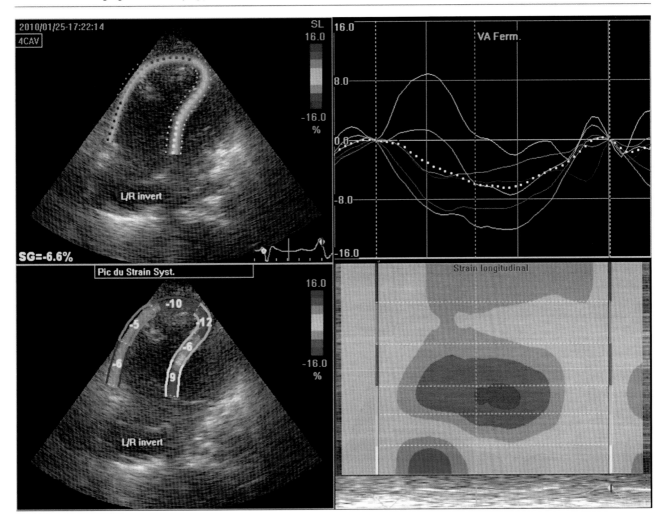

Fig. 12.5 Heterogeneous segmental contraction and dyssynchrony in a patient with pulmonary hypertension

Chest Radiography

Plain chest radiography usually provide the first clue to the presence of pulmonary hypertension. It is inexpensive and widely available. The Chest x-ray appearance of pulmonary hypertension consist of enlargement of the pulmonary arteries, rapid tapering of the vessels as they extend to the lung periphery and an enlarged heart, particularly the right sided chambers (Fig. 12.6). There is reduction of the size of the intrapulmonary vessels known as peripheral pruning, which is a distinct feature of pulmonary arterial hypertension. Transverse diameter of the proximal interlobar pulmonary artery on posterior-anterior chest radiograph that exceeds 16 mm in men and 15 mm in women is a useful measurement for enlargement of the central pulmonary arteries, likely to be due to pulmonary arterial hypertension in the absence of a left-to-right shunt [31].

Kanemoto and colleagues reviewed 59 chest radiographs in patients with primary pulmonary hypertension(PPH). They compared five measured values between normal control and PPH group. DPA/(T/2), which is an indicator of the degree of protrusion of the main pulmonary artery, where DPA is the width of the main pulmonary artery from the midline and T the thoracic diameter (divided by half thoracic diameter to eliminate differences) was significantly higher in the PPH group. The average width of the descending branch of the pulmonary artery (dPA) was more than twice that of the control group (12.1–25.1). The PL/T index (The point of union of the external border of the upper lobe artery with the pars interlobaris = point L, the sum of horizontal distances of the right and left L to the midline = Pulmonary Lobar diameter, PL) was increased in the PPH population [32]. Previously Lupi et al. had suggested that the PL/T index as a radiological index suggesting pulmonary arterial hypertension [33].

The normal values for the width of the descending branch of the right pulmonary artery has been reported as 9–13 mm by Schwedel et al. [34] 9–16 mm by Simon et al. [35] and 9–16 mm for men and 9–15 mm for women by Chang et al. [36]

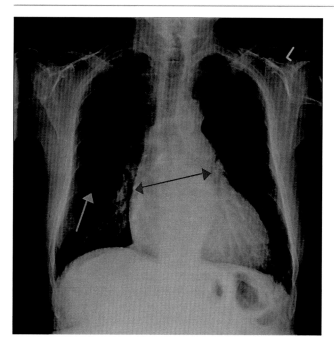

Fig. 12.6 Chest radiograph of a patient with idiopathic pulmonary arterial hypertension. There is cardiomegaly, prominent pulmonary arteries (*red arrow*) and peripheral oligaemia (*blue arrow*)

In chronic thromboembolic pulmonary hypertension apart from features of peripheral oligaemia there may be asymmetry of hilar vessels when thrombosis occurs in central pulmonary arteries. Woodruff et al. reviewed 22 chest radiographs of patients with chronic thromboembolic pulmonary hypertension. Cardiac enlargement was defined by a cardiothoracic ratio of more than 0.5 and right ventricular enlargement was defined by a retrosternal cardiac silhouette height greater than one-third the distance between the anterior cardiophrenic sulcus and the angle of Louis. All the patients in both operative and non-operative groups had abnormal chest radiographs. Nineteen patients had cardiomegaly and 13 of these had predominantly right ventricular enlargement. A value of 0.23 for the ratio of the diameter of the main pulmonary artery to the diameter of the left hemithorax (DPA/DHT) was considered normal in a previous study and all but one patient had a higher ratio in this study. Twelve patients had enlarged right descending pulmonary arteries (16 mm for men and 15 mm for women). Specific areas of diminished vascularity were found in about two third of the patients and these were confirmed by pulmonary angiography [37]. Findings of an abnormal chest radiograph in this study and in a further study by Tilkian et al. [38] were in contrast to previous studies by Moser et al. [39] and Benotti et al. [40] who concluded most patients with CTEPH have normal chest radiographs.

Chest X-ray will also provide important clues regarding the cause of pulmonary hypertension including parenchymal lung disease. Although the presence of pulmonary hypertension can be recognised in a plain chest radiograph, the characteristic findings are only likely to be visible in severe disease, which limits the role of chest radiography in diagnosing early or mild pulmonary hypertension. Assessment of peripheral pruning may be subjective and measurements of interlobar arteries are affected by variable magnification and the presence of severe parenchymal lung disease.

Ventilation Perfusion Scintigraphy

Ventilation perfusion scintigraphy (V/Q scan) is a vital investigation in the diagnostic workup of pulmonary hypertension (Fig. 12.7). The sensitivity and specificity of V/Q scanning in distinguishing chronic thromboembolic pulmonary hypertension (CTEPH) from other types of pulmonary hypertension is well documented. In a study in patients with pulmonary hypertension by Worsley et al. a high probability V/Q scan had sensitivity and specificity of 96 % and 94 % respectively in detecting patients with CTEPH [41]. When high and intermediate probability V/Q scans taken in combination the sensitivity and specificity were 100 % and 86 % respectively. In this series none of the patients with normal or low probability V/Q had CTEPH. In a larger retrospective review by Tunariu et al., when only high probability scans were considered of suggestive of CTEPH the sensitivity was 96.2 % with a specificity of 94.6 % [42]. When both high and intermediate probability scans were considered suggestive of CTEPH the specificity fell to 90 %.

These and a number of other studies demonstrated V/Q scanning to be a safe and highly sensitive test for suspected CTEPH. Grouping intermediate probability results with low probability results provide a highly sensitive and specific investigation in the diagnosis of CTEPH. It is important to note that large mismatched defects at V/Q scanning maybe seen in patients with idiopathic pulmonary arterial hypertension presumably due to thrombosis in situ. These defects may also be seen in other disease processes that affect central arteries and veins such as large vessel vasculitis [43], fibrosing mediastinitis [44], pulmonary artery sarcoma [45] and pulmonary veno-occlusive disease [46].

The introduction of multidetector CT pulmonary angiography (CTPA) has replaced V/Q scanning as first line of the investigation in the diagnosis of acute pulmonary embolism. However the role of CTPA in detecting chronic thromboembolic pulmonary hypertension is variable. Pitton et al. showed multidetector CTPA to have a sensitivity of 70.4 % for segmental and 63.6 % for subsegmental branches when compared to pulmonary digital substraction angiography (DSA) [47]. The retrospective review by Tunariu et al. confirmed that normal V/Q scintigraphy excluded CTEPH whereas normal CTPA did not [42]. In the CTEPH group in this study, CTPA was reported as showing features

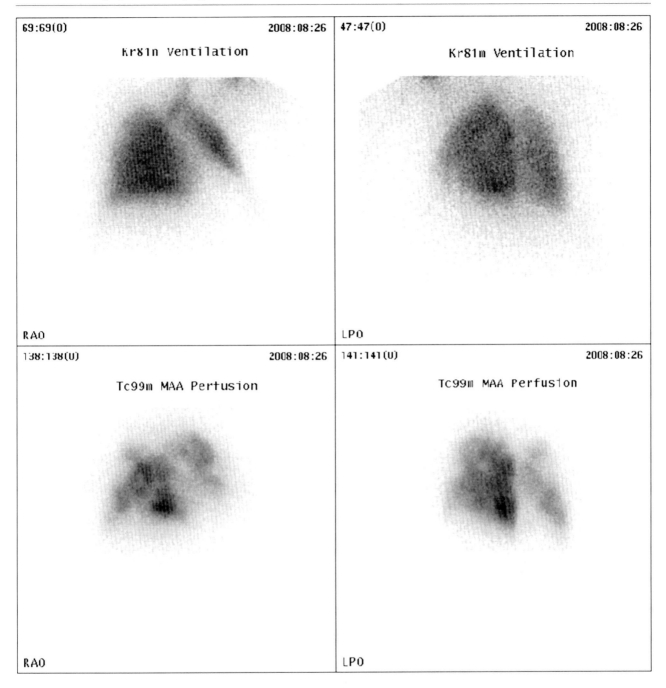

Fig. 12.7 Ventilation perfusion scintigraphy in a patient with chronic thromboembolic pulmonary hypertension showing multiple mismatched perfusion defects

suggestive of CTEPH in 40 of the 78 patients with a false negative report in 38 of the 78 (sensitivity 51 %). A CTPA report was considered as suggestive of CTEPH, if it stated visualisation of the thrombus, calcified thrombus, recanalization, sudden change of vessel calibre, strictures, poststenotic dilatation, webs or perfusion abnormality. The presence of mosaicism was also noted but its presence alone without other features was not considered diagnostic of CTPEH.

Computed Tomography

There have been dramatic technological advances in computed tomography (CT) in recent years with sub millimetre thick slices, optimal contrast enhancement and improvements in post processing power. CT also has the advantage of imaging the heart and the lung parenchyma as well as the pulmonary arteries and has a greater resolution than other imaging modalities giving a clearer view of morphological changes in the pulmonary vessels. It is also an imaging modality that is often performed as part of the early diagnostic assessment in patients presenting with chest discomfort or dyspnoea. However repeated exposure to radiation precludes CT as a routine test used in assessing disease progression and response to treatment.

The Main Pulmonary Artery Signs

The intra pericardial main pulmonary artery cannot be measured on conventional chest radiography but can be identified and measured on CT. There have been various studies over the years examining the reliability of CT in detecting pulmonary hypertension using variety of methodologies. Although right heart catheterization is gold standard in measuring pulmonary artery pressures, these studies have concentrated on providing a non-invasive surrogate of pulmonary hypertension.

In an early study of 32 patients with cardiopulmonary disease a diameter of the main pulmonary artery above 28.6 mm predicted the presence of pulmonary hypertension (Fig. 12.8). In this study the calculated cross sectional areas of main and interlobar pulmonary arteries normalised to body surface area were found to give the best estimates of PAP [48]. A study by Haimovici et al. found a similar correlation in pre lung or heart-lung transplantation patients [49].

Ng et al. measured aortic and main pulmonary artery diameters on a single defined axial scan level [50]. The level was at which the right pulmonary artery is in continuity with the main pulmonary artery and sweep across the midline. In this study both the main pulmonary artery diameter (dPA) and the ratio of the main pulmonary artery to the ascending

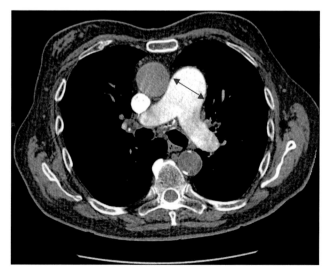

Fig. 12.8 CTPA demonstrating enlargement of the main pulmonary artery (*Arrow*) in a patient with idiopathic pulmonary arterial hypertension

aorta (rPA) were positively related to mean pulmonary artery pressure (mPAP). In patients younger than 50 years of age the mPAP correlated more with rPA than dPA and vice versa in patients older than 50 years of age. They suggested that this may be due to a gradual increase of aortic diameter with age and concluded rPA should be used as a non invasive indicator of the presence of PH. A degree of 'internal normalisation' with lack of dependence on body surface area and sex (as both variables influence pulmonary artery and aortic dimensions to a equal degree) as well as technical changes during imaging were suggested as advantages of using rPA over dPA.

In another study in patients with parenchymal lung disease or possible pulmonary vascular disease, CT determined main pulmonary artery diameter of ≥29 mm had a sensitivity of 87 %, a specificity of 89 % and a positive predictive value of 0.97 for predicting PH. The main pulmonary artery was measured at the widest portion within 3 cm of the bifurcation [51].

In a study by Mohammedi et al. the main PA was measured in 4 different ways in order to establish the method with the best correlation to mPAP. The method in which the axial diameter of the main PA, measured along the line that originates from the centre of the adjacent aorta and passes perpendicular to the long axis of the main PA at the level of PA bifurcation, was the most reproducible with the least observer variability. The study showed, a threshold of main pulmonary artery diameter (mPA)>31.5 mm was found to be 52 % sensitive and 90.2 % specific for pulmonary hypertension. In this study the main PA ratio >1 was 71 % sensitive and 76 % specific for pulmonary hypertension [52]. Truong et al. in the Framingham heart study used the transverse axial diameter of the main pulmonary artery and the ascending aorta at the level of the bifurcation of the right pulmonary artery for their measurements. They established a 90th percentile sex-specific cut off value for mPA for men of 29 mm and women of 27 mm and found an association with dyspnoea using the aforementioned cut off values. Interestingly they did not find an association with dyspnoea when using a 90th percentile cut off value of 0.9 or commonly used value of 1.0 for the pulmonary artery ratio [53].

As noted above, there is a large variation both in terms of the methodology and the reported cut-off diameter of the main pulmonary artery on CT when determining dilatation.

Beyond the Main PA

The studies that measures the calibre of right and left PA and the right interlobar artery did not appear to offer an advantage over main PA measurements on the strength of correlation with right heart catheter derived mPAP. In a study by Tan and colleagues who looked at CT determined measurements of main Pulmonary artery, right and left PA and the ratio between segmental arteries and their corresponding bronchi (ABR), a ratio of more than 1:1 in three of four lobes were higher in the PH population compared to the control group (65 % vs 22 %). The apical segmental arteries and the bronchi of the upper lobes and the posterior basal segmental arteries and the bronchi of the lower lobes were chosen for this study [51]. It is important to note that solitary segmental artery enlargement may be seen in normal patients as well as patients with regional lung abnormalities such as pulmonary fibrosis. In this study the combination of a main PA diameter of or more than 29 mm and an ABR of more than 1:1 in three or four lobes was the most specific finding for the presence of PH (specificity 100 %).

Hypertrophy of the bronchial arteries is a well-recognised radiological feature on conventional angiography and CT pulmonary angiography in patients with chronic thromboembolic pulmonary hypertension (Fig. 12.9). Although the mechanism of bronchial artery hypertrophy is not well understood its role is thought to be to maintain the viability of the lung parenchyma after pulmonary artery occlusion. Hypertrophied bronchial arteries are easily identified on CT and is usually not visualised in normal individuals. Remi-Jardin et al. defined bronchial artery hypertrophy as a curvilinear mediastinal vessel of more than 1.5 mm diameter, which is seen along the course of the proximal bronchial tree. In an earlier study of patients with primary pulmonary hypertension and chronic thromboembolic pulmonary hypertension, they suggested that visualisation of brnchopulmonary collaterals and demonstration of bronchopulmonary collateral flow to be a distinguishing feature of CTEPH from those with primary pulmonary hypertension. However more recent studies have demonstrated bronchial artery hypertrophy to occur in patients with idiopathic pulmonary arterial hypertension as well as Eisenmenger's syndrome [54].

A study by Shimizu et al. showed that in CTEPH patients the cross sectional area of bronchial arteries correlates to the extent of central pulmonary thrombus. When they grouped the CTEPH patients into main, lobar and segmental type based on the most proximal location of thrombi, they did not find any significant difference between the total area of bronchial arteries in segmental type CTPEH and pulmonary arterial hypertension patients. The cross sectional area of bronchial arteries did not have a significant correlation with mPAP or PVR but their presence predicted a better post surgical outcome [55].

Cardiac Signs

ECG gated CT can be used to obtain information regarding ventricular function and to detect congenital cardiac abnormalities but conventional CT provide information that can be used in the diagnostic workup in patients suspected of having pulmonary hypertension. An axial RV to LV ration of more than 1:1 at the mid ventricular level is indicative of right ventricular enlargement (Fig. 12.10). There may be paradoxical bulging of the inter-ventricular septum towards the left ventricle, although this is better appreciated in cine review of ECG gated studies. When CT features of PH are associated with left sided heart chamber enlargement, pulmonary venous dilation and interlobular septal thickening, this is suggestive of pulmonary venous hypertension with a possible left heart cause. Thickening and calcification of the mitral valve leaflets with associated left atrial enlargement, which is suggestive of mitral valve disease and aortic valve calcification and LV hypertrophy suggestive of aortic valve disease can be identified on conventional CT. Left atrial

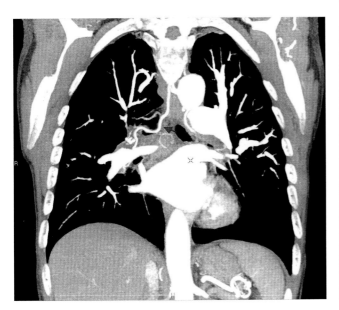

Fig. 12.9 CTPA with coronal reformatted projection showing bronchial artery hypertrophy in a patient with chronic thromboembolic pulmonary hypertension (*arrow*)

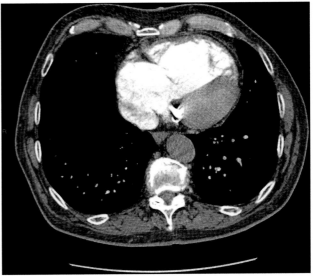

Fig. 12.10 CTPA in a patient with idiopathic pulmonary arterial hypertension demonstrating dilatation of right-sided cardiac chambers, and right ventricular hypertrophy

myxomas, by interfering with mitral valve function and pulmonary vein drainage can occasionally present with pulmonary hypertension and can be identified as a well defined intracavitary mass with low attenuation [56].

The presence of contrast in the inferior vena cava or hepatic veins during first pass contrast enhanced chest computed tomography is associated with tricuspid regurgitation. The extent of contrast reflux was associated with pulmonary artery pressures measured at right heart catheterization as well as the severity of tricuspid regurgitation by echocardiography [57]. It is important to note that although this is a specific sign of TR, the specificity decreases at higher contrast injection rates of grater than 3 ml/s [58].

Pericardial effusions are common in patients with severe pulmonary hypertension and this was demonstrated in a multicentre trial of patients with severe pulmonary hypertension on prostacyclin. The 1-year mortality in patients with small or moderate effusions was three times that of patients with trace or no effusions. The presence of effusion also correlated with right atrial size, severity of TR and reduced 6-min walk test [59]. On computed tomography pericardial effusions create an infilling of the space between the main pulmonary artery and ascending aorta which is known as the bikini bottom sign.

Lung Parenchyma

Mosaicism of the lung parenchyma is characterised by sharply demarcated areas of heterogenous attenuation that predominantly conform to the boundaries of the secondary pulmonary lobules (Fig. 12.11). In the context of pulmonary hypertension this is most commonly seen in patients with chronic thromboembolic pulmonary hypertension. In CTEPH, mosaicism corresponds to V/Q mismatch. The darker areas represent hypoperfusion while the higher attenuation areas correspond to normal or hyperperfusion. However mosaicism is not specific for CTEPH and can be seen in patients with small airways diseases as well as infiltrative lung diseases [60]. In small airways disease expiratory HRCT demonstrate air trapping which caused an increase in the conspicuity of the mosaic pattern. It was initially thought that this could be used to differentiate CTEPH from small airways disease but studies have reported air trapping as well as bronchial dilatation in patients with CTEPH [61, 62].

Computed Tomography in Chronic Thromboembolic Pulmonary Hypertension

Contrary to the findings in acute pulmonary emboli, which result in a concavity within the contrast material on angiography, CTEPH may lead to a complete vessel cut off which appears as a convex margin of contrast material on CTPA. In a complete obstruction the distal vessel diameter will be decreased and the pulmonary artery diameter may be increased at the site of the thrombus. In a partial obstruction CTPA findings include abrupt vessel narrowing, irregularity of the intimal surface contour and intravascular bands and webs. Bands are thin structures attached to the vessel wall that can be up to 20 mm in length with a free mid portion and webs are a descriptive term for a complex network of bands. These features seen in pulmonary angiography represent organising thrombi (Figs. 12.12, 12.13 and 12.14). Chronic organising thrombi can rarely be calcified. Pulmonary artery diameter may be increased with a raised main pulmonary artery to ascending aorta ratio as described earlier in the chapter. The right ventricle undergoes hypertrophy and subsequently

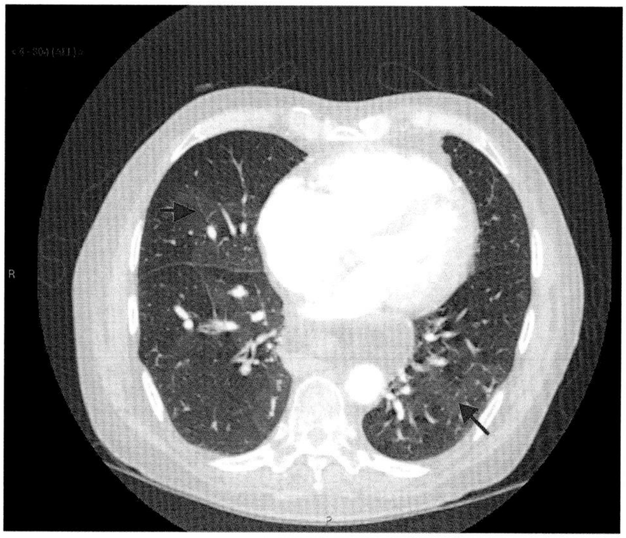

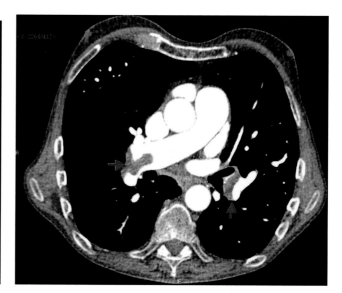

Fig. 12.11 High-resolution CT scan of chest showing subtle areas of mosaic oligaemia in a patient with CTEPH (*arrow*)

Fig. 12.12 CTPA demonstrating bilateral filling defects due to laminated thrombus in the right and left pulmonary arteries (*arrows*)

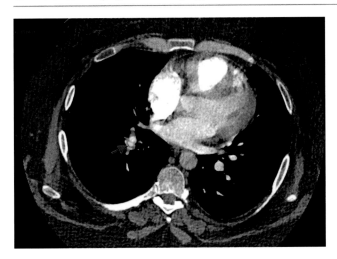

Fig. 12.13 CTPA demonstrating an arterial web in the right middle lobe pulmonary artery (*arrow*)

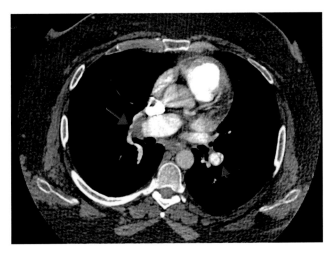

Fig. 12.14 Right sided filling defect and left pulmonary artery web (*arrow*)

dilates with right ventricular failure. There may be displacement of the interventricular septum towards the left ventricle during systole. The reflux of contrast material to the IVC or hepatic veins maybe observed which would indicate tricuspid regurgitation. Bronchial artery hypertrophy as well as enlarged non-bronchial systemic arteries are more common in patients with Chronic Thromboembolic Pulmonary Hypertension compared to other forms. The key parenchymal imaging feature of CTEPH is mosaic attenuation pattern of the lung parenchyma. Pulmonary infarcts may be visible especially at the lower parts of the lung as wedge shaped or linear, peripheral, irregular densities [63] (Fig. 12.15). They are due to occlusion of segmental and smaller pulmonary arteries and occur commonly in peripheral type CTEPH.

The morbidity and mortality from pulmonary thromboendarterecomy (PEA) has fallen significantly over the last few years. Several studies have concentrated on imaging features

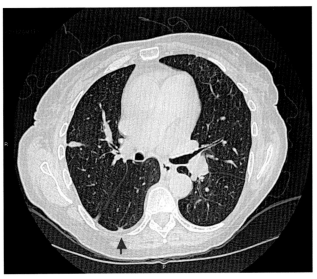

Fig. 12.15 High resolution CT showing multiple peripheral lung opacities in a patient with distal CTEPH (*arrow*)

that help predict surgical success in patients undergoing PEA. In a study by Bergin et al. CT pulmonary angiographic evidence of extensive central vessel disease and limited small vessel involvement predicted a favourable post surgical outcome [64]. In a study by Shimizu et al. the total area of bronchial arteries correlated to the central extent of thrombi and also predicted the gas exchange improvement after PEA suggesting that these patients had a lower proportion of distal vascular disease [55]. The presence of peripheral sub pleural densities, which reflect pulmonary infarcts commonly seen in peripheral type CTEPH demonstrated a positive correlation with postoperative PVR, which may lead to a poor postoperative outcome.

Computed Tomography in Pulmonary Veno-occlusive Disease

Pulmonary veno-occlusive disease is a rare cause of pulmonary hypertension where there is involvement of the post-capillary vasculature. It is difficult to make this diagnosis in vivo and a histopathological diagnosis using open surgical biopsy is usually contraindicated in these patients due to general frailty of this patient group. Two studies that retrospectively identified fifteen and eight patients with PVOD, studied the radiological features that would assist non-invasive CT assessment in these patients [65, 66]. The most common CT findings were septal lines, ground glass opacities particularly with a centrilobular distribution and lymphadenopathy. In the absence of other causes of pulmonary hypertension; e.g.; CTEPH and left sided heart disease, adenopathy was highly specific for PVOD. Normal left sided cardiac chambers and normal pulmonary capillary wedge pressure allows distinction of PVOD from pulmonary venous hypertension.

Magnetic Resonance Imaging

Although pulmonary arterial hypertension is a disease of the pulmonary vasculature, it is the subsequent right ventricular failure that is the main cause of morbidity and mortality in patients with PAH. Measurements of right ventricular structure and function have shown to be important in determining patient prognosis as well as response to treatment.

Cardiac magnetic resonance imaging is a non-invasive imaging tool and provides high-resolution three-dimensional images of the heart (Figs. 12.16, 12.17, 12.18 and 12.19).

Short axis stacks are used to reconstruct a 3D image of the right and the left ventricle and ventricular volumes and wall mass can be measured covering the entire cardiac cycle. Endocardial and epicardial contours are drawn at end-diastole and end-systole during post processing of images and ventricular volumes are calculated using the "Simpsons rule", which takes the sum of individual slice volumes and the interslice gap into account. From the volume changes of the right ventricle over time, systolic and diastolic function can be derived. New software solutions with semi automatic analysis have resulted in decreased post processing times. The inter-study reproducibility and accuracy of CMR measurements using a semiautomatic analysis have been validated in several reports [67, 68]. Velocity encoded cine MR images are used to quantify pulmonary artery flow. The aorta flow can be measured in the same plane and the ratio of pulmonary artery: aorta flow (Qp:Qs) and vice versa can be used to assess intracardiac shunts. Beerbaum et al. concluded that the calculation of Qp:Qs by cardiac MR to be quick, safe and reliable in children with cardiac defects [69]

The ability to assess right ventricular systolic function by conventional echocardiography based on volume calculations is limited. Although contrast-enhanced three-dimensional echocardiography has become available recently and has shown to be useful in assessing RV mass and RV ejection fraction, CMR remains the gold standard [26].

A large number of studies using cardiac MR imaging in patients with pulmonary arterial hypertension have been published. Many CMR measures have shown to be strongly predictive of mortality and survival thus offering potential for monitoring and assessing response to treatment.

Of these, Stroke volume (SV) is recognised as the key MR prognostic measure in PAH patients. Van Wolferen et al. investigated the prognostic significance of a variety of LV and RV structural and functional measurements in patients with idiopathic pulmonary arterial hypertension [70]. They showed that a low SV at baseline is a predictor of poor prognosis. They also showed that stroke volume rather than cardiac index to have a stronger correlation with prognosis in

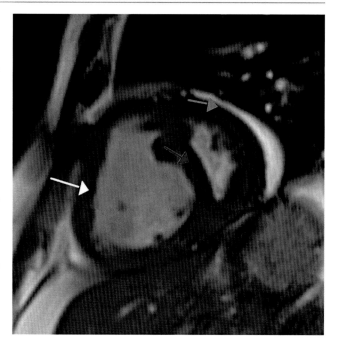

Fig. 12.16 Cardiac MR – Short axis view of a patient with IPAH demonstrating a dilated, hypertrophied right ventricle (*white arrow*), marked interventricular septal bowing (*red arrow*) and a pericardial effusion (*blue arrow*)

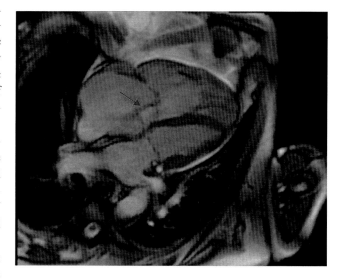

Fig. 12.17 Cardiac MR – Four-chamber view of another patient with IPAH. There is gross dilatation of the right atrium and right ventricle, increased right ventricular trabeculation and a visible tricuspid regurgitant jet (*Arrow*)

these patients, possibly explained by the fact that there may be compensatory increase in heart rate which will flaw the relationship between cardiac output and prognosis. The results in this study also suggested that a decrease in stroke volume during treatment to be an indicator of treatment failure. Although results were comparable when SV were

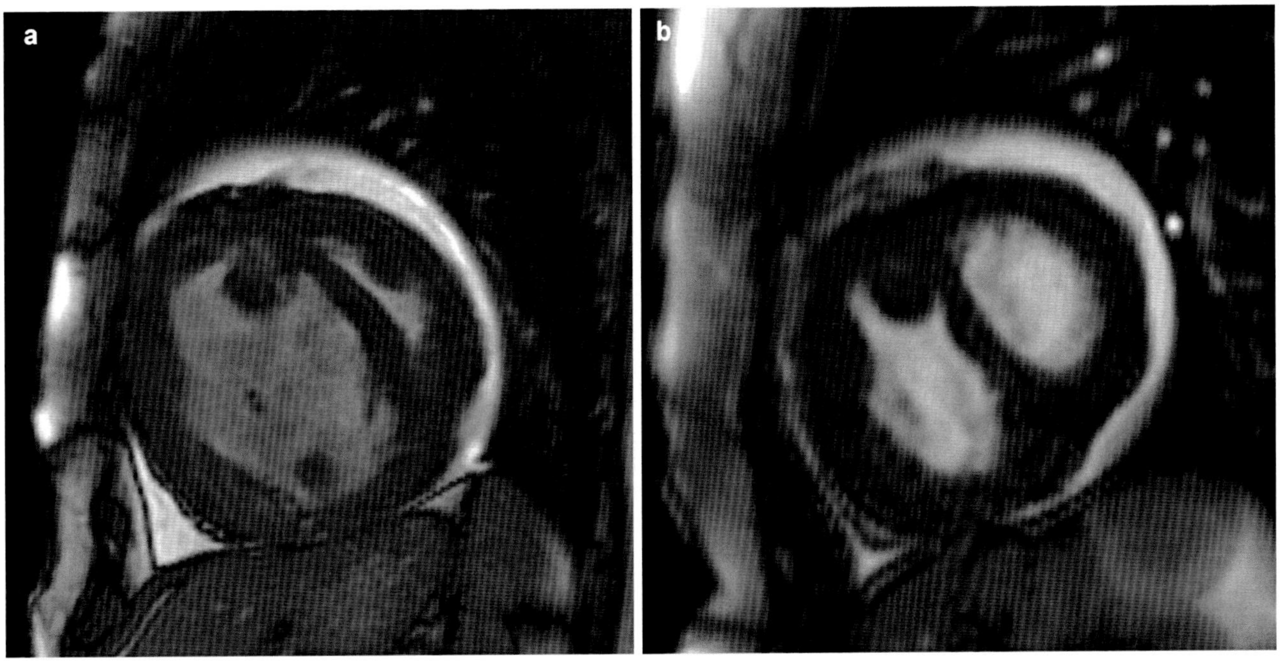

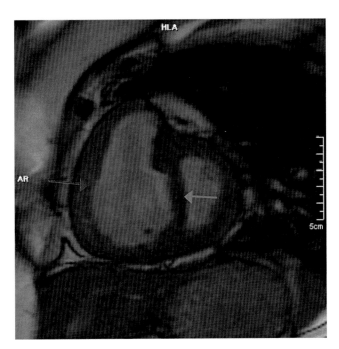

Fig. 12.18 Cardiac MR – Short axis views of a patient with IPAH at the time of diagnosis (**a**) and after 12 months of Epoprostenol and Sildenafil (**b**). Note the reduction in right ventricular dilatation, improved LV filling and resolution of the interventricular septal bowing

Fig. 12.19 Cardiac MR – Short axis view of this 33 yr old female with exertional dyspnoea. There is right ventricular dilatation and hypertrophy (*red arrow*), and interventricular septal bowing (*blue arrow*)

measured by Cardiac magnetic resonance imaging or with the Fick method, CMR underestimated stroke volume. This is probably explained by turbulent blood flow patterns observed in the main pulmonary artery. This was evident both at baseline as well as follow up.

In a large single centre cohort of patients with systemic sclerosis associated PAH stroke volume index (SVI) was a strong predictor of survival. There was twofold increased risk of mortality in patients with a SVI of 30 ml/m^2. Van Wolferen et al. evaluated 111 patients at baseline and at 1 year follow up to identify a minimally important difference in stroke volume in patients with PH. They used both an anchor based method (using 6MWT as anchor) and a distribution-based method and showed a 10 ml change in stroke volume during follow up should be considered as clinically relevant [71].

Right ventricular ejection fraction is also an important prognostic factor in patients with pulmonary hypertension and is poorly derived by conventional echocardiography. A study in a large group of WHO group 1 patients with pulmonary arterial hypertension, right ventricular ejection fraction measured at baseline was a better predictor of mortality compared to pulmonary vascular resistance (PVR) [72]. They showed, in patients who are on PAH targeted therapy that RV function can deteriorate despite reduction in PVR, which occurred in 25 % of the patients. They showed that the deterioration of RVEF was associated with poor outcome independent of any changes of PVR. They hypothesized that the deterioration in RVEF could be explained by pulmonary pressures and subsequently ventricular wall tension that was unaltered after medical treatment despite a fall in PVR. This study emphasized the importance of monitoring RV function during the course of the disease.

RV end diastolic volume is another predictor of prognosis in PAH. Kaplan-Meier survival analysis in a study by Van Wolferen et al. demonstrated that patients with a Right ventricular end diastolic volume index (RVEDVI) of <84 ml/m² at diagnosis had a significantly better survival compared to those with a RVEDVI of 84 ml/m² or more [73]. A further study by Yamada et al. showed that an increased RVEDI predicted both hospitalization and mortality in patients with IPAH but couldn't establish a significant difference between the aforementioned two groups in the previous study [74].

In a study by Mauritz and colleagues, CMR defined geometric changes during the development of RV failure [75]. They identified certain Cardiac MR derived geometric characteristics that defined non survivors (survival less than 5 years) at the beginning of the study and at 1 year follow up. They identified that the RV longitudinal shortening (distance change between end diastole and end systole of the tricuspid annulus to apex distance) and transverse shortening (change between end diastole and end systole of the RV free wall to septal distance) are already reduced at baseline in non survivors, that transverse shortening further declines over time while longitudinal shortening and RV free wall motion stay the same and that the end stage decline in RV function is due to progressive leftward septal displacement rather than further changes in RV free wall transverse or longitudinal displacement. The authors concluded that although there is a parallel decline in longitudinal and transverse shortening during progressive right ventricular failure, a floor effect is reached for longitudinal shortening. Further RV failure is due to a progressive leftward septal displacement and as transverse shortening incorporates both free wall and septal motion, it could be used as a variable of monitoring RV failure. They identified that the RV fractional area change (RVFAC) which combines the effect of both transverse and longitudinal shortening (calculated by = 100 × [(RVED area – RVES area)/RVED area]) to correlate well with RVEF. They identified that a decline in RVFAC to be an accurate measure of RV failure in patients with severe PAH.

In a multicentre study prospectively assessing the use of cardiac MR before and during PAH disease specific treatment, Peacock et al. demonstrated the importance of including both left sided and right sided variables when determining cardiac function [76]. In this EURO-MR study they highlighted that LV end-diastolic volume (LVEDV) to be more closely related to stroke volume than RV end-end diastolic volume. From previous studies it was known that poor LV output in PH patients was due to poor LV filling which was a consequence of prolonged RV contraction time. This contributed to a decreased stroke volume thus LVEDV reflected both the stroke volume and RV contraction time.

Beyond Conventional Cardiac MR

Perfusion CMR can be used to assess myocardial perfusion, thus gaining insight into right ventricular dysfunction in patients with PAH. Vogel – Claussen et al. studied the relationship between LV and RV myocardial perfusion with ventricular function and hemodynamics in patients with PAH. The subjects had stress induced with Adenosine followed by injection of gadopentate dimeglumine as the contrast agent. RV and LV myocardial perfusion values at rest and after adenosine stress was calculated. In this study they found that RV and LV myocardial perfusion reserves to be associated with elevated mPAP in patients with PAH. Reduced perfusion reserves were inversely correlated with RV workload and RV dysfunction. These findings suggested that reduced myocardial perfusion reserves may contribute to RV dysfunction in patients with PAH but concluded that further studies are required to determine the prognostic importance of these findings [77]. In another study in patients attending the Emergency department with chest pain, Cardiac MRI identified diffuse subendocardial hypoperfusion defects which were not seen in SPECT imaging. Cardiac stress perfusion MRI had a higher spatial resolution compared with both SPECT and PET imaging which may explain the higher detection of perfusion defects [78].

Contrast enhanced MR angiography may be an alternative to conventional digital subtraction angiography which is still the gold standard in the diagnosis of chronic thromboembolic pulmonary hypertension. In a study of patients with CTEPH before and after pulmonary endarterectomy breathhold MR imaging not only revealed the typical findings of CTEPH such as webs and bands, vessel cut offs and central thromboemboli but also had the added advantage of being able to assess the right ventricular volumes and function simultaneously [79].

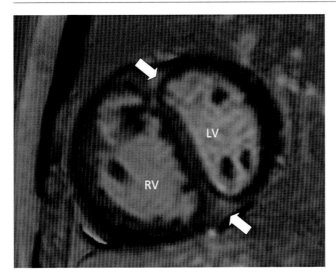

Fig. 12.20 Cardiac MR – showing late Gadolinium enhancement of the right ventricular insertion point in a patient with PH (*arrows*) (Source: Freed et al. [81], p4, Fig 1. (CC BY 2.0))

Blyth et al. used contrast enhanced Cardiac MR imaging to determine the presence and extent of delayed contrast enhancement (DCE) in patients with pulmonary hypertension. DCE was present in most patients with PH and the extent of DCE correlated with haemodynamic variables [80] (Fig. 12.20). Further studies have demonstrated the significance of right ventricular insertion point DCE as a marker for more advanced disease and poor prognosis [81].

Positron Emission Tomography

There is increasing evidence that inflammation and immune dysregulation may play a role in IPAH and elevated levels of proinflammatory cytokines have been found in the serum of these patients. There have been various efforts to develop imaging techniques to track these inflammatory changes. ^{18}F-FDG PET have been extensively used in oncology to identify primary and metastatic tumour cells and a similar increased glycolytic metabolism has been seen in endothelial cells derived

from IPAH-transplant patients. Hagan et al. hypothesized that increased FDG uptake would be present in the right ventricle, pulmonary arteries and lung parenchyma of PAH patients due to the possible pathological role of inflammation in PAH and the presence of deranged endothelial function. They demonstrated that FDG uptake (which was normalized for venous blood activity – Target background ratio) to be higher in the lung parenchyma and the right ventricle of IPAH patients compared to CTEPH or normal populations. They suggested using FDG uptake as a surrogate marker of cellular metabolism and immune activation as underlying mechanism of the disease [82] (Fig. 12.21).

In another study Wang et al. evaluated gated ^{18}F-FDG PET for the assessment of right ventricular volume and function in patients with PH and compared it to cardiac MR and cardiac CT data (Fig. 12.22). Right ventricular end diastolic and end systolic volumes and right ventricular ejection fraction were calculated. They determined ^{18}F-FDG uptake as RV corrected standardized uptake value (SUV) and the ratio of RV to left ventricular corrected standardized uptake value (Corrected SUV R/L). Their study demonstrated that gated PET correlated well with cardiac MR in assessing RV volume and function, however gated PET underestimated RVESV and RVEDV while overestimating RVEF when compared to CMR. They also found statistically significant negative correlation between RV SUV and RVEF by CMR as well as corrected SUV R/L. This study demonstrated that ^{18}F-FDG gated PET could be used in the simultaneous assessment of RV function as well as RV metabolism [83]. Previously Bokhari et al. had suggested that perfusion and metabolic PET imaging using N-NH(3) and ^{18}F-FDG respectively to be a feasible modality to quantify RV blood flow and metabolism (Figs. 12.23 and 12.24). The RV free wall myocardial glucose uptake correlated well with mean pulmonary artery pressure suggesting the possibility that this could be used as a novel early biomarker in patients with PAH [84]. Another study by Can et al. also suggested that increased FDG uptake in RV myocardium was associated with elevated systolic PAP. The myocardial FDG uptake also correlated with pre-existing prognostic markers including elevated BNP and reduced exercise capacity [85].

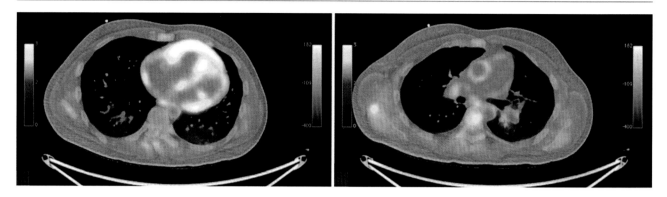

Fig. 12.21 Positron emission tomography (PET) and fused PET/computed tomography of the right ventricle and pulmonary trunk of an idiopathic pulmonary arterial hypertension subject (With permission: The University of Chicago Press, Guy Hagan et al. [82])

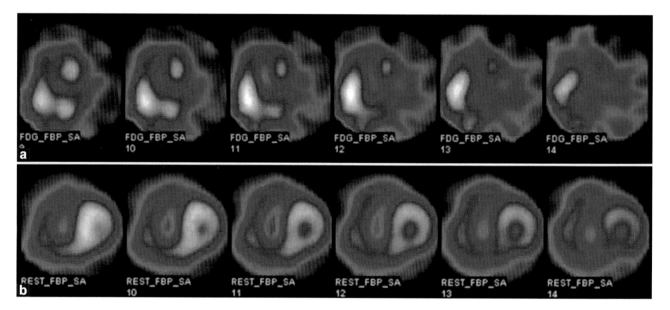

Fig. 12.22 Representative short-axis images of a patient with IPAH before (**a**) and after 6 months of treatment (**b**). Treatment resulted in a reduction of mPAP and PVR with a marked reduction in RV/LV FDG ratio (With permission: The University of Chicago Press, Fang et al. [86], p. 6, Fig 4)

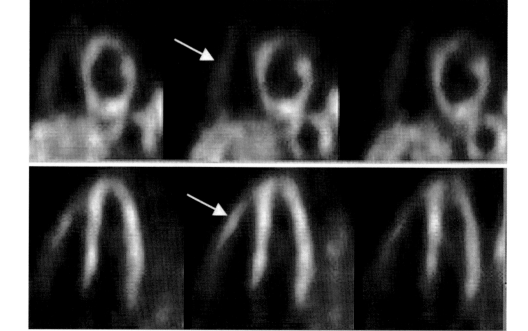

Fig. 12.23 Nitrogen 13-NH₃ resting myocardial perfusion images of the left and right ventricles, illustrating short-axis images (*top*) and horizontal long-axis images (*bottom*). *Arrows* point to the enlarged right ventricle (With permission: Wolters Kluwer Health, Bokhari et al. [84], p644)

Fig. 12.24 Fluorine
18-flurorodeoxyglucose resting myocardial
metabolism images of the left and right
ventricles, illustrating short-axis images
(*top*) and horizontal long-axis images
(*bottom*). *Arrows* point to the enlarged
right ventricle (With permission: Wolters
Kluwer Health, Bokhari et al. [84], p644)

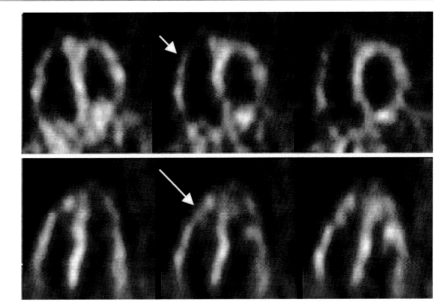

Conclusion

Although right heart catheterization is the gold standard in the diagnosis of pulmonary hypertension, imaging methods play an important role in the diagnostic process, in measuring response to treatment and determining prognosis. They are non-invasive but importantly may tell us more about RV function than we can acquire from right heart catheterization. At present there are few imaging methods, which help us understand the molecular and cellular processes occurring in the right ventricle and pulmonary circulation in patients with pulmonary hypertension. However, we hope that advances in imaging techniques such as positron emission tomography will give us greater insight into the basic pathobiology of pulmonary vascular remodeling and RV dysfunction.

Acknowledgment Echocardiography images provided by Dr. Bouchra Lamia Associate Professor chez CHU-Hôpitaux de Rouen
CXR/CT/VQ and MRI images provided by Dr. Stephen Crawley, Glasgow Royal Infirmary, Glasgow

References

1. Zenker G, Forche G, Harnoncourt K. Two-dimensional echocardiography using a subcostal approach in patients with COPD. Chest. 1985;88(5):722–5.
2. Danchin N, et al. Two-dimensional echocardiographic assessment of the right ventricle in patients with chronic obstructive lung disease. Chest. 1987;92(2):229–33.
3. Helbing WA. Right ventricular function: the comeback of echocardiography? Eur J Echocardiogr. 2004;5(2):99–101.
4. Helbing WA, et al. Comparison of echocardiographic methods with magnetic resonance imaging for assessment of right ventricular function in children. Am J Cardiol. 1995;76(8):589–94.
5. Shimada R, Takeshita A, Nakamura M. Noninvasive assessment of right ventricular systolic pressure in atrial septal defect: analysis of the end-systolic configuration of the ventricular septum by two-dimensional echocardiography. Am J Cardiol. 1984;53(8):1117–23.
6. Ryan T, et al. An echocardiographic index for separation of right ventricular volume and pressure overload. J Am Coll Cardiol. 1985;5(4):918–27.
7. Lei MH, et al. Reappraisal of quantitative evaluation of pulmonary regurgitation and estimation of pulmonary artery pressure by continuous wave Doppler echocardiography. Cardiology. 1995;86(3):249–56.
8. Nakao S, et al. Effects of positional changes on inferior vena caval size and dynamics and correlations with right-sided cardiac pressure. Am J Cardiol. 1987;59(1):125–32.
9. Kircher BJ, Himelman RB, Schiller NB. Noninvasive estimation of right atrial pressure from the inspiratory collapse of the inferior vena cava. Am J Cardiol. 1990;66(4):493–6.
10. Aessopos A, et al. Doppler-determined peak systolic tricuspid pressure gradient in persons with normal pulmonary function and tricuspid regurgitation. J Am Soc Echocardiogr. 2000;13(7):645–9.
11. McQuillan BM, et al. Clinical correlates and reference intervals for pulmonary artery systolic pressure among echocardiographically normal subjects. Circulation. 2001;104(23):2797–802.
12. Syyed R, et al. The relationship between the components of pulmonary artery pressure remains constant under all conditions in both health and disease. Chest. 2008;133(3):633–9.
13. Kitabatake A, et al. Noninvasive evaluation of pulmonary hypertension by a pulsed Doppler technique. Circulation. 1983;68(2):302–9.
14. Isobe M, et al. Prediction of pulmonary arterial pressure in adults by pulsed Doppler echocardiography. Am J Cardiol. 1986;57(4):316–21.
15. Matsuda M, et al. Reliability of non-invasive estimates of pulmonary hypertension by pulsed Doppler echocardiography. Br Heart J. 1986;56(2):158–64.
16. Gardin JM, et al. Relationship between age, body size, gender, and blood pressure and Doppler flow measurements in the aorta and pulmonary artery. Am Heart J. 1987;113(1):101–9.
17. Torbicki A, et al. Proximal pulmonary emboli modify right ventricular ejection pattern. Eur Respir J. 1999;13(3):616–21.
18. Raymond RJ, et al. Echocardiographic predictors of adverse outcomes in primary pulmonary hypertension. J Am Coll Cardiol. 2002;39(7):1214–9.
19. Tei C, et al. Doppler echocardiographic index for assessment of global right ventricular function. J Am Soc Echocardiogr. 1996;9(6):838–47.

20. Cheung MM, et al. The effects of changes in loading conditions and modulation of inotropic state on the myocardial performance index: comparison with conductance catheter measurements. Eur Heart J. 2004;25(24):2238–42.

21. Kaul S, et al. Assessment of right ventricular function using two-dimensional echocardiography. Am Heart J. 1984;107(3):526–31.

22. Karatasakis GT, et al. Prognostic significance of echocardiographically estimated right ventricular shortening in advanced heart failure. Am J Cardiol. 1998;82(3):329–34.

23. Forfia PR, et al. Tricuspid annular displacement predicts survival in pulmonary hypertension. Am J Respir Crit Care Med. 2006;174(9):1034–41.

24. Ghio S, et al. Prognostic relevance of the echocardiographic assessment of right ventricular function in patients with idiopathic pulmonary arterial hypertension. Int J Cardiol. 2010;140(3):272–8.

25. Mahapatra S, et al. The prognostic value of pulmonary vascular capacitance determined by Doppler echocardiography in patients with pulmonary arterial hypertension. J Am Soc Echocardiogr. 2006;19(8):1045–50.

26. Grapsa J, et al. Right ventricular remodelling in pulmonary arterial hypertension with three-dimensional echocardiography: comparison with cardiac magnetic resonance imaging. Eur J Echocardiogr. 2010;11(1):64–73.

27. Amaki M, et al. Usefulness of three-dimensional echocardiography in assessing right ventricular function in patients with primary pulmonary hypertension. Hypertens Res. 2009;32(5):419–22.

28. Di Bello V, et al. Advantages of real time three-dimensional echocardiography in the assessment of right ventricular volumes and function in patients with pulmonary hypertension compared with conventional two-dimensional echocardiography. Echocardiography. 2013;30(7):820–8.

29. Smith BC, et al. Three-dimensional speckle tracking of the right ventricle: toward optimal quantification of right ventricular dysfunction in pulmonary hypertension. J Am Coll Cardiol. 2014;64(1):41–51.

30. Bhave NM, et al. Three-dimensional modeling of the right ventricle from two-dimensional transthoracic echocardiographic images: utility of knowledge-based reconstruction in pulmonary arterial hypertension. J Am Soc Echocardiogr. 2013;26(8):860–7.

31. Chang CH. The normal roentgenographic measurement of the right descending pulmonary artery in 1,085 cases and its clinical application. II. Clinical application of the measurement of the right descending pulmonary artery in the radiological diagnosis of pulmonary hypertensions from various causes. Nagoya J Med Sci. 1965;28(1):67–80.

32. Kanemoto N, et al. Chest roentgenograms in primary pulmonary hypertension. Chest. 1979;76(1):45–9.

33. Lupi HE, et al. Indications and radiological measurements in the evaluation of pulmonary artery hypertension. Arch Inst Cardiol Mex. 1975;45(1):34–42.

34. Aaron RS, et al. The roentgenologic diagnosis of pulmonary hypertension in mitral stenosis. Am Heart J. 1957;53(2):163–70.

35. Arnould P, Pernot C, Simon A. Pulmonary arterial hypertension & pneumonectomy; significance of preoperative occlusion of the pulmonary artery. Rev Med Nancy. 1958;83:895–907.

36. Chang CH. Roentgenographic correlation in pulmonary venous hypertension. Prediction of pulmonary venous pressure from plain chest films. Nippon Igaku Hoshasen Gakkai Zasshi. 1968;28(9):1222–31.

37. Woodruff 3rd WW, et al. Radiographic findings in pulmonary hypertension from unresolved embolism. AJR Am J Roentgenol. 1985;144(4):681–6.

38. Tilkian AG, Schroeder JS, Robin ED. Chronic thromboembolic occlusion of main pulmonary artery or primary branches. Case report and review of the literature. Am J Med. 1976;60(4):563–70.

39. Moser KM, et al. Chronic thrombotic obstruction of major pulmonary arteries. Results of thromboendarterectomy in 15 patients. Ann Intern Med. 1983;99(3):299–304.

40. Benotti JR, et al. The clinical profile of unresolved pulmonary embolism. Chest. 1983;84(6):669–78.

41. Worsley DF, Palevsky HI, Alavi A. Ventilation-perfusion lung scanning in the evaluation of pulmonary hypertension. J Nucl Med. 1994;35(5):793–6.

42. Tunariu N, et al. Ventilation-perfusion scintigraphy is more sensitive than multidetector CTPA in detecting chronic thromboembolic pulmonary disease as a treatable cause of pulmonary hypertension. J Nucl Med. 2007;48(5):680–4.

43. Marten K, et al. Pattern-based differential diagnosis in pulmonary vasculitis using volumetric CT. AJR Am J Roentgenol. 2005;184(3):720–33.

44. Berry DF, et al. Pulmonary vascular occlusion and fibrosing mediastinitis. Chest. 1986;89(2):296–301.

45. Widera E, Sulica R. Pulmonary artery sarcoma misdiagnosed as chronic thromboembolic pulmonary hypertension. Mt Sinai J Med. 2005;72(6):360–4.

46. Weisser K, Wyler F, Gloor F. Pulmonary veno-occlusive disease. Arch Dis Child. 1967;42(223):322–7.

47. Pitton MB, et al. Chronic thromboembolic pulmonary hypertension: diagnostic impact of Multislice-CT and selective Pulmonary-DSA. Rofo. 2002;174(4):474–9.

48. Kuriyama K, et al. CT-determined pulmonary artery diameters in predicting pulmonary hypertension. Invest Radiol. 1984;19(1):16–22.

49. Haimovici JB, et al. Relationship between pulmonary artery diameter at computed tomography and pulmonary artery pressures at right-sided heart catheterization. Massachusetts General Hospital Lung Transplantation Program. Acad Radiol. 1997;4(5):327–34.

50. Ng CS, Wells AU, Padley SP. A CT sign of chronic pulmonary arterial hypertension: the ratio of main pulmonary artery to aortic diameter. J Thorac Imaging. 1999;14(4):270–8.

51. Tan RT, et al. Utility of CT scan evaluation for predicting pulmonary hypertension in patients with parenchymal lung disease. Medical College of Wisconsin Lung Transplant Group. Chest. 1998;113(5):1250–6.

52. Mahammedi A, et al. Pulmonary artery measurements in pulmonary hypertension: the role of computed tomography. J Thorac Imaging. 2013;28(2):96–103.

53. Truong QA, et al. Reference values for normal pulmonary artery dimensions by noncontrast cardiac computed tomography: the Framingham Heart Study. Circ Cardiovasc Imaging. 2012;5(1):147–54.

54. Perloff JK, et al. Proximal pulmonary arterial and intrapulmonary radiologic features of Eisenmenger syndrome and primary pulmonary hypertension. Am J Cardiol. 2003;92(2):182–7.

55. Shimizu H, et al. Dilatation of bronchial arteries correlates with extent of central disease in patients with chronic thromboembolic pulmonary hypertension. Circ J. 2008;72(7):1136–41.

56. Hoey ET, et al. Cardiac causes of pulmonary arterial hypertension: assessment with multidetector CT. Eur Radiol. 2009;19(11):2557–68.

57. Groves AM, et al. Semi-quantitative assessment of tricuspid regurgitation on contrast-enhanced multidetector CT. Clin Radiol. 2004;59(8):715–9.

58. Yeh BM, et al. Clinical relevance of retrograde inferior vena cava or hepatic vein opacification during contrast-enhanced CT. AJR Am J Roentgenol. 2004;183(5):1227–32.

59. Hinderliter AL, et al. Frequency and prognostic significance of pericardial effusion in primary pulmonary hypertension. PPH Study Group. Primary pulmonary hypertension. Am J Cardiol. 1999;84(4):481–4, A10.

60. Sherrick AD, Swensen SJ, Hartman TE. Mosaic pattern of lung attenuation on CT scans: frequency among patients with pulmonary artery hypertension of different causes. AJR Am J Roentgenol. 1997;169(1):79–82.

61. Arakawa H, et al. Chronic pulmonary thromboembolism. Air trapping on computed tomography and correlation with pulmonary function tests. J Comput Assist Tomogr. 2003;27(5):735–42.

62. Remy-Jardin M, et al. Airway changes in chronic pulmonary embolism: CT findings in 33 patients. Radiology. 1997;203(2):355–60.

63. Willemink MJ, et al. CT evaluation of chronic thromboembolic pulmonary hypertension. Clin Radiol. 2012;67(3):277–85.

64. Bergin CJ, et al. Predictors of patient response to pulmonary thromboendarterectomy. AJR Am J Roentgenol. 2000;174(2):509–15.

65. Swensen SJ, et al. Pulmonary venoocclusive disease: CT findings in eight patients. AJR Am J Roentgenol. 1996;167(4):937–40.

66. Resten A, et al. Pulmonary hypertension: CT of the chest in pulmonary venoocclusive disease. AJR Am J Roentgenol. 2004;183(1):65–70.

67. Grothues F, et al. Interstudy reproducibility of right ventricular volumes, function, and mass with cardiovascular magnetic resonance. Am Heart J. 2004;147(2):218–23.

68. Semelka RC, et al. Interstudy reproducibility of dimensional and functional measurements between cine magnetic resonance studies in the morphologically abnormal left ventricle. Am Heart J. 1990;119(6):1367–73.

69. Beerbaum P, et al. Noninvasive quantification of left-to-right shunt in pediatric patients: phase-contrast cine magnetic resonance imaging compared with invasive oximetry. Circulation. 2001;103(20):2476–82.

70. Vonk-Noordegraaf A, et al. Noninvasive assessment and monitoring of the pulmonary circulation. Eur Respir J. 2005;25(4):758–66.

71. van Wolferen SA, et al. Clinically significant change in stroke volume in pulmonary hypertension. Chest. 2011;139(5):1003–9.

72. van de Veerdonk MC, et al. Progressive right ventricular dysfunction in patients with pulmonary arterial hypertension responding to therapy. J Am Coll Cardiol. 2011;58(24):2511–9.

73. van Wolferen SA, et al. Prognostic value of right ventricular mass, volume, and function in idiopathic pulmonary arterial hypertension. Eur Heart J. 2007;28(10):1250–7.

74. Yamada Y, et al. Prognostic value of cardiac magnetic resonance imaging for idiopathic pulmonary arterial hypertension before initiating intravenous prostacyclin therapy. Circ J. 2012;76(7):1737–43.

75. Mauritz GJ, et al. Progressive changes in right ventricular geometric shortening and long-term survival in pulmonary arterial hypertension. Chest. 2012;141(4):935–43.

76. Peacock AJ, et al. Changes in right ventricular function measured by cardiac magnetic resonance imaging in patients receiving pulmonary arterial hypertension-targeted therapy: the EURO-MR study. Circ Cardiovasc Imaging. 2014;7(1):107–14.

77. Vogel-Claussen J, et al. Right and left ventricular myocardial perfusion reserves correlate with right ventricular function and pulmonary hemodynamics in patients with pulmonary arterial hypertension. Radiology. 2011;258(1):119–27.

78. Vogel-Claussen J, et al. Comprehensive adenosine stress perfusion MRI defines the etiology of chest pain in the emergency room: comparison with nuclear stress test. J Magn Reson Imaging. 2009;30(4):753–62.

79. Kreitner KF, et al. Chronic thromboembolic pulmonary hypertension: pre- and postoperative assessment with breath-hold MR imaging techniques. Radiology. 2004;232(2):535–43.

80. Blyth KG, et al. Contrast enhanced-cardiovascular magnetic resonance imaging in patients with pulmonary hypertension. Eur Heart J. 2005;26(19):1993–9.

81. Freed BH, et al. Late gadolinium enhancement cardiovascular magnetic resonance predicts clinical worsening in patients with pulmonary hypertension. J Cardiovasc Magn Reson. 2012;14:11.

82. Hagan G, et al. (18)FDG PET imaging can quantify increased cellular metabolism in pulmonary arterial hypertension: a proof-of-principle study. Pulm Circ. 2011;1(4):448–55.

83. Wang L, et al. Evaluation of right ventricular volume and ejection fraction by gated (18)F-FDG PET in patients with pulmonary hypertension: comparison with cardiac MRI and CT. J Nucl Cardiol. 2013;20(2):242–52.

84. Bokhari S, et al. PET imaging may provide a novel biomarker and understanding of right ventricular dysfunction in patients with idiopathic pulmonary arterial hypertension. Circ Cardiovasc Imaging. 2011;4(6):641–7.

85. Can MM, et al. Increased right ventricular glucose metabolism in patients with pulmonary arterial hypertension. Clin Nucl Med. 2011;36(9):743–8.

86. Fang W, et al. Comparison of 18F-FDG uptake by right ventricular myocardium in idiopathic pulmonary arterial hypertension and pulmonary arterial hypertension associated with congenital disease. Pulm Circ. 2012;2(3):365–72.

Manyoo Agarwal and Aaron B. Waxman

Right Heart Catheterization

Right heart catheterization (RHC) remains the gold standard technique for making the diagnosis of PAH. Because the catheter, a fluid filled thin hollow tube, is advanced via a central vein directly into the chambers of the right side of the heart and the pulmonary artery, it provides direct measurement of the right atrial pressure (RAP), mean pulmonary artery pressure (mPAP), and the pulmonary artery occlusion pressure (PAOP). Using various approaches the cardiac output (CO) can be determined and the total pulmonary vascular resistance (tPVR) calculated. These findings not only provide an accurate diagnosis, but also have been shown to have a strong correlation with the prognosis and survival in PAH patients. In patients studied prior to treatment in the National Institutes of Health primary pulmonary hypertension registry mPAP, RAP and cardiac index (CI) were all found to be predictive of survival. Data from the French network on pulmonary hypertension, that evaluated patients who are on current therapies showed that baseline RAP and CI were significantly associated with survival in the modern treatment era [1, 2]. RHC is recommended with pulmonary vasodilator testing to establish the diagnosis of PAH. Using an acute vasodilator such as nitric oxide (NO) and/or oxygen (O_2), vasoreactivity of the pulmonary arterial tree can be assessed. A study using multivariate analysis showed that decreases in tPVR and mPAP with inhaled NO and O_2 were independent predictors of survival in PAH patients [3].

While the RHC is considered an invasive procedure, it is relatively safe and has a very low complication rate. However, using it to serially follow patients to assess treatment response, and to decide on changes in management of therapy is expensive, and not practical. Additionally, the data obtained can be highly operator dependent resulting in potential for measurement errors from improper data acquisition and analysis. An important example of a common error is not accounting for respirophasic variation. The respirophasic changes in intra thoracic cavity can produce large swings in the atrial pressures that can lead to errors in assessing tPVR [4]. Also there is significant institutional variability in the assessment of CO. Some centers utilize an assumed oxygen consumption (VO_2) value rather than using actual measured values that require a metabolic cart. This can lead to errors in the determination of CO when using the Fick principle. Further, it is performed at rest and in the supine position when in daily life the patients' spend the majority of their time in the upright position. These changes in position can have significant impact on preload and afterload. Additionally improper leveling and, zeroing the pressure transducer to the right atrium or phlebostatic axis can influence the measurements. Because the measurements are obtained through a fluid filled catheter there can be problems with over or under damping pressure curves as a result of the position of the catheter or bubbles in the line. Adverse events related to the use of the catheter are rare, but are important. These include hematoma, pneumothorax, ventricular arrhythmias, vessel wall tear or rupture, and hypotension due to vagal stimulation. The RHC is relatively expensive and can involve the use of fluoroscopy and X-irradiation exposure.

Exercise Testing

In cardiopulmonary diseases studies have shown better correlations between exercise tolerance and peripheral abnormalities than central hemodynamic abnormalities that are a

M. Agarwal, MBBS
Pulmonary Critical Care Medicine, Center for Pulmonary Heart Disease, Brigham and Women's Hospital, Heart and Vascular Center, Boston, MA, USA

A.B. Waxman, MD, PhD, FACP, FCCP, FPVRI (✉)
Pulmonary and Critical Care Medicine, Cardiovascular Medicine, Brigham and Women's Hospital Heart and Vascular Center, Harvard Medical School, 75 Francis Street, PBB CA-3, Boston, MA 02115, USA
e-mail: abwaxman@partners.org

© Springer International Publishing Switzerland 2016
B.A. Maron et al. (eds.), *Pulmonary Hypertension: Basic Science to Clinical Medicine*, DOI 10.1007/978-3-319-23594-3_13

result of cardiac dysfunction itself. This has been suggested because peripheral changes often become more limiting factors to exercise capacity of patients [5, 6]. Thus alterations in exercise physiology in PAH can be attributed to multiple factors of the cardiopulmonary and musculoskeletal systems. Exercise intolerance in addition to being the most common symptom, is also one of the earliest symptoms experienced by PAH patients. Hence the changes in physiology and evaluation of response to therapy with exercise testing have been studied with great interest. There are a number of options of exercise testing that range from those requiring low technical expertise and are easy to perform to those which give more physiological and detailed data but demand specific expertise and are more costly. The ordering physician makes a selection among these depending on the clinical question being asked and the availability of resources.

Maximal exercise testing measures maximum oxygen consumption (VO_2max) and has been suggested as the basis for determining physical fitness [7]. VO_2max is dependent on oxygen delivery, oxygen extraction, and oxygen utilization. Maximal exercise is determined by the subject achieving a plateau of VO_2 as workload is increased along with achieving a heart rate of 80 % of age predicted maximum, and a respiratory exchange ratio (ratio of metabolic gas exchange calculated by VCO_2/VO_2) greater than 1.10. Submaximal exercise testing is attractive because even subjects, who have limited mobility because of pain, or fatigue, can easily do it in various settings. There are a number of options for submaximal testing including the six-minute walk test, and submaximal cardiopulmonary exercise testing (sCPET).

The six-minute walk test (6-MWT) has evolved as the standard approach used in clinical trials and in longitudinal follow up of patients. The combination of the ease and consistency of testing has resulted in widespread employment in the evaluation of patients. Absolute distance walked after initiation of therapy has been shown to be predictive of outcome [8]. Current treatment guidelines recommend that serial measurements be a part of longitudinal clinical care and that a 6 min walk distance (6MWD) >500 m be a goal of therapy. Lower risk patients, those who walk at least 400 m, may be considered for oral mono-therapy. Patients who walk less than 300 m fall into a higher risk group and should be considered for more complex treatments such as prostacyclin or combination therapy [9, 10]. It is important to understand that these recommendations are based primarily on experiential evidence, and the 6MWD has not been studied under these conditions. In addition, the utility of the 6MWD in PH patients who walk more than 450 m may be more limited.

The 6-MWT is attractive as it is a very simple test that correlates with CO, tPVR, changes in tPVR, RAP and also decreases in proportion to the severity of WHO FC [8, 11]. The 6MWD has been shown to have an independent correlation with survival in patients with PAH and the baseline

6MWD can act as a good index of prognosis [12]. It has been widely used to predict outcomes after commencement of therapy, and recent studies have shown that decline in 6MWD is more strongly, and significantly, associated with prognosis than improvement [13]. Exercise limitation, demonstrated by reduced 6MWD, has repeatedly been shown to be an excellent predictor of death in PAH, and the distance walked correlates strongly with peak VO_2, oxygen pulse, and VE/VCO_2 slope as measured by the maximal CPET [8].

6MWT provides additional information about oxygen desaturation with exercise, and heart rate recovery following exercise. The percentage change in oxygen saturation with exercise can be used to assess the need for supplemental oxygen, and mortality risk in patients. Paciocco et al. in 2002 assessed whether oxygen desaturation with exercise and distance achieved during a six-minute walk are associated with mortality in moderately symptomatic untreated PAH patients. They concluded that 6MWD ≤ 300 m increased the mortality risk by 2.4 while change in oxygen desaturation with exercise by more than 10 % increased the mortality risk by 2.9. Consequently, degree of oxygen desaturation was found to be a better predictor of mortality when compared with reduced 6MWD in the same study population [14].

Heart rate recovery response post exercise has been used to predict survival in PAH patients. Minai et al. calculated heart rate recovery value at 1 min (HRR1) by calculating the difference of heart rate at the end of 6MWT and at 1 min after completion of the 6MWT. They found that patients with a HRR1 <16 beats/minute were significantly more likely to have clinical worsening events (6.7 months versus 13 months) than those patients with HRR1 $\geq$16. The odds of clinical worsening were significantly greater among patients with HRR1 <16 at all time points during follow-up. HRR1 <16 was a better predictor of clinical worsening than 6MWD alone, and when combined with the 6MWD improved the ability of 6MWD to predict time to clinical worsening. They also observed that these patients were more likely to need supplemental oxygen during the 6MWT, belonged to WHO FC 4, and had more severe right ventricular dysfunction and pericardial effusion [15].

The 6-min walk test can be modified to study the age related chronotropic responses and heart rate recovery patterns. In a recent study using a modified 6MWT with a portable, signal morphology based, impedance cardiography with real-time wireless monitoring to record dynamic heart rate responses; by recording and measuring the beat-by-beat R-R intervals, heart rate (HR) acceleration and decay slopes were calculated which were then used to compare normal, PAH, and parenchymal lung diseases (with restrictive and obstructive pathologies). HR curves were less steep in PAH than both healthy and parenchymal lung disease groups. HR acceleration rates were slower in patients with PAH or other lung diseases with progression of their disease [16]. In a similar fashion, a study from the same group showed how impedance cardiography during 6 min walk test can be used to estimate hemodynamic parameters such as CI non invasively in a feasible and reliable manner. They also noted that stroke volume plays a more predominant role in the CO increase during 6MWT than heart rate in PH patients [17].

The 6-min walk distance (6MWD) has been the mainstay of evaluation of patients with PAH since 1990. Although this test provides an indirect estimate of aerobic capacity in a very convenient way, there are a number of limitations in using the 6-MWT in standard clinical practice. The 6MWT provides a global assessment of functional capacity but, it does not provide specific information on the physiological mechanisms of exercise limitation. It has limited diagnostic capability as it lacks accuracy and sensitivity. It is usually not used in an age-adjusted fashion, thereby underestimating severity of disease in younger patients. It is also subject to a "plateau effect" that limits its sensitivity for detecting improvement in patients starting with greater walk distances. Mood and motivation, age, obesity, musculoskeletal limitations, and exercise training influence the 6MWT. Hence there has been increasing enthusiasm toward creating simplified tests that allow the early detection and monitoring of PAH. Incremental sub-maximum cardiopulmonary exercise testing utilizing portable metabolic carts is one such technique. It provides information about cardiopulmonary physiology in a simple, quick and mobile way. It has the added advantage of being more objective, providing physiologic data yet being simple, and easy to perform. A recent study reported that submaximal exercise testing maybe superior to the 6-min walk test in assessing PAH disease severity. This conclusion was based on the finding that submaximal VE/VCO$_2$ correlated with WHO FC, BNP, PASP, RAP and mPAP, where as the 6MWD correlated only with WHO FC, BNP and PASP [18].

In a population where performance of a maximal test is not possible and pVO$_2$ cannot be calculated, submaximal exercise testing parameters like Oxygen Uptake Efficiency Slope (OUES) can be useful. It is a CPET-derived variable that provides a combined picture of the effects of increased ventilation and poor O$_2$ transfer and/or peripheral O$_2$ utilization. This submaximal parameter integrates the factors of pulmonary dead space ventilation and exercise-induced lactic acidosis aiming to show how effectively O$_2$ is extracted from the atmosphere and taken into the body as exercise progresses. Low OUES values have been associated with worse outcomes in PH. An ROC curve analysis in PH patients indicated a best OUES cutoff for prognostication of 0.56 L·min^{-1} per logV'$_E$ [19].

While sub maximum exercise testing can be performed quickly in an outpatient setting, providing important physiological data, it being a fairly new technique faces challenges of lack of data, validation of existing data, and need of expert skills for performance and interpretation.

Maximal Cardiopulmonary Exercise Testing

The development of non-invasive techniques like CPET has helped us to identify at risk patients or those with subtle clinical findings by detecting abnormalities in exercise physiology. It is a functional test that may elicit early and reproducible abnormalities indicative of PH. CPET generally consists of an incremental symptom-limited cycling or treadmill exercise test with measurements of ventilation and pulmonary gas exchange. It can quantify the degree of exercise impairment, rule in or out a pulmonary mechanical limit to exercise, and suggest disorders manifested by abnormal O$_2$ delivery or subsequent uptake and utilization, including PH. It is highly reproducible, with little test-to-test variability [20], which makes it a great tool to be used for serial assessment of the functional status of patients and to guide management plans. More recently PAH clinical trials have also been designed using CPET to follow patient's functional status after addition of a new drug [21] or when transitioning from one therapy to another [22].

The variables measured by this technique can largely reflect PH-related impairment of O$_2$ delivery to the exercising muscle bed, and lung ventilation-perfusion abnormalities. Additionally it allows reproducible assessment of functional capacity and treatment efficacy in PH and to predict survival. CPET can reliably demonstrate changes in VO$_2$max, rate of increase in VO$_2$, anaerobic threshold, blood pressure, O$_2$ pulse, and ventilatory efficiency slope in a reproducible and safe manner in severely decompensated patients [20] Sun et al. have shown an inverse correlation between VO$_2$max, AT, and resting pulmonary hemodynamics in PH patients [20]. Patients with a VO$_2$max value below 10.4 mL/kg/min, have been shown to have increased risk of early mortality [23].

Ventilatory inefficiency is one of the hallmarks of PH during exercise [20] and can be identified by an increased slope of the linear phase of VE/VCO$_2$ or its absolute value at the ventilatory anaerobic threshold (VE/VCO$_2$ at AT) . The ratio of VE/VCO$_2$ gives us a combined picture of the ventilatory dead space and arterial CO$_2$ levels. VE/VCO$_2$ provides a powerful marker of the abnormal pulmonary vasculature. It is calculated by the equation: VE/VCO$_2$ = (k)/ (Pa$_{CO2}$ (1 − VD/VT); where VD is dead space and VT is tidal volume. VE/VCO$_2$ is inversely related to both resting and peak CO in PH patients [20]. A sudden rise in VE/VCO$_2$ may suggest dynamic opening of a PFO and right to left shunting during exercise [24]. In a multivariate analysis, the persistence or development of an exercise-induced right-to-left shunt strongly predicted death or need for transplantation (p < 0.0001) independent of hemodynamics and all other exercise measures, including peak VO$_2$ [25].

In normal individuals exercise induces pulmonary vascular recruitment and distension. In individuals with pulmonary vascular remodeling or dysfunction, alveolar dead space fails to fall normally [26]. When $P_{ET}co_2$ at AT is <30 mmHg and especially <20 mmHg, in a patient with exertional dyspnea of unknown cause, PH should be considered. It has been shown that the $P_{ET}co_2$ [27] transition from rest to AT can distinguish between PAH and left ventricular dysfunction; $P_{ET}CO_2$ tends to decrease in PAH, whereas the $P_{ET}CO_2$ tends to increase in left ventricular dysfunction [26]. Others have also reported an association between heart rate recovery recorded during CPET to the overall response to incremental exercise. Ramos et al. showed that a preserved heart rate recovery (HRR) value of >16 beats post exercise is associated with less impaired response to incremental exercise in patients with PAH. Conversely, a delayed HRR at 1-min post exercise also had negative prognostic implications [28].

CPEt also has potential application in the management of other pulmonary vascular disease entities such as group 2 and 3 PH. In Heart failure with preserved ejection fraction (HFpEF) it can be used for assessment and management of HFpEF by quantifying the exercise impairment and ruling out a pulmonary mechanical limit. Guazzi et al. have shown that CPET variables such as VO_2max, VE/VCO_2 slope, rest and peak $P_{ET}co_2$ correlate with diastolic function in patients with HFpEF [29]. While in Group 3 PH, the two most common causes of exercise impairment are pulmonary vascular limit and pulmonary mechanical limit to exercise. This test also provides the breathing reserve index (BRI), which is the ratio of VE at peak exercise to maximum voluntary ventilation at rest. When an abnormal AT precedes a BRI of 0.70, pulmonary vascular disease can limit exercise capacity. Conversely, when a BRI of 0.70 precedes the AT, a pulmonary mechanical limit can be considered the primary impairment.

The resting pulmonary and cardiac function testing cannot reliably predict exercise performance and functional capacity. Overall health status correlates better with exercise tolerance than with resting measurements. The utility of CO and CI measured invasively to decide the management plans for PAH patients is well established, but more recently the application of inert gas rebreathing techniques to CPET has made measuring both CO and gas exchange during exercise non- invasively possible. It estimates pulmonary blood flow by using agents such as acetylene or nitrous oxide, which possess a very high solubility in blood. This methodology provides a potential tool to comment on the survival of PH patients that is more readily accessible. This technique has been widely used and studied in left heart failure patients but data in PH is lacking. Also it gives no information about pulmonary artery pressures or other aspects of right ventricular function. It's application in patients with impaired V/Q like group 3 and group 4 PH could lead to inaccurate results. This is also a concern in patients with intra-cardiac shunts.

The limitations of CPET in patients with PH are several. While generally safe, it can be difficult for some severely limited patients. It is more labor intensive than the submaximal CPET or 6MWT. It requires specific equipment, and experienced and trained personnel to operate and interpret the findings. Use of this test is also contraindicated in severe PH patients with exertional syncope, cardiac arrhythmias, or acute right ventricular failure [30]. Its utility to reliably distinguish the diagnosis of PAH from other forms of PH on its own is limited. Patients with PH have a similar pattern of response to exercise as patients with left heart failure and PH secondary to left sided heart disease. It provides information that can be used to define a management and follow up plan. For assessing right ventricular function in a simple, quick, and a non-invasive way, echocardiography has been widely used in combination with CPET.

Monitoring changes in the RV can reflect changes in the pulmonary vascular bed. Functional status and mortality in PAH is closely associated with right ventricular (RV) structure and function. Echocardiography provides us both quantitative and qualitative information about the anatomy and functional assessment of the RV and pulmonary circulation. It can record important variables including tricuspid regurgitant velocity, estimated pulmonary artery systolic pressures (PASP), Tricuspid Annular Pulmonary Systolic Excursion (TAPSE), Fractional Area change (FAC) and Tei-index, which have been shown to correlate with central hemodynamics and right heart function. In addition, it provides data about RV size, RV mass, right ventricular outflow tract structural and morphological changes that occur with disease progression. It allows noninvasive estimation of tPVR, measured as the ratio of the tricuspid regurgitant velocity to the velocity-time interval of the RV outflow tract. Each of these data makes echocardiography a great screening tool, and a tool for longitudinal follow up of patients. Unfortunately, its utility as a diagnostic tool remains limited. PASP estimated by echocardiography frequently leads to inaccurate diagnosis of pulmonary hypertension when compared with RHC results [31]. The spatial resolution, acoustic window, inter operator-variability, potential for errors in patients with challenging anatomy (obesity, associated lung diseases) and complex geometry of RV can be major limitations when using echocardiography in pulmonary vascular diseases [32].

Exercise echocardiography has increasingly been utilized to assess the response of the right ventricle and pulmonary vascular bed to exercise. It has been proposed as a reliable means to detect pathological increases in pulmonary artery pressures especially in patients at risk for pulmonary hypertension [33]. Steen et al. confirmed the presence of EiPAH by RHC in a patient group of 54 scleroderma patients. A positive exercise test result was defined as an increase of at least 20 mmHg in the RVSP with exercise. Coincident RHC with exercise was performed in those with a positive exercise test, confirming the presence of PAH in 81 % patients studied [34]. While early data are encouraging for the use of exercise echocardiography in subjects at risk of PAH, the approach is not standardized, and exercise parameters should be adjusted based on age and gender-related variations. Echocardiography is more prone to inaccuracies when performed with exercise. Moreover formal validation of non-invasive with invasive measurements during exercise has been limited. Echocardiography alone may be insufficient to include or exclude HFpEF, which can have a direct impact on PAP and PVR [35].

Invasive hemodynamic techniques can accurately characterize the changes in the pulmonary vasculature during exercise by directly measuring central hemodynamics providing data with very high specificity and sensitivity. It can be considered the gold standard approach to diagnose and differentiate various types of pulmonary vascular diseases. Although invasive in nature, it provides important data to study the pressure-flow behavior of the pulmonary circulation and provide identification of early disease states, and assessment of treatment effect.

A number of groups have studied the changes in the hemodynamics with exercise to provide prognostic information and predict changes in the exercise capacity of established PH patients. In group 1 patients, Castelain et al. [36] have shown how exercise tolerance improvement after prostacyclin therapy might be attributable to the decrease in incremental pulmonary vascular resistance during exercise. Provencher et al. [37] used changes in exercise hemodynamics to predict the changes in 6MWD on therapy. They concluded that improvement in exercise tolerance with chronic PAH therapy is independently related to improvement in pulmonary hemodynamics measured during exercise but not those measured at rest. Blumberg et al. [38] studied the application of exercise hemodynamics in a population with group 1 and group 4 PH highlighting that exercise CI and the pressure/flow relationship were significant indicators of prognosis.

Measuring the cardiac filling pressures during a resting supine RHC differentiates the diagnosis of Group 1 and Group 2 PH. Exercise hemodynamics can increase the specificity and sensitivity for the diagnosis of HfPEF. Borlaug et al. [39] demonstrated that patients with pulmonary venous hypertension showed a marked increase in PAOP during exercise, which could be used to discriminate HFpEF from PAH. Kitzman et al. [40], similarly found that compensated outpatients with HFpEF had normal resting PAOP but developed marked increase in exercise PAOP compared to resting PAH patients, suggesting that HFpEF may initially manifest with only intermittent elevations in cardiac filling pressures at rest, but with exercise the correct hemodynamics categorization can be clarified. These two sub groups of PH have also

been shown to differ at the level of systemic oxygen extraction patterns during exercise. Tolle et al. in 2008 [41] demonstrated that maximum systemic oxygen extraction ratio was highest in systolic dysfunction, intermediate in diastolic dysfunction, and lowest in PAH. Maximum Systemic oxygen extraction ratio (SER) was calculated by peak $(Ca\text{-}v^{-}O_2)$/ peak CaO_2. They also noted significant correlation of the peak CO with peak SER in PAH and systolic dysfunction in group 2 PH.

Invasive CPET (iCPET), performed with simultaneous pulmonary and radial artery catheter pressure measurements, and blood sampling every minute during the test accurately characterizes pulmonary arterial and cardiac filling pressures during exercise [32]. Performed in the upright position, it reproduces what subjects actually go through while performing daily life activities. It provides an assessment of exercise capacity, and defines the detailed contributions of any cardiac, pulmonary vascular, peripheral, skeletal or mechanical limitations leading to dyspnea.

ICPET has also been shown to have an important role in the diagnosis of exercise induced pulmonary hypertension (eiPAH). Although eiPAH was excluded from the PH clinical classification in 2008 and again in 2013, this subset of patients present with unexplained exercise intolerance, and depressed VO_2 max. They are usually placed under the category of unexplained dyspnea, after excluding all the known causes of dyspnea. They all have normal pulmonary function testing including diffusing capacity for carbon monoxide, normal radiographic imaging of the chest, and a normal resting echocardiogram. They present with a normal hemodynamic picture on resting supine RHC but when challenged with exercise they develop abnormal pulmonary vascular responses to exercise without evidence of diastolic dysfunction. Using iCPET Tolle et al. for the first time ever, showed that these patients had a significantly lower exercise capacity, as measured by VO_2max, than normal or detrained people. At peak exercise, mPAP almost doubled from resting values compared with normal. While no significant changes in RAP or PAOP were recorded, PVR, which was higher at rest compared to normal subjects, demonstrated a blunted fall with exercise. The degree of severity of the abnormal central hemodynamics, including a blunted fall in PVR, was significantly reduced, compared to patients with resting PAH. The authors suggested a PVR cut off value of 120 $dynes \cdot s \cdot cm^{-5}$ and mPAP max of >30 mmHg as the diagnostic criteria for this disease. They also showed that within the eiPAH group, mPAP response to exercise followed one of two patterns. eiPAH patients with "takeoff" physiology demonstrating significantly higher VO_2max and $Q_t$max than "plateau" eiPAH. (Fig. 13.1) The "takeoff" physiology seen in eiPAH patients resembled normal/ detrained "takeoff" physiology while the "plateau" physiology resembled the physiology seen in those with resting

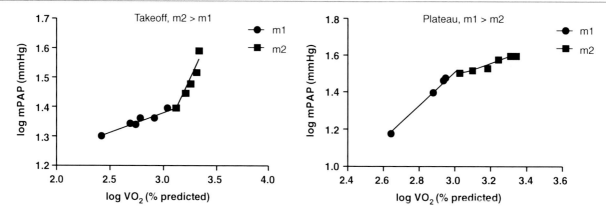

Fig. 13.1 Left panel: Representative plateau pattern of log-log plot of mPAP vs. VO₂ in eiPAH. Right: Representative "take-off" pattern of log-log plot of mPAP vs. VO₂ in eiPAH

PAH [42]. This pattern potentially identifies eiPAH as an intermediate exercise phenotype between normal subjects and those with resting PAH.

EiPAH has been described as an intermediate clinical entity by two other groups. Condliffe et al. [43] noted that 19 % of 42 systemic scleroderma (SSc- eiPAH) patients developed resting PAH when a repeat right-heart catheterization was performed. Saggar et al. [44] also noted that 3 of the 24 SSc-eiPAH patients developed resting PAH when followed serially over time. This finding was reported as part of an open label clinical trial of ambrisentan. In the same study using invasive exercise testing they also demonstrated the positive therapeutic effect of Ambrisentan on exercise hemodynamics in these subjects. In summary, iCPET can be used to diagnose disease at an earlier, milder phase. ICPET can also be used for the accurate assessment of treatment effect on pulmonary artery hemodynamics.

In Chronic thromboembolic pulmonary hypertension (CTEPH) patients, invasive exercise hemodynamics has been utilized to define the cause of persistent exertional dyspnea in post pulmonary endarterectomy patients. These subjects were found to have an abnormal pulmonary vascular response to exercise based on an abnormal PVR and pulmonary arterial compliance when the hemodynamics in spite of normal in resting hemodynamics. The increase in PVR was mild, relative to the alteration in compliance, and exercise arterial compliance was the only independent predictor of decreased exercise capacity in this group of subjects [45]. In addition to what has already been discussed, iCPET can also be used to include or exclude other causes of exercise intolerance like preload-dependent limitations to stroke volume and cardiac output, oxidative myopathies, and left to right shunting.

The limitations of exercise hemodynamic testing are significant because of its invasive nature that limits its use for serial measurements. Although rare, other potential complications include infection, vascular thrombosis, and pain at the site of catheter placement. ICPET can be costly, labor intensive, and requires technical expertise not only for accurate performance but also for recording and interpretation of the results. Consistent invasive measurements during exercise are challenging to perform and must be interpreted carefully because of the potential for large intra-thoracic pressure swings associated with increased minute ventilation during exercise. Boerrigter, et.al studied the worst possible scenario for this problem when they studied iCPET in a COPD population with esophageal balloons in place. They suggested that central hemodynamics measured using conventional end-expiration method might lead to an overestimation of intravascular pressures during exercise. To obtain exercise hemodynamic data more reliably by averaging pressures over the respiratory cycle or using the RAP waveform to correct for intra-thoracic pressure (Fig. 13.2a, b) [4].

Imaging of the Right Heart System

Functional status and mortality in patients with PAH is related primarily to RV structure and function. Direct assessment of RV function using noninvasive techniques may provide a more informative way of determining response to therapy and monitoring disease progression in PH. With constant advances in the field of imaging, we now has access to a number of non invasive imaging tools to more clearly define the interaction between the RV and pulmonary circulation. Magnetic resonance imaging (MRI) and Computed Tomographic (CT) scanning are becoming increasingly important to study the RV-PA coupling and provide detailed quantitative data with extreme quality. Prognostic markers have been identified with independent predictive value for identification of treatment failure.

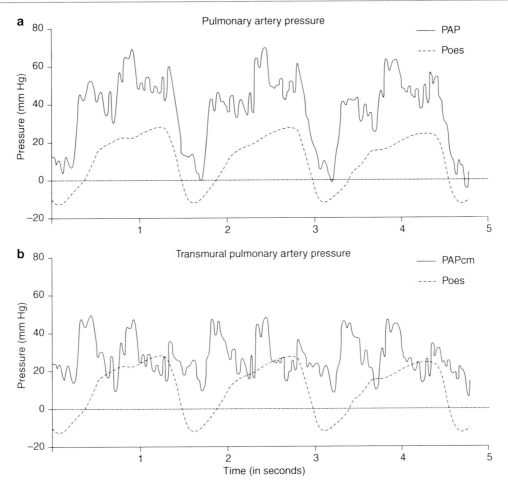

Fig. 13.2 (**a**). Example of pulmonary artery pressure before (*PAP*) and after (*PAPtm*) continuous correction for esophageal pressure (*Peso*) at maximal exercise in a patient with severe COPD (FEV1: 30 % of predicted). (**b**) Simultaneous measurement of RAP and esophageal pressure (Peso) at maximal exercise in the same patient as shown in Fig. 2.1. RAPnadir is the lowest point in RAP during expiration, which represents RAP during relaxation. Note that RAP falls towards Peso during relaxation. RAPswing was determined as the difference between inspiratory RAP and expiratory RAP

Computed Tomographic Imaging

Over the past decade, cardiac CT has evolved rapidly from the introduction of 4-detector row systems to those with 64 detectors, dual-source CT and, more recently, 320-detector systems. This has been accompanied by improvements in spatial and temporal resolution, extended longitudinal coverage and decreased scan times and radiation exposure. Current generation ECG gated multidetector CT (MDCT) scanners have a spatial resolution that ranges from 0.3 to 0.5 mm, which permits accurate and consistent assessment of the RV and PA. In addition use of the contrast agents, gives us additional information about ventricular volumes, ejection fraction, and vascular structures.

Studies have evaluated the specificity and sensitivity of CT defined dilatation of the main pulmonary artery as a marker for pulmonary hypertension. A value ≥29 mm had a sensitivity and specificity for the detection of PH of 77.4 % and 89.6 % respectively. The ratio between pulmonary artery and abdominal aorta when greater than 1, was shown to be 86.8 % sensitive and 79.2 % specific for a diagnosis of PH. This ratio correlated with RHC derived mean PA pressures and in combination with ECHO derived RV systolic pressures. The correlation was (R2 = 0.45, p < 0.001) alone, and (R2 = 0.55, p < 0.001) in combination, giving a 96 % specificity and 59 % sensitivity for PH diagnosis [46–48].

Kuriyama et al. have reported the use of cross-sectional areas of the main and inter-lobar pulmonary arteries for estimating the pulmonary artery pressures. In this study the upper limit of normal diameter for the main pulmonary artery was found to be 28.6 mm. In the PH patient group, the diameters were correlated with data from cardiac catheterization and a value greater than 28.6 mm readily predicted the presence of pulmonary hypertension. The calculated cross-sectional areas of the main and inter-lobar pulmonary arteries were also found to give the best mPAP estimates (r = 0.89, P < 0.001 and r = 0.66, P < 0.001) [49].

Groves et al. demonstrated that contrast reflux into the inferior vena cava and hepatic veins on first-pass contrast-enhanced CT was a strong marker for tricuspid regurgitation (TR), having 90.4 % sensitivity and 100 % specificity when compared to echocardiography. They further demonstrated excellent correlation between semi-quantitative grading of TR with systolic PA pressure measured by RHC ($r = 0.69$, $p < 0.001$). Subsequently, others have shown that high-grade contrast reflux was associated with a diagnosis of PH (OR 5.41, 2.95–9.94 95 % CI, $p < 0.001$) in a large retrospective cohort [50, 51].

When CT-measured PA volumetric analyses are adjusted with body surface area, they correlate highly with mean PA pressure ($r = 0.89$, $p < 0.05$) [52] A study in patients awaiting lung transplantation demonstrated that mPAP correlated strongly with the combination of cross-sectional areas of the main and left main PA indexed to body surface area ($r = 0.81$, $p = 0.0001$) [53].

Simon et al. have also shown the utility of ECG gated MDCT to detect the regional changes in RV structure and function, which may be early markers of patients at risk for developing RV failure. The increased pulmonary vascular resistance exposes the right side of the heart to chronic pressure and volume overload. The morphology of the heart compensates in the form of septal bowing into LV. When the heart contracts, the LV faces the consequences of pressure overload while during the relaxation phase, the volume changes interfere with its normal functioning. These manifest as RV hypertrophy and RV strain. This study emphasized that patients with different pulmonary and RV filling pressures display significantly different phenotypes. Even in the presence of normal RV filling pressures, RV infundibular changes might be useful to characterize regional RV remodeling and function in PH and direct therapeutic decision making early in the disease process [54].

In group 4 PH patients, pulmonary thromboendarterectomy (PTE) is the recommended treatment but the prediction of post surgical outcome remains challenging. In CTEPH patients Heinrich et al. have reported how pre operative CT scan findings can help predict hemodynamic improvement after PTE. They also concluded that absence of central thrombi is a significant risk factor for inadequate hemodynamic improvement. In a more recent study Scholzel et al. found pre-operative PA diameter indexed for body surface area as the only independent predictor for hemodynamic improvement after PTE in CTEPH [55, 56].

Although CT scan has been shown to give us important data about pulmonary vessels and morphological changes in heart structure limitations of radiation exposure, use of contrast agents, and little experience in pulmonary vascular diseases, makes its use limited.

Cardiac Magnetic Resonance Imaging

Noninvasive cMRI provides a comprehensive picture of RV structure and function with excellent resolution. It reports on markers of RV structure and function including right ventricular end-diastolic volume index (RVEDVI), left ventricular end diastolic volume index (LVEDVI), right ventricular ejection fraction (RVEF), and relative area change of the pulmonary trunk. The use of cMR in PAH is increasingly attractive as cMR is considered the gold standard for assessment of RV volume, mass, and function. In a recent pan-European study investigating the relationship between RV structure and function, and survival, a large RV end-diastolic volume, low left ventricular end-diastolic volume, and a low SV at baseline were associated with a poor prognosis. Progressive dilatation of the RV, a further decrease of LV diastolic volume, and a further decrease in SV at follow-up predicted treatment failure and a poor long-term outcome [57] MRI is ideally suited to longitudinal follow-up of patients with PAH due to its non-invasive nature, high reproducibility and has the advantage over other biomarkers in PAH due to its high sensitivity to detect changes in morphological, functional and flow related parameters.

CMRI provides details about the morphological changes in the anatomy of right ventricle, septum and related structures, which correlate with invasive pulmonary hemodynamic parameters. Saba et al. showed that Ventricular Mass Index (VMI) (ratio of right ventricular mass over left ventricular mass) had a strong correlation with mean pulmonary artery pressures ($r = 0.81$) Also the sensitivity and specificity for detecting PH were 84 and 71 % respectively for the VMI when compared with conventional commonly practiced technique of echocardiography [58]. Similarly septal curvature metrics have been used to judge the RV afterload and to assess the acute vaso-reactivity of pulmonary vasculature during vasodilator testing.

The normally cross sectional circular shape of the LV is the result of the positive pressure gradient between the LV and RV throughout the cardiac cycle. However, in PH, the LV–RV pressure gradient is less than that observed in normal population or can even be negative causing the septum to become either flattened or bow into the LV. Panda et al. have shown this septal curvature using the real time cMRI has a very strong correlation between the PAP and PVRi at baseline and during vasodilator challenge. Also others have shown the presence of a strong correlation by comparing the septal curvature parameters with the hemodynamic parameters of PASP, RVSP measured on RHC [59–61].

With the progression of the disease, the changes in the RV functioning and structure lead to the changes of LV contour. This LV deformation can be quantified using MRI, which helps to calculate echocardiographic indices such as the LV systolic and diastolic eccentricity indices (sEI, dEI). These indices correlate with mPAP and can identify the prognosis of PAH patients. Elevated RV pressures cause the inter-ventricular septum to bow to the left in patients with PH, this leftward motion of the inter ventricular septum causes the deformation of the LV, "D shape", as a result of the pressure differential between LV and RV chambers. Several investigators have quantified the paradoxical inter-ventricular septal position by measuring the curvature of the septum and have shown strong correlations with the severity of PH [61–63].

Cardiac MR can also be used to track reverse remodeling. In patients with non operable CTEPH, treated with balloon pulmonary angioplasty there was significant improvement in RV dilatation (RVEDVI and RVESVI), RV systolic function (RVEF), RV hypertrophy (RVMI and VMI), and inter ventricular septal bowing assessed by cMR. There were strong correlations between observed changes in RV remodeling, measured with cMR, and changes in invasive hemodynamic parameters. cMR has been used to demonstrate RV reverse remodeling after successful pulmonary thromboendartectomy in CTEPH patients in both early and later phases of recovery [64, 65].

Also MR angiography of the pulmonary arteries and a time resolved contrast enhanced lung perfusion scan can help in identification of CTEPH. The high signal to noise from blood flow provides good contrast within the vessel lumen and thus serves as a non-contrast enhanced angiogram, which can be useful in the delineation of adherent material in the central pulmonary arteries in CTEPH [66]. Contrast enhanced MR angiograms can provide an overview of vessel pruning in PH and the delineation of thromboembolic material in CTEPH.

While cardiac MR is considered the gold standard for measurement of cardiac function, and it offers very high spatial resolution, clinicians have been slow to utilize cardiac MRI for a number or reasons. Data on the use of cMR as an outcome measure is limited. While certain subjects cannot tolerate the claustrophobia they feel inside the magnet, some patients are too large to fit in the MRI chambers. We do not generally image patients who have implanted defibrillators or pacemakers because of heating of the tip of leads. Compared with other non-invasive approaches, cMR is more time consuming. Cardiac MR techniques are also dependent on image acquisition during repeated breath hold maneuvers of 5–10 s. If patients are unable to perform this maneuver, an important consideration in PH patients, image quality can be significantly degraded. Cardiac volumetric parameters vary with age, gender and body surface area. Hence there is also a need to adjust these measurements accordingly as they may be critical to recognize the clinical abnormalities in individual patient [67–69].

Conclusion

Since 1929 when Dr. Werner Frossman performed the first human cardiac catheterization, various tools have evolved that provide important insights about the pulmonary circulation in both clinical management and clinical research. For research we want testing that offers reliable, time sensitive information that provides clear reproducible end points in clinical trials. In contrast, tools for clinical practice need to readily provide information longitudinally to define a patients' progression of a disease state and / or response to therapy. Currently no single tool can provide comprehensive information regarding screening, diagnosis, disease progression, or prognosis in patients with pulmonary vascular disease. While RHC remains the gold standard for making the diagnosis and classification of pulmonary vascular diseases, there remains a significant gap when it comes to evaluation and quantification of symptoms, providing information about prognosis of the disease, and directing therapy. Commonly used methods such as echocardiography (screening and follow up) and 6MWT (for follow up) provide limited insight, while the use of techniques like sCPET, CPET and cMRI, have increased our understanding of the complex impact of pulmonary vascular diseases.

Because exercise intolerance is the predominant complaint in PAH and is clearly multifactorial, measuring and following changes in exercise capacity would provide important insight into disease progression and response to therapy. It is also clear that an important determinant of outcome is right ventricular function. With continued improvements in exercise testing and imaging techniques, development of an approach that combines both will result in improved understanding of the disease and provide a more reliable approach to assessment in practice and research.

References

1. Humbert M, et al. Survival in patients with idiopathic, familial, and anorexigen-associated pulmonary arterial hypertension in the modern management era. Circulation. 2010;122(2):156–63.
2. D'Alonzo GE, et al. Survival in patients with primary pulmonary hypertension. Results from a national prospective registry. Ann Intern Med. 1991;115(5):343–9.
3. Malhotra R, et al. Vasoreactivity to inhaled nitric oxide with oxygen predicts long-term survival in pulmonary arterial hypertension. Pulm Circ. 2011;1(2):250–8.
4. Boerrigter BG, et al. Measuring central pulmonary pressures during exercise in COPD: how to cope with respiratory effects. Eur Respir J. 2014;43(5):1316–25.
5. Clark AL, Poole-Wilson PA, Coats AJ. Exercise limitation in chronic heart failure: central role of the periphery. J Am Coll Cardiol. 1996;28(5):1092–102.
6. Rich S. The 6-minute walk test as a primary endpoint in clinical trials for pulmonary hypertension. J Am Coll Cardiol. 2012; 60(13):1202–3.

7. Armstrong N, et al. The peak oxygen uptake of British children with reference to age, sex and sexual maturity. Eur J Appl Physiol Occup Physiol. 1991;62(5):369–75.

8. Miyamoto S, et al. Clinical correlates and prognostic significance of six-minute walk test in patients with primary pulmonary hypertension. Comparison with cardiopulmonary exercise testing. Am J Respir Crit Care Med. 2000;161(2 Pt 1):487–92.

9. McLaughlin VV, et al. ACCF/AHA 2009 expert consensus document on pulmonary hypertension a report of the American College of Cardiology Foundation Task Force on Expert Consensus Documents and the American Heart Association developed in collaboration with the American College of Chest Physicians; American Thoracic Society, Inc.; and the Pulmonary Hypertension Association. J Am Coll Cardiol. 2009;53(17):1573–619.

10. Galie N, et al. Guidelines for the diagnosis and treatment of pulmonary hypertension: the Task Force for the Diagnosis and Treatment of Pulmonary Hypertension of the European Society of Cardiology (ESC) and the European Respiratory Society (ERS), endorsed by the International Society of Heart and Lung Transplantation (ISHLT). Eur Heart J. 2009;30(20):2493–537.

11. Groepenhoff H, et al. Exercise testing to estimate survival in pulmonary hypertension. Med Sci Sports Exerc. 2008;40(10):1725–32.

12. Barst RJ, et al. A comparison of continuous intravenous epoprostenol (prostacyclin) with conventional therapy for primary pulmonary hypertension. N Engl J Med. 1996;334(5):296–301.

13. Farber HW, et al. Predicting outcomes in pulmonary arterial hypertension based on the 6-minute walk distance. J Heart Lung Transplant. 2015;34(3):362–8.

14. Paciocco G, et al. Oxygen desaturation on the six-minute walk test and mortality in untreated primary pulmonary hypertension. Eur Respir J. 2001;17(4):647–52.

15. Minai OA, et al. Heart rate recovery predicts clinical worsening in patients with pulmonary arterial hypertension. Am J Respir Crit Care Med. 2012;185(4):400–8.

16. Tonelli AR, et al. Heart rate slopes during 6-min walk test in pulmonary arterial hypertension, other lung diseases, and healthy controls. Physiol Rep. 2014;2(6):1–11. e12038.

17. Tonelli AR, et al. Value of impedance cardiography during 6-minute walk test in pulmonary hypertension. Clin Transl Sci. 2013;6(6):474–80.

18. Neal JE, Lee AS, Burger CD. Submaximal exercise testing may be superior to the 6-min walk test in assessing pulmonary arterial hypertension disease severity. Clin Respir J. 2014;8(4):404–9.

19. Ramos RP, et al. Exercise oxygen uptake efficiency slope independently predicts poor outcome in PAH. Eur Resp J. 2013;5:5.

20. Sun XG, et al. Exercise pathophysiology in patients with primary pulmonary hypertension. Circulation. 2001;104(4):429–35.

21. Reata Pharmaceuticals I. Bardoxolone methyl evaluation in patients with pulmonary arterial hypertension (PAH) – LARIAT .In: ClinicalTrials.gov [Internet]. Bethesda (MD): National Library of Medicine (US). 2000- [cited 13 Jan 2015]. Available from: https://clinicaltrials.gov/ct2/show/NCT02036970 NLM Identifier: NCT02036970, 2014.

22. Agarwal M, De Marco T, Rischard F, Oudiz R. Protocol-Driven Transition From Parenteral Prostanoids (PP) to Inhaled Treprostinil in Pulmonary Arterial Hypertension (PAH). Chest. 2014;146(4_Meeting Abstracts):837A–A.

23. Wensel R, Opitz C, Anker S. Assessment of survival in patients with primary pulmonary hypertension. Importance of cardiopulmonary exercise testing. Circulation. 2002;106:319–24.

24. Sun XG, et al. Gas exchange detection of exercise-induced right-to-left shunt in patients with primary pulmonary hypertension. Circulation. 2002;105(1):54–60.

25. Oudiz RJ, et al. Usefulness of right-to-left shunting and poor exercise gas exchange for predicting prognosis in patients with pulmonary arterial hypertension. Am J Cardiol. 2010;105(8):1186–91.

26. Hansen JE, et al. Mixed-Expired and End-Tidal CO2 Distinguish Between Ventilation and Perfusion Defects During Exercise Testing in Patients With Lung and Heart Diseases. Chest. 2007;132(3):977–83.

27. Yasunobu Y, et al. ENd-tidal pco2 abnormality and exercise limitation in patients with primary pulmonary hypertension*. Chest J. 2005;127(5):1637–46.

28. Ramos RP, et al. Heart rate recovery in pulmonary arterial hypertension: relationship with exercise capacity and prognosis. Am Heart J. 2012;163(4):580–8.

29. Guazzi M, Cahalin LP, Arena R. Cardiopulmonary exercise testing as a diagnostic tool for the detection of left-sided pulmonary hypertension in heart failure. J Card Fail. 2013;19(7):461–7.

30. American Thoracic S, American College of Chest P. ATS/ACCP Statement on cardiopulmonary exercise testing. Am J Respir Crit Care Med. 2003;167(2):211–77.

31. Arcasoy SM, et al. Echocardiographic assessment of pulmonary hypertension in patients with advanced lung disease. Am J Respir Crit Care Med. 2003;167(5):735–40.

32. Waxman AB. Exercise physiology and pulmonary arterial hypertension. Prog Cardiovasc Dis. 2012;55(2):172–9.

33. Grunig E, et al. Stress Doppler echocardiography in relatives of patients with idiopathic and familial pulmonary arterial hypertension: results of a multicenter European analysis of pulmonary artery pressure response to exercise and hypoxia. Circulation. 2009;119(13):1747–57.

34. Steen V, et al. Exercise-induced pulmonary arterial hypertension in patients with systemic sclerosis. Chest. 2008;134(1):146–51.

35. Borlaug BA, et al. Exercise hemodynamics enhance diagnosis of early heart failure with preserved ejection fraction. Circ Heart Fail. 2010;3(5):588–95.

36. Castelain V, et al. Pulmonary artery pressure-flow relations after prostacyclin in primary pulmonary hypertension. Am J Respir Crit Care Med. 2002;165(3):338–40.

37. Provencher S, et al. Changes in exercise haemodynamics during treatment in pulmonary arterial hypertension. Eur Respir J. 2008;32(2):393–8.

38. Blumberg FC, et al. Impact of right ventricular reserve on exercise capacity and survival in patients with pulmonary hypertension. Eur J Heart Fail. 2013;15(7):771–5.

39. Borlaug BA. Mechanisms of exercise intolerance in heart failure with preserved ejection fraction. Circ J. 2014;78(1):20–32.

40. Kitzman DW, et al. Exercise intolerance in patients with heart failure and preserved left ventricular systolic function: failure of the Frank-Starling mechanism. J Am Coll Cardiol. 1991;17(5):1065–72.

41. Tolle J, Waxman A, Systrom D. Impaired systemic oxygen extraction at maximum exercise in pulmonary hypertension. Med Sci Sports Exerc. 2008;40(1):3–8.

42. Tolle JJ, et al. Exercise-induced pulmonary arterial hypertension. Circulation. 2008;118(21):2183–9.

43. Condliffe R, et al. Connective tissue disease-associated pulmonary arterial hypertension in the modern treatment era. Am J Respir Crit Care Med. 2009;179(2):151–7.

44. Saggar R, et al. Brief report: effect of ambrisentan treatment on exercise-induced pulmonary hypertension in systemic sclerosis: a prospective single-center, open-label pilot study. Arthritis Rheum. 2012;64(12):4072–7.

45. Bonderman D, et al. Right ventricular load at exercise is a cause of persistent exercise limitation in patients with normal resting pulmonary vascular resistance after pulmonary endarterectomy. Chest. 2011;139(1):122–7.

46. Chan AL, et al. Novel computed tomographic chest metrics to detect pulmonary hypertension. BMC Med Imaging. 2011;11:7.

47. Okajima Y, et al. Assessment of pulmonary hypertension what CT and MRI can provide. Acad Radiol. 2011;18(4):437–53.

48. Devaraj A, et al. Detection of pulmonary hypertension with multidetector CT and echocardiography alone and in combination. Radiology. 2010;254(2):609–16.

49. Kuriyama K, et al. CT-determined pulmonary artery diameters in predicting pulmonary hypertension. Invest Radiol. 1984; 19(1):16–22.

50. Groves AM, et al. Semi-quantitative assessment of tricuspid regurgitation on contrast-enhanced multidetector CT. Clin Radiol. 2004;59(8):715–9.

51. Aviram G, et al. Significance of reflux of contrast medium into the inferior vena cava on computerized tomographic pulmonary angiogram. Am J Cardiol. 2012;109(3):432–7.

52. Froelich JJ, et al. Relationship between pulmonary artery volumes at computed tomography and pulmonary artery pressures in patients with- and without pulmonary hypertension. Eur J Radiol. 2008;67(3):466–71.

53. Haimovici JB, et al. Relationship between pulmonary artery diameter at computed tomography and pulmonary artery pressures at right-sided heart catheterization. Massachusetts General Hospital Lung Transplantation Program. Acad Radiol. 1997;4(5):327–34.

54. Simon MA, et al. Phenotyping the right ventricle in patients with pulmonary hypertension. Clin Transl Sci. 2009;2(4):294–9.

55. Heinrich M, et al. CT scan findings in chronic thromboembolic pulmonary hypertension: predictors of hemodynamic improvement after pulmonary thromboendarterectomy. Chest. 2005;127(5): 1606–13.

56. Scholzel BE, et al. Prediction of hemodynamic improvement after pulmonary endarterectomy in chronic thromboembolic pulmonary hypertension using non-invasive imaging. Int J Cardiovasc Imaging. 2015;31(1):143–50.

57. van Wolferen SA, et al. Prognostic value of right ventricular mass, volume, and function in idiopathic pulmonary arterial hypertension. Eur Heart J. 2007;28(10):1250–7.

58. Saba TS, et al. Ventricular mass index using magnetic resonance imaging accurately estimates pulmonary artery pressure. Eur Respir J. 2002;20(6):1519–24.

59. Pandya B, et al. Real-time magnetic resonance assessment of septal curvature accurately tracks acute hemodynamic changes in pediatric pulmonary hypertension. Circ Cardiovasc Imaging. 2014; 7(4):706–13.

60. Dellegrottaglie S, et al. Pulmonary hypertension: accuracy of detection with left ventricular septal-to-free wall curvature ratio measured at cardiac MR. Radiology. 2007;243(1):63–9.

61. Roeleveld RJ, et al. Interventricular septal configuration at mr imaging and pulmonary arterial pressure in pulmonary hypertension. Radiology. 2005;234(3):710–7.

62. Lopez-Candales A, et al. Systolic eccentricity index identifies right ventricular dysfunction in pulmonary hypertension. Int J Cardiol. 2008;129(3):424–6.

63. Raymond RJ, et al. Echocardiographic predictors of adverse outcomes in primary pulmonary hypertension. J Am Coll Cardiol. 2002;39(7):1214–9.

64. Iino M, et al. Time course of reversed cardiac remodeling after pulmonary endarterectomy in patients with chronic pulmonary thromboembolism. Eur Radiol. 2008;18(4):792–9.

65. Reesink HJ, et al. Reverse right ventricular remodeling after pulmonary endarterectomy in patients with chronic thromboembolic pulmonary hypertension: utility of magnetic resonance imaging to demonstrate restoration of the right ventricle. J Thorac Cardiovasc Surg. 2007;133(1):58–64.

66. Rajaram S, et al. Diagnostic accuracy of contrast-enhanced MR angiography and unenhanced proton MR imaging compared with CT pulmonary angiography in chronic thromboembolic pulmonary hypertension. Eur Radiol. 2012;22(2):310–7.

67. Maceira AM, et al. Reference right ventricular systolic and diastolic function normalized to age, gender and body surface area from steady-state free precession cardiovascular magnetic resonance. Eur Heart J. 2006;27(23):2879–88.

68. Lorenz CH, et al. Normal human right and left ventricular mass, systolic function, and gender differences by cine magnetic resonance imaging. J Cardiovasc Magn Reson. 1999;1(1):7–21.

69. Lorenz CH. The range of normal values of cardiovascular structures in infants, children, and adolescents measured by magnetic resonance imaging. Pediatr Cardiol. 2000;21(1):37–46.

Biomarkers and Other Methods for Assessing Patient Progress

14

Nadine Al-Naamani and Ioana R. Preston

Pulmonary arterial hypertension (PAH) is associated with significant morbidity and mortality. Patients with PAH have non-specific symptoms and are often diagnosed late in the course of the disease. Patients with certain conditions, such as scleroderma or HIV infection, are at risk for PAH development. Early identification and risk stratification are necessary in disease diagnosis, evaluation of prognosis, selection of the appropriate initial treatment, and guidance of further treatment decisions. These important considerations emphasize the need for identifying biomarkers for PAH. In 1998, the National Institute of Health defined a biomarker as "a characteristic that is objectively measured and evaluated as an indicator of normal biological processes, pathogenic processes, or pharmacologic responses to a therapeutic intervention." [1] In other words, biomarkers reflect disease-associated molecular changes in body tissue and fluids [2]. Biomarkers may or may not correlate with a patient's experience and sense of well-being [3]. A useful biomarker should be reliable, reproducible, inexpensive and relatively easy to measure and interpret by clinicians. Clinical parameters have been traditionally used to assess a patient's progress and clinical course in PAH, although in recent years, several serologic markers have been investigated in PAH. However, current clinical guidelines recommend brain natriuretic peptide (BNP) or its precursor N-terminal fragment of pro-BNP (NT-pro-BNP) as the only serologic biomarkers for longitudinal follow-up of PAH patients [4]. Major impediments in the development of useful biomarkers in PAH include small sample sizes in which potential biomarkers are tested and lack of validation of associations between biomarkers and patient's health status or response to treatment.

In this chapter, we review current and potential biomarkers in PAH, emphasizing their role in the pathophysiologic

process, as well as their clinical utility and limitations (Table 14.1). Lastly, we briefly discuss other tools that are currently used in clinical context to assess patient progress.

Biomarkers in PAH can be divided into five major categories: biomarkers of endothelial dysfunction, biomarkers of inflammation and oxidative stress, biomarkers of right ventricular (RV) failure, biomarkers of pulmonary arterial remodeling, and other biomarkers.

Biomarkers of Endothelial Dysfunction

Endothelial dysfunction and eicosanoid imbalance play an integral role in the pathogenesis of PAH. Several markers of endothelial dysfunction have hence been studied as potential biomarkers in PAH.

Endothelins are a family of naturally occurring peptides that include endothelin-1 (ET-1), endothelin-2 (ET-2) and endothelin-3 (ET-3). ET-1 is abundant in the human lung and is the most potent vasoconstrictor, mainly released from the vascular endothelium [5]. ET-1 has been implicated in the pathogenesis of PAH [6, 7]. Elevated plasma ET-1 levels have been detected in patients with PAH [7–10] and in one study ET-1 levels correlated with the right atrial pressure and pulmonary artery oxygen saturation [7], both markers of prognosis. ET-1 levels have also been shown to be inversely correlated with survival of PAH patients on conventional therapy [11]. Another small study of 16 PAH patients showed that the levels of ET-1 and its precursor big ET-1 were strongly correlated with pulmonary vascular resistance (PVR), mean pulmonary artery pressure (mPAP), cardiac output (CO), cardiac index (CI) and 6-min walk distance (6MWD) [12]. In a study of 33 treatment-naïve PAH patients, the ET-1/ET-3 ratio has been shown to be positively correlated with the right atrial pressure and the New York Heart Association functional class (NYHA FC), and negatively correlated with mixed venous oxygen saturation, and associated with survival [13]. More recently, a study of 28 PAH patients evaluated

N. Al-Naamani, MD • I.R. Preston, MD (✉)
Pulmonary, Critical Care and Sleep Division, Pulmonary Hypertension Center, Tufts Medical Center, 800 Washington Street, Box 257, Boston, MA 02111, USA
e-mail: nalnaamani@tuftsmedicalcenter.org;
ipreston@tuftsmedicalcenter.org

© Springer International Publishing Switzerland 2016
B.A. Maron et al. (eds.), *Pulmonary Hypertension: Basic Science to Clinical Medicine*, DOI 10.1007/978-3-319-23594-3_14

Table 14.1 Biomarkers in PAH

Biomarker	Study endpoints
Endothelins	
Endothelin-1	Hemodynamic measurements, survival
Big ET-1	Hemodynamic measurements, 6MWD
ET-1/ET-3	Hemodynamic measurements, NYHA FC, survival
CT-pro-ET-1	Clinical severity, hospitalizations, survival
vWF	Hemodynamic measurements, survival
Angiopoietin	Hemodynamic measurements, survival
Circulating endothelial cells	Hemodynamic measurements, treatment-response
Interleukins	Survival
Osteopontin	Hemodynamic measurements, 6MWD, NYHA FC, survival
Pentraxin-3	Screening
Adiponectin	N/A
Uric acid	Hemodynamic measurements
Isoprostanes	Survival
BNP/NT-pro-BNP	Hemodynamic measurements, NYHA FC, 6MWD, treatment-response
Troponin	Hemodynamic measurements, survival
Renin-angiotensin-Aldosterone system	Hemodynamic measurements, disease progression
Pim-1	Screening, survival
Markers of renal dysfunction	Survival
Serum sodium	Survival
Hemoglobin A1c	Survival

ET endothelin, *6MWD* six-minute walk distance, *NYHA FC* New York Heart Association functional class, *CT-pro-ET-1* COOH-terminal pro-endothelin-1, *BNP* brain natriuretic peptide, *NT-pro-BNP* N-terminal fragment of pro-BNP, *Pim-1* provirus integration site for Moloney murine leukemia virus

COOH-terminal pro-endothelin-1 (CT-pro-ET-1), which is derived from the ET-1 propeptide in equal amounts as ET-1, as a potential biomarker [14]. The study found that CT-pro-ET-1 plasma levels at baseline were associated with the clinical severity of the disease and 12-months' hospitalizations due to PAH-worsening, heart/lung transplantation, or all-cause mortality. Despite these associations, endothelins have not been adopted as a valid biomarker in PAH for several reasons. First, ET-1 levels have been shown to be elevated in African ethnicity, old age and male sex and levels are reduced in individuals treated with angiotensin converting enzyme inhibitors, statins, vasodilators, or β-blockers [15]. Second, there are no studies evaluating the utility of endothelins as a screen-

ing tool for PAH. Third, in patients treated with endothelin-receptor antagonists, it is difficult to interpret changes in endothelin levels over time as attributable to treatment effect or underlying disease. Finally, endothelins have not been validated in large prospective cohorts.

Plasma von Willebrand factor (vWF) is a large glycoprotein that is produced in endothelial cells and megakaryocytes. vWF plays an important role in clot formation by stabilizing and activating factor VIII and by binding to IIb/IIIa receptors, recruiting and activating platelets. Elevated levels of vWF have been associated with worse outcomes in healthy individuals, as well as patients with congestive heart failure, coronary artery disease and acute respiratory distress syndrome [16–18]. Patients with IPAH have, on average, higher levels of vWF as compared to patients with PAH from other etiologies, such as congenital heart disease patients [19, 20]. Higher vWF levels have been associated with worse survival in patients with idiopathic, familial, anorexigen use associated- and congenital heart associated-PAH [21, 22]. A small study of 10 PAH patients showed that vWF proteolysis paralleled hemodynamic improvements after initiation of prostacyclin therapy [23]. vWF levels were also shown to be predictive of future development of elevated pulmonary artery pressures in patients with limited scleroderma, a condition recognized as a risk factor for PAH development; however, vWF levels decreased over the 3 year follow-up period of the study [24], limiting this marker only as a research tool at this time.

Angiopoietin -1 (Ang-1) and its antagonist angiopoietin-2 (Ang-2) are angiogenic factors that bind to the tyrosine kinase with immunoglobulin-like and EGF-like domains 1 (Tie) family of receptors and are responsible for vascular development, remodeling and maturation [25]. Imbalances in the angiopoetin-Tie2 receptor system have been implicated in the pathogenesis of IPAH [26, 27]. Plasma levels of Ang-1, Ang-2, soluble Tie2 and vascular endothelial growth factor (VEGF) were elevated in patients with IPAH as compared to healthy controls [28]. Ang-2 but not the other angiogenic markers correlated with CI, PVR, and mixed venous oxygen saturation and changes in Ang-2 after initiation of therapy correlated with mean right atrial pressure, PVR and mixed venous oxygen saturation [28]. Ang-2 was also an independent predictor of mortality in IPAH [28].

Circulating endothelial cells (CECs) are thought to shed in response to endothelial injury. One study found that the CECs count was increased in the serum of patients with IPAH and PAH associated with other etiologies as compared to healthy controls [29, 30]. The CECs count also correlated with hemodynamic parameters in these patients. The number of CECs decreased in response to initiation of PAH-specific therapy in children with PAH [31].

Biomarkers of Inflammation and Oxidative Stress

There is an increasing amount of evidence that implicates inflammation in the pathogenesis of PAH. There is a wide array of inflammatory cytokines that are elevated in patients with PAH, including interleukin-1 beta (IL-1 beta), IL-2, IL-4, IL-6, IL-8, IL-10, IL-12p70 and tumor necrosis factor-alpha [32, 33]. IL-6, IL-8, IL-10 and IL-12p70 levels were also shown to predict survival in patients with PAH [33]. Another study demonstrated similar findings with addition of elevated levels of vascular endothelial growth factor (VGEF), platelet-derived growth factor (PDGF), transforming growth factor-beta (TGF-beta) and IL-6 [34]. IL-6 was again shown to predict mortality. C-reactive protein (CRP), another inflammatory marker, was found to be elevated in patients with PAH and chronic thromboembolic pulmonary hypertension (CTEPH) when compared with healthy controls, it correlated with survival in patients with PAH and its normalization in response to treatment conferred a survival advantage [35]. In addition, in CTEPH patients, CRP levels decreased after pulmonary endartrectomy [35], suggesting a possible role as a biomarker for assessing the severity and response to therapy in PAH.

Osteopontin (OPN), a multicellular protein, is another cytokine involved in recruitment and retention of macrophages and T cells to sites of inflammation and has also been implicated in the pathogenesis of PAH [36–38]. Plasma OPN levels have been shown to be elevated in patients with idiopathic PAH as compared to healthy controls [39]. OPN levels correlated with hemodynamic parameters such as the right atrial pressure as well as functional parameters, including the 6MWD and NYHA FC. Moreover, baseline OPN levels were predictive of survival in patients with IPAH [39].

Human pentraxin 3 (PTX3) is one of the large proteins in the family of pentraxins, which is synthesized by dendritic cells of myelomonocytic origin in response to proinflammatory signals and Toll-like receptor engagement [40]. PTX3, a protein related to CRP and synthesized by vascular cells, as well as innate immunity cells, regulates cell proliferation, angiogenesis, inflammation, and matrix deposition [41]. In a large study of individuals free of atherosclerotic disease, PTX3 levels correlated with greater RV mass and larger RV end-diastolic volume, independent of common cardiovascular risk factors and left ventricular morphologic changes [42]. PTX3 has been recently investigated in PAH patients. In a case-control study, plasma PTX3 levels were significantly higher in PAH patients as compared to healthy age and sex-matched controls [43]. PTX3 was also shown to perform better than BNP or CRP in patients with PAH associated with connective tissue disease [43].

Adiponectin, a protein released from adipose cells, plays a role in insulin sensitivity as well as influences vascular inflammation, vascular dilation and vascular smooth muscle cell proliferation, all features of PAH pathophysiology [44–47]. In a case-control study, adiponectin levels in PAH patients were elevated compared to controls when matched for age, sex and body mass index [48].

Serum uric acid is a final product of adenine nucleotide degradation in response to tissue ischemia and hypoxia and has been shown to be elevated in several hypoxic conditions including chronic heart failure and chronic obstructive pulmonary disease [49, 50]. Serum uric acid levels were found to be elevated in PAH patients when compared to controls and the elevated uric acid levels were associated with a worse hemodynamic profile as well as increased risk of mortality [51, 52]. Similarly, elevated uric acid levels were correlated with pulmonary artery systolic pressure in patients with pulmonary hypertension (PH) associated with sickle cell disease [53].

15-F_{2t}-isoprostane derives from arachidonic acid metabolism and is a stable product of lipid peroxidation that has been linked with oxidative stress and has been shown to be elevated in both chronic left heart failure and interstitial lung disease. Urinary concentrations and more recently plasma concentrations of 15-F_{2t}-isoprostane were elevated and correlated with poor outcomes in PAH patients [54, 55].

Despite the various associations between inflammatory markers and PAH, none of these biomarkers have been adapted in clinical practice mainly due to lack of validation of their usefulness in diagnosis and prognosis. Most of these associations were derived from observational studies. Serial measurements and longitudinal follow-up are necessary before these investigational biomarkers can be incorporated into clinical practice.

Biomarkers of Right Ventricular Failure

Right ventricular adaptation is a major prognostic factor in PAH and a determinant of mortality. As a consequence, surrogate markers of RV function were investigated for their potential role as predictors of outcome in PAH. Atrial natriuretic peptide (ANP) and BNP are peptide hormones that are produced from cardiomyocytes in response to volume or pressure overload (Fig. 14.1) [56, 57]. ANP secretion is mainly driven by atrial stretch rather than ventricular stretch. On the other hand, BNP is more sensitive to ventricular overload. Natriuretic peptides have been long studied in several forms of heart failure, including RV failure. In addition to its role in assessing left ventricular failure, BNP has been shown to be useful in assessing RV dysfunction. Earlier studies have shown that BNP levels were helpful in differentiating between cardiac and pulmonary causes of dyspnea with elevated levels in patients with chronic obstructive pulmonary disease (COPD) and evidence of cor pulmonale as compared

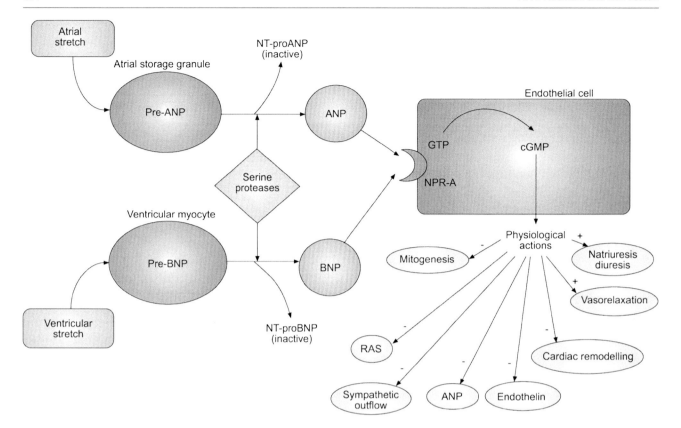

Fig. 14.1 Simplified schematic of the natriuretic peptide system. Natriuretic peptide precursors are released in response to atrial and ventricular stretch, cleaved into active molecules and inactive precursors and convert guanosine 5'-triphosphate (*GTP*) to cyclic guanosine monophosphate (*cGMP*), leading to their various physiological actions. *ANP* atrial natriuretic peptide, *NT-proANP* N-terminal pro-ANP, *NT-proBNP*

N-terminal ProBNP, *NPR-A* natriuretic peptide receptor A, *RAS* rennin-angiotensin system. This material has not been reviewed by European Respiratory Society prior to release; therefore the European Respiratory Society may not be responsible for any errors, omissions or inaccuracies, or for any consequences arising there from, in the content (Reproduced with permission of the European Respiratory Society: Willis et al. [122])

to those with COPD alone [58, 59]. Since then, BNP and NT-pro-BNP have emerged as mainstream biomarkers of RV dysfunction in several forms of PH and in acute pulmonary embolism [60–65]. The first study to demonstrate the prognostic significance of BNP levels examined 60 PAH patients at the time of diagnostic right heart catheterization and on follow-up after treatment with prostacyclin [66]. Patients with a baseline BNP level ≥150 pg/ml or ≥180 pg/ml at follow-up after treatment had significantly worse survival. BNP levels have also been shown to be related to hemodynamic parameters [63–68] and functional impairment [67]. NT-pro-BNP, a byproduct of BNP synthesis, has advantages over BNP, as it is a more stable peptide with a more accurate assay [69]. NT-pro-BNP levels correlated with hemodynamic parameters [70, 71] as well as survival in PAH [72–74]. Nevertheless, both BNP and NT-pro-BNP are affected by several factors, including renal function, weight, age and gender [75–78], which leads to difficulty in determining a single cutoff value. Improvements in NT-pro-BNP have also been shown to correlate with treatment effect in PAH [79, 80]. The significance of serial measurements of NT-pro-BNP has been studied retrospectively in patients with idiopathic

PAH [72]. A greater than 15 % decrease per year in NT-pro-BNP level was associated with improved survival. Currently, BNP or its precursor NT-pro-BNP are the only serologic markers recommended to follow and to attempt to normalize in PAH [4].

Cardiac troponin T is a biomarker of myocardial damage, which has been used as an indicator of RV dysfunction in patients with PAH and has been shown to correlate with survival in patients with PAH and CTEPH [81]. Levels of troponin T correlated with higher heart rates, lower mixed venous oxygen saturation and higher serum NT-pro-BNP. In this study of 56 patients with PAH or CTEPH, normalization of troponin T levels with treatment was associated with improved survival [81]. In the study from the National PH Registry in Ireland that included 108 PAH patients, BNP and highly sensitive troponin were independent predictors of poor outcome (hazard ratio 6.68 and 5.48, respectively) however a declining 6MWD was found to be a stronger predictor than both (hazard ratio of 12.8) [82]. The main drawback to troponin T is that it is not specific to PAH and can be elevated in patients with left ventricular dysfunction, acute coronary syndrome and patients with acute pulmonary embolism [83].

Biomarkers of Pulmonary Arterial Remodeling

Recently, activation of the renin-angiotensin-aldosterone system (RAAS) has been reported to be a contributor to cardiopulmonary remodeling in PAH similar to systemic cardiovascular diseases [84–89]. In experimental models of PAH, increased plasma and lung tissue levels of angiotensin and aldosterone have been detected and found to correlate with cardiopulmonary hemodynamics and pulmonary vascular remodeling [85, 86]. Moreover, in a cohort of 58 patients with idiopathic PAH, serum renin and angiotensin I levels were increased above the upper limit of normal in the majority of patients, whereas angiotensin II levels were elevated only in a smaller cohort [84]. With follow-up, persistently elevated levels of renin-angiotensin activity were associated with PAH disease progression assessed as a greater than 10 % decrease in the 6MWD and an increased risk of lung transplantation or death [84].

The terminal component of the RAAS, the mineralocorticoid receptor (MR), is directly activated by aldosterone. In a pilot study of patients with unexplained dyspnea, the plasma aldosterone level was increased in patients with PAH, compared with control subjects. Furthermore, aldosterone levels correlated positively with PVR and inversely with CO in a subset of patients with PAH who had severe disease [90]. We and others have shown that MR plays a direct role in the remodeling process of the pulmonary vasculature in experimental pulmonary hypertension and that MR inhibition by MR antagonists attenuates pulmonary hypertension in several experimental models [91, 92].

Collectively, these reports implicate RAAS and MR activation in PAH and suggest that renin, angiotensin and aldosterone levels have the potential to become biomarkers of disease severity.

The pathophysiology of PAH involves pulmonary artery smooth muscle cell (PASMC) proliferation and resistance to apoptosis. A tissue-specific activation of provirus integration site for Moloney murine leukemia virus (Pim-1), a protooncogene minimally expressed in healthy cells, was shown to contribute to the activation of NFAT/STAT3 signaling pathway responsible for the sustainability of this phenotype [93]. In a recent study by Renard and colleagues, Pim-1 levels were elevated in patients with IPAH (including a group with vasoreactive phenotype), PAH associated with connective tissue disease, and PAH associated with congenital heart disease, versus controls [94]. Pim-1 levels discriminated effectively between the presence vs. absence of PAH and remained an independent predictor of mortality after adjustment for hemodynamic and biochemical variables [94]. Serum Pim-1 level has, therefore, emerged as a promising biomarker of pulmonary vascular remodeling although these findings need to be replicated in larger trials.

Other Biomarkers

PAH has been associated with metabolic and systemic derangements including renal impairment, hyponatremia and impaired glucose tolerance.

Renal dysfunction has been associated with worse survival in a variety of clinical conditions including PH. In a study of 500 PAH patients, renal dysfunction defined by an elevated creatinine was associated with a worse hemodynamic profile and was an independent predictor of mortality [95]. Another study investigated several markers of renal function and their prognostic significance in a cohort of PH patients (WHO Groups 1, 3, and 4) and found that creatinine, cystatin C and blood urea nitrogen were superior to neutrophil-gelatinase-associated lipocalin (NGAL), fibroblast growth factor 23 (FGF-23) and α-Klotho in predicting prognosis [96]. The Registry to Evaluate Early and Long-Term PAH Disease Management (REVEAL) which includes PAH patients from 54 US centers similarly reported that the presence of renal insufficiency was associated with increased mortality (hazard ratio of 1.9, p <0.01) [97].

Hyponatermia is a well-established biomarker of advance left heart failure and a predictor of poor outcomes [98, 99]. Hyponatermia, defined by a serum sodium concentration ≤136 mEq/L, was found to be associated with worse functional and hemodynamic parameters in patients with PAH and was associated with poor survival [100]. These findings have been reproduced in subsequent studies showing hyponatremia as an independent predictor of mortality in PAH [101, 102]. Of note, hyponatermia was also associated with poor outcomes (death and hospitalization) in a population of patients with PH and heart failure with preserved ejection fraction [103], suggesting that it is a biomarker of advanced heart failure.

Glycosylated hemoglobin A1c (HbA1c) is a sensitive screening test to detect diabetes mellitus and glucose intolerance. In a cohort of PAH patients without diabetes mellitus, glucose intolerance (as assessed by HbA1c ≥6.0 %) was found in 56 % and unrecognized diabetes mellitus in 15 % of the cohort [104]. In another study of therapy-naïve PAH patients, mean HbA1c level was higher than expected for an age-matched non-diabetic cohort and HbA1c was a predictor of all-cause mortality with a hazard ratio of 2.23 (95 % CI 1.06–4.70; p=0.034) per 1-unit increase of HbA1c [105].

Clinical Assessment Tools

The assessment of PAH patients and their response to therapy is performed utilizing clinical indices of patient's functional status and signs of disease progression. Patient's functional status is highly relevant to both patients and physicians. The New York Heart Association (NYHA) functional class has been used to assess patient's functional status at baseline and on follow-up visits. It is a subjective evaluation of the physician's perception of the patient's exercise tolerance and associates inversely survival in patients with IPAH [106–108]. In PAH, maintenance of NYHA FC I/II or improvement from NYHA functional class III/IV to I/II has also been shown to be associated with a survival advantage over patients who remain or advance to NYHA functional class III/IV [109, 110].

Measurement of walking distance achieved in six minutes (6MWD) is a submaximal exercise test, which is easy to perform in clinical practice. The 6MWD has long been used as a surrogate marker for patient outcomes in clinical trials of PAH. A low 6MWD was predictive of adverse outcomes in patients with PAH [111]. Nevertheless, when assessed as a single marker, it has significant limitations. Data from the REVEAL registry could not identify an improvement threshold to carry a particular prognostic value [112]. Moreover, improvement in the 6MWD was not associated with survival, but worsening of the 6MWD was strongly and significantly associated with poor prognosis [112].

Echocardiography is a useful initial screening tool for patients with suspected pulmonary hypertension. Measurement of the tricuspid annular plane systolic excursion (TAPSE), an echocardiographically derived measure of RV function, has been shown to have prognostic significance in patients with pulmonary hypertension [113]. A TAPSE of <1.8 cm was associated with greater RV systolic dysfunction, right heart remodeling, and worse survival as compared to TAPSE ≥1.8 cm. The RV Tei-index is another echocardiographic-derived measure that strongly correlated with 6MWD, BNP, cardiac index, mPAP and PVR in patients with IPAH and PAH associated with connective tissue disease [114, 115]. The major limitations of echocardiographic parameters are that they are dependent on the technician's skills and that there are technical difficulties in measuring the RV chambers with adequate reproducibility. Current PH treatment guidelines recommend achieving normal or near-normal RV size with adequate PH therapy [4].

Cardiac magnetic resonance (CMR) is the gold standard for the evaluation of right heart structure and volume; however, it's value in serial follow-up of patients with pulmonary hypertension is not well established [116, 117].

Time to clinical worsening (TTCW) is a newly investigated endpoint in clinical trials of PAH. A recent study from the REVEAL Registry defined TTCW as a 15 % reduction from baseline in the 6MWD plus worsening functional class, except for patients already in functional class IV, all-cause hospitalization, or the need for parenteral prostacyclin analog therapy [118]. In this cohort, PAH patients who experienced clinical worsening were at an increased risk of death in the subsequent 1-year as compared to those who did not experience any worsening. This study supports the use of a composite endpoint to assess clinical worsening and to inform therapeutic decisions.

Composite risk scores have been developed also as a method to predict survival in patients with PAH. The REVEAL Registry, the largest, US-based PAH registry including approximately 3500 patients, derived a risk score to predict 1- and 5-year survival in patients with PAH [97, 119]. Variables that were independently associated with increased mortality were male gender, age >60 years, hereditary PAH, PAH associated with portal hypertension, PAH associated with connective tissue disease, family history of PAH, New York Heart Association (NYHA) functional class III or IV, renal insufficiency, resting systolic blood pressure <110 mmHg, heart rate >92 beats/min, mean RAP >20 mmHg, 6MWD<165 m, BNP>180 pg/ml, PVR>32 Woods units, diffusion capacity for carbon monoxide (DLCO) ≤32 % predicted, and presence of pericardial effusion on echocardiogram. The REVEAL risk score has been validated in both newly and previously diagnosed PAH patients [119, 120]. A similar composite risk score was derived from the French Registry [121]. Despite their usefulness as a tool for clinicians in determining patient prognosis, these scores have not been yet evaluated in assessing response to treatment.

Conclusions

Several potential biomarkers in PAH have been identified over the last decade; however the studies have been fraught with methodological and design issues. Studies have been limited by sample size, retrospective nature, lack of homogeneity of populations as well as selection bias. Validation of these biomarkers is needed in large prospective cohorts of patients with a wide spectrum of PH disease. Current guidelines recommend assessing PAH severity and response to treatment using a composite of clinical, echocardiographic, hemodynamic, and serologic (BNP, NT-pro-BNP) parameters.

References

1. Biomarkers Definitions Working G. Biomarkers and surrogate endpoints: preferred definitions and conceptual framework. Clin Pharmacol Ther. 2001;69(3):89–95.
2. Poste G. Bring on the biomarkers. Nature. 2011;469(7329):156–7.
3. Strimbu K, Tavel JA. What are biomarkers? Curr Opin HIV AIDS. 2010;5(6):463–6.
4. McLaughlin VV, Gaine SP, Howard LS, Leuchte HH, Mathier MA, Mehta S, et al. Treatment goals of pulmonary hypertension. J Am Coll Cardiol. 2013;62(25 Suppl):D73–81.
5. Shao D, Park JE, Wort SJ. The role of endothelin-1 in the pathogenesis of pulmonary arterial hypertension. Pharmacol Res: Off J Ital Pharmacol Soc. 2011;63(6):504–11.
6. Giaid A, Yanagisawa M, Langleben D, Michel RP, Levy R, Shennib H, et al. Expression of endothelin-1 in the lungs of

patients with pulmonary hypertension. N Engl J Med. 1993;328(24):1732–9.

7. Nootens M, Kaufmann E, Rector T, Toher C, Judd D, Francis GS, et al. Neurohormonal activation in patients with right ventricular failure from pulmonary hypertension: relation to hemodynamic variables and endothelin levels. J Am Coll Cardiol. 1995;26(7):1581–5.

8. Cacoub P, Dorent R, Maistre G, Nataf P, Carayon A, Piette C, et al. Endothelin-1 in primary pulmonary hypertension and the Eisenmenger syndrome. Am J Cardiol. 1993;71(5):448–50.

9. Cacoub P, Dorent R, Nataf P, Carayon A, Riquet M, Noe E, et al. Endothelin-1 in the lungs of patients with pulmonary hypertension. Cardiovasc Res. 1997;33(1):196–200.

10. Stewart DJ, Levy RD, Cernacek P, Langleben D. Increased plasma endothelin-1 in pulmonary hypertension: marker or mediator of disease? Ann Intern Med. 1991;114(6):464–9.

11. Galie N, Grigioni F, Bacchi-Reggiani L, Ussia G, Parlangeli R, Catanzariti P. Relation of endothelin-1 to survival in patients with primary pulmonary hypertension. Eur J Clin Invest. 1996;26 Suppl 1:273.

12. Rubens C, Ewert R, Halank M, Wensel R, Orzechowski HD, Schultheiss HP, et al. Big endothelin-1 and endothelin-1 plasma levels are correlated with the severity of primary pulmonary hypertension. Chest. 2001;120(5):1562–9.

13. Montani D, Souza R, Binkert C, Fischli W, Simonneau G, Clozel M, et al. Endothelin-1/endothelin-3 ratio: a potential prognostic factor of pulmonary arterial hypertension. Chest. 2007;131(1):101–8.

14. Silva Marques J, Martins SR, Calisto C, Goncalves S, Almeida AG, de Sousa JC, et al. An exploratory panel of biomarkers for risk prediction in pulmonary hypertension: emerging role of CT-proET-1. J Heart Lung Transpl: Off Publ Int Soc Heart Transpl. 2013;32(12):1214–21.

15. Shah R. Endothelins in health and disease. Eur J Intern Med. 2007;18(4):272–82.

16. Chin BS, Conway DS, Chung NA, Blann AD, Gibbs CR, Lip GY. Interleukin-6, tissue factor and von Willebrand factor in acute decompensated heart failure: relationship to treatment and prognosis. Blood Coagulation Fibrinolysis: Int J Haemostasis Thrombosis. 2003;14(6):515–21.

17. Folsom AR, Wu KK, Rosamond WD, Sharrett AR, Chambless LE. Prospective study of hemostatic factors and incidence of coronary heart disease: the Atherosclerosis Risk in Communities (ARIC) Study. Circulation. 1997;96(4):1102–8.

18. Ware LB, Eisner MD, Thompson BT, Parsons PE, Matthay MA. Significance of von Willebrand factor in septic and nonseptic patients with acute lung injury. Am J Respir Crit Care Med. 2004;170(7):766–72.

19. Lopes AA, Maeda NY, Bydlowski SP. Abnormalities in circulating von Willebrand factor and survival in pulmonary hypertension. Am J Med. 1998;105(1):21–6.

20. Lopes AA, Maeda NY, Goncalves RC, Bydlowski SP. Endothelial cell dysfunction correlates differentially with survival in primary and secondary pulmonary hypertension. Am Heart J. 2000;139(4):618–23.

21. Kawut SM, Horn EM, Berekashvili KK, Widlitz AC, Rosenzweig EB, Barst RJ. von Willebrand factor independently predicts long-term survival in patients with pulmonary arterial hypertension. Chest. 2005;128(4):2355–62.

22. Lopes AA, Barreto AC, Maeda NY, Cicero C, Soares RP, Bydlowski SP, et al. Plasma von Willebrand factor as a predictor of survival in pulmonary arterial hypertension associated with congenital heart disease. Brazilian J Med Biol Res=Revista brasileira de pesquisas medicas e biologicas/Sociedade Brasileira de Biofisica [et al]. 2011;44(12):1269–75.

23. Veyradier A, Nishikubo T, Humbert M, Wolf M, Sitbon O, Simonneau G, et al. Improvement of von Willebrand factor prote-

24. Barnes T, Gliddon A, Dore CJ, Maddison P, Moots RJ, Group QUTS. Baseline vWF factor predicts the development of elevated pulmonary artery pressure in systemic sclerosis. Rheumatology. 2012;51(9):1606–9.

25. Brindle NP, Saharinen P, Alitalo K. Signaling and functions of angiopoietin-1 in vascular protection. Circ Res. 2006;98(8):1014–23.

26. Du L, Sullivan CC, Chu D, Cho AJ, Kido M, Wolf PL, et al. Signaling molecules in nonfamilial pulmonary hypertension. N Engl J Med. 2003;348(6):500–9.

27. Sullivan CC, Du L, Chu D, Cho AJ, Kido M, Wolf PL, et al. Induction of pulmonary hypertension by an angiopoietin 1/TIE2/serotonin pathway. Proc Natl Acad Sci U S A. 2003;100(21):12331–6.

28. Kumpers P, Nickel N, Lukasz A, Golpon H, Westerkamp V, Olsson KM, et al. Circulating angiopoietins in idiopathic pulmonary arterial hypertension. Eur Heart J. 2010;31(18):2291–300.

29. Bull TM, Golpon H, Hebbel RP, Solovey A, Cool CD, Tuder RM, et al. Circulating endothelial cells in pulmonary hypertension. Thromb Haemost. 2003;90(4):698–703.

30. Smadja DM, Mauge L, Sanchez O, Silvestre JS, Guerin C, Godier A, et al. Distinct patterns of circulating endothelial cells in pulmonary hypertension. Eur Respir J. 2010;36(6):1284–93.

31. Levy M, Bonnet D, Mauge L, Celermajer DS, Gaussem P, Smadja DM. Circulating endothelial cells in refractory pulmonary hypertension in children: markers of treatment efficacy and clinical worsening. PLoS One. 2013;8(6), e65114.

32. Humbert M, Monti G, Brenot F, Sitbon O, Portier A, Grangeot-Keros L, et al. Increased interleukin-1 and interleukin-6 serum concentrations in severe primary pulmonary hypertension. Am J Respir Crit Care Med. 1995;151(5):1628–31.

33. Soon E, Holmes AM, Treacy CM, Doughty NJ, Southgate L, Machado RD, et al. Elevated levels of inflammatory cytokines predict survival in idiopathic and familial pulmonary arterial hypertension. Circulation. 2010;122(9):920–7.

34. Selimovic N, Bergh CH, Andersson B, Sakiniene E, Carlsten H, Rundqvist B. Growth factors and interleukin-6 across the lung circulation in pulmonary hypertension. Eur Respir J. 2009;34(3):662–8.

35. Quarck R, Nawrot T, Meyns B, Delcroix M. C-reactive protein: a new predictor of adverse outcome in pulmonary arterial hypertension. J Am Coll Cardiol. 2009;53(14):1211–8.

36. Burke DL, Frid MG, Kunrath CL, Karoor V, Anwar A, Wagner BD, et al. Sustained hypoxia promotes the development of a pulmonary artery-specific chronic inflammatory microenvironment. Am J Physiol Lung Cell Mol Physiol. 2009;297(2):L238–50.

37. Lund SA, Giachelli CM, Scatena M. The role of osteopontin in inflammatory processes. J Cell Commun Signal. 2009;3(3-4):311–22.

38. Lund SA, Wilson CL, Raines EW, Tang J, Giachelli CM, Scatena M. Osteopontin mediates macrophage chemotaxis via alpha4 and alpha9 integrins and survival via the alpha4 integrin. J Cell Biochem. 2013;114(5):1194–202.

39. Lorenzen JM, Nickel N, Kramer R, Golpon H, Westerkamp V, Olsson KM, et al. Osteopontin in patients with idiopathic pulmonary hypertension. Chest. 2011;139(5):1010–7.

40. Doni A, Peri G, Chieppa M, Allavena P, Pasqualini F, Vago L, et al. Production of the soluble pattern recognition receptor PTX3 by myeloid, but not plasmacytoid, dendritic cells. Eur J Immunol. 2003;33(10):2886–93.

41. Mantovani A, Garlanda C, Doni A, Bottazzi B. Pentraxins in innate immunity: from C-reactive protein to the long pentraxin PTX3. J Clin Immunol. 2008;28(1):1–13.

42. Leary PJ, Jenny NS, Barr RG, Bluemke DA, Harhay MO, Heckbert SR, et al. Pentraxin-3 and the right ventricle: the

Multi-Ethnic Study of Atherosclerosis-Right Ventricle Study. Pulm Circ. 2014;4(2):250–9.

43. Tamura Y, Ono T, Kuwana M, Inoue K, Takei M, Yamamoto T, et al. Human pentraxin 3 (PTX3) as a novel biomarker for the diagnosis of pulmonary arterial hypertension. PLoS One. 2012;7(9), e45834.

44. Krenning G, Moonen JR, Harmsen MC. Pleiotropism of adiponectin: inflammation, neovascularization, and fibrosis. Circ Res. 2009;104(9):1029–31.

45. Okamoto Y, Kihara S, Funahashi T, Matsuzawa Y, Libby P. Adiponectin: a key adipocytokine in metabolic syndrome. Clin Sci. 2006;110(3):267–78.

46. Summer R, Fiack CA, Ikeda Y, Sato K, Dwyer D, Ouchi N, et al. Adiponectin deficiency: a model of pulmonary hypertension associated with pulmonary vascular disease. Am J Physiol Lung Cell Mol Physiol. 2009;297(3):L432–8.

47. Tilg H, Moschen AR. Adipocytokines: mediators linking adipose tissue, inflammation and immunity. Nat Rev Immunol. 2006;6(10):772–83.

48. Santos M, Reis A, Goncalves F, Ferreira-Pinto MJ, Cabral S, Torres S, et al. Adiponectin levels are elevated in patients with pulmonary arterial hypertension. Clin Cardiol. 2014;37(1):21–5.

49. Braghiroli A, Sacco C, Erbetta M, Ruga V, Donner CF. Overnight urinary uric acid: creatinine ratio for detection of sleep hypoxemia. Validation study in chronic obstructive pulmonary disease and obstructive sleep apnea before and after treatment with nasal continuous positive airway pressure. Am Rev Respir Dis. 1993;148(1):173–8.

50. Leyva F, Anker S, Swan JW, Godsland IF, Wingrove CS, Chua TP, et al. Serum uric acid as an index of impaired oxidative metabolism in chronic heart failure. Eur Heart J. 1997;18(5):858–65.

51. Nagaya N, Uematsu M, Satoh T, Kyotani S, Sakamaki F, Nakanishi N, et al. Serum uric acid levels correlate with the severity and the mortality of primary pulmonary hypertension. Am J Respir Crit Care Med. 1999;160(2):487–92.

52. Bendayan D, Shitrit D, Ygla M, Huerta M, Fink G, Kramer MR. Hyperuricemia as a prognostic factor in pulmonary arterial hypertension. Respir Med. 2003;97(2):130–3.

53. Joshi K, Anjum F, Gowda S, Damania D, Graham-Hill S, Gillette P, et al. Uric Acid as a potential biomarker of pulmonary arterial hypertension in patients with sickle cell disease. Indian J Hematol Blood Transfusion: Off J Indian Soc Hematol Blood Trans. 2011;27(2):96–100.

54. Cracowski JL, Degano B, Chabot F, Labarere J, Schwedhelm E, Monneret D, et al. Independent association of urinary F2-isoprostanes with survival in pulmonary arterial hypertension. Chest. 2012;142(4):869–76.

55. Zhang R, Sun ML, Fan YF, Jiang X, Zhao QH, He J, et al. Plasma 15-F2t-isoprostane in idiopathic pulmonary arterial hypertension. Int J Cardiol. 2014;175(2):268–73.

56. Yap LB, Mukerjee D, Timms PM, Ashrafian H, Coghlan JG. Natriuretic peptides, respiratory disease, and the right heart. Chest. 2004;126(4):1330–6.

57. Foris V, Kovacs G, Tscherner M, Olschewski A, Olschewski H. Biomarkers in pulmonary hypertension: what do we know? Chest. 2013;144(1):274–83.

58. Bando M, Ishii Y, Sugiyama Y, Kitamura S. Elevated plasma brain natriuretic peptide levels in chronic respiratory failure with cor pulmonale. Respir Med. 1999;93(7):507–14.

59. Morrison LK, Harrison A, Krishnaswamy P, Kazanegra R, Clopton P, Maisel A. Utility of a rapid B-natriuretic peptide assay in differentiating congestive heart failure from lung disease in patients presenting with dyspnea. J Am Coll Cardiol. 2002;39(2):202–9.

60. Elstein D, Nir A, Klutstein M, Rudensky B, Zimran A. C-reactive protein and NT-proBNP as surrogate markers for pulmonary hypertension in Gaucher disease. Blood Cells Mol Dis. 2005;34(3):201–5.

61. Kucher N, Printzen G, Doernhoefer T, Windecker S, Meier B, Hess OM. Low pro-brain natriuretic peptide levels predict benign clinical outcome in acute pulmonary embolism. Circulation. 2003;107(12):1576–8.

62. Kucher N, Printzen G, Goldhaber SZ. Prognostic role of brain natriuretic peptide in acute pulmonary embolism. Circulation. 2003;107(20):2545–7.

63. Leuchte HH, Neurohr C, Baumgartner R, Holzapfel M, Giehrl W, Vogeser M, et al. Brain natriuretic peptide and exercise capacity in lung fibrosis and pulmonary hypertension. Am J Respir Crit Care Med. 2004;170(4):360–5.

64. Nagaya N, Nishikimi T, Okano Y, Uematsu M, Satoh T, Kyotani S, et al. Plasma brain natriuretic peptide levels increase in proportion to the extent of right ventricular dysfunction in pulmonary hypertension. J Am Coll Cardiol. 1998;31(1):202–8.

65. Nagaya N, Sasaki N, Ando M, Ogino H, Sakamaki F, Kyotani S, et al. Prostacyclin therapy before pulmonary thromboendarterectomy in patients with chronic thromboembolic pulmonary hypertension. Chest. 2003;123(2):338–43.

66. Nagaya N, Nishikimi T, Uematsu M, Satoh T, Kyotani S, Sakamaki F, et al. Plasma brain natriuretic peptide as a prognostic indicator in patients with primary pulmonary hypertension. Circulation. 2000;102(8):865–70.

67. Leuchte HH, Holzapfel M, Baumgartner RA, Ding I, Neurohr C, Vogeser M, et al. Clinical significance of brain natriuretic peptide in primary pulmonary hypertension. J Am Coll Cardiol. 2004;43(5):764–70.

68. Leuchte HH, Holzapfel M, Baumgartner RA, Neurohr C, Vogeser M, Behr J. Characterization of brain natriuretic peptide in long-term follow-up of pulmonary arterial hypertension. Chest. 2005;128(4):2368–74.

69. Hammerer-Lercher A, Neubauer E, Muller S, Pachinger O, Puschendorf B, Mair J. Head-to-head comparison of N-terminal pro-brain natriuretic peptide, brain natriuretic peptide and N-terminal pro-atrial natriuretic peptide in diagnosing left ventricular dysfunction. Clinica Chimica Acta; Int J Clin Chem. 2001;310(2):193–7.

70. Andreassen AK, Wergeland R, Simonsen S, Geiran O, Guevara C, Ueland T. N-terminal pro-B-type natriuretic peptide as an indicator of disease severity in a heterogeneous group of patients with chronic precapillary pulmonary hypertension. Am J Cardiol. 2006;98(4):525–9.

71. Fijalkowska A, Kurzyna M, Torbicki A, Szewczyk G, Florczyk M, Pruszczyk P, et al. Serum N-terminal brain natriuretic peptide as a prognostic parameter in patients with pulmonary hypertension. Chest. 2006;129(5):1313–21.

72. Mauritz GJ, Rizopoulos D, Groepenhoff H, Tiede H, Felix J, Eilers P, et al. Usefulness of serial N-terminal pro-B-type natriuretic peptide measurements for determining prognosis in patients with pulmonary arterial hypertension. Am J Cardiol. 2011;108(11):1645–50.

73. Soon E, Doughty NJ, Treacy CM, Ross RM, Toshner M, Upton PD, et al. Log-transformation improves the prognostic value of serial NT-proBNP levels in apparently stable pulmonary arterial hypertension. Pulm Circ. 2011;1(2):244–9.

74. Souza R, Bogossian HB, Humbert M, Jardim C, Rabelo R, Amato MB, et al. N-terminal-pro-brain natriuretic peptide as a haemodynamic marker in idiopathic pulmonary arterial hypertension. Eur Respir J. 2005;25(3):509–13.

75. Christenson RH, Azzazy HM, Duh SH, Maynard S, Seliger SL, Defilippi CR. Impact of increased body mass index on accuracy of B-type natriuretic peptide (BNP) and N-terminal proBNP for diagnosis of decompensated heart failure and prediction of all-cause mortality. Clin Chem. 2010;56(4):633–41.

76. DeFilippi C, van Kimmenade RR, Pinto YM. Amino-terminal pro-B-type natriuretic peptide testing in renal disease. Am J Cardiol. 2008;101(3A):82–8.

77. Raymond I, Groenning BA, Hildebrandt PR, Nilsson JC, Baumann M, Trawinski J, et al. The influence of age, sex and other variables on the plasma level of N-terminal pro brain natriuretic peptide in a large sample of the general population. Heart. 2003;89(7):745–51.

78. Vickery S, Price CP, John RI, Abbas NA, Webb MC, Kempson ME, et al. B-type natriuretic peptide (BNP) and amino-terminal proBNP in patients with CKD: relationship to renal function and left ventricular hypertrophy. Am J Kidney Dis: Off J Nat Kidney Found. 2005;46(4):610–20.

79. McLaughlin VV, Benza RL, Rubin LJ, Channick RN, Voswinckel R, Tapson VF, et al. Addition of inhaled treprostinil to oral therapy for pulmonary arterial hypertension: a randomized controlled clinical trial. J Am Coll Cardiol. 2010;55(18):1915–22.

80. Galie N, Olschewski H, Oudiz RJ, Torres F, Frost A, Ghofrani HA, et al. Ambrisentan for the treatment of pulmonary arterial hypertension: results of the ambrisentan in pulmonary arterial hypertension, randomized, double-blind, placebo-controlled, multicenter, efficacy (ARIES) study 1 and 2. Circulation. 2008;117(23):3010–9.

81. Torbicki A, Kurzyna M, Kuca P, Fijalkowska A, Sikora J, Florczyk M, et al. Detectable serum cardiac troponin T as a marker of poor prognosis among patients with chronic precapillary pulmonary hypertension. Circulation. 2003;108(7):844–8.

82. Roy AK, McCullagh BN, Segurado R, McGorrian C, Keane E, Keaney J, et al. Detection of high-sensitivity troponin in outpatients with stable pulmonary hypertension identifies a subgroup at higher risk of adverse outcomes. J Card Fail. 2014;20(1):31–7.

83. Antman EM. Decision making with cardiac troponin tests. N Engl J Med. 2002;346(26):2079–82.

84. de Man FS, Tu L, Handoko ML, Rain S, Ruiter G, Francois C, et al. Dysregulated renin-angiotensin-aldosterone system contributes to pulmonary arterial hypertension. Am J Respir Crit Care Med. 2012;186(8):780–9.

85. Li G, Liu Y, Zhu Y, Liu A, Xu Y, Li X, et al. ACE2 activation confers endothelial protection and attenuates neointimal lesions in prevention of severe pulmonary arterial hypertension in rats. Lung. 2013;191(4):327–36.

86. Morrell NW, Atochina EN, Morris KG, Danilov SM, Stenmark KR. Angiotensin converting enzyme expression is increased in small pulmonary arteries of rats with hypoxia-induced pulmonary hypertension. J Clin Invest. 1995;96(4):1823–33.

87. Morrell NW, Upton PD, Higham MA, Yacoub MH, Polak JM, Wharton J. Angiotensin II stimulates proliferation of human pulmonary artery smooth muscle cells via the AT1 receptor. Chest. 1998;114(1 Suppl):90S–1.

88. Morrell NW, Upton PD, Kotecha S, Huntley A, Yacoub MH, Polak JM, et al. Angiotensin II activates MAPK and stimulates growth of human pulmonary artery smooth muscle via AT1 receptors. Am J Physiol. 1999;277(3 Pt 1):L440–8.

89. Zhang F, Hu Y, Xu Q, Ye S. Different effects of angiotensin II and angiotensin-(1-7) on vascular smooth muscle cell proliferation and migration. PLoS One. 2010;5(8), e12323.

90. Maron BA, Opotowsky AR, Landzberg MJ, Loscalzo J, Waxman AB, Leopold JA. Plasma aldosterone levels are elevated in patients with pulmonary arterial hypertension in the absence of left ventricular heart failure: a pilot study. Eur J Heart Fail. 2013;15(3):277–83.

91. Maron BA, Zhang YY, White K, Chan SY, Handy DE, Mahoney CE, et al. Aldosterone inactivates the endothelin-B receptor via a cysteinyl thiol redox switch to decrease pulmonary endothelial nitric oxide levels and modulate pulmonary arterial hypertension. Circulation. 2012;126(8):963–74.

92. Preston IR, Sagliani KD, Warburton RR, Hill NS, Fanburg BL, Jaffe IZ. Mineralocorticoid receptor antagonism attenuates experimental pulmonary hypertension. Am J Physiol Lung Cell Mol Physiol. 2013;304(10):L678–88.

93. Paulin R, Courboulin A, Meloche J, Mainguy V, Dumas de la Roque E, Saksouk N, et al. Signal transducers and activators of transcription-3/pim1 axis plays a critical role in the pathogenesis of human pulmonary arterial hypertension. Circulation. 2011;123(11):1205–15.

94. Renard S, Paulin R, Breuils-Bonnet S, Simard S, Pibarot P, Bonnet S, et al. Pim-1: a new biomarker in pulmonary arterial hypertension. Pulm Circ. 2013;3(1):74–81.

95. Shah SJ, Thenappan T, Rich S, Tian L, Archer SL, Gomberg-Maitland M. Association of serum creatinine with abnormal hemodynamics and mortality in pulmonary arterial hypertension. Circulation. 2008;117(19):2475–83.

96. Kaiser R, Seiler S, Held M, Bals R, Wilkens H. Prognostic impact of renal function in precapillary pulmonary hypertension. J Intern Med. 2014;275(2):116–26.

97. Benza RL, Miller DP, Gomberg-Maitland M, Frantz RP, Foreman AJ, Coffey CS, et al. Predicting survival in pulmonary arterial hypertension: insights from the Registry to Evaluate Early and Long-Term Pulmonary Arterial Hypertension Disease Management (REVEAL). Circulation. 2010;122(2):164–72.

98. Bavishi C, Ather S, Bambhroliya A, Jneid H, Virani SS, Bozkurt B, et al. Prognostic significance of hyponatremia among ambulatory patients with heart failure and preserved and reduced ejection fractions. Am J Cardiol. 2014;113(11):1834–8.

99. Hamaguchi S, Kinugawa S, Tsuchihashi-Makaya M, Matsushima S, Sakakibara M, Ishimori N, et al. Hyponatremia is an independent predictor of adverse clinical outcomes in hospitalized patients due to worsening heart failure. J Cardiol. 2014;63(3):182–8.

100. Forfia PR, Mathai SC, Fisher MR, Housten-Harris T, Hemnes AR, Champion HC, et al. Hyponatremia predicts right heart failure and poor survival in pulmonary arterial hypertension. Am J Respir Crit Care Med. 2008;177(12):1364–9.

101. Campo A, Mathai SC, Le Pavec J, Zaiman AL, Hummers LK, Boyce D, et al. Outcomes of hospitalisation for right heart failure in pulmonary arterial hypertension. Eur Respir J. 2011;38(2):359–67.

102. Haddad F, Peterson T, Fuh E, Kudelko KT, de Jesus PV, Skhiri M, et al. Characteristics and outcome after hospitalization for acute right heart failure in patients with pulmonary arterial hypertension. Circ Heart Fail. 2011;4(6):692–9.

103. Rabinovitz A, Raiszadeh F, Zolty R. Association of hyponatremia and outcomes in pulmonary hypertension. J Card Fail. 2013;19(8):550–6.

104. Pugh ME, Robbins IM, Rice TW, West J, Newman JH, Hemnes AR. Unrecognized glucose intolerance is common in pulmonary arterial hypertension. J Heart Lung Transpl: Off Publ Int Soc Heart Transpl. 2011;30(8):904–11.

105. Belly MJ, Tiede H, Morty RE, Schulz R, Voswinckel R, Tanislav C, et al. HbA1c in pulmonary arterial hypertension: a marker of prognostic relevance? J Heart Lung Transpl: Off Publ Int Soc Heart Transpl. 2012;31(10):1109–14.

106. D'Alonzo GE, Barst RJ, Ayres SM, Bergofsky EH, Brundage BH, Detre KM, et al. Survival in patients with primary pulmonary hypertension. Results from a national prospective registry. Ann Intern Med. 1991;115(5):343–9.

107. McLaughlin VV, Shillington A, Rich S. Survival in primary pulmonary hypertension: the impact of epoprostenol therapy. Circulation. 2002;106(12):1477–82.

108. Sitbon O, Humbert M, Nunes H, Parent F, Garcia G, Herve P, et al. Long-term intravenous epoprostenol infusion in primary pulmonary hypertension: prognostic factors and survival. J Am Coll Cardiol. 2002;40(4):780–8.

109. Barst RJ, Chung L, Zamanian RT, Turner M, McGoon MD. Functional class improvement and 3-year survival outcomes in patients with pulmonary arterial hypertension in the REVEAL Registry. Chest. 2013;144(1):160–8.
110. Hoeper MM, Huscher D, Ghofrani HA, Delcroix M, Distler O, Schweiger C, et al. Elderly patients diagnosed with idiopathic pulmonary arterial hypertension: results from the COMPERA registry. Int J Cardiol. 2013;168(2):871–80.
111. Miyamoto S, Nagaya N, Satoh T, Kyotani S, Sakamaki F, Fujita M, et al. Clinical correlates and prognostic significance of six-minute walk test in patients with primary pulmonary hypertension. Comparison with cardiopulmonary exercise testing. Am J Respir Crit Care Med. 2000;161(2 Pt 1):487–92.
112. Farber HW, Miller DP, McGoon MD, Frost AE, Benton WW, Benza RL. Predicting outcomes in pulmonary arterial hypertension based on the 6-minute walk distance. J Heart Lung Transpl: Off Publ Int Soc Heart Transpl. 2014.
113. Forfia PR, Fisher MR, Mathai SC, Housten-Harris T, Hemnes AR, Borlaug BA, et al. Tricuspid annular displacement predicts survival in pulmonary hypertension. Am J Respir Crit Care Med. 2006;174(9):1034–41.
114. Vonk MC, Sander MH, van den Hoogen FH, van Riel PL, Verheugt FW, van Dijk AP. Right ventricle Tei-index: a tool to increase the accuracy of non-invasive detection of pulmonary arterial hypertension in connective tissue diseases. Eur J Echocardiogr: J Work Group Echocardiogr Eur Soc Cardiol. 2007;8(5):317–21.
115. Ogihara Y, Yamada N, Dohi K, Matsuda A, Tsuji A, Ota S, et al. Utility of right ventricular Tei-index for assessing disease severity and determining response to treatment in patients with pulmonary arterial hypertension. J Cardiol. 2014;63(2):149–53.
116. Yamada Y, Okuda S, Kataoka M, Tanimoto A, Tamura Y, Abe T, et al. Prognostic value of cardiac magnetic resonance imaging for idiopathic pulmonary arterial hypertension before initiating intravenous prostacyclin therapy. Circ J: Off J Japan Circ Soc. 2012;76(7):1737–43.
117. van Wolferen SA, Marcus JT, Boonstra A, Marques KM, Bronzwaer JG, Spreeuwenberg MD, et al. Prognostic value of right ventricular mass, volume, and function in idiopathic pulmonary arterial hypertension. Eur Heart J. 2007;28(10):1250–7.
118. Frost AE, Badesch DB, Miller DP, Benza RL, Meltzer LA, McGoon MD. Evaluation of the predictive value of a clinical worsening definition using 2-year outcomes in patients with pulmonary arterial hypertension: a REVEAL Registry analysis. Chest. 2013;144(5):1521–9.
119. Benza RL, Gomberg-Maitland M, Miller DP, Frost A, Frantz RP, Foreman AJ, et al. The REVEAL Registry risk score calculator in patients newly diagnosed with pulmonary arterial hypertension. Chest. 2012;141(2):354–62.
120. Kane GC, Maradit-Kremers H, Slusser JP, Scott CG, Frantz RP, McGoon MD. Integration of clinical and hemodynamic parameters in the prediction of long-term survival in patients with pulmonary arterial hypertension. Chest. 2011;139(6):1285–93.
121. Humbert M, Sitbon O, Chaouat A, Bertocchi M, Habib G, Gressin V, et al. Survival in patients with idiopathic, familial, and anorexigen-associated pulmonary arterial hypertension in the modern management era. Circulation. 2010;122(2):156–63.
122. Willis VC, et al. Sputum autoantibodies in patients with established rheumatoid arthritis and subjects at risk of future clinically apparent disease. Eur Respir J. 1997;65(10):2545–54.

Pulmonary Circulatory – Right Ventricular Uncoupling: New Insights Into Pulmonary Hypertension Pathophysiology

15

David Boulate, Olaf Mercier, Julien Guihaire, Elie Fadel, Robert Naeije, Francois Haddad, and Franz Rischard

Introduction

Pulmonary arterial hypertension (PAH) is a syndrome that affects both the pulmonary circulation and the right ventricle. Three important observations in patients with precapillary pulmonary hypertension have highlighted the need to better understand right ventricular-pulmonary circulation (RV-PC) coupling: first, RV function is the main determinant of exercise limitation relative to with ventilatory function [1]; second, RV failure is one of the strongest prognosis factor [2, 3]; third, RV adaptation is significantly variable among patients with elevated pulmonary vascular resistances (PVR) [4]. From a conceptual point of view, RV-PC coupling can be defined as the matching between RV contractility and afterload and thus may be used as a marker of RV function or a marker of RV adaptation to the afterload. For example, a ventricle that can adapt well to pulmonary hypertension (PH) is able to increase its contractility to match the increase in afterload and as a consequence systolic function would be well preserved (coupled RV to PC). The objective of this chapter is to describe how the concept of ventriculo-arterial coupling can bring novel insights into the pathophysiology of pulmonary hypertension. The followings sections will discuss the practical implications in measuring RV-PC coupling as well as its value in both clinical practice and research.

The RV-PC Coupling in PAH, One Piece of the Pathophysiology Puzzle

The main function of the cardio-pulmonary system is to maintain adequate cardiac output and gas exchange both at rest and with exercise. Figure 15.1 is a schematic representation of the "unfolded" circulation highlighting the different levels of coupling and interactions determining the cardio-pulmonary function. Although the main focus of this chapter is ventriculo-arterial coupling, other important features of interactions characterize the cardio-pulmonary system such as the interventricular relation and the ventilation-perfusion matching. New features are also emerging in the right heart such as the matching between perfusion/metabolism and load, and the atrio-vantricular relationships, particularly during the diastole The importance of Fig. 15.1 is to show that ventriculo-arterial coupling is only one characteristic of the cardio-pulmonary physiology.

Historical Perspective

Suga and Sunagawa et al. were one of the first to introduce the concept of ventriculo-arterial coupling [5] derived from pressure-volume loop analysis using conductance catheterization. This method allows quantifying, in a same set of acquisition, a load-independent indice of venricular contractility, the end systolic elastance (Ees); and an integrative indices of ventricular afterload, the arterial elastance (Ea).

15

D. Boulate, MD, MSc (✉)
Thoracic, Vascular and Heart-Lung Transplantation, Marie Lannelongue Hospital, 133 avenue de la Résistance, Le Plessis-Robinson 92350, France
e-mail: d.boulate@ccml.fr

O. Mercier, MR, PhD
Surgical Research Laboratory, Marie Lannelongue Hospital, Le Plessis-Robinson, France

J. Guihaire, MD, PhD
Adult Cardiac Surgery, Centre Hospitalier Universitaire de Rennes, Rennes, France

E. Fadel, MD, PhD
Thoracic and Vascular Surgery and Heart-Lung Transplantation, Marie Lannelongue Hospital, Le Plessis-Robinson, France

R. Naeije, MD, PhD
Hypertension artérielle pulmonaire, médecine du sport, Erasme Hospital, Brussel, Belgium

F. Haddad, MD
Biomarker and Phenotype Core Laboratory, Stanford Cardiovascular Institute, Palo Alto, CA, USA

F. Rischard, MD
Pulmonary, Allergy, Critical Care and Sleep Medicine, Arizona Health Sciences Center, Tucson, AZ, USA

© Springer International Publishing Switzerland 2016
B.A. Maron et al. (eds.), *Pulmonary Hypertension: Basic Science to Clinical Medicine*, DOI 10.1007/978-3-319-23594-3_15

Fig. 15.1 Simplified representation of "unfolded circulation" with representation of right atrium (*RA*), right ventricle (*RV*), lungs, left atrium (*LA*), left ventricle (*LV*) and systemic organs. Concepts related to coupling and matching between different physiological and anatomical entities are designed and an arrow indicate their relative location (Reproduced with permission from Laboratory of Surgical Research of the Marie Lannelongue Hospital)

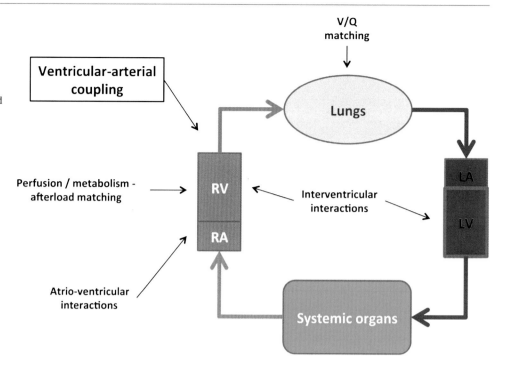

The ratio of these elastances provides a value of ventricular–arterial coupling. The major breakthrough of PV loops evaluation was to provide load independent indices of ventricular elastance using multiple pressure-volume points during acute load variations, which is the current gold standard to quantify the ventricular contractility. The end-systolic ventricular elastance is computed from a slope of linear regression of at least 2 end-systolic pressure-volume points. The linearity of the multibeat end-systolic pressure –volume relationship (ESPVR) during acute load variation was first suggested by Suga et al. from isolated heart and later verified in the clinical settings by Wallace et al. [6]. However, Kass et al. showed ESPVR being closer from a quadratic relationship [7]. The second important metric derived from PV-loop analysis was arterial elastance (Ea) which represents a measure of ventricular afterload. It is usually calculated as end-systolic pressure divided by stroke volume (Ea=ESP/SV). Other authors recommend subtracting RV end-diastolic pressure from end-systolic pressure. These differences in Ea must be considered when comparing results from different studies. Unlike impedance spectrum analysis of RV afterload, Ea is easier to quantify and relates well to lumped quantification of ventricular afterload [8].

The concept of ventriculo-arterial coupling relates to a measure of contractility corrected for afterload and is measured using the ratio of Ees/Ea. One of the points of confusion is that the term "load independency" refers to the beat-to-beat stability of the end-systolic pressure over volume ratio during acute loading variation used to measure Ees; while the contractility will adapt within 20–30 s or few minutes to an afterload variation due to homeometric

regulation, sometimes refered to as the "Anrep effect." One of the strong advantages of Ees/Ea ratio, having no dimension, is that it decreases the influence of volume and pressure calibration errors and allows comparison between individuals without requiring scaling. Initially, the ventricular-arterial coupling was referred as the ventriculo-arterial matching [9] and the value of Ees/Ea = 1 was considered as to be the perfect match. From theoretical models, the ratio Ees/Ea = 1 corresponded to the optimal mechanical coupling. Currently, there is no definition of normal values of ventriculo-arterial coupling nor is there a well-established threshold defining uncoupling. However, based on the literature the range of the right ventricular-pulmonary artery (RV-PA) coupling in healthy individuals is situated between 1 and 2 depending on the methods used for determinations of Ees and Ea, and appears to be comparable for both the right and left ventricle. Also the optimal ratio of ventricular energy production transmitted to the arterial system occurs for RV-PA coupling values of 1.5–2 [10]. In our experience in large animal model of pulmonary hypertension, the Ees/Ea values may vary from 0.3 in the setting of severe chronic pressure overload, to about 4 in the setting of dobutamine infusion in healthy animals. This range of dynamic coupling has also been shown in different experimental models as well as in several human studies.

The methodology of PV loop analysis was first introduced in the left ventricle and then applied to the right ventricle. The differences between RV- and left ventricular (LV)-PV loop interpretation are mainly due to the differences in the systolic pressure definition to determine the end-systolic elastance as well as in ventricular geometries. Due to relatively low resistance in the pulmonary circuit, normal RV ejection continues past peak pressure in contrast to the LV-systemic system (Fig. 15.2a, b). In the left ventricle, both the end-systolic-point or the peak pressure point have been shown to be valid to quantify contractility variations [11]. Dell'Italia showed using RV PV-loops in normal subjects that evaluation of RV systolic elastance was different using the systolic point of maximal pressure/volume ratio compared with the end-ejection point [12]; the end-ejection PV relationship being less correlated to the time varying elastance determined from linear regression of simultaneous acquired PV points in 3 different loading conditions. In the setting of PH, ejection occurs closer to peak pressure and the shape of beat to beat PV loops could approximates the LV [13, 14].

Several assumptions of RV-PA coupling models were tested. The linear relationship of the beat to beat RV ESPVR was verified on isolated hearts by Maughan et al. [15], and in

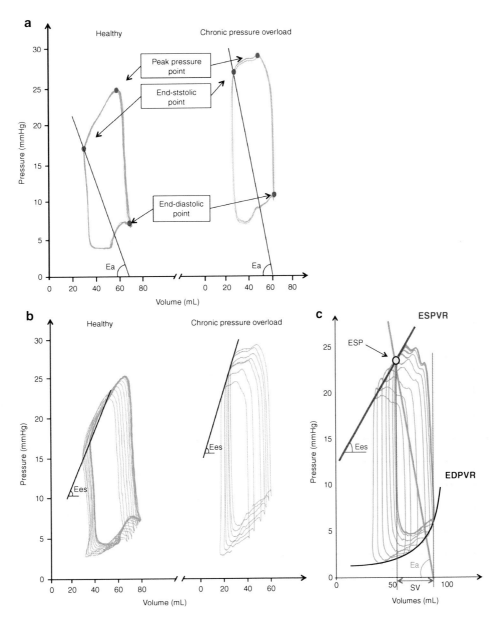

Fig. 15.2 (**a–c**) Basic representation of steady pressure-volume (PV–) loops with the right ventricular (*RV*) pressure in Y axis and RV volume in Y axis. (**a**) Representation of steady PV-loops in healthy (*left panel*) and chronic pressure overload (*right panel*) settings. End-systolic and end-diastolic points are represented in red. The peak pressure point during systole is represented in blue in both cases. The pulmonary arterial elastance (*Ea*) is the slope of the black line which represents the end-systolic pressure over stroke volume ratio. (**b**) Representation of multibeat RV-PV loops during inferior vena cava (*IVC*) occlusion in healthy (left panel) and chronic pressure overload (*right panel*). The RV end-systolic elastance (Ees) is the slope of the end-systolic pressure-volume relationship (*ESPVR*) determined from the multibeat PV-loops during IVC occlusion. (**c**) Integrative representation of PV-loops derived parameters, end-systolic pressure (ESP), ESPVR, Ees, Ea, end-diastolic pressure-volume relationship (*EDPVR*), stroke volume (*SV*) (Reproduced with permission from Laboratory of Surgical Research of the Marie Lannelongue Hospital)

dogs by Karunanithi et al. [16]. Also in humans Dell'Italia et al. [12] and Brown et al. [17] reported linear relationship of ESPVR using time varying elastance, using steady PV-loops at baseline and during different loading conditions [12]. Currently, the slope of the linear relationship of ESPVR during beat to beat pre-load reduction is the most reported for quantification of multibeat RV ESPVR. The linear relationship of RV ESPVR derived from beat-to-beat analysis during acute load variation is shown in Fig. 15.2c. Another difference between RV- and LV-PV loops analysis is the determination of ventricular volumes that may not be as accurate in RV as in LV due to the crescent shape of the RV. If volume variations may be well calibrated using stroke volume determinations with external methods such as thermodilution or echocardiography, the calibration of absolute volume values may be more difficult at time of PV loops acquisition because based on ventricular shape. As a consequence, indices based on the accurate volume values such as end-diastolic volumes, end-systolic volumes and ejection fraction are not as well quantified as in left ventricles using RV PV-loops and external methods such as MRI have been used to address this issue [13, 14].

More recently, less invasively determined indices of RV-PA coupling have been described, either based on single beat PV-loops or base on imaging analysis [18] (Fig. 15.3).

RV-PA Coupling – Which Applications?

One important question that emerges is what is the utility of measuring RV-PA coupling when more simple measures of ventricular function exist. Currently, PV loops analysis and RV-PA coupling analysis is mainly performed during pathophysiological studies or when comparing the effects of different therapeutic interventions in the experimental setting. In this context, the ability to determine the precise changes in metrics of contractility, load and coupling provides useful informations.

In the clinical setting, it is unclear whether measures of RV-PA coupling will bring additional prognostic information for the clinical care of patients with pulmonary arterial hypertension. Due to the invasive nature of multibeat PV-loops acquisitions, non-invasive surrogates of RV-PA coupling were evaluated. Recent animal studies have shown that common non-invasive measures of RV function such as RV ejection fraction (RVEF), fractional area change (RVFAC), tricuspid annular plane systolic excursion (TAPSE) or isovolumic acceleration (IVA) are more closely associated with ventriculo-arterial coupling than with RV contractility [19]. Interestingly, isovolumic indices such as the IVA are thought to be less load dependent [20] indices of contractility or coupling. As will be discussed in the next section, non-invasive single beat methods to estimate RV elastance and contractility have also been suggested. Thus, RV-PA coupling is not an esoteric concept but may rather be used daily in clinical practice in the future. Kuehne et al. validated in 2004 a single beat method for RV PV-loops acquisitions and RV-PA coupling quantification using RV catheterism for pressure measurement and MRI for volumes [21]. Sanz et al. more recently quantified the RV-PA coupling using a volumetric method with MRI using the ratio stroke volume over end-systolic volume [22]; a significant prognosis value of this indices was demonstrated in patients with PAH [23].

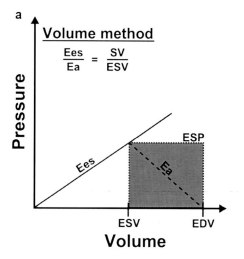
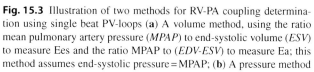
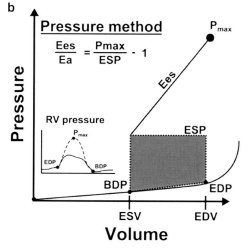

Fig. 15.3 Illustration of two methods for RV-PA coupling determination using single beat PV-loops (**a**) A volume method, using the ratio mean pulmonary artery pressure (*MPAP*) to end-systolic volume (*ESV*) to measure Ees and the ratio MPAP to (*EDV-ESV*) to measure Ea; this method assumes end-systolic pressure = MPAP; (**b**) A pressure method using Pmax measurement or extrapolation from PA clamping or RV pressure curve; the ESP may be assimilated to MPAP (method 2) or to systolic RV pressure (*sRVP*) (method 3). (Reproduced from Rebecca et al. [18], with permission from BMJ Publishing Group Ltd.)

One important pearl to keep in mind is that metrics of systolic function used in clinical practice do not reflect contractility or the potential of recovery after unloading. Quantification of contractility and recovery potential may be more complex to measure than RV-PA coupling which is only a hemodynamic parameter. Useful measurement of ventricular contractility could require correction for cardiomyocyte quantity and metabolism to provide prognostic information. Recovery potential evaluation of a right ventricle could integrate contractility and RV-PA coupling parameters associated with others such as fibrosis and capillary content or metabolic changes [4]. Thus RV-PA coupling is a part of the RV phenotyping that should be used in addition to other parameters to provide information on contractility or recovery potential.

The transition from RV adaptation to RV maladaptation may be illustrated by coupling methods. The study of Kuehne et al. shows that RV-PA coupling in patients with PAH and without overt RV failure or enlargement may be decreased relative to normal controls. This observation suggests that decreased RV-PA coupling may precede RV dilation in patients with PH. In early stage pulmonary hypertension, decreased RV-PA coupling may mainly reflect the increase in RV afterload and potentially a failure from myocardial adaptation (i.e. insufficient augmentation of ventricular contractility); in end-stage pulmonary hypertension, continued worsening RV-PA coupling may reflect more a decrease in RV contractility resulting in the clinical development of RV failure.

Practical Aspects of PV-Loops Acquisition and Interpretation

This section describes practical aspects of standard PV-loops acquisition and interpretation used to determine Ees and Ea as well as less invasive single beat methods.

Signal Acquisition and Calibration

PV loops are acquired using a conductance catheter (Fig. 15.4a) allowing concomitant, continuous and high fidelity blood pressure and volume measurements into the ventricle. The ventricular pressure is continuously measured with a micromanometer. For volume signal acquisitions, a distal electrode of the catheter emits an electrical signal transmitted through the ventricular blood to different proximal electrodes situated into the ventricle creating an axial segmentation of the ventricle along the catheter axis (Fig. 15.4b). Each volume variation of a ventricular segment is continuously acquired and the global volume variation of the ventricle is represented as a sum of each segment vol-

ume. To determine the "real" volume values, volume calibration is usually performed in 3 steps including determination of blood electrical resistivity (Rho); determination of the parallel conductance volume (Vc) which represents the volume of conducting tissues surrounding the ventricular blood (myocardium and mediastinal tissues); finally the cardiac output or the SV quantified by the conductance catheter is corrected with a factor α which is determined from external methods of CO or SV determination (thermodilution, Fick method, echocardiography or magnetic resonance imaging) [24].

Procedure for PV-Loops Acquisition

The conductance catheter is placed into the right ventricle through a jugular or femoral vein and its position at the apex and parallel to the interventricular septum is verified using fluoroscopy. Then, the distal electrodes corresponding to ventricular signals are acquired and those, more proximal corresponding to atrial signals are deactivated. The atrial ventricular segments are recognized because being in inverted phase compared to the ventricle. After obtaining optimal counterclockwise ventricular PV-loops, pressure and volume calibration is performed (Fig. 15.4b). Finally PV-loops are recorded during end-expiratory periods during baseline conditions and during inferior vena cava occlusion (Fig. 15.4c) allowing beat-to-beat determination of PV-loops variations. The "steady loops" are used to determine Ea and the loops acquired during preload variation are used to determine Ees. Usually, 3 sets of IVC occlusions are performed and analyzed for internal quality control.

Single Beat Method Estimations

To obviate Ees quantification using IVC occlusion, different single beat methods were investigated that would estimate or extrapolate an ESPVR. We listed in the Table 15.1 the different methods that have been used in humans for PV-loops acquisitions, including single beat methods. In these methods, a "real" end-systolic PV point is determined in baseline condition. There are two main methods to determine a second theoretical point to draw an end-systolic pressure volume line [25]. The Pmax method is the most used in PAH and consists in determining maximal pressure point by extrapolation from the pressure signal (Pmax) or measured during pulmonary artery clamping during one beat. In this method the end-systolic elastance is the ratio (Pmax – end-systolic pressure)/SV (Fig. 15.3). The other single beat method is the maximal elastance method where the ESPVR corresponds to the ratio of the end systolic pressure over the end systolic volume (maxima pressure over volume ratio)

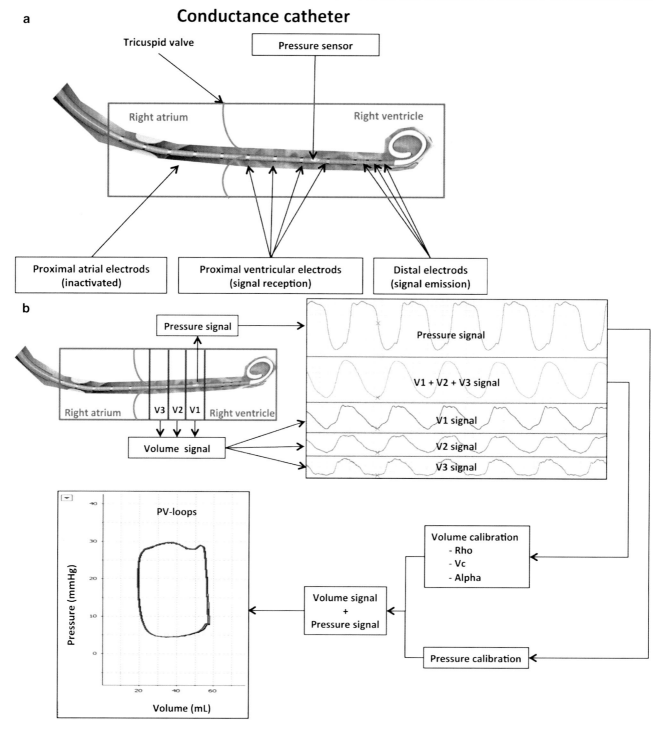

Fig. 15.4 (**a–c**) Methodological and practical aspects of RV PV-loops acquisitions. (**a**) Conductance catheter represented in the right heart cavities (*blue rectangle*). Distal electods emits an electrical signal which is conducted by the ventricular blood and surrounding tissues, proximal electrods recept the electrical signal. The pressure sensor is a micro-manometer that captures the pressure variations simultaneously with the volume signal derived from proximal electrods. Atrial proximal electrods are deactivated. (**b**) Step by step PV-loops acquisition. In the right upper corner, the conductance pressure and volume signals are transmitted a hardware and software unit providing real time pressure and volume signals (*right upper corner*). The pressure signal is the first lin (*top, green line*) and the second line (*yellow*) is the sum of the ventricular volume segments corresponding to cylindres between ventricular signal electrodes (V1, V2 and V3). In the right lower corner, volume and pres-sure calibration step. The volume calibration takes into account the blood electrical resistivity (*Rho*), the volume measured from electrical signal corresponding to tissues surrounding the ventricular blood (ventricle, mediastinum) referred as Vc (volume of the parallel conductance) and Alpha which is the ratio between the stroke volume measured from the conductance catheter and the volume measured simultaneously with an external method (echocardiography, thermodilution), it takes into account ventricular "dead space" of the ventricle not quantified with the conductance catheter such as the apex for example. (**c**) Final PV-loops used for interpretation after calibration steps. In the left panel, steady PV loops used to measure Ea for example: in the right panel, multibeat PV-loops during IVC occlusion used to measure Ees (slope of ESPVR) or β (curvature of EDPVR) (Reproduced with permission from Laboratory of Surgical Research of the Marie Lannelongue Hospital)

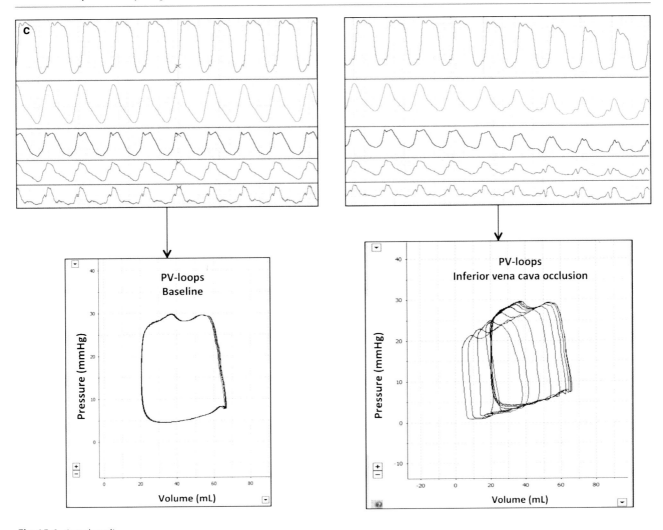

Fig. 15.4 (continued)

Table 15.1 Listing methods used to create multibeat PV-loops to determine RV-PA coupling

Invasive	Non-invasive
Pressure signal	
Micromanometer Fluid-filled catheter	Echocardiography
Volume signal	
Conductance catheter Admittance catheter Myocardial markers Cineventriculography	MRI 3D echocardiography
RV ESPVR slope determination	
IVC occlusion	Valsalva maneuver Single beat method (Pmax) Single beat method (V0)

MRI magnetic resonance imaging, *IVC* inferior vena cava, *RV* right ventricle, *ESPVR* end-systolic pressure volume relationship

and thus the extrapolated volume intercept is 0. This is often termed the volume method; this method was shown to be a poor estimate of contractility because of underestimation of Ees in sicker patients due to RV dilation [26]. There may be some advantages of the volume method, because of its ease of acquisition. Also, recent data suggest that this method to be sensitive to changes in clinical outcomes-mortality and/or transplant in patients with PAH [23].

Insights into Clinical and Experimental Pulmonary Hypertension Pathophysiology Using RV-PA Coupling Evaluation

RV-PA coupling evaluation has been used in several experimental and clinical studies providing insights into ventricular dynamics in PH including changes induced by increased RV afterload and effects of different therapeutics. Clinical studies mainly focused on RV adaptation to increased afterload in different PH groups using single beat methods. Therapeutic studies were mainly performed using animal models of acute and chronic PH, allowing evaluation of inotropic drugs and pulmonary vascular disease targeted therapies on RV-PA coupling. In animal models, RV-PA coupling evaluation provided also better characterization of the different PH models.

Changes in RV-PA Coupling with PH in Experimental and Clinical Studies

Experimental Models of PH

Table 15.2 summarizes changes in ventricular and arterial elastance as well as RV-PA coupling that were reported in the literature to characterize experimental models of acute and chronic PH. Wauthy et al. showed that RV-PA coupling was preserved after 10 min of acute hypoxia ($PaO_2 = 40$ mmHg) due to proportional increase in Ea and Ees in 3 different species (pigs, goat and dogs) [27]. This study also highlighted different hemodynamic and myocardial responses to acute hypoxia between these species. Pigs showed a worse adaptation to hypoxia with a higher increase in Ea and Ees and no increase in cardiac output, whereas dogs seemed to adapt better with a higher increase of cardiac output and lower Ea and Ees increase; goat showed an intermediate response. Rex et al. confirmed these findings in pigs [28], in their study a twofold increase in MPAP (18–36 mmHg) induced by acute hypoxia ($PaO_2 = 40$ mmHg) was associated with a significant decrease in stroke volume (47–31 mL, $P < 0.05$), a threefold increase in Ea (0.5–1.5 mmHg/mL) and a matched increase in Ees allowing RV-PA coupling to be preserved. The RV adaptation to acute pulmonary embolism was reported by Kerbaul

et al. [29]. In their study, Ea increased up to six times baseline values associated with hemodynamic compromising above 4 time increased Ea baseline values. These studies highlight that the limits of the acute RV adaptation to an acute increase in afterload is due to limits in acute contractility reserve. In pig models evaluating the chronic RV adaptation to chronic pressure overload, RV-PA coupling seemed to be preserved after 3 months of systemic to pulmonary artery shunt [30, 31], whereas after 3 months of chronic PA occlusions, RV-PA coupling seem to be decreased [19]. Also Lambert et al. showed in a pig model of pulmonary valve regurgitation associated with PA banding in pigs that Ees increased up to 3 months then decreased between 3 and 4 months [32]. In rodent models, RV-PA coupling was preserved after 1 month of PH induced by sugen-hypoxia [33] or monocrotaline [34]; whereas chronic RV-PA coupling decreased in rats between 10 and 20 weeks after aorto-caval shunt creation [35]. Taken together, these studies suggest that the RV-PA coupling is more altered secondary to an acute and massive increase in pulmonary resistances; while slowly progressive and moderate increase in RV afterload allows RV-PA coupling preservation for weeks or months due to progressive RV adaptation. In most of the models, RV-PA coupling alteration was observed after a 3 months period of RV pressure overload. Chronic

Table 15.2 RV-PA coupling characteristics of animal models of acute and chronic pulmonary hypertension

Authors (Table 15.1)	Animals	PH or RV failure model	Time of evaluation	MPAP or RVSP	Ees	Ea	Ees/Ea
Acute models							
Kerbaul et al. [38]	dogs	Acute PA constriction	Minutes/hours	RVSP 31 ± 3 (mse, n=8)	↓	↑	↓
Rex et al.[28]	Pigs	Acute hypoxia	Minutes/hours	MPAP 36 ± 6 (n=6)	↑	↑	↔
Wauthy et al. [27]	Pigs, dogs, goat	Acute hypoxia	Minutes	MPAP 40 ± 2 (8 pigs)	↑	↑	↔
		Acute PE		MPAP 43 ± 3 (10 dogs)	↑	↑	↔
		Acute PA banding		MPAP 35 ± 3 (10 dogs)	↑	↑	↔
Lambermont et al. [52]	Pigs	Acute endotoxic shock	hours	MPAP 50 mmHg (n=6)	↔	↑	↔
Missant et al. [53]	Pigs	Acute PE + RV ischemia-reperfusion injury	1 h	MPAP 41 ± 8 (18 pigs)	↓	↑	↓
Chronic models							
Lambert et al. [32]	Pigs	Chronic pulmonary valve regurgitation + pulmonary artery banding	3 months	RVSP 64 ± 11 (n=6)	↑	↑	↔
			4 months	RVSP 64 ± 11 (n=6)	↔	↑	↓ (trend)
Guihaire et al. [19]	Pigs	Chronic pulmonary artery occlusion	3 months	MPAP 35 ± 9 (n=11)	↓	↑	↓
Wauthy et al. [30]	Pigs	Chronic systemic to pulmonary artery shunt	3 months	MPAP 40 ± 1 (n=9)	↑	↑	↔ (trend↑)
Rondelet et al. [31]	Pigs	Chronic systemic to pulmonary artery shunt	3 months	MPAP 35 ± 1 (n=6)	↑	↑	↔
De Man et al. [34]	Rats	Monocrotalin	1 month	RVSP 80 ± 5 (n=8)	↑	↑	↓
Wang et al. [33]	Mice	Sugen + hypoxia	Day 21; Day J28	RVSP 41 ± 2; 45 ± 1 (n=8-9)	↑	↑	↔
Pagnamenta et al. [54]	Dogs	Heart failure induced by pacing	7 weeks	MPAP 23 ± 2 (n=14)	↔	↑	↓
Rungatscher et al. [35]	Rats	Chronic aorto-caval fistula	10 weeks	MPAP 25 ± 4 (n=10)	↔	↔	↔
			20 weeks	MPAP 44 ± 3 (n=10)	↓	↑	↓

PA pulmonary artery, *PE* pulmonary embolism, *RVSP* right ventricular systolic pressure, *MPAP* mean pulmonary artery pressure, *PH* pulmonary hypertension, *RV* right ventricular, *Ees* end-systolic elastance, *Ea* pulmonary artery elastance

models including PA banding or occlusion seemed to show earlier decrease in Ees.

Coupling in Patients with PH

Table 15.3 summarizes important clinical studies performed to better understand RV-PA coupling changes in patients with different PH etiologies and severities. McCabe et al. [13] showed that patients with chronic pulmonary artery occlusion without PH had no alteration of RV-PA coupling due to a proportional increase in Ees and Ea; whereas patients with chronic thromboembolic pulmonary hypertension (CTEPH) showed decreased coupling due to a higher increase in Ea, despite Ees was increased compared to controls. Interestingly, results from Tedford et al. [14] suggest that the cause of RV-PA uncoupling observed in patients with systemic sclerosis (Ssc) associated PH is mainly due to a lack of increase in Ees; this highlights the predominant role of lack of RV adaptation to the increased afterload in this disease. Latus et al. [36] showed that dobutamine revealed a decreased coupling reserve in patients with more delay after a Tetralogy of Fallot (TOF) repair using a method without RV out tract (OT) enlargement, compared to patients closer from their repair using RVOT enlargement methods. This study proves that RV Ees/Ea concept derived from multibeat PV-loops is applicable in clinical setting and also provides coherent and comprehensive results in congenital heart diseases evaluation. Vanderpool et al. identified the ratio stroke volume over end-systolic volume as an interesting surrogate of RV-PA coupling determined by single beat MRI imaging

in patients with PH; furthermore they showed this new index to be an independent prognostic factor of survival [23]. It remains to determine whether indices of RV hypertrophy, geometry and tissue lesions could be additional markers of RV adaptation and prognosis. In Table 15.4, we propose a potential sequence of alteration that can occur with the development of RV dysfunction with disease; first with the development of altered coupling and ventricular remodeling and dysfunction only present during exercise, then at rest; a decrease in stroke volume would only be observed at the end stage of the disease again with changes with exercise being present earlier.

The Effects of Therapeutics on RV-PA Coupling in Clinical and Experimental PH

Table 15.5 summarizes some of the key studies focusing on effects of pharmaceutical agents on RV-PA coupling in acute and chronic PH. In the acute setting, inotropic agents restore RV-PA coupling after PA occlusion or constriction [29, 37, 38]; whereas isofurane, desflurane and epoprostenol showed negative effect on Ees in acute PH induced with hypoxia thus leading to decreasing RV-PA coupling [28, 39]. In an acute hypoxia model in pigs, Rex et al. showed that pre-treatment with thoracic epidural anesthesia decreased the RV-PA coupling by reducing Ees elevation [40]. Still in PH induced by acute hypoxia, inhaled NO and sildenafil did not change significantly Ees, Ea and RV-PA coupling [41]. This group of studies suggest that only positive inotropic agents

Table 15.3 RV-PA coupling values in clinical series of patients with precapillary pulmonary hypertension

Study	Pressure acquisition	Volume acquisition	Preload variation	Ea formula	Patient cohort	MPAP (mmHg)	Ees/Ea
McCabe et al. (2013) [13]	Micromanometer	Cond.	Single beat (Pmax)	(ESP-EDP)/SV	Control (n=7), CTED, no-PH (n=7) CTEPH (n=10)	15 17 43	1.46 1.27 0.60
Tedford et al. (2013) [14]	Micromanometer	Cond.	Valsalva maneuvre	ESP/SV	SSc without PH (n=7) SScPAH (n=7) IPAH (n=5)	18 37 49	2.3 1.0 2.1
Latus et al. (2013) [36]	Micromanometer	Cond.	IVC occlusion	ESP/SV	Repaired TOF +17 years (TAP, n=11) Baseline Dobutamine +9 years (TA-TP, n=6) Baseline Dobutamine	– – – –	0.48 0.27 0.62 1.14
Herberg et al. (2013) [55]	Micromanometer	3D echo	Single beat (Pmax)	ESP/SV	CHD (n=10)	28	0.98
Kuehne et al. (2004) [21]	Fluid-filled catheter	MRI	Single beat (Pmax)	(ESP-EDP)/SV	Control (n=6) PHT (n=6)	12 57	1.9 1.1
Sanz et al. (2012) [22]	Fluid-filled catheter	MRI	Single beat (V0)	(MPAP-PCWP)/SV	No-PH (n=27) PH (n=124)	15 42	2.7 0.79

Cond. conductance catheter, *ESP* end-systolic pressure, *EDP* end-diastolic pressure, *SV* stroke volume, *CTED* chronic thrombo-embolic disease, *CTEPH* chronic thrombo-embolic pulmonary hypertension, *Ssc* systemic sclerosis, *PAH* pulmonary arterial hypertension, *PH* pulmonary hypertension, *IPAH* idiopathic PAH, *TOF* tetralogy of Fallot, *CHD* Congenital heart disease, *PHT* pulmonary hypertension, *PH* pulmonary hypertension

Table 15.4 Sequence of alteration of RV-PA coupling, RV morphology, function and stroke volume in patients with pulmonary hypertension

	Early PH	Mild PH	Moderate PH	Severe PH
Ees/Ea rest exercise	N Abnormal	Abnormal More abnormal	Abnormal More abnormal	Abnormal More abnormal
RV size	Normal/up	up	Enlarged	enlarged
RV function Rest Exercise	Normal Abnormal	Abnormal Abnormal	Abnormal Abnormal	Abnormal Abnormal
Stroke volume Rest Exercise	N N/lower	N Lower	N low	Low low

PH pulmonary hypertension, *N* normal

Table 15.5 RV-PA changes with pharmaceutical intervention in different animal models

References	Model	Animal	Drug/procedure	Ees	Ea	Ees/Ea
	Healthy					
Leather et al. (2013) [37]	Healthy animals	Pigs	Levosimendan	↑	↑	↔ (↓ higher dose)
	Acute pulmonary hypertension					
Kerbaul et al. (2004) [38]	Acute PA constriction	Dogs	Norepinephrine	↑	↓	↑
			Dobutamine	↑	↓	↑
Kerbaul et al. (2006) [29]	Acute PA constriction	Dogs	Levosimendan	↑	↓	↑
Kerbaul et al. (2004) [39]	Acute hypoxia	Dogs	Isoflurane	↓	↑	↓
			Desflurane	↓	↑	↓
Fesler et al. (2006) [41]	Acute hypoxia	Dogs	Inhaled NO	↔	↔	↔
			Sildenafil	↔	↔	↔
Rex et al. (2007) [40]	Acute hypoxia	Pigs	Thoracic epidural anesthesia	↓	↔	↓
Rex et al. (2008) [28]	Acute hypoxia	Pigs	Epoprostenol	↓↓	↓	↓
Missant et al. (2007) [53]	Acute pulmonary embolism + RV I/R injury	Pigs	Levosimendan	↑	↓	↑
	Chronic pulmonary hypertension					
Guihaire et al. (2013) [19]	Chronic pulmonary artery occlusion	Pigs	Pulmonary artery reperfusion (chronic effect)	↑	↓	↑
Wauthy et al. (2003) [30]	Chronic systemic to PA shunt	Pigs	Prostacyclin (acute effect)	↓	↓	↔
			Inhaled NO (acute effect)	↓↓	↓	↓
Rondelet et al. (2010) [31]	Chronic systemic to PA shunt	Pigs	Sildenafil + sitaxsentan (chronic effect)	↓	↓	↔
			Sitaxsentan (chronic effect)	↓↓	↓↓	↔
Rondelet et al. (2003) [42]	Chronic systemic to PA shunt	Pigs	Bosentan (chronic effect)	↑	↓↓	↑
De Man et al. (2012) [34]	Monocrotalin	Rats	Bisoprolol (chronic effect)	↑	↔	↑
	Heart failure induced pulmonary hypertension					
Pagnamenta et al. (2010) [54]	Chronic pacing	Dogs	iNO (acute effect)	↔	↔	↔
			Nitroprusside (acute effect)	↔	↔	↔
			Milrinone (acute effect)	↑	↔	↑

are able to improve the RV-PA coupling in acute PH; conversely agents targeting the pulmonary circulation or decreasing the sympathetic response do not improve or even rather decrease the RV-PA coupling in this setting.

Concerning chronic effects of therapeutics, bosentan improves RV-PA coupling in a model of chronic systemic to PA shunt [42] by decreasing RV afterload and increasing RV contractility. Conversely, in a similar model, sitaxsentan and its association with sildenafil did not improve RV-PA coupling due to both decrease in Ees and Ea [31]. Interestingly, De Man et al. showed betablockade with bisoprolol to improve RV-PA coupling in a rodent model of PH induced with monocrotaline [34]. This suggests that beta blockade therapy may have different acute versus chronic effects. In the field of chronic pulmonary artery occlusion, Guihaire et al. showed improvement of RV-PA coupling 6 weeks after surgical pulmonary artery reperfusion [43].

Perspectives

RV-PA coupling is a physiological concept that helps us to better understands systolic ventricular adaptation and represents a metric that combines measures of contractility and afterload. Consequently, RV-PA coupling is a major component of the phenotype of patients with pulmonary hypertension. We showed in this chapter that RV-PA coupling is used to quantify acute or chronic adaptation of the right ventricle in different settings including in different animal models, in different PH etiologies, and with different therapeutics. Further studies focusing on quantifying the right ventricular reserve could provide even more insights into RV pathophysiology and dysfunction stratification. Common measures that we use in practice such as RVEF, TAPSE or strain are variables related to RV-PA coupling and not measures of contractility as shown by Guihaire et al. [19]. If we consider RV chronic adaptation into stages, we can propose based on recent studies a sequence of changes in coupling that occurs at these different stages (Table 15.4). Interestingly, objective RV-PA coupling evaluation can help to provide a precise phenotyping corresponding to genetic program changes induced by chronic load variations.

Moving forward, we foresee two developments in the field of RV-PA coupling. First, PV-loop measures will likely continue to play a role in experimental studies especially when testing new medications. Multimodality imaging approaches combined heart catheterization and magnetic resonance imaging is also likely to offer more precise quantification. In clinical practice, the focus is on identifying the best marker of ventricular adaptation either by novel surrogates of RV-PA coupling [23] or by combining different prognostic indices such as RV strain and atrial dimension. Evaluation of stress imaging in PH is also likely to provide good surrogate for RV-PA coupling and will likely allow better determination of patients with moderate disease.

Some Comments of Diastolic Coupling

The common measures of RV-PA coupling mainly focus on systolic function and adaptation and diastolic function is usually not studied. There is an important difference to be made between the concepts of coupling versus adaptation. Coupling refers to matching of physiologically characteristics that allow more optimal function; whereas adaptation refers to the sum of mechanisms recruited to obtain a coupling state. This is why coupling may quantify adaptation or

maladaptation. With regards to diastolic function, it is clear that PH is associated with changes of both active relaxation constant and passive stiffness secondary to changes in pressure regimen, ventricular thickness to molecular changes in cardiomyocyte contractile apparatus, to increased ventricular hypertrophy and development of interstitial fibrosis [44, 45]. In terms of coupling, a metric describing optimal loading for function has not been clearly developed in the hemodynamic domain. In the energetic domain, Chemla et al. showed that increased right atrial pressure was associated with increased pulsatile component of RV stroke work [46], but a link between right atrial pressure and RV diastolic dysfunction has not been established. Also increased right atrial pressure and dilation were shown to be independent prognosis markers in patients with PH [47], and pulmonary artery stiffness was shown to be a major determinant of RV dysfunction in patients with PH [48] as well as an independent prognosis factor [49, 50]. Concepts such as RV stiffness quantified with PV-loops as beta (β), which represents the curvature of the end-diastolic pressure-volume relationship (EDPVR), should be quantified independently from contractility state because linear relationship between Ees and β has been shown in animal studies [51]. It is not yet determined whether a RV diastolic dysfunction may be independent from RV systolic dysfunction. Future studies should determine methods to better quantify the adaptation of RV diastolic function and right atrium remodeling in response to pulmonary arterial and ventricular changes.

Conclusion

In this chapter, we reviewed how the concept of RV-PA coupling helps understanding of the pathophysiology of RV adaptation in PH and is one of the major determinants of the phenotype of patients with PH. In the next years, much effort will be given to validating simple indices of RV-PA coupling in PH. Moreover, RV-PA coupling or its surrogate could become an integral part of new medication evaluation.

References

1. Melot C, Naeije R. Pulmonary vascular diseases. Compr Physiol. 2011;1(2):593–619.
2. Swift AJ, et al. Prognostic value of cardiovascular magnetic resonance imaging measurements corrected for age and sex in idiopathic pulmonary arterial hypertension. Circ Cardiovasc Imaging. 2014;7(1):100–6.
3. Peacock AJ, et al. Changes in right ventricular function measured by cardiac magnetic resonance imaging in patients receiving pulmonary arterial hypertension-targeted therapy: the EURO-MR study. Circ Cardiovasc Imaging. 2014;7(1):107–14.
4. Vonk-Noordegraaf A, et al. Right heart adaptation to pulmonary arterial hypertension: physiology and pathobiology. J Am Coll Cardiol. 2013;62(25 Suppl):027.

5. Suga H, Sagawa K, Shoukas AA. Load independence of the instantaneous pressure-volume ratio of the canine left ventricle and effects of epinephrine and heart rate on the ratio. Circ Res. 1973;32(3):314–22.

6. Wallace A, Lam HW, Mangano DT. Linearity, load dependence, hysteresis, and clinical associations of systolic and diastolic indices of left ventricular function in man. Multicenter Study of Perioperative Ischemia (McSPI) Research Group. J Card Surg. 1995;10(4 Suppl):460–7.

7. Kass DA, et al. Determination of left ventricular end-systolic pressure-volume relationships by the conductance (volume) catheter technique. Circulation. 1986;73(3):586–95.

8. Kelly RP, et al. Effective arterial elastance as index of arterial vascular load in humans. Circulation. 1992;86(2):513–21.

9. Sunagawa K, Sagawa K, Maughan WL. Ventricular interaction with the loading system. Ann Biomed Eng. 1984;12(2):163–89.

10. Naeije R, Manes A. The right ventricle in pulmonary arterial hypertension. Eur Respir Rev. 2014;23(134):476–87.

11. Kono A, et al. The use of left ventricular end-ejection pressure and peak pressure in the estimation of the end-systolic pressure-volume relationship. Circulation. 1984;70(6):1057–65.

12. Dell'Italia LJ, Walsh RA. Application of a time varying elastance model to right ventricular performance in man. Cardiovasc Res. 1988;22(12):864–74.

13. McCabe C, et al. Right ventricular dysfunction in chronic thromboembolic obstruction of the pulmonary artery: a pressure-volume study using the conductance catheter. J Appl Physiol. 1985;116(4):355–63.

14. Tedford RJ, et al. Right ventricular dysfunction in systemic sclerosis-associated pulmonary arterial hypertension. Circ Heart Fail. 2013;6(5):953–63.

15. Maughan WL, et al. Instantaneous pressure-volume relationship of the canine right ventricle. Circ Res. 1979;44(3):309–15.

16. Karunanithi MK, et al. Right ventricular preload recruitable stroke work, end-systolic pressure-volume, and dP/dtmax-end-diastolic volume relations compared as indexes of right ventricular contractile performance in conscious dogs. Circ Res. 1992;70(6):1169–79.

17. Brown KA, Ditchey RV. Human right ventricular end-systolic pressure-volume relation defined by maximal elastance. Circulation. 1988;78(1):81–91.

18. Vanderpool RR, et al. RV-pulmonary arterial coupling predicts outcome in patients referred for pulmonary hypertension. Heart. 2015;101(1):37–43.

19. Guihaire J, et al. Non-invasive indices of right ventricular function are markers of ventricular-arterial coupling rather than ventricular contractility: insights from a porcine model of chronic pressure overload. Eur Heart J Cardiovasc Imaging. 2013;14(12):1140–9.

20. Vogel M, et al. Validation of myocardial acceleration during isovolumic contraction as a novel noninvasive index of right ventricular contractility: comparison with ventricular pressure-volume relations in an animal model. Circulation. 2002;105(14):1693–9.

21. Kuehne T, et al. Magnetic resonance imaging analysis of right ventricular pressure-volume loops: in vivo validation and clinical application in patients with pulmonary hypertension. Circulation. 2004;110(14):2010–6.

22. Sanz J, et al. Right ventriculo-arterial coupling in pulmonary hypertension: a magnetic resonance study. Heart. 2012;98(3):238–43.

23. Vanderpool RR, et al. RV-pulmonary arterial coupling predicts outcome in patients referred for pulmonary hypertension. Heart. 2014;11(306142):2014–306142.

24. Baan J, et al. Continuous measurement of left ventricular volume in animals and humans by conductance catheter. Circulation. 1984;70(5):812–23.

25. Bellofiore A, Chesler NC. Methods for measuring right ventricular function and hemodynamic coupling with the pulmonary vasculature. Ann Biomed Eng. 2013;41(7):1384–98.

26. Trip P, et al. Accurate assessment of load-independent right ventricular systolic function in patients with pulmonary hypertension. J Heart Lung Transplant. 2013;32(1):50–5.

27. Wauthy P, et al. Right ventricular adaptation to pulmonary hypertension: an interspecies comparison. Am J Physiol Heart Circ Physiol. 2004;286(4):18.

28. Rex S, et al. Epoprostenol treatment of acute pulmonary hypertension is associated with a paradoxical decrease in right ventricular contractility. Intensive Care Med. 2008;34(1):179–89.

29. Kerbaul F, et al. Effects of levosimendan versus dobutamine on pressure load-induced right ventricular failure. Crit Care Med. 2006;34(11):2814–9.

30. Wauthy P, et al. Inhaled nitric oxide versus prostacyclin in chronic shunt-induced pulmonary hypertension. J Thorac Cardiovasc Surg. 2003;126(5):1434–41.

31. Rondelet B, et al. Sildenafil added to sitaxsentan in overcirculation-induced pulmonary arterial hypertension. Am J Physiol Heart Circ Physiol. 2010;299(4):6.

32. Lambert V, et al. Right ventricular failure secondary to chronic overload in congenital heart disease: an experimental model for therapeutic innovation. J Thorac Cardiovasc Surg. 2010;139(5):1197–204.

33. Wang Z, et al. Progressive right ventricular functional and structural changes in a mouse model of pulmonary arterial hypertension. Physiol Rep. 2013;1(7):1.

34. de Man FS, et al. Bisoprolol delays progression towards right heart failure in experimental pulmonary hypertension. Circ Heart Fail. 2012;5(1):97–105.

35. Rungatscher A, et al. Chronic overcirculation-induced pulmonary arterial hypertension in aorto-caval shunt. Microvasc Res. 2014;94:73–9.

36. Latus H, et al. Right ventricular-pulmonary arterial coupling in patients after repair of tetralogy of Fallot. J Thorac Cardiovasc Surg. 2013;146(6):1366–72.

37. Leather HA, et al. Effects of levosimendan on right ventricular function and ventriculovascular coupling in open chest pigs. Crit Care Med. 2003;31(9):2339–43.

38. Kerbaul F, et al. Effects of norepinephrine and dobutamine on pressure load-induced right ventricular failure. Crit Care Med. 2004;32(4):1035–40.

39. Kerbaul F, et al. Isoflurane and desflurane impair right ventricular-pulmonary arterial coupling in dogs. Anesthesiology. 2004;101(6): 1357–62.

40. Rex S, et al. Thoracic epidural anesthesia impairs the hemodynamic response to acute pulmonary hypertension by deteriorating right ventricular-pulmonary arterial coupling. Crit Care Med. 2007;35(1):222–9.

41. Fesler P, et al. Effects of sildenafil on hypoxic pulmonary vascular function in dogs. J Appl Physiol. 1985;101(4):1085–90.

42. Rondelet B, et al. Bosentan for the prevention of overcirculation-induced experimental pulmonary arterial hypertension. Circulation. 2003;107(9):1329–35.

43. Guihaire J, et al. Right ventricular plasticity in a porcine model of chronic pressure overload. J Heart Lung Transplant. 2014;33(2): 194–202.

44. Rain S, et al. Right ventricular diastolic impairment in patients with pulmonary arterial hypertension. Circulation. 2013;128(18):2016–25.

45. Rain S, et al. Protein changes contributing to right ventricular cardiomyocyte diastolic dysfunction in pulmonary arterial hypertension. J Am Heart Assoc. 2014;3(3):000716.

46. Chemla D, et al. Estimating right ventricular stroke work and the pulsatile work fraction in pulmonary hypertension. Chest. 2013;143(5):1343–50.

47. Austin C, et al. Echocardiographic assessment of estimated right atrial pressure and size predicts mortality in pulmonary arterial hypertension. Chest. 2014;11(10):13–3035.

48. Stevens GR, et al. RV dysfunction in pulmonary hypertension is independently related to pulmonary artery stiffness. JACC Cardiovasc Imaging. 2012;5(4):378–87.

49. Mahapatra S, et al. The prognostic value of pulmonary vascular capacitance determined by Doppler echocardiography in patients with pulmonary arterial hypertension. J Am Soc Echocardiogr. 2006;19(8):1045–50.

50. Mahapatra S, et al. Relationship of pulmonary arterial capacitance and mortality in idiopathic pulmonary arterial hypertension. J Am Coll Cardiol. 2006;47(4):799–803.

51. Chemaly ER, et al. Stroke volume-to-wall stress ratio as a load-adjusted and stiffness-adjusted indicator of ventricular systolic performance in chronic loading. J Appl Physiol. 1985;113(8):1267–84.

52. Lambermont B, et al. Effect of a novel thromboxane A2 inhibitor on right ventricular-arterial coupling in endotoxic shock. Shock. 2004;21(1):45–51.

53. Missant C, et al. Levosimendan improves right ventriculovascular coupling in a porcine model of right ventricular dysfunction. Crit Care Med. 2007;35(3):707–15.

54. Pagnamenta A, et al. Early right ventriculo-arterial uncoupling in borderline pulmonary hypertension on experimental heart failure. J Appl Physiol. 1985;109(4):1080–5.

55. Herberg U, et al. Ventricular pressure-volume loops obtained by 3D real-time echocardiography and mini pressure wire-a feasibility study. Clin Res Cardiol. 2013;102(6):427–38.

Contemporary Pharmacotherapies Involving Nitric Oxide, Prostacyclin, and Endothelin Receptor Signaling Pathways

16

Nicholas M. Furiasse and Jonathan D. Rich

Abbreviations

6MWD	Six Minute Walk Distance
BID	Dosing Twice Daily
BNP	Brain Natriuretic Peptide
cGMP	Cyclic guanosine monophosphate
CI	Cardiac Index
CTEPH	Chronic Thromboembolic Pulmonary Hypertension
ERA	Endothelin Receptor Antagonist
ET-1	Endothelin-1
ET_A	Endothelin Receptor A
ET_B	Endothelin Receptor B
FC	Functional Class
FDA	Food and Drug Administration
IPAH	Idiopathic Pulmonary Arterial Hypertension
IV	Intravenous
LFT	Liver Function Tests
Mg	Milligrams
NIH	National Institutes of Health
NO	Nitric Oxide
NT-BNP	N-Terminal Brain Natriuretic Peptide
PAH	Pulmonary Arterial Hypertension
PDE-5 Inhibitor	Phosphodiesterase Type 5 Inhibitor
PGI_2	Prostacyclin I2
PO	Oral or By Mouth
PSMCs	Pulmonary Smooth Muscle Cells
PVR	Pulmonary Vascular Resistance
RV	Right Ventricle
SC or SQ	Subcutaneous
TGF-β	Transforming Growth Factor Beta
TID	Dosing Three Times Daily

N.M. Furiasse, MD, MS • J.D. Rich, MD (✉)
Division of Cardiology, Department of Medicine, Northwestern University Feinberg School of Medicine, 676 N. St. Clair, Suite 600, Chicago, IL 60611, USA
e-mail: jonathan.rich@northwestern.edu

Introduction

Pulmonary arterial hypertension (PAH) is a progressive disorder characterized by extensive pulmonary vascular remodeling resulting in an increase in pulmonary vascular resistance, progressive right ventricular (RV) dysfunction, and an untimely death. Over the past two decades, with an improved understanding of PAH pathobiology and the development of a multitude of medical therapies, prognosis has improved, although annual mortality despite targeted PAH therapy is estimated at 15 % per year for idiopathic PAH [1]. In this chapter, we will provide a brief overview of the pathways and pathophysiologic processes implicated in PAH with a major focus on contemporary pharmacotherapies that target the prostacyclin, endothelin, and nitric oxide pathways.

Pathobiology of Pulmonary Arterial Hypertension: Fig. 16.1

Although the exact mechanisms that leads to the development and progression of idiopathic PAH remain largely elusive, there are histologic features of the disease that are common in most cases of chronic PAH [2]. Environmental factors acting through genetic mediators likely precipitate varying degrees of vasoconstriction, vascular and cellular proliferation, thrombosis, and chronic inflammation which indicate pathologic remodeling [3, 4]. The pulmonary arterial vascular system is normally a high-output circulation with low pressure and low resistance. The high vascular compliance of the pulmonary vasculature leads to a small increase in pulmonary artery pressure with increases in cardiac output that occur with exercise. Regulation of vascular tone is mediated by intracellular calcium which is influenced by adrenergic factors, calcium-dependent potassium channels, and local environmental factors (i.e. hypoxia) [5]. While fewer than 15 % of PAH patients are acutely responsive to vasodilator therapy, inappropriate pulmonary

© Springer International Publishing Switzerland 2016
B.A. Maron et al. (eds.), *Pulmonary Hypertension: Basic Science to Clinical Medicine*, DOI 10.1007/978-3-319-23594-3_16

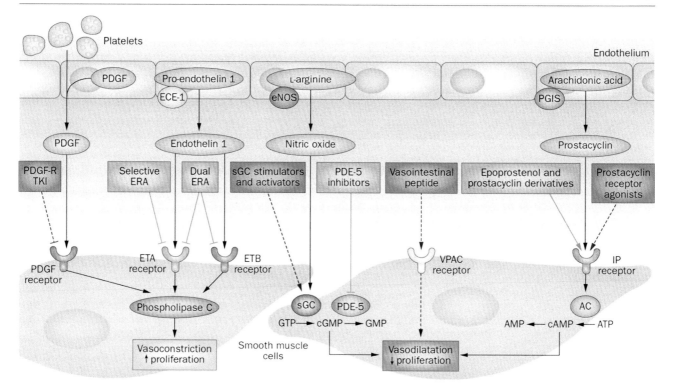

Fig. 16.1 Pulmonary artery smooth muscle cell therapeutic targets and corresponding licensed (*green boxes*) and investigational (*red boxes*) treatment approaches for pulmonary arterial hypertension. Arrows represent receptor stimulation, whereas terminated lines show receptor blockade. *Abbreviations*: *AC* adenylate cyclase, *cAMP* cyclic AMP, *cGMP* cyclic GMP, *ECE-1* endothelin converting enzyme 1, *eNOS* endothelial nitric oxide synthase, *ETA* endothelin receptor type A, *ETB* endothelin receptor type B, *ERA* endothelin receptor antagonists, *IP* prostaglandin I2, *PDE-5* phosphodiesterase type 5, *PDGF* platelet derived growth factor, *PDGF-R TKI* PDGF receptor tyrosine kinase inhibitors, *PGIS* prostaglandin I synthase, *sGC* soluble guanylate cyclase, *VPAC* vasointestinal peptide receptor (This figure is reproduced with permission from O'Callaghan et al. [115])

vasoconstriction likely contributes to PAH pathophysiology to some extent [6].

The remodeling process in PAH is marked by dysregulation of cellular proliferation, apoptosis, and angiogenesis, with some similarities to the pathologic findings in certain malignancies [7, 8]. A series of growth factors and cytokines trigger intracellular signaling pathways that alter nuclear protein expression and ultimately lead to a constitutive growth process [9–11]. PAH is a vasculitic disorder that is also notable for intraluminal thrombosis of the medium to small pulmonary arteries as noted on histologic examination [12]. Thrombin, in the setting of stressors and ongoing inflammation, appears to be a central mediator in the propagation of thrombosis [13]. Thrombin activation also leads to mitogenic and angiogenic effects in addition to direct platelet activation, potentiating the coagulation cascade [12–14].

Endothelial cells act as a central mediator in the regulation of pulmonary vascular tone through vasoactive substances, which ultimately alter pulmonary smooth muscle cells (PSMCs) [15]. In the setting of continuous or excessive activation, PSMCs demonstrate pathologic and eventually irreversible growth, proliferation, and contraction [3, 16, 17]. Prostacyclin (prostaglandin I2, PGI$_2$), through the activation

of cyclic guanosine monophosphate (cGMP) pathways, promotes vasodilation while inhibiting PSMC proliferation and platelet aggregation [15, 18]. This endogenous, potent vasodilator is decreased in idiopathic PAH patients, a finding supported by decreased expression of prostacyclin synthase and stable metabolites of PGI$_2$ noted in the endothelial cells [19, 20]. Nitric oxide (NO) is also an important mediator of vasodilation by raising cGMP intracellularly [21]. NO release occurs predominantly via the endothelial cells acting in a paracrine manner on the adjacent PSMCs [21, 22]. However, the extent of NO availability is complex with shear stress, thrombin formation, vascular injury, and toxins all mediating NO release and metabolism [23–25]. Endothelin-1 (ET-1), secreted by vascular endothelial cells, acts on endothelin receptor A (ET$_A$) and B (ET$_B$) in PSMCs to further trigger vasoconstriction and cellular proliferation [18, 26]. Additionally, the regulation of intracellular calcium through a variety of triggers and mechanisms involving local kinases and phosphatases regulates vascular tone and remodeling potential [3, 27].

Pulmonary vascular inflammation may occur in response to physical, immune, toxic, or infectious injury that initiates the recruitment of inflammatory cells. These inflammatory cells act as central propagators through immune-mediated mechanisms in an effort to resolve the perceived injury [28, 29]. Chronic inflammation appears central to the maladaptive remodeling in PAH, which is, in part, directed by the dysregulation of the immune response [30]. As mentioned above, a host of inflammatory cytokines/chemokines and growth factors can induce the proliferation and migration of endothelial and PSMCs [31, 32]. Thus, it is not entirely surprising that higher levels of inflammatory mediators have been associated with worse outcomes in PAH patients [33–37].

Central to the pathobiologic changes in PAH is a genetic predisposition to vascular and cellular injury leading to the cascade of events discussed above. Over the past two decades, the development of next-generation sequencing techniques, genome-wide association studies, carefully designed familial studies, and longitudinal data from registries have enhanced the understanding of the hereditary components of PAH [38]. As genomic research continues in the field of PAH, there will be a continued effort to define the genomics, metabolomics, and proteomics for a more robust genetic description of the disease process and predisposition to pathologic changes [39, 40]. For instance, genetic linkage analyses of patients with a known family history of PAH have elucidated the importance of the transforming growth factor beta (TGF-β) receptor and downstream signaling pathways in the pathobiologic processes [41]. Overall, the continued investigation of possible infectious, inflammatory, hypoxic, and toxic environmental triggers on a background of various genetic and genomic underpinnings will further our understanding of the complexities of PAH pathobiology and lead to additional, novel therapeutic targets.

Therapeutic Targets

Prostacyclins (Table 16.1)

Among the pathways disrupted in the pathobiology of PAH is the prostacyclin pathway leading to a relative deficiency of endogenous prostacyclin synthesis. Prostacyclins and prostacyclin analogues (prostanoids) primarily target the prostaglandin I receptor activating adenylate cyclase activity, which results in potent pulmonary (but also systemic) vasodilation, inhibition of platelet aggregation, and a blunting of certain inflammatory responses that would otherwise trigger endothelial and smooth muscle cell proliferation [15, 42, 43]. Over the past two decades, prostacyclin, the first approved therapy for PAH, has maintained its role as a cornerstone of therapy in patients with progressive PAH. The evolution of prostacyclin therapies since the original approval of intravenous epoprostenol includes the development and approval of alternative intravenous, subcutaneous, inhaled,

and oral formulations. We will review the various prostacyclin therapies with a focus on landmark clinical trials, important pharmaceutical properties, and an approach to dosing while monitoring for adverse effects and toxicity.

Parenteral Therapies: Intravenous and Subcutaneous

Intravenous Epoprostenol (Flolan™)

Epoprostenol is the intravenous formulation of prostacyclin I2 (PGI$_2$), a synthetic, stabilized compound initially approved by the FDA in 1995 for idiopathic PAH. As such, the most robust longitudinal and mortality data are available for this compound. Following a number of encouraging, smaller clinical trials of prostacyclin therapy in PAH [44–47], a pivotal, 12-week, prospective, placebo-controlled randomized trial evaluating hemodynamics, functional capacity, quality of life, and survival in 81 patients with New York Heart Association functional class (FC) III or IV idiopathic PAH (IPAH) (previously known as primary pulmonary hypertension) was performed. Patients receiving epoprostenol demonstrated significant improvements in pulmonary vascular resistance, pulmonary artery pressure, and cardiac index with marginal effects on mean systemic arterial pressure. Additionally, 6-min walk distance (6MWD) and quality of life scores improved in the epoprostenol-treated participants compared to the placebo group, with the placebo patients experiencing a worsening of quality of life and 6MWD. There were no deaths in the epoprostenol group compared to eight deaths in the placebo arm [47]. Subsequent to this trial in IPAH, similar hemodynamic and functional improvements were observed in scleroderma-related PAH treated with IV epoprostenol over a 12-week period but with similar survival rates in the IV epoprostenol group compared to the conventional therapy group [48].

Since the completion of the key epoprostenol PAH clinical trials, three additional, observational studies have compared survival in those treated with epoprostenol to historical controls from the original US National Institutes of Health registry of PAH [49, 50]. In the first study, Shapiro and colleagues prospectively followed 69 patients with FC III and IV idiopathic PAH at a single center and observed an improved survival at 1, 2, and 3 years respectively as compared to historical controls [51]. Those subjects followed for more than 1 year had additional improvements in non-invasively assessed pulmonary vascular resistance (PVR) indices, suggesting a long-term hemodynamic benefit of the therapy [51]. Similarly, a survival benefit from epoprostenol was observed by McLaughlin and colleagues in 162 patients PAH with functional class III or IV treated at a single center. With a median follow up of 31 months, a substantial survival benefit was observed in those on epoprostenol therapy at 1 year, 2 years, 3 years, and 5 years, respectively. Long-term improvements

Table 16.1 Pharmacologic and clinical points for prostacyclins in the treatment of PAH

Prostacyclin agent	Mechanism of action	Administration route(s)	Suggested dosing	Relative & absolute contraindications	Monitoring & side effects
Epoprostenol (Flolan™)	Prostaglandin I2 (PGI₂), Prostacyclin analogue Pulmonary and systemic vasodilation Inhibition of platelet aggregation Anti-proliferative properties	Intravenous via continuous pump delivery	**Initiation**: 1–2 ng/kg/min **Titration**: 1–2 ng/kg/min daily while in the hospital for 3–5 days; weekly as outpatient **Chronic**: Average dose 30–50 ng/kg/min at 1 year	Avoid abrupt discontinuation which may lead to acute rebound pulmonary hypertension and cardiogenic shock Inability to reliably manage an indwelling catheter and pump delivery system	**Catheter-related**: Sepsis, thrombosis **Drug-related**: Hypotension, nausea, vomiting, jaw pain, headache, flushing
Treprostinil (Remodulin™) (Tyvaso™) (Orenitram™)	Tricyclic benzidine analog of epoprostenol	Intravenous, Subcutaneous, Inhaled, Oral	*SQ*: **Initiation**: 2 ng/kg/min **Titration**: 2 ng/kg/min 1–2 per week as outpatient **Chronic**: Average dose 2–3× epoprostenol (i.e. 60–80 ng/kg/min) *Inhaled*: 3 breaths (18 mcg) 4 times per day; goal 9 breaths (54 mcg) per session (4 times daily); increase by 3 breaths per session every 1–2 weeks *Oral*: 0.25 mg BID; increase by 0.25 mg per dose every 3–4 days; average dose 4.2 mg BID at 1 year	IV treprostnil: See epoprostenol Oral treprostinil contraindicated in severe hepatic impairment (Child-Pugh Class C or greater)	See epoprostenol Intravenous treprostinil associated with increased risk of gram-negative bacteremia Severe site pain associated with SC Cough and throat irritation with inhaled PO administration less risk of systemic effects but frequent GI upset including nausea and diarrhea
Iloprost (Ventavis™)	Stable prostacyclin analog	Inhaled, Intravenous	*Inhaled*: 2.5 mg per inhalation 6–9 times per day; titrate to goal 5 mg per dose at least 6 times per day; do not exceed 70 mg daily	See epoprostenol Monitor closely with advanced hepatic or renal disease	See epoprostenol Additional risk of cough and throat irritation with inhalation

Abbreviations: *PGI2* prostaglandin I2, *2–3×* two to three times, *ng* nanogram, *kg* kilogram, *min* minute, *mcg* micrograms, *mg* milligrams, *BID* Twice Daily Dosing, *PO* Administration by Mouth, SC Subcutaneous, GI gastrointestinal

in symptoms and invasively measured hemodynamic parameters were demonstrated as well [52]. Around the same time, Sitbon and colleagues reported similar findings of improved symptoms, hemodynamics and survival at 1, 2, 3, and 5 years, respectively, in a French PAH cohort [53].

Pharmacologic Features and Clinical Considerations

The chemical and pharmacokinetic properties of IV epoprostenol necessitate the intricate delivery system for the drug. Epoprostenol is prepared in sterile, freeze-dried powder which requires cool storage recommended at 15 to 20 °C. The half-life of the drug is 6 min as the drug is rapidly degraded in the blood and ultimately renally excreted. Therefore, the

drug must be delivered via continuous infusion with a central catheter via a positive pressure pump (Fig. 16.2); abrupt discontinuation of therapy may lead to cardiovascular collapse and death [54]. In the hospital setting in the treatment naïve patient, epoprostenol is typically initiated via a peripherally inserted central catheter or central line. As the transition to outpatient care occurs, the placement a durable, tunneled central venous catheter is strongly advised. Additionally, the intravenous pump is converted to a battery operated portable pump (Fig. 16.2). Veletri™, a generic formulation of epoprostenol (Flolan™), is stable at room temperature and gained FDA approval in 2012. This L-arginine formulation purportedly provides a more thermally stable preparation

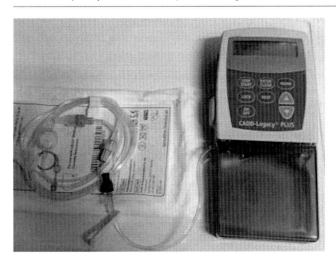

Fig. 16.2 Pictured is an actual portable, battery-powered infusion pump into which a drug cassette of epoprostenol is inserted. This set-up allows for the self-administration of a continuous infusion of prostacyclin therapy via a single lumen central venous catheter (often a Hickman catheter) (This figure is reproduced with permission from Cheryl Switzer @ PHCentral.org http://www.phcentral.org/medical/flolan-resource-page (Accessed January 2015))

with an administration time of up to 7 days after mixing the drug without a compromise in potency [55, 56].

The continuous nature of the drug infusion via central venous access, the associated equipment, and the required meticulous care can be a substantial barrier for some patients. Extensive education is required with documented competency in pump management (including alarms), sterile technique, medication preparation and storage, and awareness of pump or catheter related complications (including sepsis and thrombosis) [57]. As such, the administration and longitudinal follow up care for patients on parenteral therapy including epoprostenol should be coordinated by an experienced integrated health center expert in the management of PAH.

Dosing Recommendations and Adverse Events

Given the variability and relatively short follow-up duration in clinical trials, dosing recommendations for the long-term use of epoprostenol therapy comes from empiric clinical experience. Traditionally, epoprostenol has been initiated at a dose of 2 ng/kg/min and titrated daily to a dose that results in the initial optimization of PAH symptoms and hemodynamics while limiting side effects. In the pivotal trial by Barst and colleagues, a mean dose of 9 ng/kg/min was achieved at 8 weeks [47]. In the later studies by McLaughlin et al. and Sitbon et al., mean doses of approximately 22–27 ng/kg/min and 14 ng/kg/min respectively at 12 weeks were achieved [52, 53, 58]. Recently, McLaughlin and Palevsky provided a contemporary dosing recommendation for the initiation and dose escalation for intravenous epoprostenol therapy targeting an eventual average dose of 35–50 ng/kg/min at 1 year [57].

The off-target effect profiles are similar for all forms of prostacyclin therapies with a few exceptions. With the slow initiation of therapy, systemic vasodilation due to epoprostenol may induce a modest decrease in systemic blood pressure in addition to common side effects including flushing, headache, diarrhea, and a specific jaw discomfort that occurs with the initial mastication during a meal [52, 53]. In overdose states, patients may report extreme side effects with a predominance of diarrhea and flushing and invasive hemodynamic monitoring may even demonstrate a high cardiac output state [58]. However, many of these side effects will abate as a steady state dose is achieved and the drug is used chronically. In addition, there are potential adverse events associated with the intravenous delivery system. As with any catheter-based system, the patient and physician must remain vigilant in the monitoring of thrombotic complications and perhaps more commonly, local or systemic infections [57].

Subcutaneous and Intravenous Treprostinil (Remodulin™)

Treprostinil was the second prostacyclin therapy approved by the FDA in 2002, initially via the subcutaneous route. The subcutaneous delivery of treprostinil provided an alternative, parenteral route of prostanoid delivery given some of the limitations related to intravenous therapy. The main clinical data examining the safety and efficacy of subcutaneous treprostinil comes from a single placebo-controlled trial and a subsequent observational study. Simonneau and colleagues conducted a 12 week, multinational, double-blinded trial in four-hundred and seventy patients with PAH. The primary endpoint of 6MWD improved significantly in those treated with SC treprostinil and secondary outcomes of dyspnea scores and hemodynamic parameters also improved [59]. This study was followed by an observational study of eight-hundred sixty patients by Barst and colleagues, providing longer term follow-up data on safety and survival. Participants were followed for up to 4 years with Kaplan-Meier derived survival estimates compared to the NIH predicted mortality and suggested possible improved survival on therapy [60]. Following the approval of SC epoprostenol, the safety and efficacy of IV treprostinil was demonstrated in a prospective, open-label, 12-week trial of 16 patients with mixed etiologies of PAH (8 with idiopathic) in whom improvements in 6MWD, dyspnea scores, and hemodynamics were observed [61].

Pharmacologic Features and Clinical Considerations

The longer half-life, thermal stability at room temperature, and avoidance of a central catheter delivery system were all leveraged when developing the subcutaneous formulation. Treprostinil is a thermally stable tricyclic benzene analog of prostacyclin with peak plasma concentrations of the drug occurring within 2 to 3 h of subcutaneous delivery [62, 63].

Treprostinil also has a longer half-life of approximately 4.5 h as compared to epoprostenol. The longer half-life may mitigate the risk of cardiovascular collapse that may be seen with the acute discontinuation of epoprostenol [64, 65]. Similar to the intravenous formulations of prostacyclin therapies, the subcutaneous delivery is via a positive pressure infusion pump but with a self-inserted catheter. The initiation of subcutaneous treprostinil can be performed in the inpatient or outpatient setting with close monitoring. The initial FDA approved dose is recommended at 1.25 ng/kg/min, however there is clinical data suggesting the safety of a 2.5 ng/kg/min initial dose with rapid escalation upon demonstrating improved clinical and hemodynamic endpoints compared to a slower escalation strategy beginning at a dose of 2 ng/kg/min. When studied, those participants in the rapid titration group had a higher average dose of approximately 20 ng/kg/min at 12 weeks [59]. Particular attention to early pump and site complications should be noted by the patient and alert the care team as soon as possible [54]. Contrary to other subcutaneously-based therapies, a specific infusion pump site is not required for appropriate absorption: the abdomen is the preferred site although the buttock, flank, thigh, and upper arm are potential alternative sites. Although rotation of the administration site is recommended to occur at three day intervals, patients will often administer the drug at the same site for up to 30 days and typically rotate the site every 2–4 weeks without obvious detrimental effects. Additionally, the transition from SC to IV treprostinil (and vice versa) can be generally done safely without deterioration in clinical status as long as it is performed in an appropriate clinical setting and under expert supervision [66, 67].

Dosing Recommendations and Adverse Events

As with IV epoprostenol, IV treprostinil is typically initiated in the hospital setting at an initial dose of 2 ng/kg/min with incremental increases of 2 ng/kg/min titrated to hemodynamic and clinical endpoints and limited by tolerability. The ultimate, average dose of treprostinil achieved will typically be about two to three-times the dose of epoprostenol [61, 63]. The side effects of IV and SC treprostinil are similar to that of epoprostenol including flushing, headache, diarrhea, and jaw discomfort [54, 59, 60]. With SC treprostinil, perhaps the most limiting side effect is severe site pain, which may occur in up to 85 % of patients. Rarely, abscess formation may occur at the infusion site requiring local drainage and systemic antibiotics. With IV treprostinil, patients may be at higher risk of bacteremia, particularly gram negative rod sepsis as compared to IV epoprostenol. The concern of gram-negative systemic infections were noted in an examination of the REVEAL registry (Registry to Evaluate Early and Long Term PAH Disease Management) that demonstrated a rate of 0.36 vs. 0.12 per 1000 treatment days compared to epoprostenol therapy. A subsequent multivariate

analysis of the data adjusting for potential confounders reported an approximately 3- and 6-fold increase in the risk of bloodstream infections and gram-negative infections respectively with IV treprostinil when compared to epoprostenol [68]. Interestingly, a subsequent study demonstrated that the increased risk of gram negative bacteremia may be attenuated when epoprostenol diluent is used with IV treprostinil administration, perhaps best explained by differences in the pH between the respective diluents [69].

Inhaled Prostanoids: Iloprost (Ventavis™), Treprostinil (Tyvaso™)

The next iteration of available prostacyclin therapy moved from the pump and catheter based therapies that require continuous administration to an inhaled delivery system with frequent dosing. As with prostanoids in general, the inhaled prostacyclins induce pulmonary vascular dilation and inhibit platelet aggregation and cell proliferation [70, 71]. At their inception, inhaled prostanoids possessed some attractive theoretical characteristics that included the direct inhalation of drug directly into the alveoli and subsequently into the pulmonary capillaries. Additionally, the inhaled route avoids the need for central venous access or painful subcutaneous injections. Unfortunately, there are a number of disadvantages with inhaled prostanoids including being less potent (effective) than parenteral therapy and the requirement for multiple inhalations per day.

Pharmacologic Features and Clinical Considerations

Iloprost (Ventavis™) was the first inhaled prostacyclin to gain approval in 2004 following a 12 week, randomized, double blind, placebo-controlled trial of 203 patients with predominantly PAH but also chronic thromboembolic pulmonary hypertension (CTEPH). Patients were randomized to either 2.5 μg or 5.0 μg of iloprost versus placebo with the combined primary endpoint of improvement in at least one functional class and a 10 % improvement in 6MWD without clinical deterioration or death. By study's end, those randomized to iloprost achieved a significant improvement in the primary endpoint (17 % with iloprost versus 5 % with placebo). Improvements in secondary endpoints of dyspnea score, quality of life, and hemodynamics also favored iloprost (though it should be noted that hemodynamics were measured shortly after drug administration) [72].

A different inhaled prostanoid, inhaled treprostinil, was evaluated in two small studies of PAH and chronic thromboembolic pulmonary hypertension (CTEPH) and demonstrated encouraging clinical and hemodynamic improvements [73, 74]. These findings led the way for the Treprostinil Sodium Inhalation Used in the Management of Pulmonary Arterial Hypertension 1 (TRIUMPH-1) clinical trial of 235 patients with FC III PAH on background therapy with either bosentan or sildenafil randomized to inhaled treprostinil or placebo over a 12 week period. By study's end, a significant median improvement in peak 6MWD was seen in the inhaled treprostinil cohort although no significant improvements in secondary endpoints of time to clinical worsening or functional class were observed [75]. In a subsequent observational extension study, 118 patients who remained on inhaled treprostinil demonstrated a persistent improvement in 6MWD at 2 years. Inhaled treprostinil received FDA approval in 2009 [76].

Dosing Recommendations and Adverse Events

The short serum half-life (20–25 min for Iloprost, 3–4 h for Treprostinil) of both agents necessitates the frequent administration of the drug which is delivered through a nebulizer device [73]. The portable delivery device is battery powered with the option for monitoring of therapeutic indices of compliance and effective administration. Inhaled iloprost is particularly cumbersome, requiring 6 to 9 treatments per day at a dose of 2.5 ug or 5.0 ug per treatment for optimal benefit [77]. Treprostinil on the other hand requires 4 administrations per day with multiple breaths (3–10 per session) at an approximate dose of 6 µg per breath [54].

Aside from the inconvenience associated with the frequent dosing schedule, the inhaled prostacyclin therapies are generally well tolerated. Although some of the characteristic systemic side effects of prostanoids occur with the inhaled agents including headache, nausea, flushing, and jaw pain, these tend to be less prominent than with parenteral therapy, owed likely to its lesser relative potency and lower continuous blood concentrations. More common side effects of the inhaled formulations include cough and throat irritation [73, 78, 79]. Occasionally, a transition from parenteral to inhaled therapy is desired and can be achieved when performed carefully by an experienced clinical team at an expert PAH center [80].

Oral Prostanoids: Treprostinil (Orenitram™), Beraprost

The search for an effective oral prostanoid has been ongoing for many years in hopes of developing a therapy that might provide the benefits of prostanoid therapy while obviating the need for inconvenient drug delivery systems. While the development of oral prostanoid therapies might be considered another milestone in the treatment of PAH, its implementation has proved more difficult than anticipated [81, 82].

Pharmacologic Features and Clinical Considerations

Beraprost was the first oral prostanoid studied in the treatment of PAH via a randomized, placebo-controlled trial coined the Arterial Pulmonary Hypertension and Beraprost European Trial (ALPHABET). A total of one hundred thirty PAH patients were randomized to beraprost or placebo dosed four times per day for 12 weeks. The primary endpoint was the 6MWD which improved in those randomized to beraprost at 12 weeks [83]. Unfortunately, the drug was intolerable by a majority of patients due to severe gastrointestinal (GI) side effects. Barst and colleagues concurrently evaluated beraprost in a multicenter, randomized, placebo-controlled trial of 116 PAH patients evaluating a combined primary endpoint of disease progression or >25 % decrease in peak oxygen consumption (VO_2). While those randomized to beraprost demonstrated an improvement in 6MWD at 3 months, similar to that which was seen in the ALPHABET trial, these gains were no longer evident by 9 or 12 months and once again a similar, generally intolerable side effect profile was noted [84]. Consequently, beraprost never gained FDA approval.

More recently, oral treprostinil, a newer oral prostanoid developed in part with the goal of having a better tolerability profile than beraprost, was studied in a series of randomized, placebo-controlled trials coined the FREEDOM trials. In the FREEDOM-C (Oral Treprostinil in Combination With an ERA and/or a PDE-5 inhibitor for the Treatment of PAH) trial, PAH patients on existing, background PAH therapy were randomized to oral treprostinil (at an initial starting dose of 1 mg twice a day) or placebo for 16-weeks resulting in a nonsignificant 11 m improvement in the primary endpoint of 6MWD [85]. Notably, a high drop-out rate in those receiving oral treprostinil occurred due primarily to side effects of headache and GI upset. The FREEDOM-M trial was a randomized, double blind, placebo-controlled, clinical trial of 228 treatment naïve patients with PAH, modified to an intention to treat analysis restricted to only those with access to the 0.25 mg dose of treprostinil on the basis of intolerability of higher doses as was seen in FREEDOM-C. The primary endpoint of improvement in 6MWD at 12 weeks was achieved in the treprostinil arm, though improvements in many secondary endpoints were not achieved. Side effects of headache and GI upset were again common although use of the lower dose and a slower up titration may have helped with tolerability [86]. Finally, a third clinical trial of oral treprostinil was performed, the FREEDOM-C2 trial, which was a 16 week randomized trial of 310 patients with PAH on existing background oral therapy randomized to treprostinil (at an initial dose of 0.25 mg) versus placebo. Similar to that which was seen with the original FREEDOM-C trial, there was no significant improvement in the primary endpoint of 6MWD [87]. Ultimately on the basis of the results from these trials, oral treprostinil was approved in 2013 for use exclusively as monotherapy in the treatment of PAH.

Dosing Recommendations and Adverse Events

Sustainable blood levels for therapeutic concentrations of treprostinil have been demonstrated up to 8 to 10 h. Therefore, oral treprostinil is formulated as an extended-release tablet allowing for twice daily administration. It is recommended that patients take the medication within 10 min of consuming a meal to improve absorption [88]. In the FREEDOM-M trial noted above, the starting dose of 0.25 mg twice daily was increased every 3 days to a maximum tolerated dose, not exceeding 12 mg twice daily. The average dose at 12 weeks was 3.4 mg BID [86]. As noted, an initial low starting dose and slow up titration of oral treprostinil appears to be important for tolerability [54].

Endothelin Receptor Antagonist Therapy
(Table 16.2)

Bosentan (Tracleer™), Ambrisentan (Letairis™), and Macitentan (Opsumit™)

The pathobiology of PAH is diverse, involving multiple pathways and mechanisms of disease. A number of studies have confirmed the potent vasoconstrictor and mitogenic properties of endothelin-1 (ET-1) on the pulmonary vasculature [89, 90]. Elevated ET-1 plasma and lung levels are present in idiopathic PAH [26]. Endothelin receptors, which include endothelin receptors types A and/or B, are expressed on endothelial cells, cardiomyocytes, fibroblasts, and smooth muscle cells [91]. On the basis of biologic plausibility, the development of endothelin receptor antagonist

therapy emerged as an attractive therapeutic target in the treatment in PAH.

Pharmacologic Features and Clinical Considerations

The initial ERA to receive FDA approval was Bosentan (Tracleer™) in 2001 for patients with PAH and FC III or IV symptoms. Two randomized, double-blinded, placebo-controlled trials examined the efficacy and safety of this new class of agents. Channick and colleagues studied thirty-two patients with predominantly idiopathic PAH treated with bosentan or placebo for 12 weeks with the primary endpoint of 6MWD. Compared to placebo, the 6MWD improved significantly in those receiving bosentan with favorable changes in the secondary endpoints of PVR, cardiac index (CI), and dyspnea scores [92]. These findings led to the subsequent and larger clinical trial of 213 PAH patients in The Bosentan Randomized Trial of Endothelin Receptor Antagonist Therapy (BREATHE-1), which compared bosentan to placebo for 16 weeks and which met its primary endpoint of an improved 6MWD, while also demonstrating improvements in functional class and dyspnea scores [93].

Ambrisentan (Letairis™), a selective endothelin receptor A antagonist approved in 2007, was evaluated in two randomized, double-blinded, placebo-controlled trials of PAH patients in The Ambrisentan in Pulmonary Arterial Hypertension Randomized, Double-Blind,

Table 16.2 Pharmacologic and clinical points for ERAs in the treatment of PAH

Endothelin receptor antagonists	Mechanism of action	Administration route(s)	Suggested dosing	Relative & absolute contraindications	Monitoring & side effects
Bosentan (Tracleer™)	Nonselective endothelin receptor antagonist Pulmonary arterial vasodilation Anti-proliferative properties Anti-thrombotic properties	Oral	Initiate at 62.5 mg BID; increase to maximum dose 125 mg BID after 4 weeks	Moderate to severe hepatic disease (Child-Pugh Class B or greater) Pre-existing left sided-heart failure, fluid retention Pre-existing significant anemia Category X for pregnancy	Hepatotoxicity, peripheral edema, headache, hypotension, anemia Hepatic function testing at baseline and monthly while on therapy Effective birth control for women of child-bearing age required
Macitentan (Opsumit™)	See Bostenan	Oral	10 mg dose once daily	See Bosentan	See Bosentan Lower risk of hepatotoxicity than with bosentan
Ambrisentan (Letairis™)	Selective endothelin receptor A antagonist Similar effects as Bosentan	Oral	5 mg daily with titration to 10 mg daily in 2–4 weeks; start 2.5 mg daily if prior hepatic injury on non-selective ERA therapy	Moderate to severe hepatic disease (Child-Pugh Class B or greater) Pre-existing left heart failure, fluid retention Pre-existing significant anemia Category X for pregnancy	See Bosentan Lower risk of hepatoxicity than with bosentan

Abbreviations: mg milligrams, *ERA* endothelin receptor antagonist

Placebo-Controlled, Multicenter Efficacy Study 1 and 2 (ARIES) trials. Galie and colleagues randomized 394 FC II-IV PAH patients in a 1:1:1 design, which included placebo, ambrisentan 5 mg, or ambrisentan 10 mg in ARIES-1 and ambrisentan 2.5 mg or ambrisentan 5 mg in ARIES-2. There was a dose-related improvement in the primary endpoint of 6MWD compared to placebo that occurred at 12 weeks and which remained significant at 48 weeks in the 280 participants continuing on open label therapy [94]. Improvements in BNP, functional class, dyspnea score, and quality of life meters were also achieved at 12 weeks in those receiving ambrisentan.

The newest ERA to gain approval is macitentan (Opsumit™), which occurred in 2013 following a large, double-blinded, randomized, placebo-controlled trial the Study of Endothelin Receptor Antagonist in Pulmonary Arterial Hypertension to Improve Clinical Outcome (SERAPHIN). In this study, the PAH clinical trial of the longest duration to date, 742 patients were randomized to either macitentan 10 mg, macitentan 3 mg, or placebo to evaluate a composite primary endpoint of death, lung transplantation, atrial septostomy, initiation of subcutaneous or inhaled prostacyclin therapies, or worsening of PAH. This event-driven trial, a departure from the typical 6MWD endpoint, demonstrated a significant reduction in the combined primary endpoint in both treatment arms compared to placebo, with the primary driver being worsening of PAH. Modest improvements in secondary endpoints including exercise capacity and functional class were also observed in those receiving macitentan. Many of the patients in the study were treatment naïve but subgroup analyses found that improvements in the primary endpoint occurred in both treatment naïve patients and in those on background therapy. However, the derived benefit of the 3 mg dose was modest as compared to the 10 mg dose and ultimately only the 10 mg dose was approved [95].

Dosing Recommendations and Adverse Events
Both bosentan and macitentan are primarily hepatically metabolized and excreted by the biliary system. Macitentan is formulated as a parent drug, and, thus, compared to the 5 h half-life of bosentan, macitentan has a serum half-life of 14–19 h allowing for once daily dosing. Bosentan dosing may range from an initial dose of 62.5 mg twice daily up to a maximum dose of 250 mg twice daily, although the 250 mg dose in particular should be used with extreme caution because of the risk for hepatic dysfunction [96]. Macitentan is approved for 10 mg dosing only [95]. The serum half-life of ambrisentan allows for once daily dosing and may be administered over a range from 2.5 to 10 mg daily [97].

Arguably, the most worrisome adverse event associated with ERA therapy is hepatotoxicity and the commonest side effect is peripheral edema. Because of the hepatotoxicity risk associated with bosentan, monthly liver function testing (LFT) is mandatory for the duration of therapy and stopping the drug altogether is recommended should an elevation in LFTs above three times the upper limit of normal occur. Overall, mild elevations in aminotransferase levels occur in less than 6 % of participants receiving therapy. Additionally, co-administration of other agents metabolized via the CYP3A4 and CYP2C19 should be used with caution because of the potential for significant drug interactions to occur with concomitant bosentan use [98]. Regular monitoring of hemoglobin/hematocrit is also recommended to monitor for anemia, particularly while on chronic therapy. Peripheral edema is typically responsive to the administration of a diuretic, but the provider should remain attentive to signs of overt right ventricular failure and disease progression [96, 99].

Unlike with bosentan, ambrisentan appears to have a substantially lower risk of developing abnormal LFTs, but has similar rates of other side effects such as peripheral edema [100]. As with the other ERAs which are metabolized by the hepatic CYP system, a thorough consideration of drug interactions should be performed by the health care provider at the initiation and continuation of therapy [98]. Finally, ERAs are known to be teratogenic, therefore, therapy in women of childbearing age must include a negative pregnancy test at baseline and a discussion of appropriate contraception to avoid pregnancy while receiving treatment.

Nitric Oxide Therapies (Table 16.3)

Nitric oxide is an important contributor to the regulation of vascular tone, cellular proliferation, thrombosis, and response to injury/inflammation. The discovery of particularly high levels of phosphodiesterase type 5 in the lungs led to the development of phosphodiesterase type 5 (PDE5) inhibitors, which prevent the degradation of the second messenger cyclic guanosine monophosphate to mediate the intracellular NO signaling [101, 102]. More recently, soluble guanylate cyclase (sGC) stimulators, which have a dual mode of action to enhance sGC bioactivity, have also been developed and tested in PAH [103] (See section "Guanylate cyclase stimulators: Riociguat (Adempas™)").

Phosphodiesterase 5 Inhibitors: Sildenafil (Revatio™) and Tadalafil (Adcirca™)

Pharmacologic Features and Clinical Considerations
Sildenafil, initially studied in the treatment of erectile dysfunction, received FDA approval for the treatment of PAH in 2005. The Sildenafil Use in Pulmonary Arterial Hypertension (SUPER) study was the initial pivotal double blinded, placebo-controlled trial of 278 patients with symptomatic PAH randomized to sildenafil (dose ranged from 20 to 80 mg three

Table 16.3 Pharmacologic and clinical points for nitric oxide therapies in the treatment of PAH

Nitric oxide agent	Mechanism of action	Administration route(s)	Suggested dosing	Relative & absolute contraindications	Monitoring & side effects
Sildenafil (Revatio™)	Selective inhibitor of cyclic guanosine monophosphate (cGMP)-specific phosphodiesterase type 5 (PDE5) Smooth muscle relaxation/improve pulmonary arterial vasoconstriction Anti-proliferative and anti-inflammatory properites Anti-thrombotic properties	Oral, Intravenous	***Oral***: 20 mg TID. Off label titration to a maximum of 80 mg TID may provide added benefit ***IV***: 2.5 mg to 10 mg TID; do not exceed 10 mg TID	Avoid concomitant use with nitrate therapies or sGC stimulators due to risk of hypotension	Headache, flushing, dyspepsia, diarrhea No specific laboratory monitoring necessary
Tadalafil (Adcirca™)	See Sildenafil	Oral	40 mg daily	See Sildenafil	See Sildenafil
Riociguat (Adempas™)	Soluble guanylate cyclase stimulator Pulmonary arterial dilation Anti-proliferative, –thrombotic, and -inflammatory properties	Oral	Initiate at 0.5–1 mg TID; titrate up every 2 weeks by 0.5 mg TID; maximum dose 2.5 mg TID	Concomitant use with nitrates of PDE5 inhibitors should be avoided Category X for pregnancy	Headache, dyspepsia, peripheral edema, hypotension

Abbreviations: *cGMP* cyclic guanosine monophosphate, *PDE5* phosphodiesterase type 5, *IV* intravenous, *mg* milligrams, *TID* three times daily dosing, *sGC* Soluble guanylate cyclase

times a day) versus placebo with a primary endpoint of 6MWD at 12 weeks. By study's end, there was a significant improvement in 6MWD favoring sildenafil with a particularly notable dose-related improvement in both hemodynamics and 6MWD with escalation in sildenafil dose [104]. The SUPER-2 trial enrolled 259 patients in an open-label 3-year extension study. At 3 years, there was an overall persistent improvement in 6MWD compared to the baseline SUPER-1 indices [105].

The Pulmonary Arterial Hypertension and Response to Tadalafil (PHIRST) study enrolled 405 patients with PAH in a 16 week double-blind, placebo-controlled trial of taldalafil administered in one of four daily doses of 2.5, 10, 20, or 40 mg daily versus placebo with a primary endpoint of 6MWD. Ultimately, it was only in the higher doses of tadalafil where a significant improvement in 6MWD was achieved along with improvements in time to clinical worsening and quality of life [106]. Similar to that which was done with the SUPER trials with sildenafil, the PHIRST-2 study extended enrollment of PHIRST-1 study participants for an open-label follow up at 52 weeks showing an overall persistence in 6MWD improvements for both the 20 and 40 mg treatment arms [107]. Tadalafil was ultimately approved at the 40 mg dose.

Dosing Recommendations and Adverse Events

Despite improvements in a variety of clinical endpoints with escalating doses of sildenafil in the clinical trials, approval is for 20 mg three times daily. The longer half-life of tadalafil of upwards of 18 h allows for once daily dosing and it is prescribed at 40 mg daily [108]. The most common side effects associated with PDE5 inhibitors include headache, flushing, and nasal congestion [104, 105, 108]. One must also be aware of the quite rare but serious adverse effect of non-arteritic anterior ischemic optic neuropathy; which may present with sudden loss of vision. The co-administration of PDE5 inhibitors and nitrate therapy is contraindicated while concomitant use of other CYP3A4 inhibitors should be used with caution.

Guanylate Cyclase Stimulators: Riociguat (Adempas™)

As discussed previously, the NO pathway is a key therapeutic target in PAH. The newest therapy in the treatment of PAH targeting the NO pathway is riociguat (Adempas™), a novel soluble guanylate cyclase (sGC) stimulator. Both impaired synthesis of NO and insufficient stimulation of the NO-sGC-cGMP axis have been described in PAH. Riociguat, a stimulator of sGC, is thought to have a dual mode of action. It sensitizes sGC to endogenous NO by stabilizing NO-sGC binding and also directly stimulates sGC independently of NO [109].

Pharmacologic Features and Clinical Considerations

The FDA approval of riociguat for the treatment of both PAH and CTEPH occurred following the completion of two randomized clinical trials. The Pulmonary Arterial Hypertension Soluble Guanylate Cyclase-Stimulator Trial 1 (PATENT-1) was an international, double-blind, placebo-controlled trial which randomly assigned a total of 443 patients with underlying symptomatic PAH to one of three cohorts. Two of the cohorts were treatment arms that included a lower dose (1.5 mg three times daily) and higher dose (2.5 mg three times daily) of riociguat and the third cohort received placebo with the primary endpoint of 6MWD at 12 weeks. By study's end, those who received treatment with riociguat demonstrated a significant improvement in 6MWD compared to placebo. Improvements in secondary endpoints including NT-proBNP levels, functional capacity, dyspnea scores, time to clinical worsening, and hemodynamics also significantly favored riociguat. In fact there appeared to be a potentially important dose-response relationship between riociguat dose and cardiac output [110].

In the CTEPH population, the Chronic Thromboembolic Pulmonary Hypertension Soluble Guanylate Cyclase Stimulator Trial 1 (CHEST-1) randomized 261 patients with inoperable thromboembolic disease to riociguat versus placebo with a primary endpoint of 6MWD at 16 weeks. The same secondary endpoints from PATENT-1 were also examined. Similar to that seen in the PATENT-1 trial, riociguat was associated with a significant improvement in 6MWD as well as improved hemodynamics, NT-proBNP and functional class compared to placebo. Serious adverse events, which included right ventricular failure and syncope, occurred at rates similar to placebo [111]. It is important to emphasize that the patients with CTEPH were determined to be inoperable as the only curative treatment for CTEPH remains pulmonary thromboendarterectomy.

Dosing Recommendations and Adverse Events

The biologic effects of riociguat are demonstrable within 1.5 h of administration with an approximate terminal half-life of twelve hours. It is primarily hepatically cleared, and, thus, caution should be used in patients with advanced liver disease or with concomitant use of other CYP inhibitors. Additionally, out of concern for significant hypotension, riociguat use with nitrates or PDE5 inhibitors is contraindicated [112].

The recommended dosing of riociguat is based on the PATENT-1 trial which initiated therapy at 1 mg three times daily. The patient's systolic blood pressure and symptoms should be monitored closely with titration of therapy by 0.5 mg every 14 days as tolerated to a maximum tolerated dose of 2.5 mg three times daily. If the patient's blood pressure is marginal at baseline, a starting dose of 0.5 mg is recommended. Side effects may include headache, dyspepsia, peripheral edema, and gastrointestinal symptoms (nausea, diarrhea) [113].

Summary

In a matter of two decades, the treatment of PAH has drastically evolved with the emergence of approved therapies that target the prostacyclin, endothelin, and nitric oxide pathways. In turn, we have also observed modest improvements in both morbidity and mortality when compared to the days of the original NIH registry [1, 114]. Despite these therapeutic advances, PAH remains a devastating disease. The next generation of PAH pharmacotherapy will likely need to have potent antiproliferative and anti-inflammatory properties to directly target the adverse remodeling that is a signature of this vasculopathy. Additionally, a more individualized approach to treatment is needed given the extensive molecular heterogeneity of PAH.

References

1. Thenappan T, Shah SJ, Rich S, Tian L, Archer SL, Gomberg-Maitland M. Survival in pulmonary arterial hypertension: a reappraisal of the NIH risk stratification equation. Eur Respir J. 2010;35(5):1079–87.
2. Sakao S, Taraseviciene-Stewart L, Lee JD, Wood K, Cool CD, Voelkel NF. Initial apoptosis is followed by increased proliferation of apoptosis-resistant endothelial cells. FASEB J. 2005;19(9):1178–80.
3. Archer SL, Weir EK, Wilkins MR. Basic science of pulmonary arterial hypertension for clinicians: new concepts and experimental therapies. Circulation. 2010;121(18):2045–66.
4. Rabinovitch M. Molecular pathogenesis of pulmonary arterial hypertension. J Clin Invest. 2012;122(12):4306–13.
5. Lewis GD, Bossone E, Naeije R, Grunig E, Saggar R, Lancellotti P, et al. Pulmonary vascular hemodynamic response to exercise in cardiopulmonary diseases. Circulation. 2013;128(13):1470–9.
6. Gaine SP, Rubin LJ. Primary pulmonary hypertension. Lancet. 1998;352(9129):719–25.
7. Rai PR, Cool CD, King JA, Stevens T, Burns N, Winn RA, et al. The cancer paradigm of severe pulmonary arterial hypertension. Am J Respir Crit Care Med. 2008;178(6):558–64.
8. Voelkel NF, Cool C, Lee SD, Wright L, Geraci MW, Tuder RM. Primary pulmonary hypertension between inflammation and cancer. Chest. 1998;114(3 Suppl):225S–30.
9. Herve P, Launay JM, Scrobohaci ML, Brenot F, Simonneau G, Petitpretz P, et al. Increased plasma serotonin in primary pulmonary hypertension. Am J Med. 1995;99(3):249–54.
10. West J, Fagan K, Steudel W, Fouty B, Lane K, Harral J, et al. Pulmonary hypertension in transgenic mice expressing a dominant-negative BMPRII gene in smooth muscle. Circ Res. 2004;94(8):1109–14.
11. Yang J, Davies RJ, Southwood M, Long L, Yang X, Sobolewski A, et al. Mutations in bone morphogenetic protein type II receptor cause dysregulation of Id gene expression in pulmonary artery smooth muscle cells: implications for familial pulmonary arterial hypertension. Circ Res. 2008;102(10):1212–21.
12. White RJ, Meoli DF, Swarthout RF, Kallop DY, Galaria II, Harvey JL, et al. Plexiform-like lesions and increased tissue factor expression in a rat model of severe pulmonary arterial hypertension. Am J Physiol Lung Cell Mol Physiol. 2007;293(3):L583–90.
13. Gorlach A, BelAiba RS, Hess J, Kietzmann T. Thrombin activates the p21-activated kinase in pulmonary artery smooth muscle cells.

Role in tissue factor expression. Thromb Haemost. 2005;93(6):1168–75.

14. Benisty JI, McLaughlin VV, Landzberg MJ, Rich JD, Newburger JW, Rich S, et al. Elevated basic fibroblast growth factor levels in patients with pulmonary arterial hypertension. Chest. 2004;126(4):1255–61.

15. Humbert M, Morrell NW, Archer SL, Stenmark KR, MacLean MR, Lang IM, et al. Cellular and molecular pathobiology of pulmonary arterial hypertension. J Am Coll Cardiol. 2004;43(12 Suppl S):13S–24.

16. Richter A, Yeager ME, Zaiman A, Cool CD, Voelkel NF, Tuder RM. Impaired transforming growth factor-beta signaling in idiopathic pulmonary arterial hypertension. Am J Respir Crit Care Med. 2004;170(12):1340–8.

17. Bonnet S, Michelakis ED, Porter CJ, Andrade-Navarro MA, Thebaud B, Bonnet S, et al. An abnormal mitochondrial-hypoxia inducible factor-1alpha-Kv channel pathway disrupts oxygen sensing and triggers pulmonary arterial hypertension in fawn hooded rats: similarities to human pulmonary arterial hypertension. Circulation. 2006;113(22):2630–41.

18. Morrell NW, Adnot S, Archer SL, Dupuis J, Jones PL, MacLean MR, et al. Cellular and molecular basis of pulmonary arterial hypertension. J Am Coll Cardiol. 2009;54(1 Suppl):S20–31.

19. Christman BW. Lipid mediator dysregulation in primary pulmonary hypertension. Chest. 1998;114(3 Suppl):205S–7.

20. Tuder RM, Cool CD, Geraci MW, Wang J, Abman SH, Wright L, et al. Prostacyclin synthase expression is decreased in lungs from patients with severe pulmonary hypertension. Am J Respir Crit Care Med. 1999;159(6):1925–32.

21. Giaid A, Saleh D. Reduced expression of endothelial nitric oxide synthase in the lungs of patients with pulmonary hypertension. N Engl J Med. 1995;333(4):214–21.

22. Alderton WK, Cooper CE, Knowles RG. Nitric oxide synthases: structure, function and inhibition. Biochem J. 2001;357(Pt 3):593–615.

23. Archer SL, Djaballah K, Humbert M, Weir KE, Fartoukh M, Dall'ava-Santucci J, et al. Nitric oxide deficiency in fenfluramine- and dexfenfluramine-induced pulmonary hypertension. Am J Respir Crit Care Med. 1998;158(4):1061–7.

24. Kaneko FT, Arroliga AC, Dweik RA, Comhair SA, Laskowski D, Oppedisano R, et al. Biochemical reaction products of nitric oxide as quantitative markers of primary pulmonary hypertension. Am J Respir Crit Care Med. 1998;158(3):917–23.

25. Fagan KA, Fouty BW, Tyler RC, Morris Jr KG, Hepler LK, Sato K, et al. The pulmonary circulation of homozygous or heterozygous eNOS-null mice is hyperresponsive to mild hypoxia. J Clin Invest. 1999;103(2):291–9.

26. Giaid A, Yanagisawa M, Langleben D, Michel RP, Levy R, Shennib H, et al. Expression of endothelin-1 in the lungs of patients with pulmonary hypertension. N Engl J Med. 1993;328(24):1732–9.

27. Quinlan TR, Li D, Laubach VE, Shesely EG, Zhou N, Johns RA. eNOS-deficient mice show reduced pulmonary vascular proliferation and remodeling to chronic hypoxia. Am J Physiol Lung Cell Mol Physiol. 2000;279(4):L641–50.

28. Tamosiuniene R, Nicolls MR. Regulatory T cells and pulmonary hypertension. Trends Cardiovasc Med. 2011;21(6):166–71.

29. Tamosiuniene R, Tian W, Dhillon G, Wang L, Sung YK, Gera L, et al. Regulatory T cells limit vascular endothelial injury and prevent pulmonary hypertension. Circ Res. 2011;109(8):867–79.

30. Voelkel NF, Gomez-Arroyo J, Abbate A, Bogaard HJ, Nicolls MR. Pathobiology of pulmonary arterial hypertension and right ventricular failure. Eur Respir J. 2012;40(6):1555–65.

31. Huertas A, Perros F, Tu L, Cohen-Kaminsky S, Montani D, Dorfmuller P, et al. Immune dysregulation and endothelial dysfunction in pulmonary arterial hypertension: a complex interplay. Circulation. 2014;129(12):1332–40.

32. Hassoun PM, Mouthon L, Barbera JA, Eddahibi S, Flores SC, Grimminger F, et al. Inflammation, growth factors, and pulmonary vascular remodeling. J Am Coll Cardiol. 2009;54(1 Suppl):S10–9.

33. Dorfmuller P, Humbert M. Progress in pulmonary arterial hypertension pathology: relighting a torch inside the tunnel. Am J Respir Crit Care Med. 2012;186(3):210–2.

34. Dorfmuller P, Perros F, Balabanian K, Humbert M. Inflammation in pulmonary arterial hypertension. Eur Respir J. 2003;22(2):358–63.

35. Stacher E, Graham BB, Hunt JM, Gandjeva A, Groshong SD, McLaughlin VV, et al. Modern age pathology of pulmonary arterial hypertension. Am J Respir Crit Care Med. 2012;186(3):261–72.

36. Perros F, Cohen-Kaminsky S, Humbert M. Understanding the role of CD4+CD25(high) (so-called regulatory) T cells in idiopathic pulmonary arterial hypertension. Respir Int Rev Thorac Dis. 2008;75(3):253–6.

37. Perros F, Dorfmuller P, Montani D, Hammad H, Waelput W, Girerd B, et al. Pulmonary lymphoid neogenesis in idiopathic pulmonary arterial hypertension. Am J Respir Crit Care Med. 2012;185(3):311–21.

38. Soubrier F, Chung WK, Machado R, Grunig E, Aldred M, Geraci M, et al. Genetics and genomics of pulmonary arterial hypertension. J Am Coll Cardiol. 2013;62(25 Suppl):D13–21.

39. Ferguson JF. Omics gets personal: integrative profiling of health and disease. Circ Cardiovasc Genet. 2012;5(3):381–2.

40. Chen R, Mias GI, Li-Pook-Than J, Jiang L, Lam HY, Chen R, et al. Personal omics profiling reveals dynamic molecular and medical phenotypes. Cell. 2012;148(6):1293–307.

41. Christman BW, McPherson CD, Newman JH, King GA, Bernard GR, Groves BM, et al. An imbalance between the excretion of thromboxane and prostacyclin metabolites in pulmonary hypertension. N Engl J Med. 1992;327(2):70–5.

42. Tuder RM, Archer SL, Dorfmuller P, Erzurum SC, Guignabert C, Michelakis E, et al. Relevant issues in the pathology and pathobiology of pulmonary hypertension. J Am Coll Cardiol. 2013;62(25 Suppl):D4–12.

43. Klinger JR, Abman SH, Gladwin MT. Nitric oxide deficiency and endothelial dysfunction in pulmonary arterial hypertension. Am J Respir Crit Care Med. 2013;188(6):639–46.

44. Rubin LJ, Groves BM, Reeves JT, Frosolono M, Handel F, Cato AE. Prostacyclin-induced acute pulmonary vasodilation in primary pulmonary hypertension. Circulation. 1982;66(2):334–8.

45. Higenbottam T, Wheeldon D, Wells F, Wallwork J. Long-term treatment of primary pulmonary hypertension with continuous intravenous epoprostenol (prostacyclin). Lancet. 1984;1(8385):1046–7.

46. Rubin LJ, Mendoza J, Hood M, McGoon M, Barst R, Williams WB, et al. Treatment of primary pulmonary hypertension with continuous intravenous prostacyclin (epoprostenol). Results of a randomized trial. Ann Intern Med. 1990;112(7):485–91.

47. Barst RJ, Rubin LJ, Long WA, McGoon MD, Rich S, Badesch DB, et al. A comparison of continuous intravenous epoprostenol (prostacyclin) with conventional therapy for primary pulmonary hypertension. N Engl J Med. 1996;334(5):296–301.

48. Badesch DB, Tapson VF, McGoon MD, Brundage BH, Rubin LJ, Wigley FM, et al. Continuous intravenous epoprostenol for pulmonary hypertension due to the scleroderma spectrum of disease. A randomized, controlled trial. Ann Intern Med. 2000;132(6):425–34.

49. Rich S, Dantzker DR, Ayres SM, Bergofsky EH, Brundage BH, Detre KM, et al. Primary pulmonary hypertension. A national prospective study. Ann Intern Med. 1987;107(2):216–23.

50. Benza RL, Miller DP, Gomberg-Maitland M, Frantz RP, Foreman AJ, Coffey CS, et al. Predicting survival in pulmonary arterial hypertension: insights from the Registry to Evaluate Early and

Long-Term Pulmonary Arterial Hypertension Disease Management (REVEAL). Circulation. 2010;122(2):164–72.

51. Shapiro SM, Oudiz RJ, Cao T, Romano MA, Beckmann XJ, Georgiou D, et al. Primary pulmonary hypertension: improved long-term effects and survival with continuous intravenous epoprostenol infusion. J Am Coll Cardiol. 1997;30(2):343–9.

52. McLaughlin VV. Survival in primary pulmonary hypertension: the impact of epoprostenol therapy. Circulation. 2002;106(12): 1477–82.

53. Sitbon O, Humbert M, Nunes H, Parent F, Garcia G, Herve P, et al. Long-term intravenous epoprostenol infusion in primary pulmonary hypertension: prognostic factors and survival. J Am Coll Cardiol. 2002;40(4):780–8.

54. Orenitram (treprostinil) [Package Insert]. Research Triangle Park: United Therapeutics Corp; 2012.

55. Fuentes A, Coralic A, Dawson KL. A new epoprostenol formulation for the treatment of pulmonary arterial hypertension. Am J Health Syst Pharm AJHP Off J Am Soc Health Syst Pharm. 2012;69(16):1389–93.

56. Lambert O, Bandilla D. Stability and preservation of a new formulation of epoprostenol sodium for treatment of pulmonary arterial hypertension. Drug Des Devel Ther. 2012;6:235–44.

57. McLaughlin VV, Palevsky HI. Parenteral and inhaled prostanoid therapy in the treatment of pulmonary arterial hypertension. Clin Chest Med. 2013;34(4):825–40.

58. Rich S, McLaughlin VV. The effects of chronic prostacyclin therapy on cardiac output and symptoms in primary pulmonary hypertension. J Am Coll Cardiol. 1999;34(4):1184–7.

59. Simonneau G, Barst RJ, Galie N, Naeije R, Rich S, Bourge RC, et al. Continuous subcutaneous infusion of treprostinil, a prostacyclin analogue, in patients with pulmonary arterial hypertension: a double-blind, randomized, placebo-controlled trial. Am J Respir Crit Care Med. 2002;165(6):800–4.

60. Barst RJ, Galie N, Naeije R, Simonneau G, Jeffs R, Arneson C, et al. Long-term outcome in pulmonary arterial hypertension patients treated with subcutaneous treprostinil. Eur Respir J. 2006;28(6):1195–203.

61. Tapson VF, Gomberg-Maitland M, McLaughlin VV, Benza RL, Widlitz AC, Krichman A, et al. Safety and efficacy of IV treprostinil for pulmonary arterial hypertension: a prospective, multicenter, open-label, 12-week trial. Chest. 2006;129(3):683–8.

62. Wade M, Baker FJ, Roscigno R, DellaMaestra W, Arneson CP, Hunt TL, et al. Pharmacokinetics of treprostinil sodium administered by 28-day chronic continuous subcutaneous infusion. J Clin Pharmacol. 2004;44(5):503–9.

63. Wade M, Baker FJ, Roscigno R, DellaMaestra W, Hunt TL, Lai AA. Absolute bioavailability and pharmacokinetics of treprostinil sodium administered by acute subcutaneous infusion. J Clin Pharmacol. 2004;44(1):83–8.

64. McLaughlin VV, Gaine SP, Barst RJ, Oudiz RJ, Bourge RC, Frost A, et al. Efficacy and safety of treprostinil: an epoprostenol analog for primary pulmonary hypertension. J Cardiovasc Pharmacol. 2003;41(2):293–9.

65. McSwain CS, Benza R, Shapiro S, Hill N, Schilz R, Elliott CG, et al. Dose proportionality of treprostinil sodium administered by continuous subcutaneous and intravenous infusion. J Clin Pharmacol. 2008;48(1):19–25.

66. Rubenfire M, McLaughlin VV, Allen RP, Elliott G, Park MH, Wade M, et al. Transition from IV epoprostenol to subcutaneous treprostinil in pulmonary arterial hypertension: a controlled trial. Chest. 2007;132(3):757–63.

67. Alkukhun L, Bair ND, Dweik RA, Tonelli AR. Subcutaneous to intravenous prostacyclin analog transition in pulmonary hypertension. J Cardiovasc Pharmacol. 2014;63(1):4–8.

68. Kitterman N, Poms A, Miller DP, Lombardi S, Farber HW, Barst RJ. Bloodstream infections in patients with pulmonary arterial hypertension treated with intravenous prostanoids: insights from the REVEAL REGISTRY(R). Mayo Clin Proc. 2012;87(9):825–34.

69. Rich JD, Glassner C, Wade M, Coslet S, Arneson C, Doran A, et al. The effect of diluent pH on bloodstream infection rates in patients receiving IV treprostinil for pulmonary arterial hypertension. Chest. 2012;141(1):36–42.

70. Beghetti M, Reber G, de Moerloose P, Vadas L, Chiappe A, Spahr-Schopfer I, et al. Aerosolized iloprost induces a mild but sustained inhibition of platelet aggregation. European Respiratory Journal. 2002;19(3):518–24.

71. Olschewski H, Walmrath D, Schermuly R, Ghofrani A, Grimminger F, Seeger W. Aerosolized prostacyclin and iloprost in severe pulmonary hypertension. Ann Intern Med. 1996;124(9):820–4.

72. Olschewski H, Simonneau G, Galie N, Higenbottam T, Naeije R, Rubin LJ, et al. Inhaled iloprost for severe pulmonary hypertension. N Engl J Med. 2002;347(5):322–9.

73. Channick RN, Olschewski H, Seeger W, Staub T, Voswinckel R, Rubin LJ. Safety and efficacy of inhaled treprostinil as add-on therapy to bosentan in pulmonary arterial hypertension. J Am Coll Cardiol. 2006;48(7):1433–7.

74. Voswinckel R, Reichenberger F, Enke B, Kreckel A, Krick S, Gall H, et al. Acute effects of the combination of sildenafil and inhaled treprostinil on haemodynamics and gas exchange in pulmonary hypertension. Pulm Pharmacol Ther. 2008;21(5):824–32.

75. McLaughlin VV, Benza RL, Rubin LJ, Channick RN, Voswinckel R, Tapson VF, et al. Addition of inhaled treprostinil to oral therapy for pulmonary arterial hypertension: a randomized controlled clinical trial. J Am Coll Cardiol. 2010;55(18):1915–22.

76. Gomberg-Maitland M, Dufton C, Oudiz RJ, Benza RL. Compelling evidence of long-term outcomes in pulmonary arterial hypertension? A clinical perspective. J Am Coll Cardiol. 2011;57(9):1053–61.

77. Ventavis (iloprost) [Package Insert]. South San Francisco: Acetlion Pharmaceuticals US, Inc; 2013.

78. Channick RN, Voswinckel R, Rubin LJ. Inhaled treprostinil: a therapeutic review. Drug Des Devel Ther. 2012;6:19–28.

79. Opitz CF, Wensel R, Winkler J, Halank M, Bruch L, Kleber FX, et al. Clinical efficacy and survival with first-line inhaled iloprost therapy in patients with idiopathic pulmonary arterial hypertension. Eur Heart J. 2005;26(18):1895–902.

80. Bourge RC, Tapson VF, Safdar Z, Benza RL, Channick RN, Rosenzweig EB, et al. Rapid transition from inhaled iloprost to inhaled treprostinil in patients with pulmonary arterial hypertension. Cardiovasc Ther. 2013;31(1):38–44.

81. Waxman AB. Oral prostacyclin therapy for pulmonary arterial hypertension: another step forward. Circulation. 2013;127(5):563–5.

82. Waxman AB, Zamanian RT. Pulmonary arterial hypertension: new insights into the optimal role of current and emerging prostacyclin therapies. Am J Cardiol. 2013;111(5 Suppl):1A–16; quiz 7A–9A.

83. Galie N, Humbert M, Vachiery JL, Vizza CD, Kneussl M, Manes A, et al. Effects of beraprost sodium, an oral prostacyclin analogue, in patients with pulmonary arterial hypertension: a randomized, double-blind, placebo-controlled trial. J Am Coll Cardiol. 2002;39(9):1496–502.

84. Barst RJ, McGoon M, McLaughlin V, Tapson V, Oudiz R, Shapiro S, et al. Beraprost therapy for pulmonary arterial hypertension. J Am Coll Cardiol. 2003;41(12):2119–25.

85. Tapson VF, Torres F, Kermeen F, Keogh AM, Allen RP, Frantz RP, et al. Oral treprostinil for the treatment of pulmonary arterial hypertension in patients on background endothelin receptor antagonist and/or phosphodiesterase type 5 inhibitor therapy (the FREEDOM-C study): a randomized controlled trial. Chest. 2012;142(6):1383–90.

86. Jing ZC, Parikh K, Pulido T, Jerjes-Sanchez C, White RJ, Allen R, et al. Efficacy and safety of oral treprostinil monotherapy for the treatment of pulmonary arterial hypertension: a randomized, controlled trial. Circulation. 2013;127(5):624–33.

87. Tapson VF, Jing ZC, Xu KF, Pan L, Feldman J, Kiely DG, et al. Oral treprostinil for the treatment of pulmonary arterial hypertension in patients receiving background endothelin receptor antagonist and phosphodiesterase type 5 inhibitor therapy (the FREEDOM-C2 study): a randomized controlled trial. Chest. 2013;144(3):952–8.

88. White RJ, Torres F, Allen R, Jerjes C, Pulido T, Yehle D, et al. Pharmacokinetics of oral treprostinil sustained release tablets during chronic administration to patients with pulmonary arterial hypertension. J Cardiovasc Pharmacol. 2013;61(6):474–81.

89. Yanagisawa M, Kurihara H, Kimura S, Tomobe Y, Kobayashi M, Mitsui Y. A novel potent vasoconstrictor peptide produced by vascular endothelial cells. Nature. 1988;322:411–5.

90. Miyagawa K, Emoto N. Current state of endothelin receptor antagonism in hypertension and pulmonary hypertension. Ther Adv Cardiovasc Dis. 2014.

91. Henry PJ. Endothelin receptor distribution and function in the airways. Clin Exp Pharmacol Physiol. 1999;26(2):162–7.

92. Channick RN, Simonneau G, Sitbon O, Robbins IM, Frost A, Tapson VF, et al. Effects of the dual endothelin-receptor antagonist bosentan in patients with pulmonary hypertension: a randomised placebocontrolled study. The Lancet. 2001;358(9288):1119–23.

93. Rubin LJ, Badesch DB, Barst RJ, Galie N, Black CM, Keogh A, et al. Bosentan therapy for pulmonary arterial hypertension. N Engl J Med. 2002;346(12):896–903.

94. Galie N, Olschewski H, Oudiz RJ, Torres F, Frost A, Ghofrani HA, et al. Ambrisentan for the treatment of pulmonary arterial hypertension: results of the ambrisentan in pulmonary arterial hypertension, randomized, double-blind, placebo-controlled, multicenter, efficacy (ARIES) study 1 and 2. Circulation. 2008;117(23):3010–9.

95. Pulido T, Adzerikho I, Channick RN, Delcroix M, Galie N, Ghofrani HA, et al. Macitentan and morbidity and mortality in pulmonary arterial hypertension. N Engl J Med. 2013;369(9):809–18.

96. Tracleer (bosentan) [Package Insert]. South San Francisco: Acetlion Pharmaceuticals US, Inc; 2012.

97. Letairis (ambrisentan) [Package Insert]. Foster City: Gilead Sciences, Inc; 2014.

98. Venitz J, Zack J, Gillies H, Allard M, Regnault J, Dufton C. Clinical pharmacokinetics and drug-drug interactions of endothelin receptor antagonists in pulmonary arterial hypertension. J Clin Pharmacol. 2012;52(12):1784–805.

99. Opsumit (macitentan) [Package Insert]. South San Francisco: Acetlion Pharmaceuticals US, Inc; 2013.

100. Ben-Yehuda O, Pizzuti D, Brown A, Littman M, Gillies H, Henig N, et al. Long-term hepatic safety of ambrisentan in patients with pulmonary arterial hypertension. J Am Coll Cardiol. 2012;60(1):80–1.

101. Schermuly RT, Pullamsetti SS, Kwapiszewska G, Dumitrascu R, Tian X, Weissmann N, et al. Phosphodiesterase 1 upregulation in pulmonary arterial hypertension: target for reverse-remodeling therapy. Circulation. 2007;115(17):2331–9.

102. Archer SL, Michelakis ED. Phosphodiesterase type 5 inhibitors for pulmonary arterial hypertension. N Engl J Med. 2009;361(19):1864–71.

103. Dumitrascu R, Weissmann N, Ghofrani HA, Dony E, Beuerlein K, Schmidt H, et al. Activation of soluble guanylate cyclase reverses experimental pulmonary hypertension and vascular remodeling. Circulation. 2006;113(2):286–95.

104. Galie N, Ghofrani HA, Torbicki A, Barst RJ, Rubin LJ, Badesch D, et al. Sildenafil citrate therapy for pulmonary arterial hypertension. N Engl J Med. 2005;353(20):2148–57.

105. Rubin LJ, Badesch DB, Fleming TR, Galie N, Simonneau G, Ghofrani HA, et al. Long-term treatment with sildenafil citrate in pulmonary arterial hypertension: the SUPER-2 study. Chest. 2011;140(5):1274–83.

106. Galie N, Brundage BH, Ghofrani HA, Oudiz RJ, Simonneau G, Safdar Z, et al. Tadalafil therapy for pulmonary arterial hypertension. Circulation. 2009;119(22):2894–903.

107. Oudiz RJ, Brundage BH, Galie N, Ghofrani HA, Simonneau G, Botros FT, et al. Tadalafil for the treatment of pulmonary arterial hypertension: a double-blind 52-week uncontrolled extension study. J Am Coll Cardiol. 2012;60(8):768–74.

108. Pfizer. Revatio (sildenafil) [Package Insert]. New York: Pfizer Laboratories Div Pfizer, Inc; 2014. [updated 2014].

109. Nossaman B, Pankey E, Kadowitz P. Stimulators and activators of soluble guanylate cyclase: review and potential therapeutic indications. Crit Care Res Pract. 2012;2012:290805.

110. Ghofrani HA, Galie N, Grimminger F, Grunig E, Humbert M, Jing ZC, et al. Riociguat for the treatment of pulmonary arterial hypertension. N Engl J Med. 2013;369(4):330–40.

111. Ghofrani HA, D'Armini AM, Grimminger F, Hoeper MM, Jansa P, Kim NH, et al. Riociguat for the treatment of chronic thromboembolic pulmonary hypertension. N Engl J Med. 2013;369(4):319–29.

112. Grimminger F, Weimann G, Frey R, Voswinckel R, Thamm M, Bolkow D, et al. First acute haemodynamic study of soluble guanylate cyclase stimulator riociguat in pulmonary hypertension. Eur Respir J. 2009;33(4):785–92.

113. Adempas (riociguate) [Package Insert]. Whippany: Bayer HealthCare Pharmacueticals, Inc; 2014.

114. Benza RL, Miller DP, Barst RJ, Badesch DB, Frost AE, McGoon MD. An evaluation of long-term survival from time of diagnosis in pulmonary arterial hypertension from the REVEAL Registry. Chest. 2012;142(2):448–56.

115. O'Callaghan DS, et al. Treatment of pulmonary arterial hypertension with targeted therapies. Nature Rev Cardiol. 2011;8:526–38.

Determining the Optimal Approach to Initiating Oral, Inhaled, and Intravenous Therapies in Clinical Practice: Sequential Goal-Directed Therapy Is Best

17

Brian B. Graham

Introduction

The past 20 years have seen a revolution in the number of medications available for the treatment of pulmonary arterial hypertension (PAH). Currently available Food and Drug Administration (FDA)-approved treatments target three pathways that are each implicated in the pathogenesis of PAH: nitric oxide, endothelin, and prostacyclin. These three pathways likely have complex mutual interactions with parallel, sequential, and feedback signaling; as such, it has been proposed that concurrent therapy targeting multiple pathways can provide additive clinical benefit. However, the precise timing of combination therapy remains debated. The two potential treatment approaches to combination therapy are (Fig. 17.1):

A. **Sequential Combination Therapy**. Treatment is initiated with monotherapy and the outcome assessed. If treatment goals are not achieved, then additional, concomitant therapies are added one at a time.
B. **Up-Front Combination Therapy**. Treatment is initiated with multiple medications simultaneously.

This chapter outlines the argument for the use of sequential addition of combination therapy as opposed to up-front combination therapy.

Biologic and Practical Rationale of Sequential Combination Therapy

The application of up-front combination therapy in PAH has drawn analogies to other diseases for which this strategy is commonly used, such as malignancy and Human

Immunodeficiency Virus (HIV) infection [1, 2]. However, the molecular basis for this analogy is unclear. Monotherapy treatment for malignancy is associated with increased risk of *de novo* somatic mutations giving rise to resistant cellular clones; combination chemotherapy up-front decreases the chance of resistance, and prolongs survival in many forms of cancer [3]. Similarly, HIV may develop resistance to antiretroviral therapy, which is prevented by the use of combination therapy [4]. However, there is no evidence that aberrant pulmonary vascular cells in patients with PAH develop escape mechanisms that are, in turn, resistant to therapy, much less that such patterns of resistance may be altered by up-front combination therapy.

Alternatively, the sequential addition of therapy allows evaluation of the individual clinical response to each medication, including allowing titration of the dose to optimize the benefit versus side effect profile. If the clinical response is (a) harm or (b) inadequate with the first medication, the initial medication can be removed or substituted, and/or a second class of medication added, with further optimization of the second medication before additional advancement of therapy as required. In this manner, tolerability and benefit are systematically optimized for each patient, with a clear assessment of response to each medication.

Such personalized therapy is important, as a fraction of patients will have a suboptimal response to any single medication. This fact of biologic variability is demonstrated by the data in Fig. 17.2, which reports the change in 6 min walk distance (6MWD) reported for PAH patients treated with riociguat in the recently published PATENT-1 trial [6]. In this study, 76 % of patients had a net positive improvement in 6MWD from baseline to the last study visit at 12 weeks, while 24 % of patients had a decline in 6MWD. The heterogeneity in clinical response will be compounded with the use of multiple medications, particularly if multiple medications are started simultaneously, some of which may be beneficial and some of which may be harmful; the net result may be partial or suboptimal, with great difficulty determining if one or more medications may actually be causing harm. Thus,

B.B. Graham, MD
Program in Translational Lung Research, Department of Medicine, University of Colorado Denver, 12700 E 19th Ave, C-272, Aurora, CO 80045, USA
e-mail: brian.graham@ucdenver.edu

© Springer International Publishing Switzerland 2016
B.A. Maron et al. (eds.), *Pulmonary Hypertension: Basic Science to Clinical Medicine*, DOI 10.1007/978-3-319-23594-3_17

271

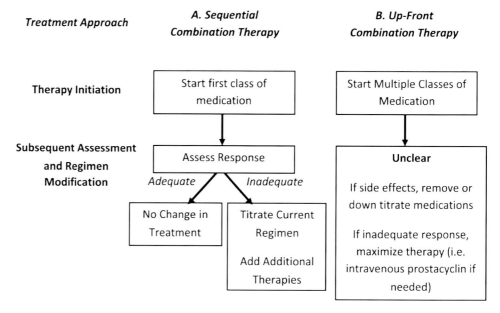

Fig. 17.1 Two approaches to initiation of therapy in PAH: sequential combination therapy or up-front combination therapy

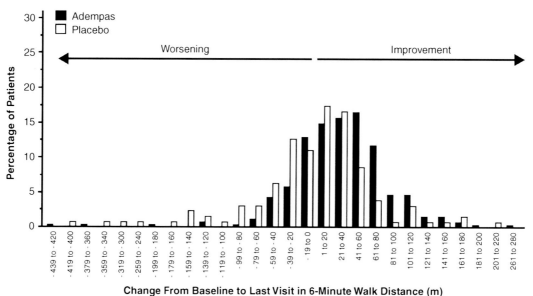

Fig. 17.2 Distribution of change in 6MWD for patients with PAH receiving riociguat in the PATENT-1 study (From the ADEMPAS monograph [5]; reproduced with permission of Bayer). Of the patients who received riociguat, 76 % experienced an improvement in 6MWD, and 24 % experienced a decrease in 6MWD

sequential combination therapy has a strong biologic and practical rationale.

Clinical Evidence in Support of Sequential Combination Therapy

To date, 14 double-blind randomized clinical trials investigating the use of combination therapy in PAH have been published. Thirteen of these studies investigated the use of medications added sequentially (Table 17.1). In these studies, sequential addition of therapy was typically performed

in the context of background PAH-specific therapy, with the exception of Iversen and colleagues, who assessed the effect of non-selective endothelin receptor antagonist therapy initiation with bosentan, followed by randomization of patients to placebo or sildenafil in a cross-over design [10].

In 3 of the 13 studies (EARLY [7], SERAPHIN [8], and PHIRST [11]), only a subset of the subjects enrolled were on background therapy. (In addition, in the imatinib phase 2 study, one patient was on calcium-channel blocker therapy alone [12].) The primary outcome in these trials was time to clinical worsening [TTCW] for SERAPHIN, and 6MWD for the remaining trials. As the overall sample size in each study

Table 17.1 Summary of results of clinical trials investigating sequential, goal-directed therapy

Study	Trial design	Number of patients	Number of weeks	Primary outcome	Subgroup on background therapy outcome
EARLY [7]	DB-RCT[a]: bosentan vs placebo; 16 % of patients on sildenafil	185	24	6MWD[b]: placebo-adjusted bosentan +19.1 m; P=0.08	Subgroup on sildenafil placebo-adjusted 6MWD: −17.3 m (P=0.85); placebo-adjusted PVR: −22.6 %; P=0.0478
SERAPHIN [8]	DB-RCT: macitentan vs placebo; 62 % on PDE5i, 5 % on inh prostacyclin	742	100	TTCW[c]: HR 0.70 for 3 mg macitentan (P=0.01); HR 0.55 for 10 mg macitentan (P<0.001)	Subgroup on background therapy: TTCW: HR 0.83 for 3 mg macitentan (P=0.27); HR 0.62 for 10 mg macitentan (P=0.009)
PACES [9]	DB-RCT: sildenafil vs. placebo; all on intravenous epoprostenol	264	16	6MWD: Placebo adjusted +28.8 m (P<0.001)	*All on background therapy by trial design*
Iversen [10]	DB-RCT: all received bosentan; 3 months later 1:1 placebo or sildenafil; 3 months later cross-over to other group	20	12	6MWD: bosentan alone +37 m (P=0.001); placebo-adjusted addition of sildenafil: +13 m (P=0.48)	*All on background therapy by trial design*
PHIRST [11]	DB-RCT: tadalafil vs placebo; 53 % on background bosentan	405	16	6MWD: placebo-adjusted tadalafil 20 mg +23 m (P=0.09); tadalafil 40 mg +44 m (P<0.01)	Subgroup on bosentan background therapy: 6MWD placebo-adjusted 40 mg dose +33 m (P=0.09)
Imatinib Phase 2 [12]	DB-RCT: imatinib vs placebo; 21 % on mono-background therapy; 65 % on dual-background therapy; 14 % on triple-background therapy	59	24	(Phase 2) 6MWD: placebo adjusted +23 m (P=0.21)	All but 1 on background therapy; outcome by number of background medications not reported.
IMPRES [13]	DB-RCT: imatinib vs placebo; 59 % on dual-background therapy; 41 % on triple background therapy	202	24	6MWD: placebo-adjusted +32 m (P=0.002)	*All on background therapy by trial design*
STEP [14]	DB-RCT: iloprost vs. placebo; on background bosentan	67	12	6MWD: placebo-adjusted +26 m (P=0.051)	*All on background therapy by trial design*
COMBI [15]	DB-RCT: iloprost vs. placebo; on background bosentan	40	12	6MWD: placebo-adjusted -10 m (P=0.49)	*All on background therapy by trial design*
TRIUMPH [16]	DB-RCT: inh treprostinil vs placebo; 70 % on background bosentan and 30 % on sildenafil	235	12	6MWD: placebo-adjusted +20 m (P<0.001)	*All on background therapy by trial design*
FREEDOM-C1 [17]	DB-RCT: po treprostinil vs. placebo; 57 % on mono-background therapy; 43 % on dual-background therapy	354	16	6MWD: placebo-adjusted +11 m (P=0.07)	*All on background therapy by trial design*
FREEDOM-C2 [18]	DB-RCT: po treprostinil vs. placebo; 59 % on mono-background therapy; 41 % on dual-background therapy	310	16	6MWD: placebo-adjusted +10 m (P=0.089)	*All on background therapy by trial design*
Selexipag Phase 2 [19]	DB-RCT: po selexipag vs placebo; 65 % mono-background therapy, 35 % dual-background therapy	43	17	(Phase 2) PVR[d]: placebo-adjusted −30.3 % (P=0.0045)	*All on background therapy by trial design*

[a]*DB-RCT* double-blind, randomized clinical trial
[b]*6MWD* 6 min walk distance
[c]*TTCW* time to clinical worsening
[d]*PVR* pulmonary vascular resistance

was powered for the primary outcome, subgroup analyses of subjects on background therapy were statistically underpowered.

Overall, of the eleven phase 3 clinical trials investigating sequential addition of combination therapies, five demonstrated a statistically significant improvement for the primary end point in the intervention group. One of the notable positive studies was the SERAPHIN trial, in which the subgroup of subjects on background therapy with sildenafil and/or inhaled or oral prostacyclin had a significant improvement in the TTCW when treated with the addition of 10 mg of macitentan, as compared to the addition of placebo (HR 0.62; P=0.009) [8].

The negative trials included the study by Iversen and colleagues, in which bosentan alone resulted in a significant clinical benefit, but the addition of sildenafil did not result in a further significant benefit as compared to the addition of placebo [10]. Only 1 of the 13 studies investigating sequential addition of combination therapy suggested possible harm from this approach: the COMBI study, which was terminated early after the addition of iloprost to patients on background therapy with bosentan resulted in a decline in 10 m relative to the addition of placebo (P=0.49) [15]. Notably, in that study, the negative results were driven almost entirely by the poor outcome of three subjects in the intervention group.

In summary, the preponderance of data of these prospective, randomized clinical trials demonstrates a clear and consistent signal indicating modest, but significant benefit associated with sequential addition of PAH therapy in appropriate circumstances. It is, therefore, appropriate that the most recent expert consensus algorithm for the treatment of PAH, from the 2013 World Symposium on Pulmonary Hypertension (Nice, France), assigned a Class 1 ("evidence and/or general agreement that a given treatment or procedure is beneficial, useful, effective") status with an "A" level of evidence ("data derived from multiple randomized clinical trials or meta-analyses") to the sequential addition of combination therapy to meet clinical goals [20].

Absence of Clinical Evidence in Support of Up-Front Combination Therapy

At the present time, the BREATHE-2 [21] trial is the only placebo-controlled randomized clinical trial designed to compare directly up-front combination therapy vs. monotherapy, and two additional non-randomized studies have been reported and are summarized collectively in Table 17.2.

In the BREATHE-2 trial, each of 33 PAH subjects were initiated on continuously infused intravenous prostacyclin therapy with epoprostenol [21]. In addition, 22 of these subjects were also initiated on bosentan (62.5 mg twice daily for 4 weeks and then increased to 125 mg twice daily thereafter)

vs. placebo for 11 subjects. The subjects were followed for 16 weeks total. In the combination therapy group, there were 4 withdrawals (18 %): 2 deaths, 1 clinical worsening (that subsequently died), and 1 adverse event (elevated hepatic transaminases). In comparison, there was one withdrawal (9 %) in the monotherapy group (elevated hepatic transaminases). The prespecificied primary outcome was total pulmonary resistance (TPR; mean pulmonary artery pressure divided by cardiac output). The TPR decreased by 22.6 % in the monotherapy group and 36.3 % in the combination therapy group (P=0.08). Between the two groups, there were no significant differences in other hemodynamic parameters between baseline and week 16 (including cardiac index, mean PA pressure, and pulmonary vascular resistance), 6 min walk distance (+68 m in combination therapy group vs. +74 m in the epoprostenol monotherapy group), or WHO functional class.

The higher withdrawal rate in the BREATHE-2 combination therapy group reinforces the concept that initiating multiple medications simultaneously may mask harm of one or more medications. Overall, it is reasonable to expect that in aggregate there will be additional benefit from multiple vasodilator medications (as suggested by a trend towards decreased TPR in BREATH-2), but care of individualized patients is optimized by the recognition of benefit and side effects of each medication in their regimen.

There have been several smaller, retrospective or non-controlled prospective trials assessing up-front combination therapy. Kemp and colleagues retrospectively analyzed 23 subjects initiated on epoprostenol plus bosentan, and compared their therapeutic response to 46 matched historical controls treated with epoprostenol alone [22]. Performance on the 6MWD improved by +134 m in the combination therapy group compared to +148 m in the historical intravenous epoprostenol subjects. The authors reported no worse side effects in the combination therapy group.

Bergot and colleagues reported findings from a prospective, non-randomized, observational series of 43 treatment-naïve subjects, initiated on epoprostenol monotherapy (N=17) or dual therapy with epoprostenol plus oral treatment (N=26) [endothelin receptor antagonist (N=16); PDE-5 (N=1); or both ERA and PDE-5 (N=9)] [23]. After 4 months of treatment, the hemodynamics improved more in the heterogeneously-treated combination therapy group (particularly the cardiac index: +1.5 versus +0.9 $L \cdot min^{-1} \ m^{-2}$; P=0.03). The 6MWD improved slightly more in the combination therapy group (+156 m versus +132 m), but this was not statistically significant, and no significant difference in transplant-free survival was observed between the two groups.

Aside from the nine patients on triple combination therapy in Bergot et al. [23] discussed above, Sitbon and colleagues also tested a protocol of up-front triple combination therapy. In this study, subjects were simultaneously initiated on intravenous epoprostenol, oral sildenafil, and oral

Table 17.2 Summary of results of clinical trials (with a comparison control group) investigating up front combination therapy

Study	Trial design	Number of patients	Duration	Primary outcome[a]
BREATHE-2 [21]	DB-RCT[b]: All started on epoprostenol, as well as Bosentan vs placebo	33	12 weeks	TPR[c]: placebo-adjusted −13.7 % (P=0.08)
Kemp [22]	Retrospective: bosentan + epoprostenol vs. epoprostenol alone	69	Mean 30 months follow up	Transplant-free survival: P=0.15; overall survival P=0.07
Bergot [23]	Retrospective: epoprostenol alone vs. epoprostenol + other oral therapy	43	Median 24 months follow up	4 months cardiac index: control adjusted +0.6 L/min/m^2 (P=0.03)

[a]Pre-specified only for double-blind, randomized clinical trials
[b]*DB-RCT* double-blind, randomized clinical trial
[c]*TPR* total pulmonary resistance (mean pulmonary artery pressure divided by cardiac output)

bosentan (n = 19), without comparison to a control group [24]. One subject underwent early heart-lung transplantation, but the other 18 subjects survived at a mean follow-up of 32 months (transplant-free survival 94 %). By the end of follow up, two of the patients had discontinued bosentan due to elevated hepatic transaminases.

Due to this insufficient, or at best equivocal, clinical trial data regarding up-front combination therapy, this approach earned a Class IIb ("usefulness/efficacy is less well established by evidence/opinion") designation with a "C" level of evidence ("consensus of opinion of the experts and/or small studies, retrospective studies, registries") in the most recent treatment guidelines [20]. In the treatment algorithm, it is suggested the up-front combination therapy be considered primarily in patients presenting with WHO functional class 3 or 4 symptoms when intravenous epoprostenol treatment is unavailable or declined due to patient preference. However, this is clearly a sub-optimal approach, as intravenous epoprostenol holds a 1A recommendation for both WHO functional classes 3 and 4.

Limitation of Sequential Goal-Directed Therapy: What's the Goal?

A major limitation to the sequential addition of combination therapy in a goal-directed approach is the lack of consensus regarding appropriate therapeutic goals. This uncertainty was highlighted in the recent consensus document on treatment goals from the 2013 Nice symposium [25]. Parameters that can be used include WHO functional class improvement, 6-min walk distance, cardiopulmonary exercise test performance, decreased B-type natriuretic peptide (BNP) concentration, or improvements to right heart function and/ or hemodynamics assessed by echocardiography, cardiac MRI, or right heart catheterization. However, it is unclear which one or combination of these parameters is most appropriate, and, furthermore, the specific goals for each parameter are also unresolved. One parameter target that is fairly

clear is the WHO functional class: patients who start in functional class 3 have a significantly improved prognosis if their functional class improves to 1 or 2 [26].

A second limitation of the sequential treatment strategy relates to methods for optimizing drug dose up titration as well as timing and class selection of add-on medications. For example, the optimal rate of dose escalation probably varies according to class, and may depend on the PAH etiology. The frequency of clinical visits for sequential treatment patients should be similar to that required for up-front combination therapy patients, to monitor clinical response and assess for side effects of therapy with either approach.

Conclusions

There is significant biologic rationale, practical experience, and clinical evidence in support of sequential addition of combination therapy in a goal-directed approach, while the evidence in support of up-front combination therapy is relatively limited and equivocal. The strength of the evidence supporting these two possible approaches is best summarized by the relative recommendations from the 2013 Nice World Symposium treatment algorithm: IA for sequential therapy if failing or inadequate response to monotherapy, versus IIbC for up-front combination therapy [20]. Pending future clinical trial results (notably the AMBITION trial [ClinicalTrials.gov NCT01178073], which is a randomized, double-blind, multicenter study of first-line combination therapy with ambrisentan alone *vs.* tadalafil alone *vs.* ambrisentan plus tadalafil therapy in patients with PAH), the current treatment approach should clearly be sequential, goal-directed therapy.

References

1. Provencher S, Jais X, Yaici A, Sitbon O, Humbert M, Simonneau G. Clinical challenges in pulmonary hypertension: Roger S. Mitchell lecture. Chest. 2005;128(6 Suppl):622S–8.
2. Sitbon O, Simonneau G. Optimal management of severe pulmonary arterial hypertension. Eur Respir Rev. 2011;20(122):254–61.

3. Bozic I, Reiter JG, Allen B, Antal T, Chatterjee K, Shah P, et al. Evolutionary dynamics of cancer in response to targeted combination therapy. Elife. 2013;2, e00747.

4. Richman DD, Havlir D, Corbeil J, Looney D, Ignacio C, Spector SA, et al. Nevirapine resistance mutations of human immunodeficiency virus type 1 selected during therapy. J Virol. 1994;68(3):1660–6.

5. ADEMPAS Monograph. Located at http://www.bayer.ca/files/ADEMPAS-PM-ENG-07APR2014-163446.pdf. Accessed 26 July 2014

6. Ghofrani HA, Galie N, Grimminger F, Grunig E, Humbert M, Jing ZC, et al. Riociguat for the treatment of pulmonary arterial hypertension. N Engl J Med. 2013;369(4):330–40.

7. Galie N, Rubin L, Hoeper M, Jansa P, Al-Hiti H, Meyer G, et al. Treatment of patients with mildly symptomatic pulmonary arterial hypertension with bosentan (EARLY study): a double-blind, randomised controlled trial. Lancet. 2008;371(9630):2093–100.

8. Pulido T, Adzerikho I, Channick RN, Delcroix M, Galie N, Ghofrani HA, et al. Macitentan and morbidity and mortality in pulmonary arterial hypertension. N Engl J Med. 2013;369(9):809–18.

9. Simonneau G, Rubin LJ, Galie N, Barst RJ, Fleming TR, Frost AE, et al. Addition of sildenafil to long-term intravenous epoprostenol therapy in patients with pulmonary arterial hypertension: a randomized trial. Ann Intern Med. 2008;149(8):521–30.

10. Iversen K, Jensen AS, Jensen TV, Vejlstrup NG, Sondergaard L. Combination therapy with bosentan and sildenafil in Eisenmenger syndrome: a randomized, placebo-controlled, double-blinded trial. Eur Heart J. 2010;31(9):1124–31.

11. Galie N, Brundage BH, Ghofrani HA, Oudiz RJ, Simonneau G, Safdar Z, et al. Tadalafil therapy for pulmonary arterial hypertension. Circulation. 2009;119(22):2894–903.

12. Ghofrani HA, Morrell NW, Hoeper MM, Olschewski H, Peacock AJ, Barst RJ, et al. Imatinib in pulmonary arterial hypertension patients with inadequate response to established therapy. Am J Respir Crit Care Med. 2010;182(9):1171–7.

13. Hoeper MM, Barst RJ, Bourge RC, Feldman J, Frost AE, Galie N, et al. Imatinib mesylate as add-on therapy for pulmonary arterial hypertension: results of the randomized IMPRES study. Circulation. 2013;127(10):1128–38.

14. McLaughlin VV, Oudiz RJ, Frost A, Tapson VF, Murali S, Channick RN, et al. Randomized study of adding inhaled iloprost to existing bosentan in pulmonary arterial hypertension. Am J Respir Crit Care Med. 2006;174(11):1257–63.

15. Hoeper MM, Leuchte H, Halank M, Wilkens H, Meyer FJ, Seyfarth HJ, et al. Combining inhaled iloprost with bosentan in patients with idiopathic pulmonary arterial hypertension. Eur Respir J. 2006;28(4):691–4.

16. McLaughlin VV, Benza RL, Rubin LJ, Channick RN, Voswinckel R, Tapson VF, et al. Addition of inhaled treprostinil to oral therapy for pulmonary arterial hypertension: a randomized controlled clinical trial. J Am Coll Cardiol. 2010;55(18):1915–22.

17. Tapson VF, Torres F, Kermeen F, Keogh AM, Allen RP, Frantz RP, et al. Oral treprostinil for the treatment of pulmonary arterial hypertension in patients on background endothelin receptor antagonist and/or phosphodiesterase type 5 inhibitor therapy (the FREEDOM-C study): a randomized controlled trial. Chest. 2012;142(6):1383–90.

18. Tapson VF, Jing ZC, Xu KF, Pan L, Feldman J, Kiely DG, et al. Oral treprostinil for the treatment of pulmonary arterial hypertension in patients receiving background endothelin receptor antagonist and phosphodiesterase type 5 inhibitor therapy (the FREEDOM-C2 study): a randomized controlled trial. Chest. 2013;144(3):952–8.

19. Simonneau G, Torbicki A, Hoeper MM, Delcroix M, Karlocai K, Galie N, et al. Selexipag: an oral, selective prostacyclin receptor agonist for the treatment of pulmonary arterial hypertension. Eur Respir J. 2012;40(4):874–80.

20. Galie N, Corris PA, Frost A, Girgis RE, Granton J, Jing ZC, et al. Updated treatment algorithm of pulmonary arterial hypertension. J Am Coll Cardiol. 2013;62(25 Suppl):D60–72.

21. Humbert M, Barst RJ, Robbins IM, Channick RN, Galie N, Boonstra A, et al. Combination of bosentan with epoprostenol in pulmonary arterial hypertension: BREATHE-2. Eur Respir J. 2004;24(3):353–9.

22. Kemp K, Savale L, O'Callaghan DS, Jais X, Montani D, Humbert M, et al. Usefulness of first-line combination therapy with epoprostenol and bosentan in pulmonary arterial hypertension: an observational study. J Heart Lung Transplant. 2012;31(2):150–8.

23. Bergot E, Sitbon O, Cottin V, Prevot G, Canuet M, Bourdin A, et al. Current epoprostenol use in patients with severe idiopathic, heritable or anorexigen-associated pulmonary arterial hypertension: data from the French pulmonary hypertension registry. Int J Cardiol. 2014;172(3):561–7.

24. Sitbon O, Jais X, Savale L, Cottin V, Bergot E, Macari EA, et al. Upfront triple combination therapy in pulmonary arterial hypertension: a pilot study. Eur Respir J. 2014;43(6):1691–7.

25. McLaughlin VV, Gaine SP, Howard LS, Leuchte HH, Mathier MA, Mehta S, et al. Treatment goals of pulmonary hypertension. J Am Coll Cardiol. 2013;62(25 Suppl):D73–81.

26. Barst RJ, Chung L, Zamanian RT, Turner M, McGoon MD. Functional class improvement and 3-year survival outcomes in patients with pulmonary arterial hypertension in the REVEAL Registry. Chest. 2013;144(1):160–8.

Determining the Optimal Approach to Initiating Oral, Inhaled, and Intravenous Therapies in Clinical Practice: Maximal Upfront Therapy Is Best

Victor F. Tapson

Introduction and Current Approaches to Therapy

Therapy for pulmonary artery hypertension (PAH) has evolved over the past two decades. While the prognosis for some PAH patients (e.g., congenital heart disease) is better than for others (e.g., scleroderma), we should still consider PAH a nearly uniformly fatal disease.

Many would argue that parenteral prostanoid therapy, the first class of PAH therapy to be FDA-approved in the U.S., remains the most effective form of therapy for patients with PAH, particularly those with advanced disease. This is based in large part upon the prospective, randomized, study of idiopathic PAH (IPAH) comparing epoprostenol to conventional therapy published in 1996, which demonstrated improved mortality with a total of only 81 patients and in a study that was conducted over only 12 weeks [1]. No study this size over such a short duration has demonstrated such results since that time. In spite of these results, and because other effective and more convenient pharmacotherapies have become available, aggressive parenteral prostanoid therapy is currently reserved for the sickest PAH patients; i.e., those with advanced functional class (FC) III or IV symptoms, very poor right ventricular (RV) function as evidenced by symptoms, signs, echocardiographic findings, and right-heart catheterization results demonstrating a very low cardiac index and high right atrial pressure. Patients with IPAH on this "best" therapy alone have been shown to have a 3-year survival of only about 63 % [2, 3], although this was in the monotherapy era. Even with improved survival suggested in scleroderma PAH based on recent registry data

(1-, 2-, and 3-year cumulative survival rates of 93 %, 88 %, and 75 %, respectively), a mortality of one in four patients at 3 years is *unacceptable* [4]. Current "aggressive therapy" consists of initiating parenteral prostanoid therapy, perhaps adding sildenafil several months later and subsequently adding additional therapies if certain goals are not met. This approach is clearly inadequate.

Reluctance to use potent parenteral prostanoids as initial therapy (except in advanced cases) is based upon the efficacy and ease of oral PAH therapies approved since the advent of epoprostenol (albeit with no solid proven mortality benefit), and the perceived potential adverse effects, expense, and inconvenience of chronic parenteral therapy. Goal-oriented therapy has become a "buzz phrase" in PAH [5]. In fact, we included a specific section on "Treatment Goals in PAH" in the NICE WSPH guidelines [6]. Although the primarily observational studies reviewed in these guidelines did not allow for definitive conclusions, we felt that reasonable goals of therapy included: (1) modified New York Heart Association (NYHA) FC I or II, (2) echocardiography/magnetic resonance imaging demonstrating normal/near-normal RV size and function, (3) hemodynamic parameters showing normalization of RV function (mean right atrial pressure <8 mmHg and cardiac index >2.5–3.0 l/min/m^2, (4) 6MWD of >380–440 m, (5) cardiopulmonary exercise testing, including peak oxygen consumption >15 ml/min/kg and ventilator equivalent for carbon dioxide <45 l/min/l/min, and (6) normal brain natriuretic peptide (BNP) levels [6]. Patients achieving these goals, regardless of the specific therapy or approach used, appear to have a better prognosis than those who do not. In the Nice document, we suggested that "a more aggressive approach to goal-oriented therapy may help us shift the survival curves farther to the right." So, a more fundamental question might be: Should we consider an even *more* aggressive approach to therapy that *does not wait to see if initial goals are achieved? Should we be offering upfront, multi-agent "induction" therapy?* Based upon the potential benefit and the relatively low risk, I believe we should.

V.F. Tapson, MD, FCCP, FRCP
Pulmonary and Critical Care Division, Clinical Research for the Women's Guild Lung Institute, Cedars-Sinai Medical Center, Los Angeles, CA, USA

Cedars-Sinai Medical Center, LeDoux Building, 8536 Wilshire Blvd Suite 201, Beverly Hills, CA 90211, USA
e-mail: victor.tapson@cshs.org

© Springer International Publishing Switzerland 2016
B.A. Maron et al. (eds.), *Pulmonary Hypertension: Basic Science to Clinical Medicine*, DOI 10.1007/978-3-319-23594-3_18

Aggressive, Upfront Therapy:
Why We Need It

One argument for aggressive, upfront parenteral "induction" therapy in this disease involves consideration of the cancer model of PAH pathobiology. Many have suggested the common features of IPAH and malignancy [7, 8]. The cancer paradigm has been characterized as integrating certain specific cancer-defining mechanisms. These include angiogenesis, loss of apoptosis, a self-sufficient growth signaling system, insensitivity to *anti*growth signals, tissue invasion and metastasis, and unlimited replicative potential [9]. For example, the balance of anti-apoptotic and pro-apoptotic factors may be upset, with damaged cells continuing to replicate in spite of being programmed to die.

The lesions in IPAH are angiogenic. They do not possess apoptotic cells [10–12], and antiapoptotic proteins are expressed in the abnormal pulmonary vasculature. While the lesions in PAH are not truly neoplastic, they clearly have malignant characteristics in that there is a process of uncontrolled cellular proliferation. The precise therapy for *bona fide* malignancy hinges on the specific tumor type and extent, but there are general approaches. Neither surgical resection, nor radiation therapy apply to PAH but chemotherapy has a valid analogy in PAH. In advanced non-small cell lung cancer (NSCLC), for example, standard first-line chemotherapy (i.e. induction therapy) with four to six cycles of platinum-based chemotherapy results in a modest increase in survival and improvement in cancer-related symptoms [13]. With chemotherapy, long-term survival for patients with advanced NSCLC is still poor, with mortality rates of 95 % reported at 5 years. Thus, aggressive, potentially toxic therapy is standard care with certain malignancies, with subsequent consideration given to longer-term chemotherapy [13, 14].

In NSCLC, two effective single-agent maintenance strategies evolved, including continuation maintenance therapy and switch maintenance therapy. Continuation maintenance is the continuation of one or more drugs used in the induction regimen. Switch maintenance introduces an additional agent immediately after completion of four to six cycles of induction chemotherapy. Both strategies were shown to improve progression-free survival and/or overall survival for patients with stable/responsive disease after completion of induction chemotherapy. We already utilize "continuation maintenance." Should we consider switch strategies or more likely, "addition strategies" earlier in the treatment schedule for PAH patients?

Mortality with NSCLC is higher than for PAH, justifying aggressive toxic induction therapy which includes adverse effects such as nausea, vomiting, alopecia, anemia, febrile neutropenia, thrombocytopenia, nephrotoxicity, and sensory neuropathy. Adverse effects of chemotherapy are potentially fatal [14]. The adverse effects even with our most aggressive PAH therapies are very rarely life-threatening, although it is inconvenient to have continuous intravenous therapy.

It should be emphasized, that prostacyclins have antiproliferative effects. Aggressive upfront "induction" therapy for PAH would be markedly less toxic than that offered in NSCLC. We have three pathways, the prostanoid pathway, the nitric oxide pathway, and the endothelin pathway which have proven to be crucial in the pathophysiology of PAH. We have shown in large, well-designed, prospective randomized trials that these drugs are effective [15]. There is essentially no toxic death rate. Adverse effects are addressed with dose reduction or discontinuation of a drug with institution of another one. *So why don't we utilize "induction therapy?"*

We try our best in medicine to be evidence based. We want data. We have an expanding evidence base in PAH therapy, which has moved into the realm of combination therapy. We have learned that combinations of PAH therapies when added in sequence, may be more effective than single agents in certain settings, although some such combination studies have not proven beneficial. Difficulty proving benefit may be due to inadequate doses of a drug, or inadequate time on the therapy being tested. Or, it could be that certain combinations of drugs are simply not synergistic or even additive with regard to clinical benefit. Furthermore, PAH medications are expensive. Triple therapy aimed at the prostanoid, nitric oxide, and endothelin pathways could cost well over $200,000 per year. It may, however, be feasible that upfront combination therapy, if beneficial, could lower the cost of long-term therapy, and perhaps reduce hospitalizations. Thus, an induction therapy approach could be more or less expensive. We cannot be certain without data.

Maximal upfront combination therapy has not been studied. Upfront aggressive therapy with prostanoid therapy has generally been the standard of care for severe PAH characterized by a high mean right atrial pressure and very low cardiac index. Based on the data from the PACES trial, adding sildenafil to parenteral epoprostenol therapy in PAH proved an effective strategy, but the sildenafil was added to long-term intravenous epoprostenol therapy (on infusion at least 3 months, and with a stable dose for at least 4 weeks before randomization. Patients with a 6-min walk distance less than 100 m or greater than 450 m or those whose 6-min walk distance was affected by conditions other than PAH were excluded. Thus, this study, which showed benefit, was clearly not as aggressive as an upfront induction-type approach would have been [16].

Another recently-completed study offers insight. The preliminary data available thus far from the AMBITION trial suggest that combination upfront therapy, even *without* including a prostanoid, may be beneficial in treatment-naïve patients with PAH. The results of this international, prospective, randomized, double-blind trial were presented at the European Respiratory Society meeting in September 2014

[17]. Prior to the results of AMBITION, preclinical studies in a rat model had demonstrated that ambrisentan and tadalafil act synergistically to relax endothelin-1-constricted pulmonary arteries, and suggested that the endothelial ET_B receptor is required for this synergism [18].

The study design for AMBITION included three arms. Five hundred patients were randomized (2:1:1) to receive the ambrisentan and tadalafil combination upfront (n = 253) or monotherapy with ambrisentan (n = 126) or tadalafil (n = 121), titrated from 5 to 10 mg once-daily and from 20 to 40 mg once-daily for ambrisentan and tadalafil, respectively. It should be understood that "upfront" did not mean the drugs were initiated within a few days or even a few weeks of each other. They were initiated much more slowly, but addition of the second therapy was part of the protocol, and was added in all patients. It was not based upon, for example, a poor walk distance or echocardiogram result.

The primary endpoint was time to first clinical failure event and the combination arm showed superiority compared with the monotherapy arms. The length of time before patients experienced clinical failure was significantly prolonged for those receiving first-line combination compared to monotherapy. The risk of clinical failure was reduced by 50 % compared with the *pooled* ambrisentan and tadalafil monotherapy arm (hazard ratio = 0.502; p = 0.0002). The combination was also statistically significant versus the *individual* ambrisentan and tadalafil monotherapy arms for the primary endpoint of time to first clinical failure event. Three secondary endpoints also showed statistically significant improvements in this trial, including 6 min walk distance, percentage of patients with satisfactory clinical response, and change from baseline in BNP. The remaining two secondary endpoints (FC and Borg dyspnea index) did not meet statistical significance. Rates of serious adverse events and events leading to study discontinuation were similar across the treatment arms. Thus, we now have data that starting two non-prostanoid therapies at once is beneficial in PAH, and this was proven using a time to first clinical failure event endpoint [17].

Thus, it would appear that patients with PAH could potentially benefit from even more aggressive upfront therapy, utilizing each of our three lines of therapy; i.e., w*hy not add an upfront prostanoid?* And how would such a protocol look and how would it be instituted?

Ideally, every PAH patient receiving aggressive, upfront therapy would first undergo right-heart catheterization and vasodilator testing. This would ensure that vasodilator responders would have the option of also receiving calcium channel blocker therapy, since such responders have been shown to have better outcomes on this therapy than nonresponders. Volume status would be optimized prior to this procedure. Patients would not have the entire "induction therapy" regimen started the same day. Enough time would be allowed to characterize obvious early adverse effects such as severe headache, nausea, lightheadedness, cough, hypotension, etc. Drugs would be introduced sequentially, but quickly. An example of a potential induction therapy approach is offered in Fig. 18.1.

The initial drug offered might be the parenteral prostanoid, followed by two additional oral agents. First, a phosphodiesterase inhibitor (PDE-5I) or soluble guanylate cyclase stimulator, could be added, followed by an endothelin receptor antagonist (ERA) or *vice versa*. These would ideally be spaced by at least 3 days to allow for assessment of adverse effects. The three drugs would be initiated over a period of 7–10 days as adverse effects permitted. Based upon the AMBITION trial, it would appear logical to include tadalafil and ambristentan as the PDE-5I and ERA, respectively. Some might argue that based on the success of the SERAPHIN study that macitentan would be a good ERA candidate [19]. Still, others might argue that based upon expense and the efficacy of bosentan, that this drug (generic in November 2015, and thus cheaper) would be appropriate.

Inpatient versus outpatient initiation of the parenteral prostanoid would generally be in the hospital, although it is feasible that an experienced PH center with adequate infrastructure and personnel, could accomplish this protocol in the outpatient clinic setting, except in more advanced cases. Finally, the parenteral prostanoid could be initiated after oral therapy, although initiation and tolerance of the prostanoid might be deemed more crucial especially in advanced cases.

How long would parenteral prostanoid therapy be continued? In patients with less severe PAH, for example, slow weaning of the IV prostanoid could be initiated after 6 months, so that a patient would be off of the IV therapy in 9 months. There are several potential permutations that could be applied with such an aggressive upfront approach.

One approach in patients that would not ordinarily be considered advanced enough to be treated aggressively with IV prostanoid therapy would be to treat for 6 months and then, based upon certain criteria, wean the prostanoid off. This would be a true, albeit prolonged "induction" therapy approach. There are a number of potential permutations that could be applied with such an aggressive upfront approach.

What Are the Disadavantages of a Multiagent Induction Approach?

Adverse effects occur with all PAH therapies. Clearly however, benefit outweighs the risk when initiating single-agent PAH therapy, regardless of the class of drug. Patients are generally followed closely, and PAH drug doses are decreased or the drugs are discontinued if adverse effects are intolerable. Severe adverse effects leading to hospitalization, and particularly to death are distinctly unusual. Even when

Fig. 18.1 Example of a potential induction therapy protocol. If a similar protocol were to be transformed into a clinical trial, an additional arm could include dual oral therapy. A third arm could substitute inhaled therapy for intravenous therapy. *If severe PAH requiring hospital stay, then more prolonged observation/dose titration required in the inpatient setting. **Based upon AMBITION study (REF). †Either ambrisentan, based on AMBITION study, or macitentan, based upon recent SERAPHIN trial. *Abbreviations*: *PH* pulmonary hypertension, *PAH* pulmonary arterial hypertension, *IV* intravenous, *ERA* endothelin receptor antagonist, *IPAH* idiopathic PAH, *BNP* brain natriuretic peptide, *6MWD* 6-min walk distance, *RHC* right-heart catheterization

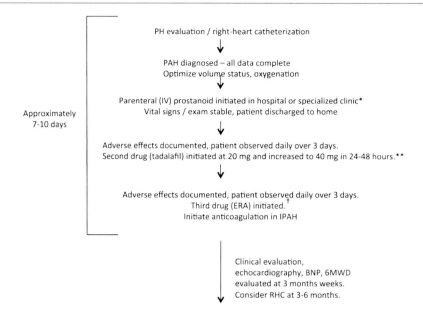

*If severe PAH requiring hospital stay, then more prolonged observation / dose titration required in the inpatient setting.
**Based upon AMBITION study (REF).
† Either ambrisentan, based on AMBITION study, or macitentan, based upon recent SERAPHIN trial.
Abbreviations: PH = pulmonary hypertension; PAH= pulmonary arterial hypertension; IV = intravenous; ERA = endothelin receptor antagonist; IPAH = idiopathic PAH; BNP = brain natriuretic peptide; 6MWD = six-minute walk distance; RHC = right-heart catheterization.

intravenous therapy is undertaken, fatal sepsis from line infections, or other severe line complications are rare when patients are treated by experts and followed closely [1, 20–24].

In the 81 patient, randomized, epoprostenol trial, 41 patients received this drug [1]. Adverse effects included jaw pain, diarrhea, flushing, headaches, nausea, and vomiting. Serious complications were usually due to the delivery system and included four episodes of nonfatal, catheter-related sepsis. There were 26 episodes of malfunction of the drug-delivery system resulting in temporary interruption of the infusion. These included occlusions, perforations, and dislodgements of the catheter and pump malfunction. When epoprostenol therapy was interrupted, patients experienced an increase in PAH symptoms. Irritation or infection at the catheter site occurred in seven patients, bleeding at the catheter site in four, and catheter-site pain in four. More than 20 years have passed since this study was initiated. PH centers now have substantial experience in preventing and addressing adverse effects.

More recently, we studied the transition from epoprostenol to IV treprostinil and found no serious adverse events that could be attributed to treprostinil [20]. When we examined *de novo* therapy with IV treprostinil, side effects were mild and consistent with those reported with prostacyclin treatment [21]. Finally, we conducted a long-term (48-week), multicenter, prospective, open-label, uncontrolled, study of continuous IV treprostinil in 16 patients on no prior PAH specific therapy at baseline and 31 patients transitioned at

baseline from IV epoprostenol [22]. During the study, 5 patients died of causes not considered related to the therapy, and 7 discontinued due to adverse events.

With regard to inhaled prostanoid therapy, common adverse effects following administration of inhaled treprostinil in the double-blind trial included cough (54 %), headache (41 %), nausea (19 %), flushing (15 %) and throat irritation (14 %) or pain (11 %) [23]. Over a 2-year treatment period in the TRIUMPH trial extension, adverse events resulting in drug discontinuation occurred in 19 % of patients; these included worsening PAH, cough, headache, throat discomfort and pneumonia [24].

A number of clinical trials have included a study drug and one or two background therapies, and while on multi-agent therapy an increase in adverse effects would be expected, these studies have shown that severe, life-threatening adverse events in patients on three PAH therapies including a parenteral or inhaled prostanoid would be appear to be unusual.

Clinical Protocol or Research Protocol?

Ideally, in any setting, when a novel therapeutic approach is considered, particularly when it involves added patient inconvenience or potential discomfort and expense, as much preparation and preliminary data collection should be undertaken as possible. A randomized trial comparing the above-described protocol with a standard goal-oriented approach would be ideal. Such a trial could be undertaken. In an ideal world, an additional arm could substitute an inhaled prostanoid arm (perhaps combined with an oral prostanoid; i.e., treprostinil) for the IV prostanoid. A second option would be to randomize less severely ill patients to the aggressive three-drug protocol, while proceeding with the protocol in more advanced cases of PAH who would ordinarily undergo upfront parenteral prostanoid therapy. That way, patients with more severe PAH would be getting the most aggressive therapy possible. Finally, once the data for oral prostanoid receptor agonists are available, it could be judged if such therapy could substitute for parenteral/inhaled prostanoid therapy in an upfront, multi-agent protocol perhaps reducing adverse effects and offering a more convenient approach.

In any setting in which randomization is not done, prospective data should at least be collected, either in the form of a pilot study, or as a long-term single-arm study in which detailed data are collected. There is always a concern that triple-combination therapy could conceivably have antagonistic effects, but this does not appear to be evident in the limited PH literature thus far.

Several studies have suggested that patients on background PAH therapy, however, may have less robust responses than patients who had been untreated when a new therapy was initiated [25, 26]. In the FREEDOM C study evaluating oral treprostinil, more than 40 % of patients were on both a PDE-5I and an ERA, and most of the remainder of the patients were on one or the other [27]. In this study, the primary end point (6MWD at week 16) did not achieve significance. Other possible explanations for this were the premature discontinuation of the study drug due to adverse events associated with higher-dose tablets. A 1-mg twice-daily dose of oral treprostinil is approximately equivalent to 10 ng/kg/min of infused treprostinil and dose increases of 0.5 or 1 mg were poorly tolerated by most patients [28–30]. No patient with access to the 0.25-mg tablets discontinued because of adverse events. In the follow-up study, FREEDOM C2, again essentially all patients were on either one or two background therapies, and again the primary endpoint was not met [30]. It is notable, however, that patients receiving oral treprostinil combined with background PDE-5I therapy were found to have approximately twice the 6MWD treatment effect (15.0 m) as those receiving background ERA therapy (7.7 m). This potential effect was *not*, however, demonstrated in patients receiving *both* ERA and PDE-5I background therapy (4.0 m). In FREEDOM C2, the 6MWD treatment effect tended to be greater in patients receiving a more recent diagnosis (28 m for patients with PAH diagnosed within the first year) than in patients with a longer disease duration (−2 m if the diagnosis was made ≥3.6 years prior to therapy). It is possible that these data reflect a survivor effect, with favorable responders to their current PAH therapy having less room for response to additional therapies. The patients who received intensive PAH-specific treatment

for a longer period could simply be less responsive to the addition of new therapy. While there is the possibility that earlier initiation of multi-agent PAH therapy could result in a patient "using up" their therapeutic options, there is no clear data clinical supporting this.

Finally, a small, retrospective, nonrandomized study of upfront triple combination therapy has been piloted in France. Sitbon, and colleagues, published data from 18 newly diagnosed functional class III and IV PAH patients initiated on upfront intravenous epoprostenol, bosentan and sildenafil [31]. Significant improvements in 6 min walk distance and hemodynamics were observed after 4 months of this triple therapy combination. This pilot study provides preliminary evidence of the potential for long-term benefit from upfront triple combination therapy in patients with severe PAH. A carefully thought out combination approach needs to now be studied in a randomized trial and should include patients with less advanced disease.

Conclusions

We have seen improvement in survival in PAH since the advent of therapy for this disease. However, the disease remains a fatal one and the current mortality rate remains unacceptable.

We need forward-thinking treatment approaches and when possible, the evidence base should be expanded with additional clinical trials. Unfortunately, acquisition of such data will take years. In the meantime, more patients will die. Aggressive, upfront "induction" therapy with triple therapy that includes parenteral prostanoid therapy should be considered in treatment naïve PAH patients. This is particularly true in the setting of clinically advanced disease.

References

1. Barst RJ, Rubin LJ, Long WA, McGoon MD, Rich S, Badesch DB, Groves BM, Tapson VF, Bourge RC, Brundage BH, Koerner SK, Langleben D, Keller CA, Murali S, Uretsky BF, Clayton LM, Jobsis MM, Blackburn SD, Shortino D, Crow JW. A comparison of continuous intravenous epoprostenol (prostacyclin) with conventional therapy for primary pulmonary hypertension. N Engl J Med. 1996;334:296–301.
2. Sitbon O, Humbert M, Nunes H, et al. Long-term intravenous epoprostenol infusion in primary pulmonary hypertension: prognostic factors and survival. J Am Coll Cardiol. 2002;40:780–8.
3. McLaughlin VV, Shillington A, Rich S. Survival in primary pulmonary hypertension: the impact of epoprostenol therapy. Circulation. 2002;106:1477–82.
4. Chung L, Domsic RT, Lingala B, Alkassab F, Bolster M, Csuka ME, Derk C, Fischer A, Frech T, Furst DE, Gomberg-Maitland M, Hinchcliff M, Hsu V, Hummers LK, Khanna D, Medsger Jr TA, Molitor JA, Preston IR, Schiopu E, Shapiro L, Silver R, Simms R, Varga J, Gordon JK, Steen VD. Survival and predictors of mortality in systemic sclerosis-associated pulmonary arterial hypertension: outcomes from the pulmonary hypertension assessment and

recognition of outcomes in scleroderma registry. Arthritis Care Res. 2014;66(3):489–95.

5. Hoeper MM, Markevych I, Spiekerkoetter E, Welte T, Niedermeyer J. Goal-oriented treatment and combination therapy for pulmonary arterial hypertension. Eur Respir J. 2005;26:858–63.

6. McLaughlin VV, Gaine SP, Howard LS, et al. Treatment goals in pulmonary arterial hypertension. JACC. 2013;62(25):D73–81.

7. Rai PR, Cool CD, King JAC, Stevens T, Burns N, Winn RA, Kasper M, Voelkel NF. The cancer paradigm of severe pulmonary arterial hypertension. Am J Respir Crit Care Med. 2008;178(6):558–64.

8. Voelkel NF, Cool C, Lee SD, Wright L, Geraci MW, Tuder RM. Primary pulmonary hypertension between inflammation and cancer. Chest. 1998;114:225S–30.

9. Hanahan D, Weinberg R. The hallmarks of cancer. Cell. 2000;100:57–70.

10. Levy M, Maurey C, Celermajer DS, Vouhe PR, Danel C, Bonnet D, Israel-Biet D. Impaired apoptosis of pulmonary endothelial cells is associated with intimal proliferation and irreversibility of pulmonary hypertension in congenital heart disease. J Am Coll Cardiol. 2007;49:803–10.

11. Yeager ME, Halley GR, Golpon HA, Voelkel NF, Tuder RM. Microsatellite instability of endothelial cell growth and apoptosis genes within plexiform lesions in primary pulmonary hypertension. Circ Res. 2001;88:E2–11.

12. McMurtry MS, Archer SL, Altieri DC, Bonnet S, Haromy A, Harry G, Bonnet S, Puttagunta L, Michelakis ED. Gene therapy targeting survivin selectively induces pulmonary vascular apoptosis and reverses pulmonary arterial hypertension. J Clin Invest. 2005;115:1479–91.

13. D'Addario G, Pintilie M, Leighl NB, Feld R, Cerny T, Shepherd FA. Platinum-based versus non-platinum-based chemotherapy in advanced non-small-cell lung cancer: a meta-analysis of the published literature. J Clin Oncol. 2005;23:2926–36.

14. Bahl A, Sharma DN, Julka PK, Rath GK. Chemotherapy related toxicity in locally advanced non-small cell lung cancer. Cancer Res Ther. 2006;2(1):14–6.

15. Galiè N, Corris PA, Frost A, Girgis RE, Granton J, Jing ZC, et al. Updated treatment algorithm of pulmonary arterial hypertension. J Am Coll Cardiol. 2013;62(25):D60–72.

16. Simonneau G, Rubin L, Galiè N, et al. Addition of sildenafil to longterm intravenous epoprostenol therapy in patients with pulmonary arterial hypertension. Ann Intern Med. 2008;149:521–30.

17. Galiè N, et al. AMBITION. European Respiratory Society. Munich; 2014 (Abstract #2916).

18. Liang F, Yang S, Yao L, Belardinelli L, Shryock J. Ambrisentan and tadalafil synergistically relax endothelin-induced contraction of rat pulmonary arteries. Hypertension. 2012;59(3):705–11.

19. Pulido T, Adzerikho I, Channick RN, et al. Macitentan and morbidity and mortality in pulmonary arterial hypertension. N Engl J Med. 2013;369:809–18.

20. Gomberg-Maitland M, Tapson VF, Benza RL, et al. Transition from intravenous epoprostenol to intravenous treprostinil in pulmonary hypertension. Am J Respir Crit Care Med. 2005;172(12):1586–9.

21. Tapson VF, Gomberg-Maitland M, McLaughlin VV, et al. Safety and efficacy of IV treprostinil for pulmonary arterial hypertension: a prospective, multicenter, open-label, 12-week trial. Chest. 2006;129(3):683–8.

22. Benza RL, Tapson VF, Gomberg-Maitland M, Poms A, Barst RJ, McLaughlin VV. One-year experience with intravenous treprostinil for pulmonary arterial hypertension. J Heart Lung Transplant. 2013;32(9):889–96.

23. McLaughlin VV, Benza RL, Rubin LJ, et al. Addition of inhaled treprostinil to oral therapy for pulmonary arterial hypertension: a randomized controlled clinical trial. J Am Coll Cardiol. 2010;55(18):1915–22.

24. Benza RL, Seeger W, McLaughlin VV, et al. Long-term effects of inhaled treprostinil in patients with pulmonary arterial hypertension: the Treprostinil Sodium Inhalation Used in the Management of Pulmonary Arterial Hypertension (TRIUMPH) study open-label extension. J Heart Lung Transplant. 2011;30(12):1327–33.

25. Galiè N, Brundage BH, Ghofrani HA, et al; Pulmonary Arterial Hypertension and Response to Tadalafil (PHIRST) Study Group. Tadalafil therapy for pulmonary arterial hypertension [published correction in Circulation. 2011;124(10):e279]. Circulation. 2009;119(22):2894–903.

26. McLaughlin VV, Oudiz RJ, Frost A, et al. Randomized study of adding inhaled iloprost to existing bosentan in pulmonary arterial hypertension. Am J Respir Crit Care Med. 2006;174(11):1257–63.

27. Tapson VF, Torres F, Kermeen F, Keogh AM, Allen RP, Frantz RP, Badesch DB, Frost AE, Shapiro SM, Laliberte K, Sigman J, Arneson C, Galiè N. Oral treprostinil for the treatment of pulmonary arterial hypertension in patients on background endothelin receptor antagonist and/or phosphodiesterase type 5 inhibitor therapy (the FREEDOM-C study): a randomized controlled trial. Chest. 2012;142(6):1383–90.

28. White RJ, Torres F, Allen R, Jerjes C, Pulido T, Yehle D, Howell M, Laliberte K, Marier JF, Tapson VF. Pharmacokinetics of oral treprostinil sustained release tablets during chronic administration to patients with pulmonary arterial hypertension. J Cardiovasc Pharmacol. 2013;61(6):474–81.

29. Wade M, Baker FJ, Roscigno R, DellaMaestra W, Hunt TL, Lai AA. Absolute bioavailability and pharmacokinetics of treprostinil sodium administered by acute subcutaneous infusion. J Clin Pharmacol. 2004;44(1):83–8.

30. Tapson VF, Jing ZC, Xu KF, Pan L, Feldman J, Kiely DG, Kotlyar E, McSwain CS, Laliberte K, Arneson C, Rubin LJ, FREEDOM-C2 Study Team. Oral treprostinil for the treatment of pulmonary arterial hypertension in patients receiving background endothelin receptor antagonist and phosphodiesterase type 5 inhibitor therapy (the FREEDOM-C2 study): a randomized controlled trial. Chest. 2013;144(3):952–8.

31. Sitbon O, Jaïs X, Savale L, Cottin V, Bergot E, Macari EA, Bouvaist H, Dauphin C, Picard F, Bulifon S, Montani D, Humbert M, Simonneau G. Upfront triple combination therapy in pulmonary arterial hypertension: a pilot study. Eur Respir J. 2014;43(6):1691–7.

Surgery, Devices, Transplantation and Other Interventional Options for the Treatment of Advanced Pulmonary Hypertension

Christian Bermudez and Balakrishnan Mahesh

Introduction

Pulmonary hypertension (PH) is a progressive disease characterized by high pulmonary arterial pressures. PH occurs as a result of multiple clinical conditions with differing histopathological abnormalities and clinical course depending on the etiology [1]. The cause of PH can also be multifactorial, presenting a diagnostic and management dilemma. Historically, a myriad of surgical options have been available and considered in the management of PH [2]. In this chapter, we will review current surgical techniques, including transplantation, thromboendarterectomy, mechanical circulatory support, and other interventional options used in patients with PH.

Classification of PH

The recently updated World Health Organization (WHO) classification of PH, put forth at the 5th World Symposium on Pulmonary Hypertension (Nice, France 2013), represents a valid attempt to classify patient phenotypes and assist clinicians in differentiating the diverse etiologies of PH [3]. It provides the ability to differentiate pulmonary arterial hypertension (PAH) from other forms of PH with different clinical manifestations and prognoses. Identifying the form of PH that is primarily responsible for the patient's clinical presentation is a priority when considering surgical interventions. Current treatment algorithms recommend certain medical and surgical interventions for specific WHO groups, while

C. Bermudez, MD (✉)
Division of Cardiovascular Surgery, Hospital of the University of Pennsylvania, 3400 Spruce Street, 6th Floor Silverstein, Philadelphia, PA 19104, USA
e-mail: christian.bermudez@uphs.upenn.edu

B. Mahesh, MD, FRCS, PhD
Division of Cardiothoracic Transplantation, Department of Cardiothoracic Surgery, University of Pittsburgh Presbyterian Medical Center, Pittsburgh, PA, USA

cautioning against the same interventions in other forms of PH [3].

Group 1 PH

Pulmonary arterial hypertension (PAH) is defined as group 1 PH. PAH develops as the result of vascular remodeling and proliferation that leads to increased pulmonary vascular resistance, right ventricular (RV) strain and hypertrophy, and eventually, over a prolonged period of time, RV failure [1, 2]. Patients with PAH have seen a notable improvement in the medical management of PAH over the last two decades, especially patients with idiopathic PAH (IPAH). Targeted therapies include prostacyclin analogs, endothelin receptor antagonists, phosphodiesterase-5 inhibitors, and soluble guanylate cyclase activators [3–9]. There is no doubt that the natural course of this disease has been altered by advances in medical management [8, 10]. Early and mid-term survival rates are *currently* 88 %, 73 % and 64 % at 1, 3 and 5 years, respectively, based on data from the Registry to Evaluate Early and Long-Term Pulmonary Arterial Hypertension Management (REVEAL) [11], a drastic improvement as compared with historical NIH data demonstrating survival of 68 % at 1 year, 48 % at 3 years, and 34 % at 5 years, with a median survival of 2.8 years [12]. However, the annual estimated mortality is still very high at 15 % [2, 3, 11, 12].

The relative success of medical treatments in patients with PAH and their relatively low urgency for transplantation as compared with patients listed for other disease processes relegated lung transplantation to consideration as a second-line therapeutic option. Frequently, patients are subjected to sequential combination therapies and are only referred for lung transplantation after failing maximal medical treatment. These patients typically present in advanced stages of their disease with significant multi-organ involvement in the presence of severe RV failure and arrhythmias [13]. There have been an increasing number of temporizing strategies to allow these patients a successful lung transplantation including percutaneous atrial septostomy (AS) and the use of mechanical circulatory support (MCS) including extracorporeal membrane oxygenation (ECMO), Novalung (Novalung GmbH, Germany), and most recently right ventricular assist devices (RVADs).

Group 2 PH

In patients with Group 2 PH, PH is secondary to left-sided heart disease. These patients have been offered different therapeutic strategies depending on the etiology of the PH. There is no specific treatment for Group 2 PH, and management focuses on treatment of the heart failure with the use of diuretics, beta-blockers, angiotensin-converting-enzyme (ACE) inhibitors, and occasionally intravenous inotropes [2]. Medications used in the management of PAH have shown either negative or neutral effects in patients with Group 2 PH [14–18]. Cardiac resynchronization therapy (CRT) has shown some potential benefit [19]. Group 2 PH is present in 6–12 % of patients with mitral stenosis and 25–30 % of patients with aortic stenosis, and established surgical interventions, including mitral valve and aortic valve repair and replacement, have been associated with improvements in the degree of PH. The effective prosthetic or residual valvular functional area is directly related to the reversibility of the PH in the vast majority of these patients [20, 21]. Heart valve repair and replacement can be performed using standard open techniques or percutaneous techniques with excellent outcomes and frequently with improvement in symptoms and signs of PH [22–24].

The presence of PH in patients with non-valvular left-sided heart failure has a negative impact in the patients' functional status and survival [25, 26]. In patients with a poor response to medical treatment, mechanical left ventricular support using left ventricular assist devices (LVADs), heart transplantation, and heart-lung transplantation have been considered viable alternatives. The use of LVADs has been associated with improvement of PH in 70–80 % of patients presenting with Group 2 PH and may permit heart transplantation following the improvement of PH observed after prolonged left ventricular unloading [27–30].

Group 3 PH

For more than two decades, lung transplantation has been considered an established treatment strategy for patients with advanced lung disease and PH (Group 3 PH). The presence of significant PH in this patient population may be associated with a more rapid progression of symptoms and decreased survival. There is no evidence that therapy directed at PH alters the course of the underlying lung disease. This is especially valid in patients with different types of fibrotic lung disease and chronic obstructive lung disease [31].

Group 4 PH

In cases of PH associated with thromboembolic disease (Group 4 PH), bilateral thromboendarterectomy (PTE) has become the standard of care for symptomatic patients with operable disease with excellent long-term outcomes [32–36]. Chronic thromboembolic pulmonary hypertension (CTEPH) is a chronic occlusive disease of the pulmonary arterial vasculature as a result of a single episode or recurrent episodes of venous thromboembolism that affects 0.5–3.8 % of patients presenting with an acute pulmonary embolism (PE); systolic pulmonary artery pressure (PAP) >50 mmHg at time of admission or discharge and large or bulky PE are predictors of CTEPH [37, 38].

Group 5 PH

Group 5 PH comprises PH caused by etiologies not classifiable into the other WHO groups. Patients with Group 5 PH are encountered infrequently. Lung transplantation is occasionally the only surgical treatment available.

Medical Management of PH

Medical treatment of PAH was revolutionized with the discovery of the pulmonary vasodilator prostacyclin. Initial experience [4] and subsequently, a landmark randomized control trial demonstrated that epoprostenol (a prostacyclin analog delivered intravenously) improved exercise capacity and hemodynamics and decreased pulmonary arterial pressure and pulmonary vascular resistance, culminating in improved survival in patients with PAH and New York Heart Association (NYHA) functional class III or IV heart failure [10]. Improvements in medical therapy for chronic PAH are discussed in detail in other chapters.

Despite innovative medical therapies, the prognosis of patients with advanced PH remains poor, as evident by a mortality of 15 % per year in PAH [2, 39]. Predictors of a poor prognosis include advanced NYHA functional class, poor exercise capacity as measured by six-minute walk test (6MWT) or cardiopulmonary exercise test, high right atrial (RA) pressures, significant right ventricular (RV) dysfunction, evidence of right-sided heart failure (RHF), low cardiac index, elevated brain natriuretic peptide (BNP), and an underlying diagnosis of scleroderma [2, 39]. These predictors must be considered to refer patients for advanced surgical therapies in a timely fashion. Not infrequently, these changes can occur rapidly with patients presenting with acute and profound cardiopulmonary failure.

Medical Management of Patients with PH Presenting with Acute Decompensation

The management of patients with PH presenting with advanced disease and acute decompensation is challenging. Acute decompensation is not infrequently the trigger for surgical evaluation. The clinical assessment is often confounded by the presence of RV failure, and the management of the primary PH pathology may have detrimental effects on RV function. For example, hypotension associated with use of pulmonary vasodilators may lead to worsening RV dysfunction due to decreased myocardial perfusion. Invasive hemodynamic evaluation is frequently necessary to understand the patient's physiologic derangement and assess the patient's pulmonary vascular resistance (PVR) and systemic vascular resistance (SVR). The simultaneous assessment of fluid status, degree of RV involvement, and whether or not an intra-atrial shunt is present is useful to the clinician to determine a plan of action.

In general, inotropes and vasoconstrictors should be carefully selected in patients with acutely decompensated PH. It is important to maintain the SVR higher than the PVR, as RV perfusion occurs in these patients during systole and diastole and may be greatly reduced in patients with elevated right ventricular end diastolic pressure (RVEDP) in association with hypotension. Shorter acting inotropes with a pulmonary vasodilatory effect (e.g. dobutamine or milrinone) can be administered with vasopressors for this objective. Inhaled nitric oxide (iNO) and other direct inhaled pulmonary vasodilators (such as epoprostenol) have shown efficacy in these acute situations but may be associated with rebound PH especially in the absence of other replacement therapy. If mechanical ventilation (MV) is needed, careful intubation should be conducted to avoid an abrupt increase in PVR that can result in hemodynamic collapse due to RV pressure overload. MV should be maintained using protective lung ventilation strategies and minimizing positive end expiratory pressure (PEEP).

Surgery and Other Interventions

Conventional surgery has a well-established role in PH. Because the specific management of left-sided heart lesions that result in secondary PH is out of the scope of this review, we will focus in other causes of PH.

The most accepted surgical procedures are PTE for the management of CTEPH and lung transplantation or heart-lung transplantation for patients with PAH or patients with PH associated with advanced parenchymal disease. Both PTE and transplantation are associated with acceptable mid- and long-term outcomes in patients with advanced disease. More recently, different alternatives of mechanical support have been utilized with success to temporize patients with PH to lung transplantation and, in certain cases, to recovery. Other percutaneous interventions (AS, Pott's shunt) continue to have a role in centers with limited access to transplantation or as a temporizing measure in nonoperative candidates.

Pulmonary Thromboendarterectomy

With more than 600,000 new cases of PE estimated every year in the US and considering that two-thirds of these patients will have the history of a previous PE, it is counter-intuitive to assume that CTEPH continues to be underdiagnosed [40]. The natural history of CTEPH, in the absence of medical or surgical treatment, has been previously reported with survival of <50 % at 5 years in patients with severe PH and with mortality as high as 90 % in patients with an initial PAP >50 mmHg [37, 41]. CTEPH should be considered in patients with a mean PAP ≥ 25 mmHg, with symptoms including dyspnea and history of previous PE or deep vein thrombosis.

Only 200–250 PTE cases are performed every year in the United States—a reflection of the lack of clinical suspicion for CTEPH in the overall medical community. The procedure can be performed with low mortality (2–11 %), with excellent resolution of PH, and marked improvement in hemodynamic parameters and functional capacity [32, 33, 35]. The indications for PTE include NYHA functional class III–IV heart failure; $PVR > 300$ dyn·sec·cm^5; surgically accessible thrombi in the main, lobar or segmental pulmonary arteries; and the absence of other major comorbidities [33, 42]. More recently, the indications for PTE have been extended to patients in NYHA functional class II (i.e. with exertional dyspnea) with increased PVR at rest or exertion. Although a clear survival benefit has not been reported for patients in NYHA functional class II, PTE is associated with clinical and symptomatic improvement and theoretically could decrease the risk of developing secondary pulmonary arteriopathy. Among patients with CTEPH, 20–40 % are considered inoperable, though it has become recently evident that this can be heavily influenced by the center's experience with PTE [33–36, 42].

Medical management has a limited role in patients with CTEPH and has included diuretics, anticoagulation therapy, and oxygen therapy. Long-term anticoagulant therapy has been shown to reduce *in situ* pulmonary artery thrombosis and recurrent thromboembolism [32, 38]. Inferior vena caval filters have been used to prevent the recurrence of new PE but have not been uniformly adopted due to the long-term complications of these devices [43]. The use of PH therapy prior to PTE has been associated with a delay in referral, with patients who have been treated presenting with only minimal improvement in PAP and 6MWT. Only limited data is available supporting medical management in high-risk patients to improve hemodynamics and surgical success [44, 45]. Despite the lack of scientific evidence, more than 60 % of patients with CTEPH will be referred for surgical evaluation while on therapy for PH [38].

The preoperative assessment is important to define operability and perioperative risks and includes an echocardiogram, right-heart catheterization (RHC), ventilation/perfusion scan (VQ scan), computerized tomography (CT) angiography, and pulmonary angiography [32, 33, 35, 36, 42]. More recently magnetic resonance angiography has been suggested as a useful tool in the assessment of this patient population. Anatomic considerations and the extent of vascular involvement play major roles in candidate selection. Although age has not been considered a contraindication per se, the need for circulatory arrest to complete the operation theoretically excludes patients of very advanced age with deconditioning or with significant cerebrovascular disease. The combination of very distal disease, especially microvascular disease, and a PVR > 1200 dyn·sec·cm^5 has been considered an important risk factor for poor outcome [45].

Jamieson and colleagues [36] have proposed an intraoperative classification for CTEPH (Fig. 19.1). In this classification, type I (central thrombus present) and type II (thickened intima, fibrous webs and bands) represent the typical condition of surgical patients, and are present in up to 80 % of cases. Type III occlusions in the segmental and subsegmental branches require adequate surgical experience with dissection within the peripheral pulmonary arteries. Type IV disease represents secondary *in situ* thrombosis in patients with primary pulmonary hypertension (PPH) and cannot be treated by PTE; lung transplantation is an option for these patients [36].

The surgical technique of sequential PTE with circulatory arrest was developed and standardized at the University of California San Diego (UCSD) and requires the use of cardiopulmonary bypass or extracorporeal circulation under conditions of deep hypothermia at 20 °C with briefs periods of circulatory arrest (limited to 20 min on each side). The procedure can be performed safely in patients with previous interventions including patients who have undergone previous coronary artery bypass grafting with patent bypass grafts [34].

The most relevant perioperative complication associated with PTE is pulmonary edema in the early postoperative period. Edema occurs in up to 20 % of patients who undergo PTE, particularly in patients presenting with high postoperative cardiac output. Careful fluid administration and restriction, reduction of cardiac output, and diuretics are important components of the perioperative management in patients with edema after PTE. Pulmonary hemorrhage is seen in up to 3 % of patients and is frequently associated with technical complications resulting in disruption of the vasculature during the endarterectomy, especially in cases with high PVR. Patients with pulmonary hemorrhage may require the use of postoperative ECMO support to allow stabilization. The most feared complication is the absence of surgically removable disease (Type IV); this may be associated with unchanged PVR and postoperative progression of RV dysfunction and is associated with poor early outcome [46].

PTE is a curative procedure with excellent long-term outcomes. A systematic review demonstrated 5-year survival ranging from 74 to 89 % [47]. A recent analysis of the UCSD experience in more than 1400 patients followed longitudinally

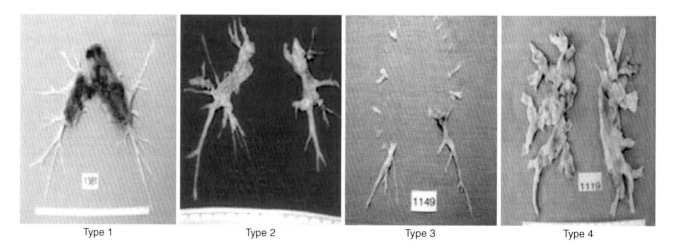

Type 1   Type 2   Type 3   Type 4

Fig. 19.1 Jamieson surgical classification of chronic thromboembolic disease (Reprinted from [36] with permission from Elsevier)

found that PTE was associated with a 10-year survival close to 70 % [33] (Fig. 19.2). Seventy-five percent of the patients who underwent PTE presented with NYHA functional class III–IV heart failure; almost 90 % of these patients were in functional class I–II at follow-up after intervention [35]. Despite these clinical and survival improvements, a subset of patients (10–30 %) will present with residual PH. Recently, a phase 3 study investigated the efficacy and side-effect profile of riociguat (a soluble guanylate cyclase stimulator) in patients with CTEPH who were ineligible for surgery or who had persistent or recurrent PH after PTE [48]. The study demonstrated hemodynamic and functional (6MWT) improvement, stimulating the use of medical management in patients with recurrent PH after PTE and patients ineligible for surgery.

Atrial Septostomy

The creation of an atrial septal defect without a thoracotomy using catheter and balloon-based techniques for patients with complete transposition of the great arteries was first introduced by Rashkind and Miller in 1966 and was then modified using blade septostomy by Park and colleagues in 1978 [49–51]. The first application of an atrial septostomy (AS) in patient with PAH was described by Rich and Lam in 1983 in a 22-year old woman with severe PH and RHF who was unresponsive to medical treatment with vasodilators. An AS was created percutaneously to offload her failing heart. The procedure was successful, but the patient died the following day due pulmonary edema and refractory hypoxemia

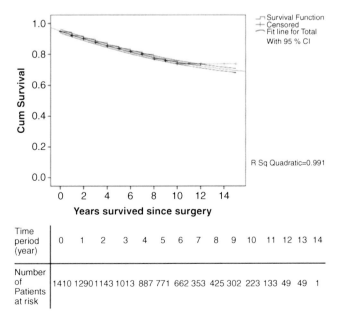

Fig. 19.2 Long-term survival following PTE (From [33] with permission from Elsevier)

[52]. Subsequently, the technique underwent several refinements. Although initial attempts were unsuccessful, they were followed by series demonstrating the efficacy of the technique with clinical and hemodynamic improvement (Fig. 19.3) [53, 54].

AS is based on the concept that survival of patients with PAH is closely correlated with the functional status of the RV, and that RV failure and syncope are associated with poor short-term outcomes [12, 55–57]. This rationale for AS is supported by the observation that patients with PAH with a patent foramen ovale (PFO) have better survival as compared with those who lack a PFO [58]. It has also been established that patients with Eisenmenger syndrome (a condition in which a congenital shunt and elevated pulmonary pressures result in deoxygenated blood in the left ventricle) have improved survival as compared with patients with IPAH, with a 3-year survival of 77 % vs. 35 % due to better cardiac output and lower RA pressures, despite higher pulmonary artery pressures [59]. Experimental work by Austen and colleagues in a canine model of PH showed that the creation of an AS decompressed the RV and increased the cardiac output on exertion [60].

The deterioration of the patient's clinical condition and ultimately mortality caused by PAH are associated with the progressive dilation and dysfunction of the RV and the coexistent decrease of systemic output. The main predictors for decreased survival in PH are high RA pressure, high pulmonary artery pressure, and a low cardiac index [12, 56]. Creation of an AS allows a right-to-left arterial shunt, increasing the systemic cardiac output and oxygen transport to the periphery, despite a decrease in SaO_2 (systemic arterial oxygen saturation), while allowing simultaneous decompression of the RV and improvement of RV function.

AS was initially performed using a blade balloon (BB) technique [53, 54]. Subsequently, the graded balloon dilatation (GBD) technique was popularized. The GBD technique provides more control over the size of the septostomy, with similar clinical and hemodynamic results as BB septostomy and a possible reduction of periprocedural risks [57, 61–63]. However, higher rate of spontaneous closure has been reported with the GBD technique [57]. Other techniques of creating a right-to-left shunt have been described that are based on the creation of a shunt between the descending aorta and the left pulmonary artery. These include the surgical creation of a Pott's shunt (an anastomosis between the descending aorta and the left pulmonary artery), percutaneous creation of an aortopulmonary shunt, and percutaneous placement of a shunt following dilatation of a small probe-patent ductus arteriosus [64]. None of these techniques have been widely accepted. Most recently, mechanical cardiopulmonary support, including ECMO and Novalung, has been used in association with AS in decompensated patients with PH as bridge to lung transplantation, though the rapid and

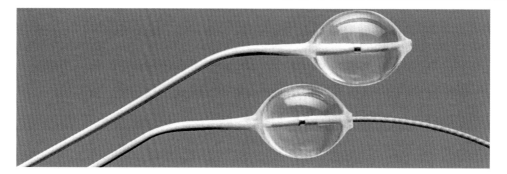

Fig. 19.3 Balloon dilators used for atrial septostomy

complete hemodynamic and respiratory support provided by ECMO and Novalung is decreasing the use of AS in patients with PH as a population [65].

The indications for AS in patients with PH lack strong evidence and are based primarily on limited single-institution series [61–63, 66]. The benefits and risks of AS were reported in an analysis of 64 cases published in the literature [67]. The main indication for AS is persistent RHF or recurrent syncope despite maximal medical therapy. Due to high periprocedural mortality in high-risk patients, AS should be avoided in patients *in extremis*. More recently AS has been used in patients with PH as a bridge to lung transplantation [63, 68]. AS has also been associated with the use of VV ECMO as a bridge to lung transplantation to avoid the thromboembolic and vascular complications present with VA ECMO [69, 70]. Occasionally, AS can be used as palliation, if lung transplantation is not an option.

Prior to the AS procedure, the candidate should have an adequate oxygen saturation (saturation of peripheral oxygen $(SpO_2) > 90$ %) on room air or relatively low supplemental oxygen) to avoid profound desaturation once the right-to-left shunt is created. A hematocrit >35 % should be present to assure adequate oxygen-carrying capacity. Left ventricular (LV) function should be sufficient to tolerate the sudden in increase in blood return and volume overload [56, 57]. A left ventricular ejection fraction (LVEF) of >45 %, defined by echocardiogram, is preferable, and preconditioning patients with severe LV or RV dysfunction using inotropes and diuretics is recommended. Although severe RV failure remains a contraindication to AS, improving RV filling pressure using inotropes may allow the procedure [57]. Furthermore, the size of the septostomy should be carefully tailored. An AS that is too large can cause excessive shunting of blood away from pulmonary circulation, inadequate oxygenation, and excessive systemic desaturation. The excessive blood flow to the LV can precipitate LV failure and pulmonary edema further exacerbating desaturation and hypoxemia [57]. AS should be avoided in patients with left ventricular end diastolic pressure (LVEDP) >12 mmHg [52, 71]. Precautions for undertaking AS are outlined in Table 19.1.

The technique utilized to perform the AS (BB or GBD) will depend on the surgeon's experience. Both techniques follow the same catheterization protocols using the left femoral artery and vein, followed by simultaneous right- and left-heart catheterization. The BB technique utilizes the Park blade. The GBD technique initially punctures the interatrial septum with a Brockenbrough needle followed with a stepwise, transseptal balloon dilation, beginning at 4 mm using the Inoue dilator followed by successive balloon dilation to 8, 12, and 16 mm. The final size of the AS is determined based on any of occurrence of (a) an increase of LVEDP to 18 mmHg, (b) reduction of SaO_2 to ~80 %, (c) 10 % change from baseline or (d) diameter of 16 mm. This criteria is used to decrease the risk of excessive LV overload and refractory hypoxemia, which was identified as the most important cause of mortality in many studies [52, 67, 71]. Intraprocedural and postprocedural echocardiograms are useful to assess changes in the LV and RV and to determine final size of the AS, typically about 80 % of the diameter of the largest balloon utilized [52, 67, 71].

Limited single-institution series have provided insight into the immediate-term and long-term effects of AS in patients with PH. Sandoval and colleagues described the creation of AS in 15 patients with severe PPH with mean PA pressure of 66 ± 13 mmHg. They defined the basic requirements of $SaO_2 > 80$ %, hematocrit >35 %, and reasonable RV function before undergoing AS. AS was created percutaneously and dilated progressively to 8–16 mm, keeping $SaO_2 > 75$ % and LVEDP <18 mmHg. Postprocedure, there was an immediate and significant decrease in RV end-diastolic pressure and SaO_2 and an increase in cardiac index. One patient died, and 14 survived the procedure and significantly improved their mean NYHA functional class and 6MWT [57]. Similar improvements in cardiac index and mid-term survival were observed by others [56]. In the first overall analysis of the worldwide experience with AS, the early postprocedural mortality after AS in patients with PH was 16 %, but implementation of the guidelines to minimize the procedure-related mortality of AS (Table 19.1) decreased this rate to 5.4 % [46, 67]. The immediate effects of the AS

Table 19.1 Recommendations for minimizing procedure-related mortality of atrial septostomy

Criteria	Recommendation
Location	Only perform in a center experienced in pulmonary hypertension
Actions to take before the procedure	Optimize cardiac function with adequate right heart filling pressure and additional inotropic support if needed
	Optimize oxygen delivery to maintain adequate hemoglobin (>15) with transfusion of packed red blood cells or darbepoetin alfa
Actions to take during the procedure	Monitor variables (LAP, SaO_2%, and mRAP)
	Tailor the defect to <10 % decrease in O_2 saturation
Actions to take after the procedure	Optimize oxygen delivery to maintain adequate hemoglobin (>15 g/dL) with transfusion of packed red blood cells or darbepoetin alfa
Contraindications to atrial septostomy	Avoid atrial septostomy if the following contraindications are present:
	Severe right ventricular failure on cardiorespiratory support
	mRAP >20 mmHg
	PVRI >55 U/m²
	Resting O_2 saturation <90 % on room air
	LVEDP >18 mmHg

Modified from [72]

LAP left atrial pressure, *LVEDP* left ventricular end diastolic pressure, *mRAP* mean right atrial pressure, *PVRI* pulmonary vascular resistance index, *SaO2* arterial oxygen saturation

on resting pulmonary hemodynamics were variable. The mean RA pressure declined by 3 mmHg; the cardiac index increased by 0.7 l/min/m₂. Baseline mean RA pressure is the best indicator of hemodynamic response, and the best hemodynamic and clinical responses are obtained when mean RA pressure is between 10 and 20 mmHg. Patients with mean RA pressure > 20 mmHg may also present adequate hemodynamic response but with a higher risk of mortality [57, 67].

The long-term results of the AS have not been well documented. Kerstein and colleagues noticed an improvement in the RV function with improvement in diastolic PAP and cardiac index in patients studied 7–27 months after AS [53]. Long-term clinical response seems to have a close correlation with the immediate response including cardiac index and oxygen transport [63]. In this study, patients with greater increases in cardiac index (52 % vs 15 %) and systemic oxygen transport (37 % vs 4 %) shortly after the AS procedure had an improved clinical response. The median long-term survival of 54 patients surviving AS was 19.5 months. Progression of the underlying pulmonary vascular disease was the main factor associated with late mortality.

Transplantation

Lung transplantation is an established therapeutic option for patients with advanced respiratory failure caused by many etiologies including restrictive and obstructive diseases, infectious complications, and pulmonary vascular complications as in the case of PAH. The first lung transplantation in a human was performed by Hardy in 1963 in a patient with advanced lung cancer who died soon after the intervention

due to renal failure [73]. The first heart-lung transplant was successfully performed at Stanford University by Norman Shumway, John Wallwork, and Bruce Reitz in 1981 for PAH [74]. Joel Cooper reported the first successful single lung transplant for pulmonary fibrosis in 1983, followed by the first series of bilateral lung transplants in 1986 [75–77]. Since 1995, more than 47,000 lung transplants and 3700 heart-lung transplants have been performed [78, 79].

Although PAH was recognized as a clinical entity in the early 1950s, the medical community lacked effective treatments for decades, with a median survival of only 2.8 years [12, 80]. Thirty years later, the treatment and prognosis of patients with PAH was notably improved with the introduction of heart-lung transplantation and subsequently lung transplantation as a valid treatment alternative. Due to technical considerations and concerns regarding postoperative RV performance, heart-lung transplantation was considered the procedure of choice in patients with PAH, whereas lung transplantation was used mostly for other forms of end-stage lung disease [81]. After the efficiency of prostacyclin analogs, endothelin receptor antagonists, and PDE5 inhibitors became evident, transplantation remained a second-line treatment for years. As medical therapy improved, we observed an important decrease in pulmonary vascular disease as indication for transplantation—representing 10–15 % of patient undergoing transplantation initially but only 4 % in more contemporary reports [78, 79]. Most recently, with improvements in surgical techniques and outcomes in lung transplantation and the understanding that despite optimal medical therapy up to 30 % of patients will progress rapidly or respond poorly to medical treatment, transplantation has regained attention in the management of PAH [81, 82].

Indication and Timing for Transplantation

The indications and patient selection for lung or heart-lung transplantation have been previously stated by International Society for Heart and Lung Transplantation (ISHLT) consensus [83]. In general, patients are considered for transplant if they have advanced end-stage lung disease, NYHA functional class III–IV heart failure, have a life expectancy of <2 years, and have no contraindications [83]. The indications for lung transplantation referral in patients with PH are summarized in Table 19.2.

In patients with PAH, an adequate response to medical treatment occurs in the majority of patients and may be responsible for a delay in referral for lung transplantation. However, there are other factors that need to be considered at the time of referral. The development of the lung allocation scoring (LAS) system, implemented in 2005 with the intention to increase access to lung transplantation in higher risk patients, may not accurately reflect risk in patients with IPAH [11, 84]. The LAS is a scoring system, developed from demographic and clinical characteristics, that takes into account waiting list urgency and probability of post-transplant survival [84]. After implementation of the LAS system, deaths while on the waiting list for a lung transplant decreased for all diagnosis groups except for patients with IPAH, which remained unchanged. Patients with IPAH were less likely receive a transplant than patients with idiopathic pulmonary fibrosis (IPF) or cystic fibrosis (CF) and more likely to die on the waiting list than patients with chronic obstructive pulmonary disease (COPD) or CF [83, 85, 86].

Some variables associated with worse prognosis in patients with PAH, as studied in the REVEAL cohort, are not represented in the LAS. These variables include right atrial pressure (RAP) >14 mmHg and 6MWT <300 m [11]. Recent

analyses have suggested that current prediction models that utilize the LAS may overestimate the survival of patients listed with IPAH. New statistical models that consider other variables, including 6MWT, resting O_2, invasive cardiac output testing, and NYHA functional class, have been suggested to help guide clinical decision-making [11, 87]. For this reason, the United Network for Organ Sharing (UNOS) now considers LAS appeal in lung transplant candidates with PAH [82]. If certain criteria related to declining right ventricular function are met (including deterioration in clinical condition on optimal medical therapy, right atrial pressure >15 mmHg, and cardiac index <1.8 L/min/m²), an LAS is assigned such that the patient is placed in the 90th percentile on the wait list.

Debate still exists regarding outcomes on the wait list and posttransplantation survival after implementation of the LAS score. Schaffer and colleagues in a recent review of the UNOS registry found that after LAS implementation, the incidence of transplantation increased and wait-list mortality decreased in patients with IPAH, and that both heart-lung transplantation and lung transplantation are predictive of survival, as is being listed at a medium- to high-volume center [88]. This report provided a positive perspective of the problem. Unfortunately, we continue to see patients coming late for referral for transplantation, and in some circumstances, they are not able to be considered for a transplant due to their advanced disease and multi-organ involvement. Patients with PAH who are listed continue to have a high mortality while on the wait list—as high as 34 % in recent analyses by UNOS and others [89]. This has forced experienced transplant centers to suggest early referral of patients with PH for transplant evaluation. Despite the availability of advanced circulatory support systems, including ECMO and Novalung, to bridge patients to transplantation, advanced circulatory support is only possible in selected and experienced centers [90–96]. It does not seem appropriate to wait until advanced right-sided heart failure, liver failure, frequent arrhythmias, and syncope are present to consider referral.

Lung transplantation generally is offered to patients with PH who do not respond to optimal vasodilator therapy [82]. Updated treatment algorithms have been proposed in patients with PAH in NYHA class IV [97]. In an attempt to prevent late referral for lung transplantation, some experienced centers consider initiation of treatment with intravenous epoprostenol to be a better time to perform an initial lung transplantation evaluation [89]. Due to the difficulty in predicting the clinical course of patients with PAH and associated PAH (APAH; PAH resulting from another disease), early referral is recommended even for a preliminary evaluation. The inadequate response of a patient with PAH to monotherapy should prompt physicians to consider a lung transplantation evaluation in parallel with initiation of sequential combination therapy. Failure of the combination

Table 19.2 ISHLT guidelines for transplantation referral

1. NYHA functional class III or IV, on maximal medical therapy
2. Rapidly progressing disease with low (<350 m) or declining 6 min walk distance
3. Syncope
4. Additional risk factors for poor outcome in PAH
(a) Hyponatremia
(b) Hyperbilirubinemia
5. Right ventricular dysfunction:
(a) Cardiac index <2 l/min/m²
(b) Right atrial pressure >15 mmHg
(c) Tricuspid annular plane systolic excursion <1.8 cm
6. Underlying connective tissue disease (e.g. scleroderma)
7. Chronic obstructive pulmonary disease
8. Sarcoidosis
9. Pulmonary fibrosis
10. Combined emphysema, pulmonary fibrosis, and PAH

Modified from [82]

therapy should then trigger the activation of the patient on the transplant wait list [97].

Sitbon and colleagues identified a high-risk subset of patients with PH who are likely to have a poor outcome without transplantation. These include patients with a history of right-sided heart failure, who remained in NYHA functional class III or IV after 3 months on epoprostenol, who showed a 6MWT <250 m, and who had high RAP (>12 mmHg) along with the absence of a decrease in total pulmonary resistance of >30 %, relative to baseline. These patients should be prioritized for lung transplantation [8].

It is worth mentioning that patients with PH associated with underlying lung disease, such as COPD, pulmonary fibrosis, or sarcoidosis, are also at increased risk of mortality, and patients with combined emphysema, interstitial lung disease and PH have a particularly high mortality risk with 1-year survival in only 60 % [98–101]. In these patients with lung disease and PH, the variable effects of oral and inhaled vasodilators with the potential to worsen symptoms frequently indicate the need of an expedited lung transplantation evaluation [82].

Considering the implications of severe PAH in the management and prognosis of patients being considered for transplantation, it is advisable that these patients are cared for during the mid-late phase of the clinical course of their disease by an experienced and multidisciplinary group with the ability to provide lung and heart-lung transplantation, mechanical respiratory and circulatory support, and other temporizing strategies.

Type of Transplantation

With the utilization of cyclosporine and better immunosuppressive regimens beginning in the early 1980s, the survival of patients after heart-lung transplantation improved markedly [102, 103], and heart-lung transplantation became the accepted treatment for patients with advanced PAH and other advanced cardiopulmonary diseases. The acceptable outcomes of various single-center experiences were published [81, 104, 105]. PAH remains an important indication for heart-lung transplantation with 27.6 % of heart-lung transplants being performed for PAH, second in frequency only to heart-lung transplantation performed for cyanotic congenital heart disease [106]. As the overall number of patients listed for transplantation increased and the organ scarcity became evident, single-lung transplantation and double-lung transplantation were considered as alternatives to heart-lung transplantation in patients with PH. More recently, double-lung transplantation has been favored over single-lung transplantation [81, 107–109].

In the 1990s, our group at the University of Pittsburgh demonstrated that single-lung transplantation could be done with survival comparable with double-lung transplantation [107, 108], suggesting that single-lung transplantation could

be considered the procedure of choice in patients with PAH to increase organ utilization. Gammie and co-workers reviewed the results of 58 lung transplants performed for PPH or secondary PH; 37 double-lung transplants and 21 single-lung transplants were performed. As expected, cardiopulmonary bypass times were longer in patients who underwent double-lung transplantation as compared with those who underwent single-lung transplantation. Recipients with PH had similar functional status and similar early- and mid-term survival after single-lung transplantation or double-lung transplantation [109]. We have recently observed patients surviving more than 20 years after single-lung transplant who occasionally require redo transplantation.

A recent report from the Cleveland Clinic concluded that the use of single-lung transplantation in older patients (>65 years) with secondary PH was associated with similar outcomes as double-lung transplantation. Murthy and colleagues presented a series of single-lung transplant recipients that compared 36 patients with PH (mean PAP 30.4 mmHg) and 48 patients with no PH. Survival at 3 years was similar, 70 % and 72 % respectively, with patients with PH having only a longer hospital stay (24 days vs 16 days; $p = 0.015$). This study suggested that single-lung transplantation could be an acceptable solution to minimize the surgical intervention and increase organ utilization [110].

Other series have associated double-lung transplantation with better outcomes than single-lung transplantation, however, and perioperative management of patients after double-lung transplant may be more straightforward. In a series of patients with PH, including 27 patients with PAH and 30 patients with Eisenmenger syndrome, Bando and co-workers from our institution found that double-lung transplantation and heart-lung transplantation provided a better option than single-lung transplantation in reducing pulmonary arterial pressure, improving cardiac index, and providing better functional outcomes and better early and mid-term survival [107, 108]. Subsequently, Conte and colleagues, in a study that included patients with PPH (n = 15) and secondary PH (n = 40), observed a significant improvement in survival in patients with PPH who underwent double-lung transplantation as compared with single-lung transplantation in patients with PPH as the indication for transplantation [111].

The combined clinical experience of many groups has demonstrated the complexity of the perioperative management needed for single-lung transplantation because the majority of the cardiac output (80–90 %) perfuses the newly implanted lung. There is an increased likelihood of needing ECMO support due to the increased risk of severe primary graft dysfunction (PGD) in patients with PH [106, 112]. Using double-lung transplantation may also eliminate the risk of recurrent PH seen occasionally after single-lung transplantation [81]. Thus, double-lung transplantation may be a safest alternative. Since this realization, the use of single-lung transplantation has decreased rapidly with fewer than 5 % of patients with PAH undergoing single-lung transplantation, as per ISHLT transplantation registry reports [106, 112].

Double-lung transplantation is currently the preferred choice worldwide over heart-lung transplantation for patients with PH, especially considering the importance of organ scarcity. Double-lung transplantation offers comparable outcomes as heart-lung transplantation in patients with PAH with the advantage of better organ sharing [113]. A recent meta-analysis used nine selected studies to answer the question, "Should we perform double-lung transplantation or heart-lung transplantation in patients with PH?" Reviewing 1189 lung transplants (67 %) and 578 heart-lung transplants, the authors concluded that neither procedure had an overall survival benefit over the other [113]. Interestingly, the same study corroborated that heart-lung transplantation is associated with excellent functional and survival outcomes in patients with congenital heart disease and Eisenmenger syndrome, severe right ventricular dysfunction (EF < 10–25 %) or left ventricular dysfunction (EF < 35–55 %), and those who are chronically inotrope-dependent. In all other patients with PH, double-lung transplantation offered similar outcomes with better organ utilization [113]. Supporting the use of heart-lung transplantation in the situations mentioned above, some authors have reported a lower PGD rate and better survival without bronchiolitis obliterans syndrome (BOS) when heart-lung transplantation was performed [81]. Dartevelle and colleagues reviewed their experience with lung transplantation and heart-lung transplantation in patients with severe PH with an extensive analysis of 219 patients: 152 who underwent heart-lung transplantation and 67 who underwent lung transplantation for end-stage PH (including 147 patients with PAH) over a 22-year period (1986–2008). They concluded that in patients with end-stage PH, good long-term outcomes were obtained with both protocols as indicated by a 43 % survival after double-lung transplantation and 39 % survival after heart-lung transplantation at 10 years posttransplant (p = 0.9) (Fig. 19.4). These similar survival outcomes were obtained despite the fact that the heart-lung transplantation group was composed of sicker patients with worse NYHA functional class heart failure, worse kidney and liver function, and a higher need for preoperative inotropes as compared with the double-lung transplantation group [81]. Heart-lung transplantation was associated with lower postoperative morbidity, shorter MV time, lower rates of bronchial complications and postoperative PGD, and greater freedom from BOS-related death at follow-up. Heart-lung transplantation has been associated with a certain degree of immunologic

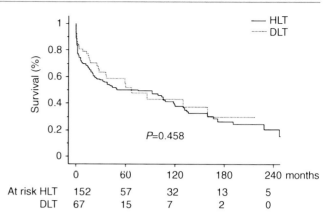

Fig. 19.4 Outcomes of double-lung transplantation vs heart-lung transplantation. *DLT* double-lung transplant, *HLT* heart-lung transplant (Reprinted from [81] with permission by Oxford University Press)

protection to the lung, which the authors put forth to explain the lower rate of BOS after heart-lung transplantation as compared with double-lung transplantation in this study [81]. This theory has not been supported by other studies [114–116].

Heart-lung transplantation continues to be an excellent alternative in patients with a complex congenital systemic-to-pulmonary shunt (e.g. Eisenmenger syndrome), with intra-cardiac lesions that require complex repair (e.g. a ventricular septal defect), or with profound RV dysfunction and dilation. In an analysis of transplantation for Eisenmenger syndrome, survival was significantly better after heart-lung transplantation than after lung transplantation, a difference that was not apparent for recipients with IPAH [117]. This benefit was more pronounced when the congenital defect was a ventricular septal defect (VSD).

Although double-lung transplantation may be doable in the majority of patients, even those with severe RV dysfunction, a careful consideration should be made in patients with extreme cardiac dilation, as severe compression of the vascular structures on the left-side of the chest may occur as a consequence of cardiac-left chest cavity mismatch or cardiac herniation, leading occasionally to a loss of the allograft requiring redo transplantation [118]. We have experienced a similar situation following double-lung transplantation (Fig. 19.5).

Despite its potential benefits in certain high-risk situations, heart-lung transplantation is only occasionally possible due to logistic considerations and organ availability. Double-lung transplantation has become, for most transplant centers, the procedure of choice in patients with PAH. In an analysis by the ISHLT, double-lung transplantation was performed in 1073 of 1160 cases operated between 1995 and 2012, constituting 4.6 % of all the double-lung transplants done during this interval [78].

The surgical techniques for lung and heart-lung transplantation have been previously published [77, 119, 120]. Lung transplantation and heart-lung transplantation require the use of sternotomy or clamshell incision (bilateral thoracosternotomy) and the use of circulatory support in the form of cardiopulmonary bypass or ECMO to support and stabilize the patient during the procedure.

Outcomes

Despite the increasing use of double lung transplantation in patients with PAH, PAH has been long considered a major risk factor for severe PGD [121–123]. The relief of the elevated PAP in patients with RV hypertrophy may be associated with a high output requiring careful dosage of inotropes to minimize pulmonary overflow. The opposite situation may be present in patients with severe RV dysfunction; the surgical procedure may unmask a dynamic RV outflow obstruc-

tion caused by RV hypertrophy and worsened by inotropes [112]. Another complication, not infrequently seen in the early postoperative period and frequently during attempts of extubation, is dysfunction of the LV (systolic and/or diastolic) associated with elevated LV filling pressures and pulmonary pressures in the setting of a small LV cavity trying to adapt to the hemodynamic changes. This can be accompanied by the presence of transient severe mitral regurgitation and pulmonary edema, increasing the risk of allograft dysfunction and severe PGD [124] (Fig. 19.6). Careful hemodynamic management—avoiding high doses of inotropes, weaning from cardiopulmonary bypass, slow and gradual weaning from MV in the ICU, and avoiding increased afterload (systemic hypertension)—is of major importance in this patient population. The use of posttransplant ECMO for PGD may be necessary and should be considered early in the presence of severe and rapidly progressive pulmonary deterioration [125–129], with an observed 96 % ECMO wean rate, 82 % 30-day survival and 64 % 1-year survival [125].

As previously noted, immediately postoperatively following double-lung transplantation, there is a marked reduction in PA pressure, RV dimensions, RV pressure and RV stroke work. In one study, PA systolic and mean pressures markedly decreased after transplantation in patients with severe pulmonary hypertension (from 115 to 45 mmHg for the systolic pressure and from 76 to 31 mmHg for the diastolic pressure) [130]. This effect of double-lung transplantation on PA pressure persists long-term. In another study examining the impact of lung transplantation on PH, 100 lung transplant recipients were followed; mean PA pressure decreased from 64 to 22 mmHg when measured 5 years posttransplant [114]. These rapid changes in the PA pressure will produce an immediate and remarkable response of the RV seen as early as in the operating room.

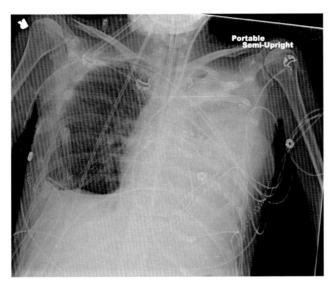

Fig. 19.5 Left lung infarct following double-lung transplant in a patient with PAH

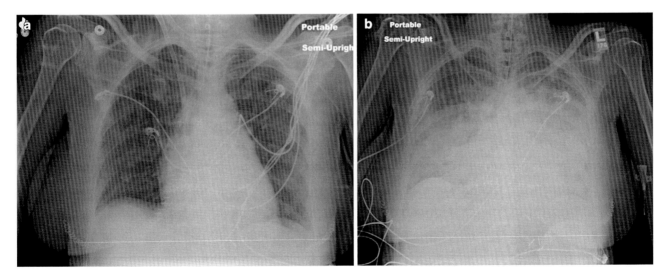

Fig. 19.6 (**a**) Rapidly progression of pulmonary edema in a patient with double-lung transplant for PAH. (**a**) Prior to onset. (**b**) 2 h later

Despite the acceptable results obtained with double-lung transplantation in patients with PAH, mid-term outcomes following double-lung transplantation remain inferior in recipients with PAH as compared with patients who undergo lung transplant for other pathologies [78] (Fig. 19.7). Posttransplant 5-year survival was 57 %, along with marked improvement in functional capacity [114]. According to the ISHLT transplantation registry, the median survival after transplant is 5.5 years in patients with IPAH vs 8.3 years in patients with CF and 6.4 years in patients with alpha 1-antitrypsin deficiency, although patients with IPAH have significantly better outcomes than patients with IPF (4.7 years) [78]. Patients with IPAH have a greater risk of early mortality and, in a multivariate analysis, the diagnosis of IPAH was the greatest categorical risk factor for 1-year mortality with a two- to threefold increase in mortality risk. Long-term survival after double-lung transplantation is inferior in recipients with PAH as compared with patients with other pulmonary pathologies with 10-year survival of 42 % in recipients with PPH as compared with 70 % in patients with other pulmonary pathologies [89]. Similar findings were reported using the ISHLT transplantation registry data, and PAH was identified as an independent predictor of increased early and late mortality [106]. The reason for this decrease in early and late survival was thought to be due to a higher risk of PGD in PAH recipients after double-lung transplantation, as PGD was an independent predictor of increased early and late mortality [121].

Devices

Options for mechanical circulatory support (MCS) in patients with severe PH are limited and associated with significant complications. Patients with PH secondary to left-sided heart failure can be managed with different types of support devices

at the time of LVAD implantation including implantable and percutaneous RVADS in the absence or presence of an oxygenator (oxyRVAD). Patients with PAH or PH secondary to lung disease in the absence of left-sided heart failure present an enormous challenge for the clinicians who care for them. Historically in cases of profound decompensation and shock, peripheral or central veno-arterial (VA) ECMO or peripheral or central Novalung have been used to treat patients until they can receive a lung transplant, heart-lung transplant, or more recently, until recovery in selected cases [90, 131–133].

MCS in Patients with PH Secondary to an LVAD

Patients with PH secondary to LV dysfunction (Group 2) with chronically elevated filling pressure will typically respond to LV unloading with the use of an LVAD. In these patients, fixed PH and other hemodynamic parameters seem to improve early after LVAD implantation and for up to 6 months following the procedure [27, 30, 134]. This positive response is seen in the majority of patients (70–80 %) and is sustained following heart transplantation. Survival after heart transplantation is strictly related to the reversibility of PVR and the transpulmonary gradient following LVAD implantation [30]. With better patient selection and perioperative management, the use of an RVAD due to severe RV dysfunction at the time of LVAD implantation is only necessary in a small subset of patients (6–8 % of elective LVAD implants) [135]. In patients with LV dysfunction requiring an LVAD, PH is not considered a risk factor per se for RV failure. To the contrary, the inability of the RV to generate elevated pulmonary artery pressure in the presence of severe RV dysfunction, severe tricuspid regurgitation, elevated right atrial pressure and a decreased PAP/CVP (central venous pressure) ratio (<0.6) has been considered a risk factor for RV failure and the need

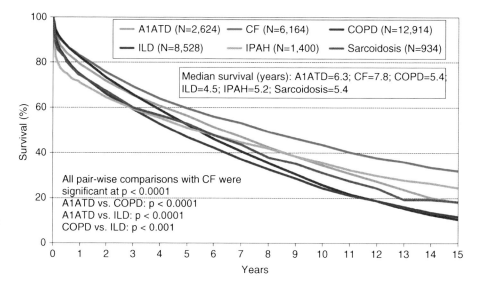

Fig. 19.7 Lung transplant survival by disease. *A1ATD* alpha-1 antitrypsin deficiency, *CF* cystic fibrosis, *COPD* chronic obstructive pulmonary disease, *ILD* interstitial lung disease, *IPAH* idiopathic pulmonary hypertension (Reprinted from [78] with permission from Elsevier)

for mechanical support [135]. There are different alternatives for mechanical support to assist the RV in these situations including the Centrimag pump (Thoratec, Pleasanton, CA), which requires open surgical implantation, and two percutaneously implanted options: the Impella RP (Abiomed, Danvers MA) and the TandemHeart (TandemHeart, Pittsburgh, PA) pump coupled with the Protek Duo Cannula (TandemHeart, Pittsburgh, PA).

The Centrimag is a bearingless centrifugal pump that is United States Food and Drug Administration (FDA)-approved and has been used extensively for RV support

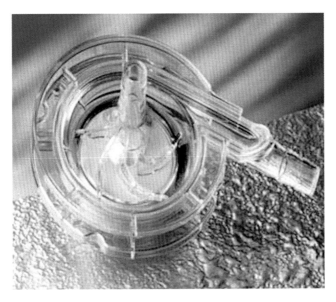

Fig. 19.8 Centrimag Pump used for right ventricular support

(Fig. 19.8). Cannulas must be implanted into the right atrium and pulmonary artery during open surgery. Different studies have demonstrated excellent outcomes with survival ranging from 50 to 80 % [136, 137]. More recently the Impella RP, a percutaneous axial flow pump implanted through the right femoral vein into the proximal PA, was approved for use in the United States after a successful trial with ~80 % survival in patients in whom the device was used for RV dysfunction following LVAD implantation [138] (Fig. 19.9). Another alternative for percutaneous use is the TandemHeart pump in association with the Protek Duo cannula, a dual-lumen cannula that allows support with a single cannula implanted through the right internal jugular vein into the proximal PA (Fig. 19.10).

MCS in Patients with PAH and PH Secondary to Lung Disease

In contrast to patients with PH secondary to LVAD implantation (Group 2), patients with PAH (Group 1) or PH secondary to intrinsic lung disease (Group 3) are considered for MCS during the late stages of acute decompensation, generally with severe acute heart failure, RV dysfunction, hypoxemia, ventricular arrhythmias, and syncope. In these cases, PAH is associated with profound RV dysfunction and generally preserved LV function. Although RVADs alone have been considered, and anecdotally implanted in this situation, there is absence of scientific evidence to support RVAD use in treating PAH and no proven role for RVAD use in patients with PH and intrinsic lung disease. In experimental compu-

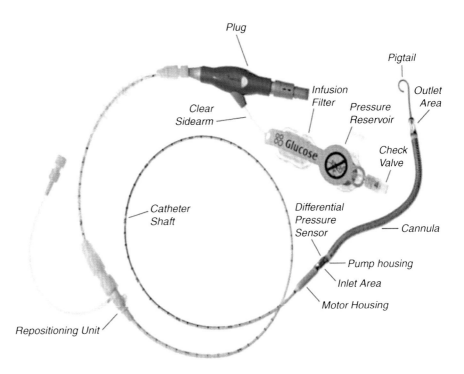

Fig. 19.9 Impella RP used for right ventricular support

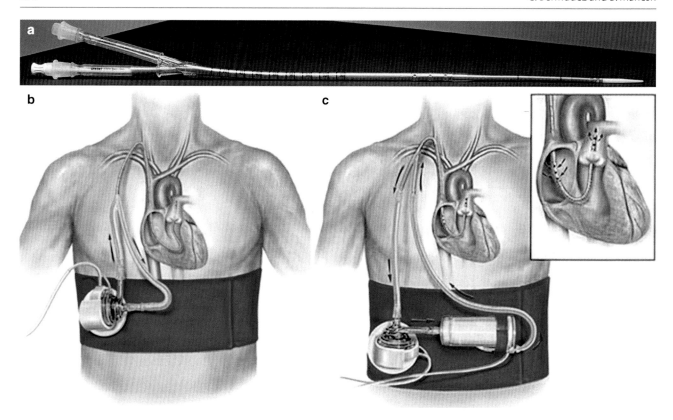

Fig. 19.10 (**a**) Protek Duo cannula. (**b**) Percutaneous RVAD and (**c**) RVAD/ECMO (oxyRVAD) using TandemHeart pump and Protek-Duo cannula

tational models, the use of an RVAD has been associated with important elevations of the pulmonary pressure and left atrial pressure with an increased risk of pulmonary hemorrhage [131, 139], a phenomenon also anecdotally observed in clinical situations [131]. For this reason, although conceptually attractive, there has been limited interest in the use of durable or short-term RVAD support in patients with PAH.

VA ECMO is the most commonly used MCS in patients with severe PAH or PH secondary to lung disease presenting with profound decompensation unable to be sustained on MV or presenting with cardiogenic shock due to RV collapse. VA ECMO is used generally as a bridge to lung transplantation (Fig. 19.11). VA ECMO can be applied in a central (surgical implantation) or peripheral configuration as a bridge to lung transplantation ([90, 140], and personal experience) and occasionally considered as a bridge to recovery in patients presenting in acute decompensation with the absence of previous pulmonary vasodilator treatment and without an intrinsic lung disease (patients with IPAH) [133].

In patients with an established history of severe PH, VA ECMO should be considered the most straightforward alternative to provide full hemodynamic and ventilator support. Peripheral groin cannulation (femoral artery and vein) and upper body perfusion (subclavian artery and right internal jugular vein) have both been used successfully. Central cannulation (right atrium to aorta) is rarely utilized but can be useful in patients

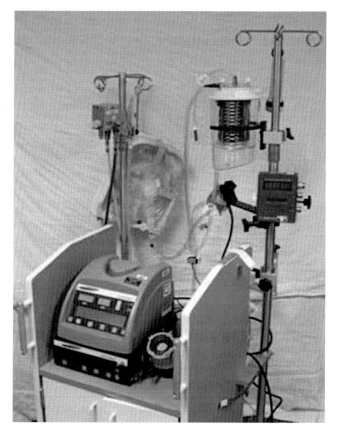

Fig. 19.11 Extracorporeal membrane oxygenation (ECMO) system

with difficult distal peripheral vascular access or patients of small stature. ([141] and personal experience) When a femoral approach is use, the femoral artery and veins are cannulated using the Seldinger technique after heparinization, and ECMO flows are maintained between 3 and 5 L/min (Fig. 19.12). This technique is associated with vascular complications of the lower extremities, which are seen in up to 15 % of patients, For this reason, distal cannulation should be evaluated frequently to avoid vascular complications that can restrict future treatment options. Certain groups have favored the use of subclavian artery cannulation (Fig. 19.13) with the objective to prevent lower extremity vascular complications and avoid upper body desaturation as seen in some cases of femoral VA ECMO with potentially catastrophic implications. Rosenzweig and colleagues presented six patients using these techniques. Two patients underwent lung transplantation, and four received aggressive pulmonary vasodilator therapy as a bridge to recovery. Three of the four survived to decannulation, and two survived to discharge [133]. This technique is considered with the intention to extubate patients, allow ambulation and physical therapy, and minimize the impact of MV on RV function. Abrams and colleagues described the technique of upper body VA ECMO in detail [142]. Despite potential benefits, upper body VA ECMO requires careful surgical technique using an 8–10 mm Dacron graft anastomosed to the subclavian artery and, in our experience, has been associated with significant bleeding, upper extremity hyperperfusion syndrome, and a higher rate of stroke than femoral VA ECMO. An awake and extubated ECMO strategy (with VV or VA ECMO) was popularized by the lung transplantation group in Hannover Germany, and in a series comparing 26 patients on ECMO versus 34 patients on MV, VA ECMO was associated with better posttransplantation outcomes, shorter MV duration, and shorter hospital stay as compared with maintaining patients on MV [91]. In an earlier series of nonintubated patients with PH by Olsson and colleagues, peripheral VA ECMO was used as a bridge to lung transplant in five patients; three patients survived to discharge (more than 3 months) [95] (Fig. 19.14). Subsequent series have supported the benefit of extubation or early tracheostomy and rehabilitation in patients supported on ECMO as a bridge to lung transplantation [143, 144].

Venovenous (VV) ECMO has also been used successfully to support patients with profound respiratory failure secondary to lung disease [145], but has a limited role or no role in patients with severe PH because VV ECMO does not pro-

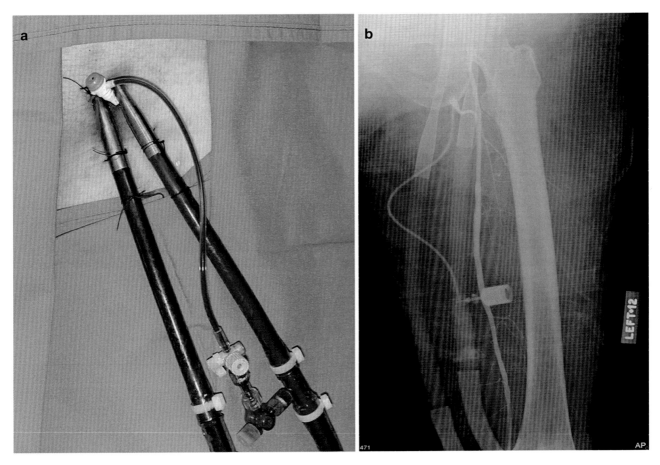

Fig. 19.12 (a) Peripheral VA ECMO (femoral vein and femoral artery). (b) Fluoroscopy confirming adequate distal perfusion using a 5–7 Fr distal perfusion cannula

Fig. 19.13 Peripheral subclavian veno-arterial ECMO (right internal jugular vein to right subclavian/axillary artery). (**a**) Schematic of the cannulation strategy. (**b**) Cannula placement

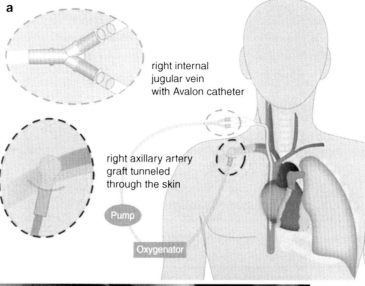

right internal
jugular vein
with Avalon catheter

right axillary artery
graft tunneled
through the skin

Pump

Oxygenator

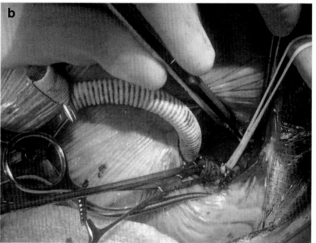

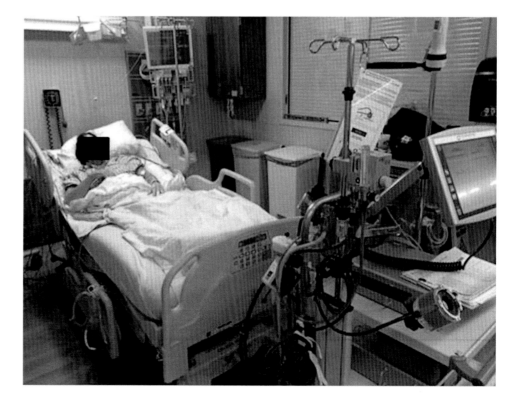

Fig. 19.14 Awake-extubated
veno-arterial ECMO

vide adequate RV and hemodynamic support, which is frequently needed in the acute decompensation stage or for shock. VV ECMO should only be considered in the presence of large intra-atrial communication allowing a right-to-left shunt, including a PFO, atrial septal defect (ASD), or following the creation of an AS [133, 146] (Fig. 19.15). The rapid changes in size of a percutaneously created AS may complicate the management of patients requiring redilatation of the AS. Small anecdotal series have been published with the use of single, dual-lumen cannula (AVALON) used in combination with AS or an ASD as bridge to lung transplantation or recovery with acceptable outcomes [93, 133].

We recently administered successful long-term support (3 weeks) using VV ECMO as a low-flow oxyRVAD (RVAD pumping capability with an oxygenator included in the circuit) using the TandemHeart pump with a dual-lumen cannula (Fig. 19.16) in a patient with sarcoidosis and severe systemic PH who presented with cardiac arrest but in whom femoral VA ECMO was unsuccessful. Although complex initial management required prolonged nitric oxide use, we were able to successfully mobilize the patient with stable cardiopulmonary support as a bridge to lung transplantation.

Worldwide, an important experience has been gained bridging patients on ECMO with end-stage lung disease to lung transplantation. More than 250 cases of ECMO used as a bridge to lung transplantation have been performed in the United States, and 1–2 % of patients are on ECMO at the time of lung transplantation, according to the Scientific Registry of Transplant Recipients [148, 149]. The majority of series describing the use of ECMO as a bridge to lung transplantation have concentrated on the basic strategies of

ECMO implementation and outcomes of patients who underwent lung transplantation including all diagnoses. These series have confirmed that in high-volume centers with MCS expertise, ECMO (VA and VV) can be used safely as a bridge to lung transplantation with adequate survival, ranging from 60 to 100 % at 1 year [91, 96, 148, 150–153]. Limiting the time on support has been deemed crucial to prevent complications (especially in patients on VA ECMO) with 50 % mortality in patients supported for more than 15 days vs no mortality in patients supported ≤14 days in a small series of 17 patients [154].

Here at the University of Pittsburgh Medical Center, we initiated the consistent use of ECMO as a bridge to lung transplantation in 2008 following important improvements in pump and cannula technologies and experience gained in the lung transplantation program. We reported consecutive series in 2010 and 2013 confirming acceptable outcomes of patients with ECMO as a bridge to lung transplantation as compared with non-supported patients with 2-year survival of 74 % in the pre-lung transplantation ECMO group (24 patients) and in the control group. Of these 24 patients, 15 patients were on VV ECMO—10 via femoral venous and right internal jugular venous cannulas and 5 via the right internal jugular vein using the Avalon Elite bicaval dual-lumen cannula [Avalon laboratories LLC, Rancho Dominguez, CA]. The remaining 9 patients were on VA ECMO—4 via a femoral veno-arterial route, 4 via a right atrial and ascending aortic route, and 1 via the right internal jugular vein and femoral arterial route. The patients on VA ECMO were supported with this strategy primarily due to severe PH secondary to lung disease; one patient had

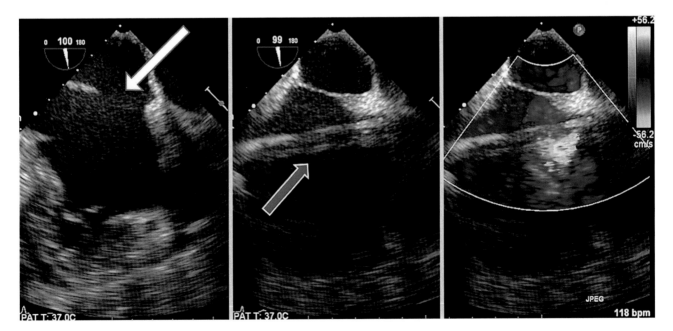

Fig. 19.15 VV ECMO in a patient with an ASD. The right atrial infusion port (*blue arrow*) shunts oxygenated blood across the ASD (*white arrow*) (Reprinted from [147] with permission from Elsevier)

PAH. There were four deaths (17 %) in the ECMO group as compared with 9 % in the control group (a nonsignificant difference). Therefore, bridging to double-lung transplantation using ECMO offers a chance for high-risk patients, who may be deteriorating rapidly, to undergo double-lung transplantation with good outcomes instead of dying on the waiting list. Our results compared favorably with the original UNOS series, in which only 57 % of patients on ECMO survived [96].

Our most recent series was presented at the ISHLT meeting in 2014; we examined 48 patients supported with ECMO as bridge to lung transplantation. Thirteen patients were supported on VA ECMO due to presence of severe PH (9 peripheral cannulation and 4 central cannulation). The diagnoses of

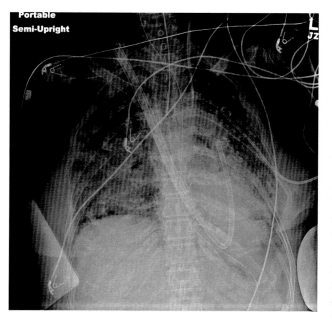

Fig. 19.16 Protek-Duo cannula placement in a patient supported with percutaneous RVAD/ECMO using the TandemHeart

the patients with PH included PAH (2 patients), scleroderma (5 patients), and other restrictive diseases (2 patients). The mean time of ECMO support was 199 h, and all these patients received double-lung transplantation. There was no difference in survival between the VA ECMO group and the VV ECMO group, with a 1- and 3-year survival of 88 % for the VA group and 78 % and 72 %, respectively, in the VV ECMO group (p=0.59). If we consider the entire series by the presence of severe PH (mean PAP>40 mmHg), we observed a lower transplant rate, lower survival, and a higher incidence of early mortality (p=0.04) with the use of ECMO with the intention to treat in patients with PH as compared with those with no PH. In the PH group, the patients have higher chances of dying while on ECMO support before getting a lung transplant due to vascular and thromboembolic complications.

Another alternative for circulatory support in patients with PH is the lung assist device (iLA; Novalung, Heilbronn, Germany), a pumpless oxygenator that provides an alternative to full VA ECMO and allows a controlled passive left-to-right shunt using smaller cannulas (15–18 Fr) in a central (left atrium to pulmonary artery) or peripheral configuration (femoral artery to femoral vein) [90, 140]; the iLA is used in patients with PAH as a bridge to lung transplantation (Fig. 19.17). This efficient, low-gradient oxygenator, which was originally considered as a CO_2 removal system, relies on a pressure gradient to allow blood passage through the fibers. With its effect on CO_2 removal and slight secondary effect on oxygenation, the iLA has been used extensively in patients with ARDS to minimize the deleterious effects of high-volume MV with acceptable outcomes [3]. In these cases, the femoral implantation technique was used with 15–18 F femoral arterial and venous cannulas receiving ~20 % of the cardiac output, and for this reason, it cannot be used in patients with LV dysfunction [140, 156, 157]. Flows will usually range between 1.2 and 2.0 L/min. Use of the iLA requires

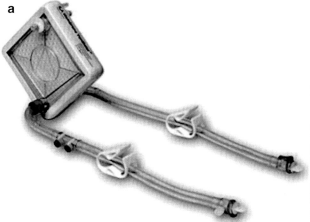

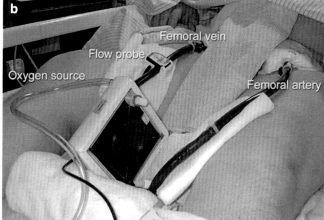

Fig. 19.17 Interventional Lung Assist (iLA, Novalung). (**a**) iLA device. (**b**) Novalung device used with femoral (FA-FV) cannulation (From Fischer and Strueber [155]. Copyright 2012, used with permission from CTSNet (www.ctsnet.org). All rights reserved.)

anticoagulation with heparin to prevent systemic thrombosis. The use of the iLA in patients with PH, specifically PAH, was first reported by Schmid and colleagues [156]. The iLA was used as a bridge to lung transplantation for 62 days before the patient underwent successful double-lung transplantation. Other limited series with peripheral iLA have been reported in patients with PH as a bridge to lung transplantation with improvement in hemodynamics, inotrope requirements, and gas exchange [157]. Some of these patients required the addition of a pump to the oxygenator (i.e. conversion to VA ECMO), which reflects the limitations of this strategy in high-risk patients, a limitation our experience confirms.

The surgeons at Toronto University presented a novel approach to the use of the iLA with central, surgical placement from the pulmonary artery to the left atrium (Fig. 19.18) in patients with severe PH. The concept was that this strategy would provide a controlled right-to-left shunt allowing unloading of the RV while maintaining certain oxygenation (systemic level) via the shunt. De Perrot published the first series of four patients bridged to lung transplantation through the use of this technique with the iLA; all four patients survived to lung transplantation [90]. The time of support was prolonged with 9–69 days on the iLA device. Further experience with this technique using the Novalung iLA and with VA ECMO allowed this group to minimize mortality on the waitlist in patients listed with PAH [89].

In our experience with similar use of the Novalung iLA system, the low flows maintained (1.5–2 L/min) in the absence of a high-speed pump (as seen in VA ECMO) increased the chances of systemic thrombosis despite adequate anticoagulation. When used in a central configuration (PA-left atrium), this may be associated with an increased risk of thromboembolism and cerebrovascular accident (CVA).

MCS in Acute Pulmonary Embolism and Chronic Thromboembolic Disease

For patients with an acute pulmonary embolism (PE) and chronic thromboembolic disease (Group 4 PH), VA ECMO has been used to provide initial hemodynamic support. In the case of acute PE, ECMO has also been used to support patients presenting in severe right-heart failure with circulatory collapse as a bridge to surgical embolectomy, partial thrombolysis, or heparin treatment with adequate success [158]. Additionally, VA ECMO has been used in patients with CTEPH experiencing acute decompensation and shock as a bridge to PTE [159]. In our local experience at the University of Pittsburgh Medical Center, five of six patients in profound cardiogenic shock survived with the use of emergent peripheral VA ECMO without the need for surgical intervention. Thrombolysis was performed in four patients and one patient received only heparin due to a recent, large CVA. In a study by Maggio and colleagues, 21 patients were placed on ECMO for massive PE, and subsequently anticoagulated; 20 % of the patients underwent PTE. The overall survival rate was 62 % (13/21) [160]. Occasionally, ECMO may be necessary following PTE in cases of severe pulmonary flow redistribution with ventilation/perfusion (VQ) mismatch or pulmonary hemorrhage [33].

Summary

Despite improvements in the medical treatment of PH, there is an inevitable progression of the disease. In the advanced phases of clinical deterioration, a combination of surgical and medical options becomes available. It is critical for those involved in the management of patients with PH to have a

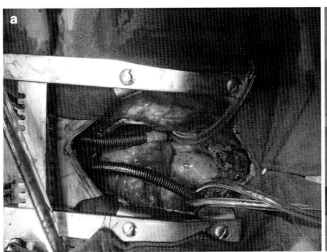 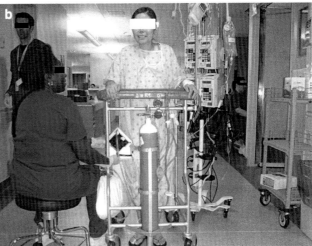

Fig. 19.18 Interventional Lung Assist (iLA, Novalung) used with central LA-PA cannulation in a patient with PAH. (**a**) Cannula placement in the operating room. (**b**) Patient mobilization on the ward during support (Reprinted from [90] with permission from Elsevier)

clear understanding of the alternatives and their results for specific groups of patients with PH. Surgical options include less invasive modalities, such as percutaneous balloon AS, Pott's shunt, and stenting of a patent ductus arteriosus; and more definitive invasive options, such as pulmonary endarterectomy, double-lung transplantation, and heart-lung transplantation, and most recently, the use of mechanical circulatory support as a bridge to transplant and in selected cases, to recovery.

References

1. Norfolk SG, Lederer DJ, Tapson VF. Lung transplantation and atrial septostomy in pulmonary arterial hypertension. Clin Chest Med. 2013;34:857–65.
2. McLaughlin VV, Archer SL, Badesch DB, et al. ACCF/AHA 2009 expert consensus document on pulmonary hypertension a report of the American College of Cardiology Foundation Task Force on Expert Consensus Documents and the American Heart Association developed in collaboration with the American College of Chest Physicians; American Thoracic Society, Inc.; and the Pulmonary Hypertension Association. J Am Coll Cardiol. 2009;53:1573–619.
3. Zamanian RT, Kudelko KT, Sung YK, de Jesus Perez V, Liu J, Spiekerkoetter E. Current clinical management of pulmonary arterial hypertension. Circ Res. 2014;115:131–47.
4. Higenbottam T, Wheeldon D, Wells F, Wallwork J. Long-term treatment of primary pulmonary hypertension with continuous intravenous epoprostenol (prostacyclin). Lancet. 1984;1:1046–7.
5. Hoeper MM, Schwarze M, Ehlerding S, et al. Long-term treatment of primary pulmonary hypertension with aerosolized iloprost, a prostacyclin analogue. N Engl J Med. 2000;342:1866–70.
6. Rubin LJ, Badesch DB, Barst RJ, et al. Bosentan therapy for pulmonary arterial hypertension. N Engl J Med. 2002;346:896–903.
7. Simonneau G, Barst RJ, Galie N, et al. Continuous subcutaneous infusion of treprostinil, a prostacyclin analogue, in patients with pulmonary arterial hypertension: a double-blind, randomized, placebo-controlled trial. Am J Respir Crit Care Med. 2002;165:800–4.
8. Sitbon O, Humbert M, Nunes H, et al. Long-term intravenous epoprostenol infusion in primary pulmonary hypertension: prognostic factors and survival. J Am Coll Cardiol. 2002;40:780–8.
9. Galie N, Ghofrani HA, Torbicki A, et al. Sildenafil citrate therapy for pulmonary arterial hypertension. N Engl J Med. 2005;353:2148–57.
10. Barst RJ, Rubin LJ, Long WA, et al. A comparison of continuous intravenous epoprostenol (prostacyclin) with conventional therapy for primary pulmonary hypertension. N Engl J Med. 1996;334:296–301.
11. Benza RL, Miller DP, Barst RJ, Badesch DB, Frost AE, McGoon MD. An evaluation of long-term survival from time of diagnosis in pulmonary arterial hypertension from the REVEAL Registry. Chest. 2012;142:448–56.
12. D'Alonzo GE, Barst RJ, Ayres SM, et al. Survival in patients with primary pulmonary hypertension. Results from a national prospective registry. Ann Intern Med. 1991;115:343–9.
13. McGoon M, Gutterman D, Steen V, et al. Screening, early detection, and diagnosis of pulmonary arterial hypertension: ACCP evidence-based clinical practice guidelines. Chest. 2004;126:14S–34.
14. Angel Gomez-Sanchez M, Saenz De La Calzada C, Escribano Subias P, et al. Pilot assessment of the response of several pulmo-

nary hemodynamic variables to sublingual sildenafil in candidates for heart transplantation. Eur J Heart Fail. 2004;6:615–7.
15. Califf RM, Adams KF, McKenna WJ, et al. A randomized controlled trial of epoprostenol therapy for severe congestive heart failure: The Flolan International Randomized Survival Trial (FIRST). Am Heart J. 1997;134:44–54.
16. Cotter G, Kaluski E, Stangl K, et al. The hemodynamic and neurohormonal effects of low doses of tezosentan (an endothelin A/B receptor antagonist) in patients with acute heart failure. Eur J Heart Fail. 2004;6:601–9.
17. Guazzi M, Tumminello G, Di Marco F, Fiorentini C, Guazzi MD. The effects of phosphodiesterase-5 inhibition with sildenafil on pulmonary hemodynamics and diffusion capacity, exercise ventilatory efficiency, and oxygen uptake kinetics in chronic heart failure. J Am Coll Cardiol. 2004;44:2339–48.
18. Hare JM, Shernan SK, Body SC, Graydon E, Colucci WS, Couper GS. Influence of inhaled nitric oxide on systemic flow and ventricular filling pressure in patients receiving mechanical circulatory assistance. Circulation. 1997;95:2250–3.
19. Healey JS, Davies RA, Tang AS. Improvement of apparently fixed pulmonary hypertension with cardiac resynchronization therapy. J Heart Lung Transplant. 2004;23:650–2.
20. Gamra H, Zhang HP, Allen JW, Lou FY, Ruiz CE. Factors determining normalization of pulmonary vascular resistance following successful balloon mitral valvotomy. Am J Cardiol. 1999;83:392–5.
21. Malouf JF, Enriquez-Sarano M, Pellikka PA, et al. Severe pulmonary hypertension in patients with severe aortic valve stenosis: clinical profile and prognostic implications. J Am Coll Cardiol. 2002;40:789–95.
22. Bishu K, Suri RM, Nkomo VT, et al. Prognostic impact of pulmonary artery systolic pressure in patients undergoing transcatheter aortic valve replacement for aortic stenosis. Am J Cardiol. 2014;114:1562–7.
23. Sinning JM, Hammerstingl C, Chin D, et al. Decrease of pulmonary hypertension impacts on prognosis after transcatheter aortic valve replacement. EuroIntervention. 2014;9:1042–9.
24. Smith CR, Leon MB, Mack MJ, et al. Transcatheter versus surgical aortic-valve replacement in high-risk patients. N Engl J Med. 2011;364:2187–98.
25. Butler J, Chomsky DB, Wilson JR. Pulmonary hypertension and exercise intolerance in patients with heart failure. J Am Coll Cardiol. 1999;34:1802–6.
26. Ghio S, Gavazzi A, Campana C, et al. Independent and additive prognostic value of right ventricular systolic function and pulmonary artery pressure in patients with chronic heart failure. J Am Coll Cardiol. 2001;37:183–8.
27. Nair PK, Kormos RL, Teuteberg JJ, et al. Pulsatile left ventricular assist device support as a bridge to decision in patients with end-stage heart failure complicated by pulmonary hypertension. J Heart Lung Transplant. 2010;29:201–8.
28. Atluri P, Fairman AS, MacArthur JW, et al. Continuous flow left ventricular assist device implant significantly improves pulmonary hypertension, right ventricular contractility, and tricuspid valve competence. J Card Surg. 2013;28:770–5.
29. Gupta S, Woldendorp K, Muthiah K, et al. Normalisation of haemodynamics in patients with end-stage heart failure with continuous-flow left ventricular assist device therapy. Heart Lung Circ. 2014;23:963–9.
30. Mikus E, Stepanenko A, Krabatsch T, et al. Reversibility of fixed pulmonary hypertension in left ventricular assist device support recipients. Eur J Cardiothorac Surg. 2011;40:971–7.
31. Andersen CU, Mellemkjaer S, Nielsen-Kudsk JE, Bendstrup E, Hilberg O, Simonsen U. Pulmonary hypertension in chronic obstructive and interstitial lung diseases. Int J Cardiol. 2013;168:1795–804.

32. Jenkins DP, Madani M, Mayer E, et al. Surgical treatment of chronic thromboembolic pulmonary hypertension. Eur Respir J. 2013;41:735–42.

33. Madani MM, Auger WR, Pretorius V, et al. Pulmonary endarterectomy: recent changes in a single institution's experience of more than 2,700 patients. Ann Thorac Surg. 2012;94:97–103; discussion 103.

34. Mahesh B, Nwaejike N, Dunning JJ, Jenkins DP. A novel technique for pulmonary endarterectomy in the presence of patent coronary artery bypass grafts. Eur J Cardiothorac Surg. 2012;42:175–7.

35. Mayer E, Jenkins D, Lindner J, et al. Surgical management and outcome of patients with chronic thromboembolic pulmonary hypertension: results from an international prospective registry. J Thorac Cardiovasc Surg. 2011;141:702–10.

36. Thistlethwaite PA, Mo M, Madani MM, et al. Operative classification of thromboembolic disease determines outcome after pulmonary endarterectomy. J Thorac Cardiovasc Surg. 2002;124:1203–11.

37. Fedullo P, Kerr KM, Kim NH, Auger WR. Chronic thromboembolic pulmonary hypertension. Am J Respir Crit Care Med. 2011;183:1605–13.

38. Ozsu S, Cinarka H. Chronic thromboembolic pulmonary hypertension: medical treatment. Pulm Circ. 2013;3:341–4.

39. Thenappan T, Shah SJ, Rich S, Gomberg-Maitland M. A USA-based registry for pulmonary arterial hypertension: 1982–2006. Eur Respir J. 2007;30:1103–10.

40. Moser KM, Auger WR, Fedullo PF. Chronic major-vessel thromboembolic pulmonary hypertension. Circulation. 1990;81:1735–43.

41. Riedel M, Stanek V, Widimsky J, Prerovsky I. Longterm follow-up of patients with pulmonary thromboembolism. Late prognosis and evolution of hemodynamic and respiratory data. Chest. 1982;81:151–8.

42. Pepke-Zaba J, Delcroix M, Lang I, et al. Chronic thromboembolic pulmonary hypertension (CTEPH): results from an international prospective registry. Circulation. 2011;124:1973–81.

43. Jamieson SW, Nomura K. Indications for and the results of pulmonary thromboendarterectomy for thromboembolic pulmonary hypertension. Semin Vasc Surg. 2000;13:236–44.

44. Bresser P, Pepke-Zaba J, Jais X, Humbert M, Hoeper MM. Medical therapies for chronic thromboembolic pulmonary hypertension: an evolving treatment paradigm. Proc Am Thorac Soc. 2006;3:594–600.

45. de Perrot M, Thenganatt J, McRae K, et al. Pulmonary endarterectomy in severe chronic thromboembolic pulmonary hypertension. J Heart Lung Transplant. 2015;34:369–75.

46. Klepetko W, Mayer E, Sandoval J, et al. Interventional and surgical modalities of treatment for pulmonary arterial hypertension. J Am Coll Cardiol. 2004;43:73S–80.

47. Rahnavardi M, Yan TD, Cao C, Vallely MP, Bannon PG, Wilson MK. Pulmonary thromboendarterectomy for chronic thromboembolic pulmonary hypertension: a systematic review. Ann Thorac Cardiovasc Surg. 2011;17:435–45.

48. Ghofrani HA, D'Armini AM, Grimminger F, et al. Riociguat for the treatment of chronic thromboembolic pulmonary hypertension. N Engl J Med. 2013;369:319–29.

49. Rashkind WJ, Miller WW. Creation of an atrial septal defect without thoracotomy. A palliative approach to complete transposition of the great arteries. JAMA. 1966;196:991–2.

50. Watson H, Rashkind WJ. Creation of atrial septal defects by balloon catheter in babies with transposition of the great arteries. Lancet. 1967;1:403–5.

51. Park SC, Zuberbuhler JR, Neches WH, Lenox CC, Zoltun RA. A new atrial septostomy technique. Cathet Cardiovasc Diagn. 1975;1:195–201.

52. Rich S, Lam W. Atrial septostomy as palliative therapy for refractory primary pulmonary hypertension. Am J Cardiol. 1983;51:1560–1.

53. Kerstein D, Levy PS, Hsu DT, Hordof AJ, Gersony WM, Barst RJ. Blade balloon atrial septostomy in patients with severe primary pulmonary hypertension. Circulation. 1995;91:2028–35.

54. Nihill MR, O'Laughlin MP, Mullins CE. Effects of atrial septostomy in patients with terminal cor pulmonale due to pulmonary vascular disease. Cathet Cardiovasc Diagn. 1991;24:166–72.

55. Kanemoto N. Natural history of pulmonary hemodynamics in primary pulmonary hypertension. Am Heart J. 1987;114:407–13.

56. Law MA, Grifka RG, Mullins CE, Nihill MR. Atrial septostomy improves survival in select patients with pulmonary hypertension. Am Heart J. 2007;153:779–84.

57. Sandoval J, Gaspar J, Pulido T, et al. Graded balloon dilation atrial septostomy in severe primary pulmonary hypertension. A therapeutic alternative for patients nonresponsive to vasodilator treatment. J Am Coll Cardiol. 1998;32:297–304.

58. Rozkovec A, Montanes P, Oakley CM. Factors that influence the outcome of primary pulmonary hypertension. Br Heart J. 1986;55:449–58.

59. Hopkins WE, Ochoa LL, Richardson GW, Trulock EP. Comparison of the hemodynamics and survival of adults with severe primary pulmonary hypertension or Eisenmenger syndrome. J Heart Lung Transplant. 1996;15:100–5.

60. Austen WG, Morrow AG, Berry WB. Experimental studies of the surgical treatment of primary pulmonary hypertension. J Thorac Cardiovasc Surg. 1964;48:448–55.

61. Kothari SS, Yusuf A, Juneja R, Yadav R, Naik N. Graded balloon atrial septostomy in severe pulmonary hypertension. Indian Heart J. 2002;54:164–9.

62. Reichenberger F, Pepke-Zaba J, McNeil K, Parameshwar J, Shapiro LM. Atrial septostomy in the treatment of severe pulmonary arterial hypertension. Thorax. 2003;58:797–800.

63. Rothman A, Beltran D, Kriett JM, Smith C, Wolf P, Jamieson SW. Graded balloon dilation atrial septostomy as a bridge to lung transplantation in pulmonary hypertension. Am Heart J. 1993;125:1763–6.

64. Bhamra-Ariza P, Keogh AM, Muller DW. Percutaneous interventional therapies for the treatment of patients with severe pulmonary hypertension. J Am Coll Cardiol. 2014;63:611–8.

65. Lordan JL, Corris PA. Pulmonary arterial hypertension and lung transplantation. Expert Rev Respir Med. 2011;5:441–54.

66. Hayden AM. Balloon atrial septostomy increases cardiac index and may reduce mortality among pulmonary hypertension patients awaiting lung transplantation. J Transpl Coord. 1997;7:131–3.

67. Sandoval J, Rothman A, Pulido T. Atrial septostomy for pulmonary hypertension. Clin Chest Med. 2001;22:547–60.

68. Trulock EP. Lung transplantation and atrial septostomy for pulmonary arterial hypertension. In: Hill NS, Farber HW, editors. Pulmonary hypertension. Totowa: Humana Press; 2008. p. 383–403.

69. Biscotti M, Sonett J, Bacchetta M. ECMO as bridge to lung transplant. Thorac Surg Clin. 2015;25:17–25.

70. Hayanga AJ, Aboagye J, Esper S, et al. Extracorporeal membrane oxygenation as a bridge to lung transplantation in the United States: an evolving strategy in the management of rapidly advancing pulmonary disease. J Thorac Cardiovasc Surg. 2015;149:291–6.

71. Rich S, Dodin E, McLaughlin VV. Usefulness of atrial septostomy as a treatment for primary pulmonary hypertension and guidelines for its application. Am J Cardiol. 1997;80:369–71.

72. Keogh AM, Mayer E, Benza RL, et al. Interventional and surgical modalities of treatment in pulmonary hypertension. J Am Coll Cardiol. 2009;54:S67–77.

73. Hardy JD, Webb WR, Dalton Jr ML, Walker Jr GR. Lung homotransplantation in man. JAMA. 1963;186:1065–74.

74. Reitz BA. The first successful combined heart-lung transplantation. J Thorac Cardiovasc Surg. 2011;141:867–9.

75. Cooper JD, Pearson FG, Patterson GA, et al. Technique of successful lung transplantation in humans. J Thorac Cardiovasc Surg. 1987;93:173–81.

76. Kaiser LR, Pasque MK, Trulock EP, Low DE, Dresler CM, Cooper JD. Bilateral sequential lung transplantation: the procedure of choice for double-lung replacement. Ann Thorac Surg. 1991;52:438–45. discussion 45–6.

77. Patterson GA, Cooper JD, Goldman B, et al. Technique of successful clinical double-lung transplantation. Ann Thorac Surg. 1988;45:626–33.

78. Yusen RD, Christie JD, Edwards LB, et al. The Registry of the International Society for Heart and Lung Transplantation: Thirtieth Adult Lung and Heart-Lung Transplant Report – 2013; focus theme: age. J Heart Lung Transplant. 2013;32:965–78.

79. Yusen RD, Edwards LB, Kucheryavaya AY, et al. The registry of the International Society for Heart and Lung Transplantation: thirty-first adult lung and heart-lung transplant report – 2014; focus theme: retransplantation. J Heart Lung Transplant. 2014;33:1009–24.

80. Dresdale DT, Schultz M, Michtom RJ. Primary pulmonary hypertension. I. Clinical and hemodynamic study. Am J Med. 1951;11:686–705.

81. Fadel E, Mercier O, Mussot S, et al. Long-term outcome of double-lung and heart-lung transplantation for pulmonary hypertension: a comparative retrospective study of 219 patients. Eur J Cardiothorac Surg. 2010;38:277–84.

82. George MP, Champion HC, Pilewski JM. Lung transplantation for pulmonary hypertension. Pulm Circ. 2011;1:182–91.

83. Orens JB, Estenne M, Arcasoy S, et al. International guidelines for the selection of lung transplant candidates: 2006 update – a consensus report from the Pulmonary Scientific Council of the International Society for Heart and Lung Transplantation. J Heart Lung Transplant. 2006;25:745–55.

84. Egan TM, Murray S, Bustami RT, et al. Development of the new lung allocation system in the United States. Am J Transplant. 2006;6:1212–27.

85. Chen H, Shiboski SC, Golden JA, et al. Impact of the lung allocation score on lung transplantation for pulmonary arterial hypertension. Am J Respir Crit Care Med. 2009;180:468–74.

86. Davis SQ, Garrity Jr ER. Organ allocation in lung transplant. Chest. 2007;132:1646–51.

87. Chan KM. Idiopathic pulmonary arterial hypertension and equity of donor lung allocation in the era of the lung allocation score: are we there yet? Am J Respir Crit Care Med. 2009;180:385–7.

88. Schaffer JM, Singh SK, Joyce DL, et al. Transplantation for idiopathic pulmonary arterial hypertension: improvement in the lung allocation score era. Circulation. 2013;127:2503–13.

89. de Perrot M, Granton JT, McRae K, et al. Outcome of patients with pulmonary arterial hypertension referred for lung transplantation: a 14-year single-center experience. J Thorac Cardiovasc Surg. 2012;143:910–8.

90. de Perrot M, Granton JT, McRae K, et al. Impact of extracorporeal life support on outcome in patients with idiopathic pulmonary arterial hypertension awaiting lung transplantation. J Heart Lung Transplant. 2011;30:997–1002.

91. Fuehner T, Kuehn C, Hadem J, et al. Extracorporeal membrane oxygenation in awake patients as bridge to lung transplantation. Am J Respir Crit Care Med. 2012;185:763–8.

92. Haneya A, Philipp A, Mueller T, et al. Extracorporeal circulatory systems as a bridge to lung transplantation at remote transplant centers. Ann Thorac Surg. 2011;91:250–5.

93. Javidfar J, Brodie D, Iribarne A, et al. Extracorporeal membrane oxygenation as a bridge to lung transplantation and recovery. J Thorac Cardiovasc Surg. 2012;144:716–21.

94. Mason DP, Thuita L, Nowicki ER, Murthy SC, Pettersson GB, Blackstone EH. Should lung transplantation be performed for patients on mechanical respiratory support? The US experience. J Thorac Cardiovasc Surg. 2010;139:765–73. e1.

95. Olsson KM, Simon A, Strueber M, et al. Extracorporeal membrane oxygenation in nonintubated patients as bridge to lung transplantation. Am J Transplant. 2010;10:2173–8.

96. Toyoda Y, Bhama JK, Shigemura N, et al. Efficacy of extracorporeal membrane oxygenation as a bridge to lung transplantation. J Thorac Cardiovasc Surg. 2013;145:1065–70. discussion 70–1.

97. Galie N, Corris PA, Frost A, et al. Updated treatment algorithm of pulmonary arterial hypertension. J Am Coll Cardiol. 2013;62:D60–72.

98. Chaouat A, Bugnet AS, Kadaoui N, et al. Severe pulmonary hypertension and chronic obstructive pulmonary disease. Am J Respir Crit Care Med. 2005;172:189–94.

99. Cottin V, Le Pavec J, Prevot G, et al. Pulmonary hypertension in patients with combined pulmonary fibrosis and emphysema syndrome. Eur Respir J. 2010;35:105–11.

100. Lettieri CJ, Nathan SD, Barnett SD, Ahmad S, Shorr AF. Prevalence and outcomes of pulmonary arterial hypertension in advanced idiopathic pulmonary fibrosis. Chest. 2006;129:746–52.

101. Palmero V, Sulica R. Sarcoidosis-associated pulmonary hypertension: assessment and management. Semin Respir Crit Care Med. 2010;31:494–500.

102. Reitz BA, Gaudiani VA, Hunt SA, et al. Diagnosis and treatment of allograft rejection in heart-lung transplant recipients. J Thorac Cardiovasc Surg. 1983;85:354–61.

103. Reitz BA, Wallwork JL, Hunt SA, et al. Heart-lung transplantation: successful therapy for patients with pulmonary vascular disease. N Engl J Med. 1982;306:557–64.

104. Bolman 3rd RM, Shumway SJ, Estrin JA, Hertz MI. Lung and heart-lung transplantation. Evolution and new applications. Ann Surg. 1991;214:456–68. discussion 69–70.

105. Toyoda Y, Thacker J, Santos R, et al. Long-term outcome of lung and heart-lung transplantation for idiopathic pulmonary arterial hypertension. Ann Thorac Surg. 2008;86:1116–22.

106. Christie JD, Edwards LB, Kucheryavaya AY, et al. The Registry of the International Society for Heart and Lung Transplantation: 29th adult lung and heart-lung transplant report-2012. J Heart Lung Transplant. 2012;31:1073–86.

107. Bando K, Armitage JM, Paradis IL, et al. Indications for and results of single, bilateral, and heart-lung transplantation for pulmonary hypertension. J Thorac Cardiovasc Surg. 1994;108:1056–65.

108. Bando K, Keenan RJ, Paradis IL, et al. Impact of pulmonary hypertension on outcome after single-lung transplantation. Ann Thorac Surg. 1994;58:1336–42.

109. Gammie JS, Keenan RJ, Pham SM, et al. Single- versus double-lung transplantation for pulmonary hypertension. J Thorac Cardiovasc Surg. 1998;115:397–402; discussion –3.

110. Brown CR, Mason DP, Pettersson GB, Murthy SC. Outcomes after single lung transplantation in older patients with secondary pulmonary arterial hypertension. J Heart Lung Transplant. 2013;32:134–6.

111. Conte JV, Borja MJ, Patel CB, Yang SC, Jhaveri RM, Orens JB. Lung transplantation for primary and secondary pulmonary hypertension. Ann Thorac Surg. 2001;72:1673–9. discussion 9–80.

112. Christie JD, Edwards LB, Aurora P, et al. Registry of the International Society for Heart and Lung Transplantation: twenty-fifth official adult lung and heart/lung transplantation report – 2008. J Heart Lung Transplant. 2008;27:957–69.

113. Olland A, Falcoz PE, Canuet M, Massard G. Should we perform bilateral-lung or heart-lung transplantation for patients with pul-

monary hypertension? Interact Cardiovasc Thorac Surg. 2013;17:166–70.

114. Mendeloff EN, Meyers BF, Sundt TM, et al. Lung transplantation for pulmonary vascular disease. Ann Thorac Surg. 2002;73:209–17. discussion 17–9.

115. Mikhail G, al-Kattan K, Banner N, et al. Long-term results of heart-lung transplantation for pulmonary hypertension. Transplant Proc. 1997;29:633.

116. Moffatt-Bruce SD, Karamichalis J, Robbins RC, Whyte RI, Theodore J, Reitz BA. Are heart-lung transplant recipients protected from developing bronchiolitis obliterans syndrome? Ann Thorac Surg. 2006;81:286–91. discussion 91.

117. Waddell TK, Bennett L, Kennedy R, Todd TR, Keshavjee SH. Heart-lung or lung transplantation for Eisenmenger syndrome. J Heart Lung Transplant. 2002;21:731–7.

118. Mohite PN, Sabashnikov A, Rao P, Zych B, Simon A. Single lung retransplantation for graft infarction due to herniation of heart. Thorac Cardiovasc Surg Rep. 2013;2:40–2.

119. Hayanga JW, D'Cunha J. The surgical technique of bilateral sequential lung transplantation. J Thorac Dis. 2014;6:1063–9.

120. Vouhe PR, Dartevelle PG. Heart-lung transplantation. Technical modifications that may improve the early outcome. J Thorac Cardiovasc Surg. 1989;97:906–10.

121. Diamond JM, Lee JC, Kawut SM, et al. Clinical risk factors for primary graft dysfunction after lung transplantation. Am J Respir Crit Care Med. 2013;187:527–34.

122. Fang A, Studer S, Kawut SM, et al. Elevated pulmonary artery pressure is a risk factor for primary graft dysfunction following lung transplantation for idiopathic pulmonary fibrosis. Chest. 2011;139:782–7.

123. Kuntz CL, Hadjiliadis D, Ahya VN, et al. Risk factors for early primary graft dysfunction after lung transplantation: a registry study. Clin Transplant. 2009;23:819–30.

124. Bermudez CA, Rocha RV, Katz WE, Toyoda Y. Novel mechanism of mitral regurgitation after lung transplantation in a patient with scleroderma and pulmonary hypertension. J Thorac Cardiovasc Surg. 2011;141:e1–3.

125. Castleberry AW, Hartwig MG, Whitson BA. Extracorporeal membrane oxygenation post lung transplantation. Curr Opin Organ Transplant. 2013;18(5):524–30.

126. Fischer S, Bohn D, Rycus P, et al. Extracorporeal membrane oxygenation for primary graft dysfunction after lung transplantation: analysis of the Extracorporeal Life Support Organization (ELSO) registry. J Heart Lung Transplant. 2007;26:472–7.

127. Hartwig MG, Appel 3rd JZ, Cantu 3rd E, et al. Improved results treating lung allograft failure with venovenous extracorporeal membrane oxygenation. Ann Thorac Surg. 2005;80:1872–9. discussion 9–80.

128. Hartwig MG, Snyder LD, Finlen-Copeland A, et al. Lung transplantation at Duke University. Clin Transpl. 2009;197–210.

129. Mason DP, Boffa DJ, Murthy SC, et al. Extended use of extracorporeal membrane oxygenation after lung transplantation. J Thorac Cardiovasc Surg. 2006;132:954–60.

130. Katz WE, Gasior TA, Quinlan JJ, et al. Immediate effects of lung transplantation on right ventricular morphology and function in patients with variable degrees of pulmonary hypertension. J Am Coll Cardiol. 1996;27:384–91.

131. Gregoric ID, Chandra D, Myers TJ, Scheinin SA, Loyalka P, Kar B. Extracorporeal membrane oxygenation as a bridge to emergency heart-lung transplantation in a patient with idiopathic pulmonary arterial hypertension. J Heart Lung Transplant. 2008;27:466–8.

132. Mohite PN, Sabashnikov A, Reed A, et al. Extracorporeal life support in "awake" patients as a bridge to lung transplant. Thorac Cardiovasc Surg. 2015 [Epub ahead of print March 5, 2015].

133. Rosenzweig EB, Brodie D, Abrams DC, Agerstrand CL, Bacchetta M. Extracorporeal membrane oxygenation as a novel bridging strategy for acute right heart failure in group 1 pulmonary arterial hypertension. ASAIO J. 2014;60:129–33.

134. Alba AC, Rao V, Ross HJ, et al. Impact of fixed pulmonary hypertension on post-heart transplant outcomes in bridge-to-transplant patients. J Heart Lung Transplant. 2010;29:1253–8.

135. Kormos RL, Teuteberg JJ, Pagani FD, et al. Right ventricular failure in patients with the HeartMate II continuous-flow left ventricular assist device: incidence, risk factors, and effect on outcomes. J Thorac Cardiovasc Surg. 2010;139:1316–24.

136. Bhama JK, Kormos RL, Toyoda Y, Teuteberg JJ, McCurry KR, Siegenthaler MP. Clinical experience using the Levitronix CentriMag system for temporary right ventricular mechanical circulatory support. J Heart Lung Transplant. 2009;28:971–6.

137. John R, Long JW, Massey HT, et al. Outcomes of a multicenter trial of the Levitronix CentriMag ventricular assist system for short-term circulatory support. J Thorac Cardiovasc Surg. 2011;141:932–9.

138. Clinical trial results for impella RP right ventricular heart failure trial. Recover Right. Released at TCT 2014. 2014.

139. Punnoose L, Burkhoff D, Rich S, Horn EM. Right ventricular assist device in end-stage pulmonary arterial hypertension: insights from a computational model of the cardiovascular system. Prog Cardiovasc Dis. 2012;55:234–43. e2.

140. Fischer S, Hoeper MM, Tomaszek S, et al. Bridge to lung transplantation with the extracorporeal membrane ventilator Novalung in the veno-venous mode: the initial Hannover experience. ASAIO J. 2007;53:168–70.

141. Biscotti M, Vail E, Cook KE, Kachulis B, Rosenzweig EB, Bacchetta M. Extracorporeal membrane oxygenation with subclavian artery cannulation in awake patients with pulmonary hypertension. ASAIO J. 2014;60:748–50.

142. Abrams DC, Brodie D, Rosenzweig EB, Burkart KM, Agerstrand CL, Bacchetta MD. Upper-body extracorporeal membrane oxygenation as a strategy in decompensated pulmonary arterial hypertension. Pulm Circ. 2013;3:432–5.

143. Hayes Jr D, Galantowicz M, Preston TJ, Lloyd EA, Tobias JD, McConnell PI. Tracheostomy in adolescent patients bridged to lung transplantation with ambulatory venovenous extracorporeal membrane oxygenation. J Artif Organs. 2014;17:103–5.

144. Hayes Jr D, McConnell PI, Preston TJ, Yates AR, Kirkby S, Galantowicz M. Active rehabilitation with venovenous extracorporeal membrane oxygenation as a bridge to lung transplantation in a pediatric patient. World J Pediatr. 2013;9:373–4.

145. Peek GJ, Mugford M, Tiruvoipati R, et al. Efficacy and economic assessment of conventional ventilatory support versus extracorporeal membrane oxygenation for severe adult respiratory failure (CESAR): a multicentre randomised controlled trial. Lancet. 2009;374:1351–63.

146. Hoopes CW, Gurley JC, Zwischenberger JB, Diaz-Guzman E. Mechanical support for pulmonary veno-occlusive disease: combined atrial septostomy and venovenous extracorporeal membrane oxygenation. Semin Thorac Cardiovasc Surg. 2012;24:232–4.

147. Javidfar J, Brodie D, Sonett J, Bacchetta M. Venovenous extracorporeal membrane oxygenation using a single cannula in patients with pulmonary hypertension and atrial septal defects. J Thorac Cardiovasc Surg. 2012;143:982–4.

148. Cypel M, Keshavjee S. Extracorporeal life support as a bridge to lung transplantation. Clin Chest Med. 2011;32:245–51.

149. Valapour M, Skeans MA, Heubner BM, et al. OPTN/SRTR 2012 annual data report: lung. Am J Transplant. 2014;14 Suppl 1:139–65.

150. Bermudez CA, Rocha RV, Zaldonis D, et al. Extracorporeal membrane oxygenation as a bridge to lung transplant: midterm outcomes. Ann Thorac Surg. 2011;92:1226–31. discussion 31–2.

151. Chiumello D, Coppola S, Froio S, Colombo A, Del Sorbo L. Extracorporeal life support as bridge to lung transplantation: a systematic review. Crit Care. 2015;19:19.

152. Hoopes CW, Kukreja J, Golden J, Davenport DL, Diaz-Guzman E, Zwischenberger JB. Extracorporeal membrane oxygenation as a bridge to pulmonary transplantation. J Thorac Cardiovasc Surg. 2013;145:862–7. discussion 7–8.

153. Lang G, Taghavi S, Aigner C, et al. Primary lung transplantation after bridge with extracorporeal membrane oxygenation: a plea for a shift in our paradigms for indications. Transplantation. 2012;93:729–36.

154. Crotti S, Iotti GA, Lissoni A, et al. Organ allocation waiting time during extracorporeal bridge to lung transplant affects outcomes. Chest. 2013;144:1018–25.

155. Fischer S, Strueber M. The Novalung(R) iLA membrane ventilator: technical aspects. http://www.ctsnet.org/portals/thoracic/newtechnology/article-9. Published 19 July 2012. Accessed 9 Apr 2015.

156. Schmid C, Philipp A, Hilker M, et al. Bridge to lung transplantation through a pulmonary artery to left atrial oxygenator circuit. Ann Thorac Surg. 2008;85:1202–5.

157. Strueber M, Hoeper MM, Fischer S, et al. Bridge to thoracic organ transplantation in patients with pulmonary arterial hypertension using a pumpless lung assist device. Am J Transplant. 2009;9:853–7.

158. Deehring R, Kiss AB, Garrett A, Hillier AG. Extracorporeal membrane oxygenation as a bridge to surgical embolectomy in acute fulminant pulmonary embolism. Am J Emerg Med. 2006;24:879–80.

159. Mydin M, Berman M, Klein A, et al. Extracorporeal membrane oxygenation as a bridge to pulmonary endarterectomy. Ann Thorac Surg. 2011;92:e101–3.

160. Maggio P, Hemmila M, Haft J, Bartlett R. Extracorporeal life support for massive pulmonary embolism. J Trauma. 2007;62:570–6.

Patient Registries in Pulmonary Arterial Hypertension: the Role of Survival Equations and Risk Calculators

20

Colleen A. McEvoy, Mayank Sardana, Matthew Moll, Harrison W. Farber, and Murali M. Chakinala

Abbreviations

6 MW	6 minute walk
CHD	Congenital heart disease
CI	Cardiac index
COMPERA	Comparative Prospective Registry of Newly Initiated Therapies for Pulmonary Arterial Hypertension
CTD	Connective tissue disease
CTEPH	Chronic thromboembolic pulmonary hypertension
DLCO	Diffusing capacity of the lung for carbon monoxide
ERA	Endothelin receptor antagonist
HIV	Human immunodeficiency virus
HPAH	Heritable pulmonary arterial hypertension
IPAH	Idiopathic pulmonary arterial hypertension
LAS	Lung Allocation Score
LVEDP	Left ventricular end-diastolic pressure
MAI	Million adult inhabitants
NIH	National Institutes of Health
NYHA	New York Heart Association
PAH	Pulmonary arterial hypertension
PAP	Pulmonary arterial pressure
PAWP	Pulmonary arterial wedge pressure
PDE5	Phosphodiesterase 5
PHC	Pulmonary Hypertension Connection
PVOD	Pulmonary veno-occulsive disease
PVR	Pulmonary vascular resistance
QuERI	Quality Enhancement Research Initiative
RAP	Right atrial pressure
REHAP	Spanish Registry of Pulmonary Arterial Hypertension
REVEAL	Registry to evaluate early and long-term pulmonary arterial hypertension management
RHC	Right heart catheterization
ROC	Receiver operator characteristic
SMR	Scottish Morbidity Record
SPVU	Scottish Pulmonary Vascular Unit
WHO	World Health Organization

C.A. McEvoy, MD
Pulmonary and Critical Care Division, Washington University School of Medicine, St. Louis, MO, USA

M. Sardana, MBBS
Department of Medicine, Boston Medical Center, Boston, MA, USA

M. Moll, MD
Internal Medicine, Boston Medical Center, Boston, MA, USA

H.W. Farber, MD
Division of Pulmonary, Allergy, Sleep and Critical Care Medicine, Pulmonary Hypertension Center, Boston University School of Medicine, Boston Medical Center, Boston, MA, USA

M.M. Chakinala, MD (✉)
Pulmonary and Critical Care Division, Washington University School of Medicine, St. Louis, MO, USA

Internal Medicine, Washington University, St. Louis, MO, USA
e-mail: chakinalam@wustl.edu

Pulmonary arterial hypertension (PAH) is a rare and incurable disease with an estimated prevalence of 10–25 cases per million. As a consequence of chronically elevated right ventricular afterload, patients develop progressive right-sided heart failure, which is the primary mode of death. Many advances have been appreciated with PAH during the last three decades, thanks to improved awareness, more refined classification schemes, better understanding and management of right-sided heart failure and, most importantly, the availability of numerous PAH-specific therapies.

During this period, many observational registries have been conducted in different parts of the world, providing a global perspective of this rare disease. These efforts have characterized the presentation of PAH, documented the changing phenotype of PAH patients, updated survival rates and identified predictors of death. Some registries have also developed predictive equations that estimate survival rates; and when eventually validated, could assist clinicians with patient assessment and clinical decision-making.

© Springer International Publishing Switzerland 2016
B.A. Maron et al. (eds.), *Pulmonary Hypertension: Basic Science to Clinical Medicine*, DOI 10.1007/978-3-319-23594-3_20

In this chapter, some general aspects of patient registries will be introduced, followed by a review of some of the major PAH registries conducted in the last 30 years, emphasizing observations on survival and associated risk factors. Discussion will center on several predictive equations developed from four different large registries – National Institutes of Health (NIH), French National, Pulmonary Hypertension Connection (PHC), and Registry to Evaluate Early and Long-term Pulmonary Arterial Hypertension Disease Management (REVEAL). Next, the challenges of applying these predictive equations in clinical practice will be covered. Lastly, lessons learned from PAH registries and survival equations, as they pertain to improving the allocation of lungs for transplantation of PAH patients, will be introduced.

Observational Patient Registries

Registries provide information about a select group of patients, who ideally, represent individuals with similar disease characteristics in the general population. A major aim of clinical registries is to provide information about the natural history and prognosis of the patient cohort. Such registries have high generalizability and are especially useful for characterizing populations, assessing the burden of illness, and developing prognostic models [1, 2]. However, the observational nature of registries means that there is neither randomization nor a rigorous way to compare effectiveness of therapies, and it is difficult to account for confounding variables [3]. Furthermore, there are no hypotheses at the initiation of a registry, but the breadth of clinical information collected makes registries a rich medium for generating new hypotheses.

Registries can be used to complement randomized controlled trials in determining outcomes. The Effective Health Care Program of the Agency for Healthcare Research and Quality defines a patient registry as "an organized system that uses observational study methods to collect uniform data (clinical and other) to evaluate specified outcomes for a population defined by a particular disease, condition or exposure and that serves a predetermined scientific, clinical or policy purpose(s)" [1]. Registries describe the natural history of the disease and can help determine clinical effectiveness. The European Medicine Agency also defines registry as "an organized system that uses observational methods to collect uniform data on specified outcomes in a population defined by a particular disease, condition or exposure" [4].

Registries examine the epidemiology of *prevalent* or *incident* cases. Prevalent cases comprise individuals who have previously been diagnosed. The term incident refers to cases that are newly diagnosed during a pre-defined time period. Generally, patients are considered incident on the day of

diagnosis and prevalent the following day [3]. But, registries can differ even in their definition of incident and prevalent cases. Methodological differences can account for some variation in incidence and prevalence across registries. For example, the allowable time elapsed between the diagnostic right heart catheterization (RHC) and enrollment in a registry can vary when differentiating an incident from a prevalent case. Prevalent patients are enrolled after enduring the disease for varying periods of time. This may lead to underestimation of true mortality since the sickest patients may have already died and not had the opportunity to be enrolled, while less severely affected patients survive the pre-enrollment period to become eligible for a registry. In essence, patients who die before study initiation are precluded from enrollment and patients who survive to study initiation are included, leading to an *immortal time bias*, which is a form of survivor bias that potentially inflates survival estimates. If the mortality rate for a condition were constant over time, as might be encountered in a natural history study of a condition without any available interventions, then the differentiation between prevalent and incident cases may not impact the estimation of mortality. But active treatment of PAH patients through management of right ventricular failure and PAH-specific medications, has impacted survival for many, but not all, individuals. Therefore, it is important to understand if a particular registry includes incident and prevalent cases because information derived from incident cases may not be generalizable to prevalent patients and vice versa.

Each registry defines specific *inclusion and exclusion criteria*. Although there are no standard inclusion and exclusion criteria amongst registries, the goal is to maximize generalizability, identify clear objectives for data collection, and minimize bias [2, 3]. These criteria vary depending on the objective of the registry, such as evaluating only Idiopathic Pulmonary Arterial Hypertension (IPAH) or including PAH associated with other conditions as most modern PAH registries have done (Table 20.1). The definition of PAH and World Health Organization (WHO) classification of PAH has evolved over time, leading to modifications in the inclusion-exclusion criteria across registries in different eras. For example, the NIH registry used a PAWP ≤ 12 mmHg with a PAP > 25 mmHg; whereas the REVEAL registry used a pulmonary arterial wedge pressure (PAWP) or left ventricular end-diastolic pressure (LVEDP) ≤ 18 mmHg as an inclusion criteria [5, 6]. And even though RHC is the gold standard for diagnosis, some have used echocardiographic measurement of pulmonary pressures for diagnosis as RHC may be infrequently performed within a region [7]. These factors are important to recognize when applying the results of a particular registry to another patient population.

Another key distinguishing design aspect of registries is the *method of data collection* – prospective, retrospective, or a mixture of the two. Clearly prospective and standardized

Table 20.1 Major PAH registries conducted over the last 30 years

Registry	Time period	Year of publication	Method of data collection	Location (number of centers)	Number of patients
NIH* [5]	1981–1985	1987	prospective	United States (32)	187
French National* [10]	2002–2003	2006	prospective	France (17)	674
PHC* [8]	1982–2004	2007	retrospective	United States (3)	578
	2004–2006		prospective		
Scottish – SMR [11]	1986–2001	2007	retrospective	Scotland	374
Chinese (pre-modern) [7]	1999–2004	2007	prospective	China (1)	72
REVEAL* [6]	2006–2009	2010	prospective	United States (55)	3515
Mayo [9]	1995–2004	2011	prospective	United States (1)	484
Swiss [15]	1999–2004	2011	prospective	Switzerland (9)	222
Chinese (modern) [14]	2008–2011	2011	prospective	China (9)	956
United Kingdom & Ireland [16]	2001–2009	2012	prospective	United Kingdom & Ireland (8)	482
Spanish [12]	1998–2006	2012	retrospective	Spain (31)	PAH: 866 CTEPH: 162
	2007–2008		prospective		
PAH QuERI [18]	2005–2007	2013	prospective	United States (60)	791
COMPERA [27]	2007–2016	2013	prospective	Western Europe (28)	1283

Registry	Study Cohort	Prevalent cases included	Prevalence of PAH (per MAI)	Prevalence of IPAH (per MAI)
NIH*	IPAH, HPAH, Anorexigen- PAH	No	–	–
French National*	Group 1 PH, age > 18 years	Yes	15	5.9
PHC*	Group 1 PH, age > 18 years IPAH 48 %, CTD 30 %, CHD 11 %	Yes	–	–
Scottish – SMR	Group 1 PH, age 16–65	Yes	26	9
Chinese (pre-modern)	IPAH and HPAH	Yes	–	–
REVEAL*	Group 1 PH, age > 3 months IPAH 46 %, CTD 25 %, CHD 10 %	Yes	10.6	0.9
Mayo	Group 1 PH, age > 18 years IPAH/HPAH 56 %, CTD 24 %, other 20 %	No	–	–
Swiss	Group 1 PH, Group 3 PH, CTEPH	Yes	–	–
Chinese (modern)	Group 1 PH, age > 18 years IPAH 35 %, CTD 19 %, CHD 43 %	No	–	–
United Kingdom & Ireland	IPAH, HPAH, Anorexigen-PAH	No	6.6	–
Spanish	Group 1 PH, CTEPH, age > 14 years IPAH 30 %, CTD 25 %, CHD 16 %	Yes	16	4.6
PAH QuERI	Group 1 PH IPAH/HPAH 38 %, CTD 29 %, CHD 7 %, Drug-exposure 5 %	Yes	–	–
COMPERA	Group 1 PH, age > 18 years	No	–	–

Registries listed by the year of publication. (*) Registries that developed survival prediction equations. *NIH* National Institutes of Health, *PHC* pulmonary hypertension connection, *SMR* Scottish Medical Record, *REVEAL* Registry to evaluate early and long-term pulmonary arterial hypertension disease management, *COMPERA* comparative, prospective registry of newly initiated therapies for pulmonary hypertension, *IPAH* idiopathic pulmonary arterial hypertension, *HPAH* heritable pulmonary arterial hypertension, *PAH* pulmonary arterial hypertension, *CTD* connective tissue disease, *CHD* congenital heart disease, *CTEPH* chronic thromboembolic pulmonary hypertension, *MAI* million adult inhabitants

data collection is superior, in order to minimize biases and missing or inaccurate data, but requires a much greater investment in time and resources.

PAH Registries

PAH Registries have a number of distinguishing characteristics, including the population recruited, the method of data collection, allowance of prevalent patients, era and region of data collection, timing of diagnosis, and period of observation. Table 20.1 displays the major PH registries conducted during the last 30 years. Starting with the landmark NIH registry of the early 1980s, PAH registries have been analyzed across the globe, allowing for comparison between populations in different eras and regions [3]. Important prognostic information has also been obtained. Systematic clinical surveillance of PAH is important especially as the field advances the knowledge of pathophysiology and therapeutics. Registries have importantly identified the changing phenotype of PAH over time. The continual reassessment of patient demographics and survival are essential in the aging population and in the ever-changing climate of improved PAH targeted therapies. New assessments of survival in the modern era helped develop predictive survival equations. Furthermore, epidemiological data and practice patterns from different countries with diverse healthcare systems and variable availability to expert cen-

ters and drugs provide a more widespread view of the current management of PAH.

Several registries that are either historically relevant or provide vital survival data in PAH will be spotlighted, including ones that have generated equations for predicting survival [5, 6, 8–13]. Fundamental information about other registries, from China, Switzerland, United Kingdom-Ireland, and the United States (PAH-QuERI) are also listed in Tables 20.1 and 20.2 [7, 14–18].

National Institutes of Health (NIH) Registry

The Patient Registry for the Characterization of Primary Pulmonary Hypertension was the first national registry [5]. This landmark registry, sponsored by the NIH, began in 1981 and prospectively collected clinical data on 194 patients from 32 centers in the United States with primary pulmonary hypertension (corresponding to idiopathic PAH in recent classification schemes), familial PAH (now heritable PAH), or anorexigen-induced PAH. Prior to the registry, there were many questions regarding the epidemiology and natural history of the disease. Data were collected on patients prospectively according to standardized protocol from July 1981 to Sept 1985 and patients were followed through August 1988. The registry did not address prevalence of PAH. Pulmonary hypertension was defined by catheterization as a mean pulmonary arterial pressure of >25 mmHg at rest or >30 mmHg

Table 20.2 Demographic, clinical & hemodynamic characteristics of PAH registries

Registry	Age (years)	Female (%)	FC III-IV (%)	6 MW distance (meters)	RAP (mmHg)	Mean PAP (mmHg)	PVRI (WU·m²)
PAH patients							
PHC	48 ± 14	77	80	–	11 ± 7	52 ± 14	–
Scottish-SMR	52 ± 12	70	–	–	–	–	–
French National	50 ± 15	65	75	329 ± 109	8 ± 5	55 ± 15	21 ± 10
REVEAL	50 ± 14	80	56	366 ± 126	9 ± 6	51 ± 14	21 ± 13
Spanish	45 ± 17	71	69	363 ± 120	9 ± 5	54 ± 16	–
Chinese (modern)	36 ± 13	70	54	378 ± 125	8 ± 5	63 ± 20	25 ± 14
Mayo	52 ± 15	76	55	329 ± 125	13 ± 6	53 ± 14	–
IPAH patients							
NIH	36 ± 15	63	75	–	10 ± 6	60 ± 18	26 ± 14
PHC	45 ± 14	75	80	–	11 ± 7	56 ± 13	–
Scottish-SMR	49 ± 11	62	–	–	–	–	–
French National	52 ± 15	62	81	328 ± 112	9 ± 5	56 ± 14	23 ± 10
Chinese (pre-modern)	36 ± 12	71	61	–	13 ± 6	69 ± 19	–
REVEAL	50 ± 15	83	55	374 ± 129	10 ± 6	52 ± 13	23 ± 11
Spanish	46 ± 18	73	70	382 ± 117	8 ± 5	55 ± 15	–
Chinese (modern)	38 ± 13	70	66	353 ± 127	8 ± 6	63 ± 15	27 ± 12
Mayo	52 ± 15	76	56	344 ± 125	13 ± 6	55 ± 12	–
COMPERA	65 ± 15	60	91	293 ± 126	8 ± 5	44 ± 12	–

FC functional class, *6MWD* six minute walk distance, *RAP* right atrial pressure, *PVRI* pulmonary vascular resistance index, *mmHg* millimeters of mercury, *WU·m2* Wood Units × meters²

with exercise. Primary pulmonary hypertension was only diagnosed after exclusion of other potential causes of pulmonary hypertension, including collagen vascular disease and elevated left-sided filling pressures, defined as pulmonary capillary wedge pressure >12 mmHg. Demographic data, hemodynamic measures, pulmonary function, and gas exchange variables were obtained at baseline and assessed at 6-month intervals.

There were 187 patients with mean age of 36 ± 15 years with a female to male ratio of 1.7:1. Five percent had a history of appetite suppressant use and 6 % were familial pulmonary hypertension. Female patients tended to have more severe symptoms at presentation with 75 % being in New York Heart Association (NYHA) functional class III or IV compared with 64 % of male patients. The median time from onset of symptoms to diagnosis was 2.0 ± 4.9 years (median 1.27). This landmark registry helped correlate hemodynamic findings to severity of symptoms and survival. As expected, patients with NYHA functional class III or IV symptoms had higher mean pulmonary artery pressures, higher right atrial pressures and lower cardiac indices compared to less symptomatic patients. By the time of diagnosis, the clinical and hemodynamic findings were advanced in most cases.

The NIH registry also characterized mortality and identified factors associated with survival for this select group of PAH patients. Because only incident cases were recruited and catheterizations were part of the initial evaluation, the date of diagnostic catheterization served as the baseline from which survival was measured. The estimated median survival was 2.8 years [19]. Variables associated with poor survival included NYHA functional class III or IV, presence of Raynaud's phenomenon, elevated right atrial pressure (RAP), elevated mean pulmonary artery pressure (PAP), decreased cardiac index (CI) and decreased diffusing capacity (of the lung) for carbon monoxide (DLCO) (Table 20.3). Estimated survival rates at 1-, 3- and 5-years were 68 %, 48 % and 34 % respectively. By the end of the registry, 106 of the 194 patients had died, including 26 % with sudden or unexpected death and 47 % from right ventricular failure. Symptom duration did not correlate with disease severity implying that disease progression differs among patients. Of the 36 patients (19 %) receiving long-term (non PAH-specific) medication at study entry, there was no significant difference in survival time compared with patients not receiving therapy. However, the design of the study did not allow for valid assessment of differences in therapeutic interventions. This study certainly confirmed the poor prognosis of patients with pulmonary arterial hypertension.

The NIH registry gave the first national characterization of a rare disease with detailed evaluation of symptoms, labo-

Table 20.3 Predictors of mortality

		NIH	PHC	French	REVEAL	Spanish	United Kingdom	Mayo	COMPERA
Demographics	Male			X	X	X	X	X	X
	Age		X		X		X	X	X
PAH etiology	Connective tissue disease		X		X	X	X	X	
	Porto-pulmonary hypertension				X	X			
	Heritable PAH				X				
	Veno-occlusive disease					X	X		
Functional assessment	↑ NYHA or WHO functional class		X		X	X		X	X
Pulmonary function test	↓ 6 MW distance			X	X			X	
	↓ DLCO				X			X	
Hemodynamics	↑ RAP	X	X		X	X	X	X	
	↑ mean PAP	X							
	↓ Cardiac output or index	X	X	X		X	X	X	X
	↑ PVR or PVRI				X			X	
Biomarkers	↑ BNP or NT-Pro BNP				X				
	Renal insufficiency				X				
	Pericardial effusion				X			X	

(X) indicates that a particular demographic, diagnosis, objective measure, etc. was identified as a predictor of mortality in the corresponding registry. *NYHA* New York Heart Association, *WHO* World Health Organization, *6 MW* six minute walk, *DLCO* diffusing capacity for carbon monoxide, *RAP* right atrial pressure, *PAP* pulmonary arterial pressure, *PVR* pulmonary vascular resistance, *PVRI* pulmonary vascular resistance index, *BNP* brain natriuretic peptide, *NT* N-terminus

ratory, imaging and hemodynamic findings as well as providing prognostic indicators. This registry provided the foundation for subsequent studies of PAH.

French National Registry

The French National Registry is considered the first PAH registry in the modern treatment era. Disease-specific therapies were absent at the time of the NIH registry and the classification of pulmonary hypertension had changed since the late 1980s. In the nearly two decades since the NIH registry, prostanoids, endothelin receptor antagonists (ERA) and phosphodiesterase-5 (PDE5) inhibitors became specifically available for PAH. Despite these significant advances, there had not been a large-scale, national-level registry to update clinical and hemodynamic parameters of patients, prevalence of the disease or estimates of survival.

The prospective registry included 17 university hospitals with a total of 674 patients (121 incidence cases, 553 prevalent cases) through the French Network on PAH with 3-year follow-up [10]. Adult PAH patients, including idiopathic, familial, anorexigen-induced, or PAH associated with CTDs, congenital heart diseases (CHD), portal hypertension and HIV were seen between October 2002 and October 2003. Diagnosis was considered to be the time of RHC, which was a pre-requisite for enrollment. Because prevalent cases were catheterized before study entry, Humbert et al. accounted for immortal time bias by using survival estimates and a Cox proportional hazards model from the time of diagnosis. In addition, prevalent cases were entered into the risk set in delayed fashion (i.e. left truncation), by the same amount of time that had elapsed between diagnostic catheterization and registry entry. For example, if 12 months had elapsed between an individual's diagnostic catheterization and recruitment into the registry, that individual's subsequent time alive in the registry and contribution to the cohort's survival estimate did not begin until the 12 month point of the cohort's survival curve and was not included in the first 12 months. There were also 121 incident cases (newly diagnosed), who were patients diagnosed during the registry's recruitment phase and none of these patients were lost to follow-up.

Mean age was 50 ± 15 years, much older than in the NIH registry due to a more diverse group of enrolled PAH patients; female to male ratio was 1.9. The delay between the onset of symptoms and diagnosis was still 27 months. At diagnosis, 75 % of patients had NYHA functional class III or IV symptoms. Hemodynamic evaluation demonstrated severe compromise with RAP 8 ± 5 mmHg, mean PAP 55 ± 15 mmHg and pulmonary vascular resistance index 20.5 ± 10.2 WU·m^2 with correlation to the NYHA functional class. IPAH comprised 39.2 % of patients and familial cases represented

3.9 % of the population. At that time, epoprostenol, bosentan, iloprost and sildenafil were the available approved therapies. No mandatory specific treatment algorithm was used; thus, use of PAH targeted therapies was at the discretion of the treating physician.

Prevalence in France was calculated to be 15.0 cases per million adults, although a significant range (5–25 cases per million population) was noted across regions of the country. Unfortunately, this registry identified that despite the increased awareness of PAH since the NIH registry 20 years prior, patients were still being diagnosed with clinical impairment as severe as during the time of the NIH registry.

The French PAH network followed patients for 3 years after study entry and demonstrated 1-, 2- and 3- year survival of 87 %, 76 % and 67 %, respectively in the overall cohort [20]. In a combined incident and prevalence (i.e. diagnosed <3 years from study entry) cohort of idiopathic, familial and anorexigen-associated PAH cases, survival for 1-, 2-, and 3-year survival rates were slightly lower, 83 %, 67 % and 58 % respectively, but still considerably better than NIH registry's estimates [19]. The prevalent patients with idiopathic, familial and anorexigen associated PAH had higher survival rates than incident patients. Even though the registry made efforts to eliminate survivor bias (as described earlier), this finding may still reflect such a bias. There was better 3-years survival rate in patients with congenital heart disease, but poorer survival in CTD; these observations were subsequently confirmed by the REVEAL registry [21]. Multivariate analysis identified female sex, higher six minute walk distances, and higher cardiac output at time of diagnosis as independent prognostic factors for survival (Table 20.3).

Pulmonary Hypertension Connection (PHC) Registry

The Pulmonary Hypertension Connection registry (PHC) was a large U.S. based registry conducted at three sites by essentially one group of researchers. From 1982 to 2006, 578 patients with WHO Group 1 Pulmonary Arterial Hypertension were included [8]. The goal was to define clinical characteristics and prognosis of WHO Group 1 PAH patients and compare groups by etiology and across treatment eras.

Patients were segregated into prevalent (1982–2004) versus incident (2004–2006) groups, with only the latter group's data being collected prospectively. Patients were also compared by treatment era: pre-1996 (before approved therapies), 1996–2002 (only IV epoprostenol) and post-2002 (IV, subcutaneous or inhalational prostacyclins, ERAs and PDE5 inhibitors). Seventy-seven percent of the PHC cohort was female, confirming again the female predominance of PAH; the only subgroup without female predominance was Human

Immunodeficiency Virus (HIV) -associated PAH. The PHC registry again recognized that patients with PAH are referred to specialty centers far into the disease course, as 80 % of patients had NYHA functional class III or IV symptoms at presentation.

PHC included all types of Group 1 PAH patients, including 44 % idiopathic, 4 % heritable PAH (HPAH) and 3 % anorexigen, along with several associated PAH groups – 30 % CTD, 11 % CHD, 7 % porto-pulmonary hypertension and 1 % HIV-associated PAH. These frequencies were similar to the French registry, but differed from the NIH registry which only included IPAH, HPAH and anorexigen-related PAH. Compared with other subgroups, patients with connective tissue disease (CTD) had more severe disease: poorer exercise capacity, a worse functional class, a higher mean PAP, higher pulmonary vascular resistance (PVR) and lower CI. Meanwhile, higher functional class, better exercise capacity, lower mean PAP, lowered PVR and higher CI were seen with porto-pulmonary hypertension and congenital heart disease (CHD) -associated PAH.

For the entire cohort, median survival time was 3.6 years. The 1-, 3-, and 5- year survival rates were 84 %, 67 % and 58 %, respectively. The 1-year survival for the incident cohort was 85 %, which is similar to the French registry (88 % 1 year survival) but improved from NIH registry [10, 19]. Using Cox proportional hazards analysis, increasing age, CTD as the etiology for PAH, higher functional class, higher RAP and lower CI were identified as significant and independent predictors of mortality (Table 20.3) [22]. In essence, PHC confirmed some of the NIH findings but once again highlighted how advancements in care had improved survival.

Scottish Registry

The Scottish registry described the epidemiologic features of PAH in a population over a prolonged period of time (1986–2001), by reporting data from the Scottish Morbidity Record (SMR) and the Scottish Pulmonary Vascular Unit (SPVU) [11]. This retrospective population cohort study used records from a national hospitalization database for Scotland; the SMR relied on systematic coding of hospital admissions and assembled a cohort of 374 incident patients, aged 16–65 years with diagnosis of IPAH, CTD-PAH or CHD-PAH. The overall population prevalence was 52 cases per million. The median survival of incident patients with IPAH was 3.8 years in females and 5.6 years in males, which is contrary to the poorer survival in male patients in the NIH, French, PHC and REVEAL registries [8, 19, 20, 23]. These lengthier survival times cast doubt on the PAH diagnosis in some of the patients from the SMR group.

The incidence and prevalence was also examined from the SPVU (1997–2005), which is a national specialist center for PAH management and is responsible for diagnosis and treatment of all cases of PAH in Scotland. All patients with PAH were diagnosed by standardized protocol, including RHC. The prevalence was 26 cases per million adult inhabitants.

The Scottish registry collected epidemiologic data from two perspectives. The SMR identified patients simply by ICD-9 code. The accuracy of the diagnosis was not confirmed by standardized protocol, like the SPVU data. As a result, there was a lower prevalence of PAH from the SPVU than from the SMR analysis (52 versus 26 cases per million adult inhabitants). Even though the data from SMR represents a survey of inexpert diagnoses, it still suggests that registries conducted at specialized centers may underestimate prevalence rates due to numerous challenges precluding some individuals from being evaluated at distant expert-based referral centers. In addition, the lower prevalence rate from SPVU is still significantly higher than the French National Registry (26 versus 15 cases per million) [10]. Considering these two large national experiences, differences in prevalence likely exist in various regions of the world, but also depend on the method of case identification and data collection [24].

Spanish Registry of PAH (REHAP)

The Spanish Registry of Pulmonary Arterial Hypertension (REHAP) examined the prevalence, incidence and survival of PAH and chronic thromboembolic pulmonary hypertension (CTEPH) in Spain from January 1998 to June 2008 [12]. One of its objectives was to assess the applicability of recently developed predictive equations (for survival). Demographic, functional and hemodynamic variables were evaluated in 866 PAH and 162 patients with CTEPH. Patients were diagnosed as incident if diagnostic RHC took placed within 6 months of the Registry's inception. PAH prevalence was estimated to be 16 cases per million. The prevalence for CTEPH was only 3.2 cases per million. With incident PAH cases, the delay between the onset of symptoms and diagnosis was 2.2 years and in previously diagnosed patients was 3.7 years, possibly suggesting some improvement in disease awareness over the period of the recruitment. Sixty-nine percent of patients in the PAH group were in WHO functional class III or IV, which was similar to the 77 % of the CTEPH group. Interestingly, only 30 % of CTEPH patients underwent pulmonary thromboendarterectomy, the treatment of choice for CTEPH. This was also the first registry to describe pulmonary veno-occlusive disease (PVOD) within a larger PAH cohort. PVOD only made up 1.5 % of the cohort and prevalence was estimated to be 0.16 cases per million adults; but the authors speculated an underestimation of true prevalence. Patients with PVOD had more severe hypoxemia, lower DLCO, absence of vasodilator response and poorer survival compared with patients with IPAH.

Observed survival at 1- and 3- years was 87 % and 75 %, respectively with no significant differences between the PAH and CTEPH cohorts. Corresponding survival in IPAH patients was 89 % and 77 % at 1- and 3- years respectively. In multivariate analysis, PAH associated with connective tissue disease, portal hypertension and pulmonary veno-occlusive disease were independently associated with death. Again, males, higher WHO functional class, higher mean RAP and lower CI were also independent predictors of death in PAH (Table 20.3). As defined in their objectives, Spanish investigators explored the accuracy of predictive equations from NIH, PHC, French National and REVEAL. While estimates from the PHC equation fit fairly well with the REHAP observations, significant differences between projected and observed survival were noted with the NIH, French, and REVEAL equations.

Registry to Evaluate Early and Long-Term Pulmonary Arterial Hypertension Disease Management (REVEAL)

REVEAL is the largest PAH registry to date and provided updated WHO Group 1 patient demographics in the U.S. The observational REVEAL registry also characterized the landscape of PAH in the modern era, by enrolling ~3500 patients from 54-centers between 2006 and 2009 [6]. Of note, the publication of REVEAL was prior to the fourth World Symposium on Pulmonary Hypertension; therefore, PAH was diagnosed based on criteria from third World Symposium on Pulmonary Hypertension (i.e. mean PAP > 25 mmHg at rest or >30 mmHg with exercise; PAWP or LVEDP ≤ 15 mmHg and PVR > 240 dyne/s/cm⁵).

Importantly, REVEAL only included 14 % recently-diagnosed (incident) cases, whereas 86 % were previously-diagnosed (prevalent) patients, most of whom were already receiving PAH-specific treatment at enrollment. Patients must have been diagnosed by catheterization, but REVEAL did expand the PAWP cut-off for enrollment to 18 mmHg. The higher PAWP facilitated enrollment of a more typical 'real-world' population of PH patients, thus separating it from previous registries.

REVEAL explored questions of whether population demographics in the current era differ from those encountered in previous registries. The registry included 2,955 patients with IPAH, HPAH and PAH- associated with other disorders, in contrast to the NIH registry. Prospectively collected data illustrated an older cohort (mean age at diagnosis 47 years) with an even greater female predominance (3.6:1) compared to the NIH registry (mean age 36 years and 1.7:1

female to male ratio). Compared to the French registry, the REVEAL cohort had a higher percentage of obesity (32.5 % versus 14.8 % with body mass index ≥ 30 kg/m²) [25]. REVEAL also recruited a larger percentage of anorexigen-related PAH than the NIH or French registries (15.3 % versus 5 % versus 9/5 %, respectively), which may reflect the increasing obesity epidemic in the United States, availability of anorexigen compounds in the 1990s and the potential latent effects of anorexigen exposure on PAH pathogenesis. Hemodynamic parameters at time of diagnosis had not changed significantly since the NIH registry. Despite increased physician awareness, there was little change in severity of PAH at time of diagnosis: 72 % classified as being in NYHA functional class III/IV similar to the 70–80 % range of other registries, including NIH. REVEAL essentially followed a large cohort of diverse PAH patients in the modern treatment era.

Survival in REVEAL was determined from the date of the diagnostic catheterization, similar to the French National Registry. Immortal time bias was also addressed in a manner similar to the French National Registry, i.e. left-truncation of prevalent cases during survival analysis. But unlike the French National Registry, REVEAL investigators incorporated factors for their multivariable predictor analysis from the time of registry enrollment and not the time of diagnosis (or catheterization) [6, 10, 23, 26]. One-, 3-, 5- and 7- year survival estimates were 85 %, 68 %, 57 % and 49 % respectively. In addition, survival in the IPAH/HPAH subset, which was matched to NIH registry entry criteria, was 91 %, 74 %, 65 % and 59 % at 1-, 3-, 5-, 7- years, which was considerably higher at all time points than the projected survival from the NIH equation [26]. REVEAL identified 19 prognostic variables, some favorable and some unfavorable, such as subtype of PAH, age, PVR, RAP, renal insufficiency, resting systolic blood pressure, resting heart rate, brain natriuretic peptide, presence of pericardial effusion and DLCO. Similar to the French registry, sex, functional class and 6-minute walk distance were significant predictors (Table 20.3) [23]. It is noteworthy that PVR, and not mean PAP or cardiac output was a significant predictor of survival; even though PVR is a derived measure (i.e. the ratio of pressure and flow) with potential for inaccuracy in certain clinical condition such as a low cardiac output state, severe tricuspid regurgitation, etc.

Mayo Clinic Registry

The Mayo Clinic registry prospectively evaluated 484 patients with WHO group 1 pulmonary hypertension from January 1995 to December 2004 followed at the Mayo Clinic pulmonary hypertension specialty clinic in Rochester, MN [9]. The objective was to evaluate survival patterns in patients with PAH and establish clinical and hemodynamic prognostic factors. Unlike other modern registries, only newly diagnosed or incident cases were included. The time of diagnosis was the date of evaluation by the PH physician and generally corresponded to the date of the pre-requisite heart catheterization. The mix of PAH patients was broad and similar to other contemporary registries, including 56 % percent idiopathic, familial or anorexigen-related PAH, 24 % PAH associated with CTD and remaining 20 % were congenital systemic to pulmonary shunts, portal hypertension and HIV. Mean age was 52 years and similar for men and women. The mean disease duration from onset of symptoms to Mayo Clinic evaluation was 1.8 years. Seventy-one percent of patients were in NYHA functional class III/IV. Patients with CTDs were older, predominately female, exhibited greater markers of disease severity and worse hemodynamic parameters than IPAH patients.

Overall cohort's mean survival was 4.56 years with 1-, 3-, and 5-year survival rates of 81.1 %, 61.1 %, 47.9 %, respectively. Males had a poorer prognosis and mortality increased by 27 % with every decade of increasing age. Patients with PAH associated with CTD had two-fold higher risk of death compared to other PAH sub-groups. Higher WHO functional class, lower CI and higher RAP were associated with mortality. Renal insufficiency (serum creatinine level >1.5 mg/dL) was also associated with a higher mortality rate. Interestingly, the Mayo Registry showed that survival predictions were enhanced when the functional class was supplemented by additional factors, such as demographics and objective measures (i.e. labs, 6MW distance, pulmonary function testing, echocardiogram, and heart catheterization) (Table 20.3).

Comparative, Prospective Registry of Newly Initiated Therapies for Pulmonary Hypertension (COMPERA)

COMPERA is an ongoing European registry started in July 2007. A total of 1283 PAH patients, including 800 IPAH, have been enrolled from 41 pulmonary hypertension centers from 7 European countries (Germany, Belgium, Netherlands, Italy, Austria, Switzerland, and United Kingdom) [13, 27]. All patients were newly diagnosed with PAH and no one diagnosed prior to May 2007 was entered. Interestingly, median ages of the entire cohort (68 years [IQR 55–75]) and the IPAH/HPAH/drug-associated subgroups (71 years [IQR 55–87]) were considerably higher than other historic or even contemporary registries, which in part reflects the changing demographics of the PAH population or that COMPERA may also be including patients with heart failure with preserved ejection fraction (Group 2 PH) rather than traditional PAH (or Group 1 PH) patients. The registry also evaluated initial PAH treatment and found that the majority of patients received PDE5 inhibitors (58 %). Forty-four percent of

patients were treated with ERAs and 2 % of patients were receiving prostacyclin analogues. Forty-five percent of patients were treated with combination therapy during follow-up. In multivariable analysis, males, increasing age and NYHA functional class IV were independent predictors of poor prognosis in IPAH (Table 20.3). COMPERA also utilized registry data to compare survival rates in patients with IPAH and other forms of PAH stratified by the use of anticoagulation [27].

Considering all these registries collectively, several points and trends are apparent. PAH remains a very serious and lethal condition with the majority of patients being in functional class III or IV at the time of diagnosis. PAH afflicts women much more than men. The largest PAH subgroups remain IPAH and CTD-PAH. The mean age of PAH cohorts has increased considerably, partly due to inclusion of a more heterogeneous patients, but perhaps also because of a burgeoning group of older individuals diagnosed with IPAH. The severity of initial cardiopulmonary hemodynamics has changed very little over time. Consistent and significant predictors of survival include demographic factors (age, males), hemodynamics (RAP, CI) and functional assessments (NYHA or WHO functional class, 6MW distance). In particular CTD-PAH and porto-pulmonary PAH patients have the poorest survival. Most importantly, survival from the registries has improved over time, presumably due to the availability of PAH-specific therapies; but a significant caveat is the inclusion of prevalent patients into registries and the resulting impact of immortal time bias.

Survival Prediction and Prognosis

One potential use of registry data is to develop risk equations that predict mortality or, stated differently, forecast survival. Ideally, a predictive equation should have broad applicability to diverse patients with the same diagnosis and at different times in an individual's course. And, since some components of an equation may not be available, the equation should still be usable in the face of some missing data. An equation should exhibit good *calibration* for estimating survival in cohorts of patients. But for clinical practice, a survival equation also needs to reliably *discriminate* between survivors and non-survivors.

PAH registries have generally collected a wide range of clinical data, including demographics, physiologic variables (e.g. right-heart catheterization data, DLCO), laboratory measurements (e.g. BNP), and co-morbidities. These data have then been used to create multivariate equations for predicting survival. The NIH and PHC equations are based entirely on the hemodynamic parameters mean PAP, mean RAP, and CI [5, 8, 19, 22]. By contrast, the French survival equation also included 6 MW distance and sex along with the cardiac output [10, 20]. The REVEAL equation also includes hemodynamic measures, but instead of the mean PAP or cardiac output, PVR and mean RAP were incorporated. Importantly, the REVEAL equation also factors in numerous non-hemodynamic variables, including demographics, etiologies of PAH, functional class, laboratory markers, renal insufficiency and presence of a pericardial effusion among others; all items were found to be significant to the model through a multivariate Cox proportional hazards analysis (Table 20.4) [21, 23, 28]. Additional details of the four equations, efforts at their validation, and their respective strengths and weaknesses are described below and summarized in Table 20.5.

NIH Equation

As noted earlier, the NIH registry enrolled patients with IPAH in an era before modern therapies for pulmonary hypertension were available. This model was developed by multivariate regression analysis of the variables that independently predicted mortality. Estimated percentages of patient survival at 1, 3, and 5 years using this equation are 68 %, 48 %, and 34 %, respectively [19].

$$P(t)=\left[H(t)\right]^{A(xyz)}$$

$$H(t)=\left[0.88-0.14t+0.01t^2\right]$$

$$A(x\,v\,z)=e^{(0007325x+00526y-0.3275z)}$$

P (t) indicates the patient's chances of survival and t = 1, 2 or 3 years

x = mean pulmonary artery pressure

y = mean right atrial pressure

z = cardiac index

Sandoval et al. demonstrated good correlation between survival estimates from the NIH equation and observed survival in an external cohort of IPAH patients from Mexico in essentially the same treatment era as the NIH registry. The NIH equation appeared to have greater accuracy when applied to the sub-group of patients that were not acutely responsive to vasodilators [29]. A number of clinical trials have subsequently utilized NIH equation-predicted survival as the comparator to the observed survival on that specific medication [14, 30–34]. But when applied to more contemporary cohorts, the NIH equation has underestimated survival, even when limited to cohorts of IPAH, HPAH and anorexigen patients [14, 23, 35, 36]. This has been attributed to change in awareness, updated management strategies, availability of PAH-specific therapies, and possibly a change in the phenotype of pulmonary hypertension [3].

Table 20.4 Predictors of mortality from the REVEAL registry: variable coefficients for the linear component of the Cox model and weighted values for the REVEAL risk calculator

WHO Group 1 subgroup	Heritable PAH		Porto-pulmonary hypertension		CTD-PAH	
	+0.7737	+2	+1.2801	+2	+0.4624	+1
Demographics and co-morbid conditions	Male > 60 years		Renal insufficiency			
	+0.7779	+2	+0.6422	+1		
NYHA/WHO functional class	FC I		FC III		FC IV	
	−0.8740	−2	+0.3454	+1	+1.1402	+2
Vital signs	SBP < 110 mmHg		Heart rate > 92 bpm			
	+0.5128	+1	+0.3322	+1		
6 MW distance	≥440 m		<165 m			
	−0.5455	−1	+0.5210	+1		
BNP	BNP < 50 pg/ml or NT-Pro BNP < 300 pg/ml		BNP > 180 pg/ml or NT-Pro BNP > 1500 pg/ml			
	−0.6922	−2	+0.6791	+1		
Echocardiogram	Any pericardial effusion					
	+0.3014	+1				
Pulmonary function test	% predicted DLCO ≥ 80 %		% predicted DLCO ≤ 32 %			
	−0.5317	−1	+0.3756	+1		
Right heart catheterization	RAP > 20 mmHg within 1 year		PVR > 32 wood units			
	+0.5816	+1	+1.4062	+2		

(+) and (−) numbers are additions and subtractions to the linear component of the REVEAL survival equation. Italicized numbers represent the corresponding weighted value for a particular variable in the REVEAL risk calculator. (+) values indicate increased risk of mortality and (−) values indicate decreased risk of mortality. *CTD* connective tissue disease, *FC* functional class, *SBP* systolic blood pressure, *6 MW* six minute walk, *BNP* brain natriuretic peptide, *NT* N-terminus, *pg/ml* pictograms/milliliter, *DLCO* diffusion capacity for carbon monoxide, *RAP* right atrial pressure, *PVR* pulmonary vascular resistance

Table 20.5 Strengths and limitations of the various predictive equations

		NIH	French National	PHC	REVEAL
Strengths		First national registry	17 expert centers	Large center over extended period of time	National registry (>50 centers)
		Prospective data collection	Derivation cohort similar to NIH	Derivation cohort similar to NIH	Included all PAH groups
		First characterization of the disease	Uniform diagnostic criteria	Equation allows survival prediction over extended time	Modeling with clinical objective variables
		Modeling with clinical objective variables	Modeling with clinical objective variables	Modeling with clinical objective variables	Usefulness for cohort
		Usefulness for cohort	Usefulness for cohort	Usefulness for cohort	Incident and prevalent cases
			Incident and prevalent cases		
			Equation allows survival prediction over extended time		
Weaknesses		Different standard of care	Potential for bias since data set included prevalent patients diagnosed up to 3 years prior to study entry	Only uses hemodynamics	Industry sponsored
		Lack of advanced imaging modalities		Retrospective and prospective chart review	Included all PAH groups
		Only uses hemodynamics		Single center	Prevalence may be underestimated as not all patients enrolled at every site
		Not updated over time	Limited usefulness for individual patient	Limited usefulness for individual patient	Only valid to predict 1-year survival
		Limited usefulness for individual patient	Not adaptive or able to predict the trajectory	Not adaptive or able to predict the trajectory	
		Not adaptive or able to predict the trajectory			Not adaptive or able to predict the trajectory

Adapted with permission from Thenappan et al. [35]

Improvements to the NIH equation have been proposed from data collected by recent PH registries [22, 35].

French National Registry Equation

Although the French National Registry included patients with all types of Group 1 PAH, the equation was developed from a subset of incident and prevalent cohorts (diagnosed less than 3 years before enrollment) with idiopathic, familial or anorexigen-associated PAH (n = 190 – 56 incident and 134 prevalent), and importantly left out patients with CTD, congenital heart disease, portal hypertension, and HIV [10, 20]. This subset of patients was chosen to better control for the presence or absence of associated conditions that would independently affect mortality. For this PAH subgroup, 1-, 2-, and 3- year survival was 83 %, 67 % and 58 % respectively. The French equation included factors which independently influenced survival as determined by the multivariate regression model. Probability of survival with this equation is estimated as:

$$P(t)=\exp\left(-0.02-0.28t\right)^{\exp(-(0.004x+0.98y+0.28z))}$$

t = time since diagnosis
x = 6MWD at diagnosis
y = 1 if female, y = 0 if male
z = cardiac output at diagnosis

The French registry has been prospectively validated and shown to have adequate predictive power when tested in a matched cohort from the U.S.-based REVEAL registry [37]. But when tested in the U.K. and Spanish Registries, the French equation tended to overestimate the risk of death [12, 38].

Pulmonary Hypertension Connection (PHC) Equation

Similar to the French equation, the PHC equation was developed to predict survival in a subgroup of patients with idiopathic, familial or anorexigen-associated PAH enrolled in the PHC Registry [8, 22]. For this subgroup, 1-, 3-, and 5-year survival was 91 %, 75 % and 65 % respectively, whereas survival predicted by NIH equation was 65, 43 and 32 %, respectively. Again, these mortality differences likely represent the recent availability of targeted PAH therapies. PHC equation predicts the probability of survival primarily by hemodynamic values:

$$P(t) = e^{-A(x,y,z)t}$$

$A(x,y,z) = e^{(-1.270-0.0148x+0.0402y-0.361z)}$ in non-responders to calcium-channel blocker

$A(x,y,z) = e^{(-3.012-0.0148x+0.0402y-0.361z)}$ in responders to calcium-channel blocker

t = time since diagnosis

x = mean pulmonary arterial pressure (mean PAP)

y = mean right atrial pressure

z = cardiac index

Although only seen in approximately 3 % of patients, an acute vasodilator response was noted to be a strong prognostic indicator. Thenappan et al. externally validated the PHC and the French equations in a dataset of 449 patients with IPAH, HPAH or anorexigen-PAH prospectively assembled from four different clinical trials of investigational prostanoid therapy [35].

REVEAL Prognostic Equation and Risk Score

The REVEAL prognostic equation was derived from variables independently associated with mortality through multivariable analysis (with Cox proportional hazards) in 2716 patients enrolled in the REVEAL registry [21, 23, 28]. Because REVEAL's enrollment was several-fold larger than the other registries, the predictor analysis was much more robust, leading to quite a few more predictors. The equation predicts 1- year survival as:

$$P = S0(1)^{\exp(Z'\beta\gamma)}$$

S0(1) = baseline survivor function (0.9698)

γ = shrinkage coefficient (0.939)

$Z'\beta$ = linear component.

The linear component of this complex equation is dependent on 19 variables (Table 20.4). Variables that add to the linear component are risk factors (total 15), whereas the ones which subtract from it are protective factors (total 4).

Benza et al. validated the prediction equation in a subgroup of 504 recently diagnosed PAH patients (catheterization <3 months of registry enrollment) from REVEAL. Survival estimates from the REVEAL equation were stratified into 5 groups, ranging from low to very high risk of death; and the model calibrated extremely well with observed 1-year survival [21]. The full REVEAL survival equation also showed good external calibration for predicting 1-year survival in a relatively small cohort of PAH patients from a single U.S. center [39]. Furthermore, the REVEAL risk calculator was developed by assigning weighted values to the independent prognostic variables of the full survival equation (Table 20.4), in order to develop a more facile tool for routine clinical practice. The simplified risk calculator was also shown to have excellent calibration for predicting 1- year survival across the same 5 risk groups [40]. Prognostic abilities of the REVEAL risk calculator has also been externally validated in a cohort of matched patients from the French Registry [39, 41, 42].

Applying Survival Equations

An important aspect of a risk equation is its intended use – projecting survival estimates for cohorts or an individual. As described above, the French, PHC and REVEAL predictive equations have been shown through external validation to provide accurate survival estimates in cohorts of PAH patients. However, reliability of these equations for predicting the survival of an individual patient is not robust. For example, Sandoval's analysis demonstrated that the NIH equation was highly predictive of which individuals would survive (i.e. highly sensitive) but struggled to identify which individuals would die (i.e. low specificity) when using a rigid survival prediction cutoff of 50 % [29]. In Thenappan's analysis, the PHC equation also had high sensitivity for predicting individual's survival, but again lacked specificity (i.e. identifying likely deaths). The NIH equation had high specificity at the expense of low sensitivity. Meanwhile, the French equation predicted individual survival with intermediate sensitivity and specificity. Moreover, the area under the receiver operator characteristic (ROC) curve for all 3 equations was similar (only ~0.55), indicating a lack of predictive accuracy. The authors concluded that none of these three equations could be applied to predicting an individual patient's survival [35].

Benza et al. demonstrated better discrimination of survivors and non-survivors by the REVEAL survival equation and the REVEAL risk score through a validation cohort from within the REVEAL registry. The probability of concordance (or c-index) was 0.72, thus confirming good discrimination (of survivors from non-survivors at 1 year) for both tools [21]. The c-index, which approximates the area under an ROC curves, is a different statistical evaluation of an equation's discriminatory capability. In essence, an equation's c-index is the probability that a randomly chosen survivor will have a higher projected survival estimate than a randomly chosen deceased subject; a c-index equaling 1.0 is perfectly discriminatory, while 0.5 represents chance prediction [43]. The REVEAL equation was also able to discriminate effectively when tested for specific subgroups of maximally treated patients (i.e. on parenteral prostanoids), newly diagnosed patients, patients with a pulmonary capillary wedge pressure ≤ 12 mmHg (NIH registry definition), as well as IPAH/HPAH or other forms of PAH. Cogswell et al. demonstrated very good discrimination of 1-year survival, using the original REVEAL equation, in their single-center cohort of 140 PAH patients with a reported c-index of 0.77. The concordance index held up even though there were significant differences in the composition of PAH sub-types (from REVEAL) and a substantial number of patients with missing data for some key variables in the equation [39]. Meanwhile, Kane et al. studied the REVEAL risk score in the much larger Mayo cohort and determined a comparable c-index of 0.71 [9]. Therefore, the REVEAL risk calculator has discriminatory power similar to the full survival equation and has the potential to be used in everyday clinical practice (pending further studies and validation).

Another important test characteristic of predictive equations is the time-frame for predicting survival. While the NIH, French, and PHC equations may not offer as strong discriminatory power as the REVEAL equation or the risk score, these older equations are designed to estimate survival as a function of time. Therefore, an individual's survival can be estimated at 1, 2 and 3 years, etc. The REVEAL equation and simplified risk calculator were designed to estimate survival 1 year from the point of acquisition of the variables entered into the risk calculator. One analysis of the Mayo registry cohort did note good discrimination of 5 year survival with the REVEAL risk score [9]. In another report though, the discriminatory ability of the full REVEAL equation for predicting 5 year survival was not as good as the 1 year projection, and particularly overestimated risk in patients in the intermediate risk category [39]. Additional experience is needed before the REVEAL equation or risk calculator can be used reliably to forecast survival beyond 1 year, especially as therapeutic options in PAH continue to expand.

In total, numerous analyses demonstrate that currently available modern survival equations, notwithstanding the NIH equation, are best suited to estimate survival in cohorts of patients. In addition, the REVEAL survival equation and risk score, which are also able to discriminate between survivors and non-survivors, can be used at the individual level but are best limited to predicting short term or 1-year survival.

Challenges to Applying Survival Equations in Clinical Practice

Heterogeneity of PAH

At its core, PAH is a heterogeneous group of disorders that share some common pathologic features and, presumably, underlying mechanisms of disease. But PAH disorders have largely been linked together by a clinical classification system based on the severity of hemodynamic derangements, clinical presentation, and disease course in the late stages. Given the rarity of Group 1 PAH conditions, such as IPAH, HPAH, and HIV-associated PAH, it is understandable to aggregate data from potentially diverse subgroups. By assembling a larger cohort of patients, a registry's statistical power increases and predictive value enhanced. Modern PAH registries have incorporated several hundred to several thousand PAH patients with the majority of patients having either IPAH or CTD-associated PAH, while less frequent representation from rarer subgroups such as porto-pulmonary HTN, HIV-PAH and CHD-PAH. But, these subgroups behave quite differently and exhibit different survival curves, especially in the long-term [21]. Accordingly, caution has to be exercised when applying survival equations to rarer PAH sub-groups, which sorely need dedicated registries.

Age is an important discriminator of outcome in PAH, with older adults faring worse [9, 13, 16, 22, 26]. Furthermore, PAH subgroups can also be differentiated by age at PAH diagnosis. In the NIH registry of the 1980s, patients with IPAH typically presented in the third or fourth decade of life with an average age of 36 ± 15 years [5]. PAH patients with CHD are often recognized during childhood or present in young adulthood, depending on the complexity and size of the defect [44]. On the other end of the spectrum, patients with systemic sclerosis, which is the most common form of CTD-PAH, present much later in life as one large series from the United Kingdom demonstrated (mean age of 63.9 ± 10.5 years) [45]. With more diverse enrollment, modern PAH registries typically report an average age in the fifties, which is much older than the average age of the more homogeneous cohort of IPAH patients entered into the NIH registry 30 years ago [5, 6, 8, 10]. Age alone challenges the use of older survival equations as the population of PAH evolves.

Co-morbidities, which are often associated with the underlying disorder implicated in PAH pathogenesis, also factor into survival and are often not captured in large registry efforts. For example, renal dysfunction appears to be an important predictor of outcome in PAH; in fact, the relatively crude creatinine value (as an estimate of renal function) is part of the REVEAL risk calculator [9, 21, 46]. However, other registries have failed to capture information on renal function. Patients with systemic sclerosis not infrequently exhibit concomitant pulmonary conditions, such as interstitial lung disease, or cardiac issues, including diastolic dysfunction, arrhythmias and valvular disease, that may impact response to PAH therapies and survival [45, 47–49]. Individuals with CHD, ultimately develop Eisenmenger's physiology with irreversible pulmonary vasculopathy leading to right-to-left circulatory shunting and severe chronic hypoxemia. Eisenmenger's syndrome is a multi-system disorder with intrinsic cardiac, hematologic, musculoskeletal, renal, and cerebrovascular manifestations [50]. Similarly, non-PAH manifestations of liver disease and portal hypertension, certainly impact the course of patients with portopulmonary hypertension and likely lead to the noticeably poor survival of that PAH sub-group [21, 51]. This level of comorbidity detail has not been captured in large-scale PAH registries and therefore challenge the ability of predictive equations to equally forecast survival in diverse PAH subgroups, many of which only make up a small portion of registry enrollment.

Measurement of Predictors and the Use of Survival Equations

The REVEAL survival equation and risk calculator represent a significant advancement from earlier risk equations. Thanks to a richer body of variables that are entered in the REVEAL equations, a more thorough assessment of an individual is undertaken, leading to better discrimination of individual's short-term survival. But the cost of implementing the equation in routine clinical practice cannot be overlooked, as the full dataset requires recent data from an echocardiogram, laboratory tests, pulmonary function tests, and RHC. This burden of testing will limit use of the equation or the risk calculator on a repetitive and longitudinal basis. Developers of the risk equation and calculator note that absence of some data does not hinder the equation's ability to provide reliable predictions, but its discriminatory value does diminish with incremental missing data [23]. Efforts are underway to simplify the REVEAL risk calculator without compromising its predictive power, but additional validation will be needed [41].

Once data are collected, the operational aspects of the various equations come into play. None of the equations is particularly user-friendly in the routine clinical environment and require a fair degree of computation. For this reason, the REVEAL risk calculator is much more ideally suited for routine clinical use as the weighted values for individual risk factors can be easily calculated.

Another challenge to applying survival equations stems from inaccuracy and variability of the actual variables needed to compute survival. The NIH, French, and PHC equations rely heavily on hemodynamic measures, such as the cardiac output (or index), RAP and PAP. Even the elaborate REVEAL risk calculator relies on two key hemodynamic measures, RAP and PVR. Although RHC remains critical for diagnosing PAH and assessing prognosis, there are concerns about the accuracy and consistency of these fundamental measurements as routine clinical practices vary considerably [52–54]. Efforts to better standardize hemodynamic measurement in PAH have been published [55]. The 6 MW distance is

another important variable in the French and REVEAL equations. While the 6 minute walk test is designed to measure an individual's exercise capacity and thereby providing an inferential assessment of one's pulmonary vascular disease and right ventricular function, co-morbidities can influence the test's output. This is particularly relevant in older patients with peripheral musculoskeletal impairments (e.g. individuals with systemic sclerosis), whose walk distance is limited by more than just cardio-pulmonary issues. Other factors, such as patient's motivation and cognitive abilities can also influence the six minute walk test output. Another frequently cited measure is the NYHA or WHO functional class, which is a subjectively assigned measure based on somewhat vague definitions. One study demonstrated poor inter-grader agreement, even among experts, for assigning functional class in PAH patients [56]. As a result of challenges in measuring some of these variables that are incorporated into survival equations, the generalizability of survival equations into diverse clinical settings may be impacted.

Newer and promising measures of cardiac function obtained from echocardiography (e.g. tricuspid annular systolic plane excursion, right ventricular strain, etc.) or cardiac MRI (e.g. RV ejection fraction, stroke volume index, myocardial mass, etc.), as well as other exercise indices, such as peak oxygen consumption and the heart rate recovery (after the 6MWT) among others, have not yet been investigated as predictors of survival in large-scale registries. These non-invasive measures might improve the predictive power and discriminatory capabilities of survival prediction equations and, in some cases, are more easily attained [57–61].

All of the survival equations and risk calculators rely on measurements at a single time-point. None of the equations is adaptive and incorporate favorable or unfavorable time-dependent changes of key clinical measures, e.g. improvement in functional class, % decline in six minute walk distance, change in key hemodynamic measures etc., even though clinical experience suggests that changes to these dynamic measures offer predictive value [59, 62–65]. Using relevant trends of key variables in predictive models, intuitively, should better track an individual's or cohort's trajectory over time.

Rapidly Evolving PAH Field Leads to Antiquated Survival Equations

An important impediment to applying registry-derived prediction equations to clinical practice is the out-datedness of registry data, which is especially relevant when a condition's management evolves rapidly. PAH management has been transformed dramatically in the last 20 years and most of the registries in listed Table 20.1 observed patients in earlier eras. PAH-specific therapies were non-existent during the time of the NIH registry. Then, intravenous epoprostenol followed by early oral agents had just become treatment options during the period of the PHC and French registries. More contemporary registries, such as REVEAL and COMPERA, mark the beginning of the era of sequential (or "add-on") combination therapy. Accordingly survival rates were dismal in the NIH registry with median survival of 2.8 years; but the REVEAL Registry reported a median survival of 7 years [19, 21, 23]. While inclusion of prevalent patients in REVEAL (as opposed to only incident cases enrolled in the NIH registry) likely accounted for some of the improvement in median survival, the availability of PAH therapies and a better general approach to right-sided heart failure also likely influenced the improved survival shown in REVEAL [26].

As of 2015, there are 12 approved PAH therapies in the United States, including approval of three new agents between late 2013 and early 2014. Moreover, another shift in the treatment paradigm will likely occur in 2015, based on the increasing number of oral agents and the positive results of a large, rigorous study that demonstrated a reduction in the risk of "Clinical Failure" with upfront dual oral therapies as opposed to (traditional) monotherapy in newly diagnosed and treatment naive PAH patients [66]. There is even early experience with upfront triple therapy with agents from each of the major classes of therapy – prostanoid, ERA, and PDE5-inhibitor in functional class IV patients [67]. Beyond the use of PAH specific therapies, management of right ventricular failure and more appropriate use of background therapies, including diuretics, inotropes, anticoagulants and calcium-channel blockers have also evolved over the last few decades. Therefore, survival estimates displayed in registries and their derived prediction equations are pertinent to their respective eras, but quickly become outdated as the PAH therapeutic landscape continues to evolve with new classes of medications and treatment strategies. Accordingly, more modern registries have shown that the older NIH equation significantly underestimates observed survival [15, 22]. These reports should inform clinicians and researchers that a survival equation's clinical application should be in the same era of the equation's originating Registry, in order to assure similar therapeutic options and management approaches.

PAH Is a Global Condition

PAH is a global problem but its makeup is not the same around the world. In the U.S., Canada, and Europe, IPAH and CTD-related PAH predominate in large patient cohorts and in clinical practice. But, CHD-PAH and Schistosomiasis-associated PAH are much more relevant in under-developed regions of the world, including Latin America, Africa, China and India. Even though all of these conditions are still viewed as PAH under the Nice Classification, PAH cohorts from

these regions are distinct and their natural history and response to treatment are not likely similar [68]. And with the exception of two reports from China, all registry-based published experiences emanate from the United States or Europe (Table 20.1) [7, 14].

PAH patients in under-developed regions of the world also face numerous obstacles that patients in more developed areas generally do not face, such as access to health-care (let alone experienced PH physicians) and availability of expensive and complicated PAH medications. Most Western countries, including France, United Kingdom, and Canada, have developed a few national PH referral centers, staffed by PH experts that have concentrated the care of PAH patients originating throughout their respective countries. In the United States, such a program is in its infancy, but there are many large and small PH Centers throughout the country that offer expert management of PH patients [69]. In most under-developed countries, expert PH care is offered at only a handful of locations; unfortunately, geography and economics greatly hinder access to these specialized care centers. As a result, early disease recognition and appropriate comprehensive evaluations, including catheterization, are significant challenges [7]. Finally, PAH-specific therapies are quite expensive and advanced therapies, namely parenteral prostanoids, are extremely complex to administer. Even though parenteral prostanoids have tremendous potential and are often the treatment of choice for the most compromised PAH individuals or for patients failing simpler therapies, prostanoid usage is essentially nil in under-developed regions of the world due to a combination of exorbitant costs, limited understanding of safe infusion practices, or lack of prerequisite infrastructure to safely administer [70].

Many of these points are nicely corroborated by efforts in China and illustrated through two separate registries, spanning altogether a 10 year period from 1999 to 2009 [7, 14]. In the first registry, 72 incident or prevalent IPAH and HPAH patients were recruited from two facilities between 1999 and 2004. The majority of patients were diagnosed by echocardiogram and 90 % of patients received calcium-channel blocker therapy even though acute vaso-responsiveness was only confirmed in a few individuals. Survival estimates at 1, 3, and 5 years were 68.0 %, 38.9 %, 20.8 % respectively [7]. In essence, this early Chinese Registry provided natural history data (i.e. without PAH-specific therapy) on a sub-population of PAH patients, similar to the NIH Registry conducted 15 years earlier. By 2007, a number of PH referral centers were established throughout China [14]. Zhang subsequently provided a more modern account of PAH in China by reporting on 276 IPAH and CTD-PAH patients, recruited from five centers throughout the country between 2007 and 2009. Even though data collection was retrospective, all patients underwent a standardized and comprehensive evaluation including RHC. Importantly, the mean age for the

IPAH cohort in both Chinese registries was in the low 30s, similar to the NIH registry but far younger than COMPERA [5, 27]. This finding may stem from regional population differences but probably also indicates a referral bias against older individuals being evaluated at the few PH referral centers in China. Majority of patients in the modern Chinese registry received PAH specific therapy, either a PDE5-I or an ERA and only a handful of patients received a calcium channel blocker, but prostanoids were not utilized due to reasons mentioned earlier [14]. Survival estimates for IPAH patients improved considerably in the second registry to 92.1 % and 75.1 % at 1 and 3 years, respectively. Zhang also confirmed poorer survival estimates for the CTD-PAH cohort, as opposed to IPAH, which has also been shown in other registries [14].

Significant obstacles, including accuracy of diagnosis, limited access to expert PH care and limited availability of PAH-specific therapies, especially advanced prostanoids, hinder the use of modern survival equations generated from resource-laden countries to regions of the world without similar resources.

Use of Risk Calculators for Allocating Lung Transplants in PAH

Advances in medical therapies have dramatically improved the mortality and quality of life for PAH patients [14, 30–34, 62, 71–74]. However, the disease remains uniformly fatal, and the only curative measure is lung transplantation [75]. Scarce donor organs and chronic rejection necessitates that resources be carefully allocated to patients with the most urgent need and greatest likelihood of successful lung transplantation. For this reason, the Lung Allocation Score (LAS) was developed and weighs both wait-list urgency and post-transplant survival based on disease severity, physiologic reserve, and disease subgroup [76].

Evaluations of the LAS system indicate that overall wait times and wait-list mortality have decreased, and the total number of transplants has increased [77]. However, amongst IPAH patients, transplant rates are lower and wait-list mortality higher [78]. This likely reflects the fact that the LAS does not include many of the key variables that predict mortality in PAH, such as mean RAP and CI [19, 21, 22, 29]. Additionally, the 6 MW distance is included in LAS, but at a threshold level so low that it applies to few patients. The inability of the LAS to distinguish low- and high-risk IPAH patients at least partially reflects the difficulty in clinically identifying the sickest IPAH patients.

To address these issues, attempts have been made to modify the LAS by including key clinical and physiologic variables [79]. To study the effectiveness of modified prediction equations in a transplant population, data were analyzed

from the Scientific Registry of Transplant Recipients files to compare wait-list mortality with predicted mortality. The PHC equation and LAS-predicted mortality were compared to observed mortality in 827 PAH patients, divided into pre- and post-2006 cohorts; the post-2006 cohort was substantially sicker than the pre-2006 cohort. The PHC equation underestimated and overestimated survival in the pre- and post-2006 cohorts, respectively; the LAS had similar accuracy. The authors developed a new equation that included elements of the LAS along with 6-MWD, resting oxygen requirements, invasive cardiac output, and functional class. The new equation outperformed the PHC equation. Among CTD-associated and secondary PAH patients, the new equation outperformed the LAS, but performed similarly in a subgroup analysis of IPAH patients [80]. These results point to the fact that including more relevant variables in predictive models of survival can indeed lead to higher accuracy in actual transplantable populations. This is similar to what was observed in the transformation from earlier PAH survival equations to the REVEAL prediction models. However, fine tuning of these transplant allocation equations for the PAH group and prospective validation are still needed. More research is needed to ensure that PAH patients in need of lung transplantation are appropriately ranked on wait-lists, as transplant offers the greatest chance of survival for the most advanced PAH patients, even in patients with systemic multi-organ diseases such as scleroderma [81].

Conclusion

Registries conducted around the world over the last 30 years have provided a wealth of information about PAH, including epidemiologic data, prevalence estimates, survival statistics, and risk factors for important long-term outcomes. These registries have chronicled remarkable improvement in outcomes, including survival, but have also reaffirmed the ongoing struggles of this incurable disease. Survival equations and risk calculators are important by-products of registry efforts and, when used in the appropriate sub-groups and therapeutic era, have proven adept at predicting outcomes of sizable cohorts and for producing comparator data to judge various therapeutic interventions. But application of these prediction equations is challenged by the global nature of PAH that leads to disparities in care, a rapidly evolving therapeutic landscape, and the equations' limitations for predicting outcomes at an individual patient level. Progress has been made with the development and validation of a more robust and clinically relevant REVEAL risk calculator, but additional enhancements and validation is needed. Given how rapidly the PAH field is evolving though, it is unclear if a valid and reliable survival prediction tool will ever be widely implemented in clinical practice.

References

1. Gliklich R, Dreyer N, editors. Registries for evaluating patient outcomes: a user's guide. 2nd ed. (Prepared by Outcome DEcIDE Center [Outcome Sciences, Inc. d/b/a Outcome] under Contract No. HHSA290200500351 TO3.) AHRQ Publication No. 10-EHC049. Rockville: Agency for Healthcare Research and Quality; 2010.

2. Dreyer NA, Schneeweiss S, McNeil BJ, Berger ML, Walker AM, Ollendorf DA, et al. GRACE principles: recognizing high-quality observational studies of comparative effectiveness. Am J Manag Care. 2010;16(6):467–71. PubMed.

3. McGoon MD, Benza RL, Escribano-Subias P, Jiang X, Miller DP, Peacock AJ, et al. Pulmonary arterial hypertension: epidemiology and registries. J Am Coll Cardiol. 2013;62(25 Suppl):D51–9. PubMed.

4. Guidelines on Pharmacovigilance for Medicinal Products for Human Use. http://www.ema.europa.eu/docs/en_GB/document_library/Scientific_guideline/2013/05/WC500143294.pdf. European Medicines Agency; 2013 [cited 25 Aug 2014].

5. Rich S, Dantzker DR, Ayres SM, Bergofsky EH, Brundage BH, Detre KM, et al. Primary pulmonary hypertension. A national prospective study. Ann Intern Med. 1987;107(2):216–23. PubMed.

6. Badesch DB, Raskob GE, Elliott CG, Krichman AM, Farber HW, Frost AE, et al. Pulmonary arterial hypertension: baseline characteristics from the REVEAL Registry. Chest. 2010;137(2):376–87. PubMed.

7. Jing ZC, Xu XQ, Han ZY, Wu Y, Deng KW, Wang H, et al. Registry and survival study in chinese patients with idiopathic and familial pulmonary arterial hypertension. Chest. 2007;132(2):373–9. PubMed.

8. Thenappan T, Shah SJ, Rich S, Gomberg-Maitland M. A USA-based registry for pulmonary arterial hypertension: 1982–2006. Eur Respir J. 2007;30(6):1103–10. PubMed.

9. Kane GC, Maradit-Kremers H, Slusser JP, Scott CG, Frantz RP, McGoon MD. Integration of clinical and hemodynamic parameters in the prediction of long-term survival in patients with pulmonary arterial hypertension. Chest. 2011;139(6):1285–93. PubMed.

10. Humbert M, Sitbon O, Chaouat A, Bertocchi M, Habib G, Gressin V, et al. Pulmonary arterial hypertension in France: results from a national registry. Am J Respir Crit Care Med. 2006;173(9):1023–30. PubMed.

11. Peacock AJ, Murphy NF, McMurray JJ, Caballero L, Stewart S. An epidemiological study of pulmonary arterial hypertension. Eur Respir J. 2007;30(1):104–9. PubMed.

12. Escribano-Subias P, Blanco I, Lopez-Meseguer M, Lopez-Guarch CJ, Roman A, Morales P, et al. Survival in pulmonary hypertension in Spain: insights from the Spanish registry. Eur Respir J. 2012;40(3):596–603. PubMed.

13. Hoeper MM, Huscher D, Ghofrani HA, Delcroix M, Distler O, Schweiger C, et al. Elderly patients diagnosed with idiopathic pulmonary arterial hypertension: results from the COMPERA registry. Int J Cardiol. 2013;168(2):871–80. PubMed.

14. Zhang R, Dai LZ, Xie WP, Yu ZX, Wu BX, Pan L, et al. Survival of Chinese patients with pulmonary arterial hypertension in the modern treatment era. Chest. 2011;140(2):301–9. PubMed.

15. Fischler M, Speich R, Dorschner L, Nicod L, Domenighetti G, Tamm M, et al. Pulmonary hypertension in Switzerland: treatment and clinical course. Swiss Med Wkly. 2008;138(25–26):371–8. PubMed.

16. Ling Y, Johnson MK, Kiely DG, Condliffe R, Elliot CA, Gibbs JS, et al. Changing demographics, epidemiology, and survival of incident pulmonary arterial hypertension: results from the pulmonary hypertension registry of the United Kingdom and Ireland. Am J Respir Crit Care Med. 2012;186(8):790–6. PubMed.

17. Khanna D, Tan M, Furst DE, Hill NS, McLaughlin VV, Silver RM, et al. Recognition of pulmonary hypertension in the rheumatology community: lessons from a Quality Enhancement Research Initiative. Clin Exp Rheumatol. 2014;32:s-21–7.

18. McLaughlin VV, Langer A, Tan M, Clements PJ, Oudiz RJ, Tapson VF, et al. Contemporary trends in the diagnosis and management of pulmonary arterial hypertension: an initiative to close the care gap. Chest. 2013;143(2):324–32. PubMed.

19. D'Alonzo GE, Barst RJ, Ayres SM, Bergofsky EH, Brundage BH, Detre KM, et al. Survival in patients with primary pulmonary hypertension. Results from a national prospective registry. Ann Intern Med. 1991;115(5):343–9. PubMed.

20. Humbert M, Sitbon O, Yaici A, Montani D, O'Callaghan DS, Jais X, et al. Survival in incident and prevalent cohorts of patients with pulmonary arterial hypertension. Eur Respir J. 2010;36(3):549–55. PubMed.

21. Benza RL, Miller DP, Barst RJ, Badesch DB, Frost AE, McGoon MD. An evaluation of long-term survival from time of diagnosis in pulmonary arterial hypertension from the REVEAL Registry. Chest. 2012;142(2):448–56. PubMed.

22. Thenappan T, Shah SJ, Rich S, Tian L, Archer SL, Gomberg-Maitland M. Survival in pulmonary arterial hypertension: a reappraisal of the NIH risk stratification equation. Eur Respir J. 2010;35(5):1079–87. PubMed.

23. Benza RL, Miller DP, Gomberg-Maitland M, Frantz RP, Foreman AJ, Coffey CS, et al. Predicting survival in pulmonary arterial hypertension: insights from the Registry to Evaluate Early and Long-Term Pulmonary Arterial Hypertension Disease Management (REVEAL). Circulation. 2010;122(2):164–72. PubMed.

24. McLaughlin VV, Suissa S. Prognosis of pulmonary arterial hypertension: the power of clinical registries of rare diseases. Circulation. 2010;122(2):106–8. PubMed.

25. Frost AE, Badesch DB, Barst RJ, Benza RL, Elliott CG, Farber HW, et al. The changing picture of patients with pulmonary arterial hypertension in the United States: how REVEAL differs from historic and non-US Contemporary Registries. Chest. 2011;139(1):128–37. PubMed.

26. Benza RL, Gomberg-Maitland M, Frost AE, Frantz RP, Humbert M, McGoon MD. Development of prognostic tools in pulmonary arterial hypertension: lessons from modern day registries. Thromb Haemost. 2012;108(6):1049–60. PubMed.

27. Olsson KM, Delcroix M, Ghofrani HA, Tiede H, Huscher D, Speich R, et al. Anticoagulation and survival in pulmonary arterial hypertension: results from the Comparative, Prospective Registry of Newly Initiated Therapies for Pulmonary Hypertension (COMPERA). Circulation. 2014;129(1):57–65. PubMed.

28. McGoon MD, Krichman A, Farber HW, Barst RJ, Raskob GE, Liou TG, et al. Design of the REVEAL registry for US patients with pulmonary arterial hypertension. Mayo Clin Proc Mayo Clin. 2008;83(8):923–31. PubMed.

29. Sandoval J, Bauerle O, Palomar A, Gomez A, Martinez-Guerra ML, Beltran M, et al. Survival in primary pulmonary hypertension. Validation of a prognostic equation. Circulation. 1994;89(4):1733–44. PubMed.

30. Rubin LJ, Badesch DB, Barst RJ, Galie N, Black CM, Keogh A, et al. Bosentan therapy for pulmonary arterial hypertension. N Engl J Med. 2002;346(12):896–903. PubMed.

31. McLaughlin VV, Shillington A, Rich S. Survival in primary pulmonary hypertension: the impact of epoprostenol therapy. Circulation. 2002;106(12):1477–82. PubMed.

32. McLaughlin VV, Sitbon O, Badesch DB, Barst RJ, Black C, Galie N, et al. Survival with first-line bosentan in patients with primary pulmonary hypertension. Eur Respir J. 2005;25(2):244–9. PubMed.

33. Provencher S, Sitbon O, Humbert M, Cabrol S, Jais X, Simonneau G. Long-term outcome with first-line bosentan therapy in idiopathic pulmonary arterial hypertension. Eur Heart J. 2006;27(5):589–95. PubMed.

34. Barst RJ, Galie N, Naeije R, Simonneau G, Jeffs R, Arneson C, et al. Long-term outcome in pulmonary arterial hypertension patients treated with subcutaneous treprostinil. Eur Respir J. 2006;28(6):1195–203. PubMed.

35. Thenappan T, Glassner C, Gomberg-Maitland M. Validation of the pulmonary hypertension connection equation for survival prediction in pulmonary arterial hypertension. Chest. 2012;141(3):642–50. PubMed.

36. Humbert M, Sitbon O, Chaouat A, Bertocchi M, Habib G, Gressin V, et al. Survival in patients with idiopathic, familial, and anorexigen-associated pulmonary arterial hypertension in the modern management era. Circulation. 2010;122(2):156–63. PubMed.

37. McGoon M, Benza R, Frost A. External validation of the French predictive model to estimate PAH survival: a REVEAL analysis (abstr). Eur Respir J. 2012;40(41S).

38. Lee WT, Ling Y, Sheares KK, Pepke-Zaba J, Peacock AJ, Johnson MK. Predicting survival in pulmonary arterial hypertension in the UK. Eur Respir J. 2012;40(3):604–11. PubMed.

39. Cogswell R, Kobashigawa E, McGlothlin D, Shaw R, De Marco T. Validation of the Registry to Evaluate Early and Long-Term Pulmonary Arterial Hypertension Disease Management (REVEAL) pulmonary hypertension prediction model in a unique population and utility in the prediction of long-term survival. J Heart Lung Transplant. 2012;31(11):1165–70. PubMed.

40. Benza RL, Gomberg-Maitland M, Miller DP, Frost A, Frantz RP, Foreman AJ, et al. The REVEAL Registry risk score calculator in patients newly diagnosed with pulmonary arterial hypertension. Chest. 2012;141(2):354–62. PubMed.

41. Cogswell R, Pritzker M, De Marco T. Performance of the REVEAL pulmonary arterial hypertension prediction model using noninvasive and routinely measured parameters. J Heart Lung Transplant. 2014;33(4):382–7. PubMed.

42. Sitbon O, Humbert M, Simonneau G. External validation of the REVEAL risk score calculator for PAH survival: a French pulmonary hypertension network analysis (abstr). Eur Respir J. 2012;40(41S).

43. Pencina MJ, D'Agostino RB. Overall C as a measure of discrimination in survival analysis: model specific population value and confidence interval estimation. Stat Med. 2004;23(13):2109–23. PubMed.

44. Duffels MG, Engelfriet PM, Berger RM, van Loon RL, Hoendermis E, Vriend JW, et al. Pulmonary arterial hypertension in congenital heart disease: an epidemiologic perspective from a Dutch registry. Int J Cardiol. 2007;120(2):198–204. PubMed.

45. Condliffe R, Kiely DG, Peacock AJ, Corris PA, Gibbs JS, Vrapi F, et al. Connective tissue disease-associated pulmonary arterial hypertension in the modern treatment era. Am J Respir Crit Care Med. 2009;179(2):151–7. PubMed.

46. Shah SJ, Thenappan T, Rich S, Tian L, Archer SL, Gomberg-Maitland M. Association of serum creatinine with abnormal hemodynamics and mortality in pulmonary arterial hypertension. Circulation. 2008;117(19):2475–83. PubMed.

47. de Groote P, Gressin V, Hachulla E, Carpentier P, Guillevin L, Kahan A, et al. Evaluation of cardiac abnormalities by Doppler echocardiography in a large nationwide multicentric cohort of patients with systemic sclerosis. Ann Rheum Dis. 2008;67(1):31–6. PubMed.

48. Meune C, Avouac J, Wahbi K, Cabanes L, Wipff J, Mouthon L, et al. Cardiac involvement in systemic sclerosis assessed by tissue-doppler echocardiography during routine care: a controlled study of 100 consecutive patients. Arthritis Rheum. 2008;58(6):1803–9. PubMed.

49. Tongers J, Schwerdtfeger B, Klein G, Kempf T, Schaefer A, Knapp JM, et al. Incidence and clinical relevance of supraventricular tachyarrhythmias in pulmonary hypertension. Am Heart J. 2007;153(1):127–32. PubMed.

50. Vongpatanasin W, Brickner ME, Hillis LD, Lange RA. The Eisenmenger syndrome in adults. Ann Intern Med. 1998;128(9):745–55. PubMed.

51. Kawut SM, Taichman DB, Ahya VN, Kaplan S, Archer-Chicko CL, Kimmel SE, et al. Hemodynamics and survival of patients with portopulmonary hypertension. Liver Transpl. 2005;11(9):1107–11. PubMed.

52. Halpern SD, Taichman DB. Misclassification of pulmonary hypertension due to reliance on pulmonary capillary wedge pressure rather than left ventricular end-diastolic pressure. Chest. 2009;136(1):37–43. PubMed.

53. Ryan JJ, Rich JD, Thiruvoipati T, Swamy R, Kim GH, Rich S. Current practice for determining pulmonary capillary wedge pressure predisposes to serious errors in the classification of patients with pulmonary hypertension. Am Heart J. 2012;163(4):589–94. PubMed.

54. Pugh ME, Hemnes AR, Trammell A, Newman JH, Robbins IM. Variablity in hemodynamic evalution of pulmonary hypertension at large referral centers. Pulmonary circulation. 2014;2014:4(4).

55. Hoeper MM, Bogaard HJ, Condliffe R, Frantz R, Khanna D, Kurzyna M, et al. Definitions and diagnosis of pulmonary hypertension. J Am Coll Cardiol. 2013;62(25 Suppl):D42–50. PubMed.

56. Taichman DB, McGoon MD, Harhay MO, Archer-Chicko C, Sager JS, Murugappan M, et al. Wide variation in clinicians' assessment of New York Heart Association/World Health Organization functional class in patients with pulmonary arterial hypertension. Mayo Clin Proc Mayo Clin. 2009;84(7):586–92. PubMed Pubmed Central PMCID: 2704130.

57. Forfia PR, Fisher MR, Mathai SC, Housten-Harris T, Hemnes AR, Borlaug BA, et al. Tricuspid annular displacement predicts survival in pulmonary hypertension. Am J Respir Crit Care Med. 2006;174(9):1034–41. PubMed.

58. van Wolferen SA, Marcus JT, Boonstra A, Marques KM, Bronzwaer JG, Spreeuwenberg MD, et al. Prognostic value of right ventricular mass, volume, and function in idiopathic pulmonary arterial hypertension. Eur Heart J. 2007;28(10):1250–7. PubMed.

59. van de Veerdonk MC, Kind T, Marcus JT, Mauritz GJ, Heymans MW, Bogaard HJ, et al. Progressive right ventricular dysfunction in patients with pulmonary arterial hypertension responding to therapy. J Am Coll Cardiol. 2011;58(24):2511–9. PubMed.

60. Wensel R, Opitz CF, Anker SD, Winkler J, Hoffken G, Kleber FX, et al. Assessment of survival in patients with primary pulmonary hypertension: importance of cardiopulmonary exercise testing. Circulation. 2002;106(3):319–24. PubMed.

61. Minai OA, Gudavalli R, Mummadi S, Liu X, McCarthy K, Dweik RA. Heart rate recovery predicts clinical worsening in patients with pulmonary arterial hypertension. Am J Respir Crit Care Med. 2012;185(4):400–8. PubMed.

62. Sitbon O, Humbert M, Nunes H, Parent F, Garcia G, Herve P, et al. Long-term intravenous epoprostenol infusion in primary pulmonary hypertension: prognostic factors and survival. J Am Coll Cardiol. 2002;40(4):780–8. PubMed.

63. Nickel N, Golpon H, Greer M, Knudsen L, Olsson K, Westerkamp V, et al. The prognostic impact of follow-up assessments in patients with idiopathic pulmonary arterial hypertension. Eur Respir J. 2012;39(3):589–96. PubMed.

64. Hoeper MM, Markevych I, Spiekerkoetter E, Welte T, Niedermeyer J. Goal-oriented treatment and combination therapy for pulmonary arterial hypertension. Eur Respir J. 2005;26(5):858–63. PubMed.

65. Tiede H, Sommer N, Milger K, Voswinckel R, Bandorski D, Schermuly RT, et al. Short-term improvement in pulmonary hemodynamics is strongly predictive of long-term survival in patients with pulmonary arterial hypertension. Pulm Circ. 2013;3(3):523–32. PubMed Pubmed Central PMCID: 4070816.

66. Galie N, Barbera JA, Frost AE, Ghofrani HA, Hoeper MM, McLaughlin VV, et al. Initial use of Ambrisentan plus Tadalafil in Pulmonary Arterial Hypertension. N Eng J Med. 2015;373(9):834–44.

67. Sitbon O, Jais X, Savale L, Cottin V, Bergot E, Macari EA, et al. Upfront triple combination therapy in pulmonary arterial hypertension: a pilot study. Eur Respir J. 2014;43(6):1691–7. PubMed.

68. Simonneau G, Gatzoulis MA, Adatia I, Celermajer D, Denton C, Ghofrani A, et al. Updated clinical classification of pulmonary hypertension. J Am Coll Cardiol. 2013;62(25 Suppl):D34–41. PubMed.

69. Chakinala MM, McGoon M. Pulmonary hypertension care centers. Adv Pulm Hyper. 2014;12(4):175–8.

70. Hiremath J, Thanikachalam S, Parikh K, Shanmugasundaram S, Bangera S, Shapiro L, et al. Exercise improvement and plasma biomarker changes with intravenous treprostinil therapy for pulmonary arterial hypertension: a placebo-controlled trial. J Heart Lung Transplant. 2010;29(2):137–49. PubMed.

71. Galie N, Olschewski H, Oudiz RJ, Torres F, Frost A, Ghofrani HA, et al. Ambrisentan for the treatment of pulmonary arterial hypertension: results of the ambrisentan in pulmonary arterial hypertension, randomized, double-blind, placebo-controlled, multicenter, efficacy (ARIES) study 1 and 2. Circulation. 2008;117(23):3010–9. PubMed.

72. Galie N, Ghofrani HA, Torbicki A, Barst RJ, Rubin LJ, Badesch D, et al. Sildenafil citrate therapy for pulmonary arterial hypertension. N Engl J Med. 2005;353(20):2148–57. PubMed.

73. Ghofrani HA, Galie N, Grimminger F, Grunig E, Humbert M, Jing ZC, et al. Riociguat for the treatment of pulmonary arterial hypertension. N Engl J Med. 2013;369(4):330–40. PubMed.

74. Awdish RL, Cajigas HR. Early initiation of prostacyclin in portopulmonary hypertension: 10 years of a transplant center's experience. Lung. 2013;191(6):593–600. PubMed.

75. Orens JB. Lung transplantation for pulmonary hypertension. Int J Clin Pract Suppl. 2007;158:4–9. PubMed.

76. Davis SQ, Garrity Jr ER. Organ allocation in lung transplant. Chest. 2007;132(5):1646–51. PubMed.

77. Hachem RR, Trulock EP. The new lung allocation system and its impact on waitlist characteristics and post-transplant outcomes. Semin Thorac Cardiovasc Surg. 2008;20(2):139–42. PubMed.

78. Chen H, Shiboski SC, Golden JA, Gould MK, Hays SR, Hoopes CW, et al. Impact of the lung allocation score on lung transplantation for pulmonary arterial hypertension. Am J Respir Crit Care Med. 2009;180(5):468–74. PubMed Pubmed Central PMCID: 2742763.

79. Benza RL, Miller DP, Frost A, Barst RJ, Krichman AM, McGoon MD. Analysis of the lung allocation score estimation of risk of death in patients with pulmonary arterial hypertension using data from the REVEAL Registry. Transplantation. 2010;90(3):298–305. PubMed.

80. Gomberg-Maitland M, Glassner-Kolmin C, Watson S, Frantz R, Park M, Frost A, et al. Survival in pulmonary arterial hypertension patients awaiting lung transplantation. J Heart Lung Transplant. 2013;32(12):1179–86. PubMed.

81. Khan IY, Singer LG, de Perrot M, Granton JT, Keshavjee S, Chau C, et al. Survival after lung transplantation in systemic sclerosis. A systematic review. Respir Med. 2013;107(12):2081–7. PubMed.

Support Care for the Pulmonary Hypertension Patient

Abby Poms, Mary Bartlett, Traci Housten,
Martha Kingman, and Glenna L. Traiger

Introduction

Pulmonary arterial hypertension (PAH) is a rare disease with complex treatments, and, therefore, patients require a comprehensive care plan that often includes education, support and frequent clinical assessment. In order to meet the unique challenges specific to patients afflicted with PAH, many pulmonary vascular disease centers rely on pulmonary hypertension (PH) clinical care coordinators (PHCs) to ensure effective monitoring and support of patients and their families at each stage of disease trajectory. Indeed, PH center accreditation by the Pulmonary Hypertension Association (PHA), for example, requires access to a dedicated PHCC.

Overview of Pulmonary Hypertension Clinical Care Coordinator Role

Understanding PH classification and pathophysiology is complex and, therefore, proper education regarding these issues is uniformly required for newly diagnosed patients.

A. Poms, BS, RRT, CCRP (✉)
Department of Pulmonary and Critical Care Medicine, Duke University Pulmonary Vascular Disease Center, Durham, NC, USA
e-mail: abby.poms@duke.edu

M. Bartlett, MSN, FNP
Department of Pulmonary Medicine, Winthrop University Hospital, Mineola, NY 11501, USA

Division of Pulmonary and Critical Care, Department of Medicine, Winthrop University Hospital, Mineola, NY USA

T. Housten, RN, MS
Pulmonary and Critical Care Medicine, Johns Hopkins University Pulmonary Hypertension Program, Baltimore, MD 21287, USA

M. Kingman, BSN, DNP, FNP-C
Pulmonary and Critical Care, Heart and Lung Center, University of Texas Southwestern Medical Center, Dallas, TX 75390, USA

G.L. Traiger, RN, MSN, CNS-BC
Division of Pulmonary and Critical Medicine, David Geffen School of Medicine at UCLA, Los Angeles, CA 957035, USA

Often, there is insufficient time in the initial encounter to address fully each question raised by patients. More commonly, questions or concerns will arise following point of care. Therefore, it is crucial to refer patients to the abundant array of educational material that is available online and as pamphlet handouts. For example, the PH Survival Guide, a comprehensive book written by a patient and edited by PAH professionals, is available from the PHA at a modest cost. The PHA website (phassociation.org) maintains a plethora of information about PH, and should be the recommended resource for patients, as all information has been validated by experts as accurate and up to date.

Additionally, pharmaceutical companies have produced both branded and unbranded educational materials, which can be utilized to augment education provided by the PH treatment team, the Specialty Pharmacy (SP), and the PHA. Branded materials are medication-specific and outline the method of action and side effects, while unbranded materials intend to provide education regarding disease awareness, diagnostic testing, optimal nutrition, and lifestyle guidelines. These materials are provided to clinicians at no cost for distribution to patients.

Patients with PAH require close monitoring; a minor illness or adverse event may be life threatening. Much of the care provided to this patient population occurs in between office visits through phone contact, and, therefore, face-to-face encounters comprise a fraction of overall care by establishing a platform to guide management remotely. Although survival has improved, PAH remains an incurable disease [1]. As patients approach end of life, there are additional educational needs that must be considered: palliative care or hospice may be appropriate and each destination involves transitional changes to PAH medical therapy (including discontinuation). This, in turn, is likely to introduce substantial anxiety and uncertainty. The PHC, having an established relationship with the patient, is well positioned to explain the ramifications of palliation, help locate social services, and provide emotional support (Fig. 21.1).

© Springer International Publishing Switzerland 2016
B.A. Maron et al. (eds.), *Pulmonary Hypertension: Basic Science to Clinical Medicine*, DOI 10.1007/978-3-319-23594-3_21

A. Poms et al.

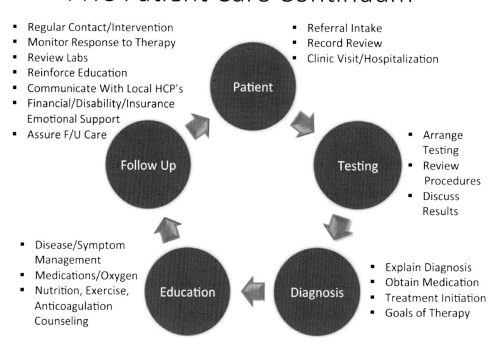

Fig. 21.1 The pulmonary hypertension clinical patient care continuum. The Pulmonary Hypertension Clinical (*PHC*) care coordinator plays a pivotal role in coordinating each element of the treatment plan individualized to each patient. *HCP* health care provider, *F/U* follow up

PHC Patient Care Continuum

- Regular Contact/Intervention
- Monitor Response to Therapy
- Review Labs
- Reinforce Education
- Communicate With Local HCP's
- Financial/Disability/Insurance Emotional Support
- Assure F/U Care

Patient
- Referral Intake
- Record Review
- Clinic Visit/Hospitalization

Follow Up

Testing
- Arrange Testing
- Review Procedures
- Discuss Results

- Disease/Symptom Management
- Medications/Oxygen
- Nutrition, Exercise, Anticoagulation Counseling

Education

Diagnosis
- Explain Diagnosis
- Obtain Medication
- Treatment Initiation
- Goals of Therapy

Supporting PAH Patient Vulnerabilities

The PHC is critical to discovering factors that may influence unexpected test results, such as musculoskletal pain, inter-current illness, or improved footwear may be critical to interpreting unfavorable results on exercise testing. Additionally, PHC reinforcement of daily body weight monitoring, peripheral edema self-assessment, medication adherence, low sodium/PAH healthy diet, fluid restriction if appropriate, and notifying their healthcare provider in the event of progressive symptoms are all critical areas of opportunity for improved outcome. Along these lines, the PHC often provides technical training with respect to home vital sign monitoring including proper self-assessment by home blood pressure cuff, weight scale, and pulse oximetry as well as use of telemonitoring [2], each of which are vital to keep a continuous record of clinical status between clinic visits.

Medication Education

Once a diagnosis of PAH is established, a treatment plan in which oral, inhaled, subcutaneous, and/or intravenous therapies is considered. The provider, patient, family, and PHC are often involved in this decision making process owing to the complexity and unique safety profile of many PAH-specific therapies.

Endothelin Receptor Antagonists

There are three U.S. Food and Drug Administration (FDA) approved medications in this class including bosentan (Tracleer), ambrisentan (Letairis), and macitentan (Opsumit). All ERAs are considered to be teratogenic based on animal studies. Importantly, women of child-bearing potential (WCBP) taking an ERA must be taught about pregnancy avoidance and acceptable forms of birth control. A negative pregnancy test is required prior to starting therapy, monthly while on therapy and 1 month after discontinuation of therapy. Patients should use two reliable forms of birth control while on therapy and up to 1 month after discontinuing therapy. Should pregnancy be suspected while on therapy, patients must contact their PH provider immediately.

Bosentan (Tracleer) was approved by the FDA in 2001 and was the first available oral therapy for the treatment of PAH. Because of the risks of hepatotoxicity and teratogenicity, bosentan is available only through the restricted Tracleer Access Program (T.A.P.), which is a component of the Tracleer Risk Evaluation and Mitigation Strategy (REMS). Tracleer REMS requires the prescribers, patients, and pharmacies must enroll in the program. Patients must be counseled that co-administration of cyclosporine A and glyburide are contraindicated with bosentan. Other drug-drug interactions can occur with ritonavir, ketaconozole, sildenafil, rifampin, tacromilus, simvastatin and other statins, requiring close surveillance of patients' medication regimens.

Providing a list of potential drug-drug interactions to patients may be useful. The recommended starting dose of bosentan is 62.5 mg twice daily with a maximum approved dosage of 125 mg twice daily. It carries a black box warning for liver injury, therefore any patient on this medication will require education about monthly liver function testing (liver aminotransferases [ALT and AST] [3]. Dependent upon results of liver function tests, dose reduction or discontinuation may be necessary. A decrease in hemoglobin concentration has been associated with the use of bosentan; therefore, monitoring hemoglobin is recommended prior to starting, after 1 and 3 months, and quarterly thereafter [4].

The second ERA to gain approval through the FDA for PAH was ambrisentan (Letairis) in 2007. Because of the risk of embryo-fetal toxicity, females can only receive ambrisentan through a restricted program called the Letairis REMS program. Because co-administration of ambrisentan with cyclosporine has been shown to increase ambrisentan exposure in healthy volunteers; the ambrisentan dosage should be limited to 5 mg once daily when administered together. Ambrisentan is supplied as a 5 mg or 10 mg tablet. The recommended starting dose is 5 mg daily, and if tolerated, up-titration to 10 mg daily can be considered. WCBP require a negative pregnancy test prior to therapy initiation, monthly pregnancy tests while on therapy and 1 month after discontinuation of therapy. Providers must obtain and review pregnancy tests monthly. Though elevations of liver function tests have been reported with ambrisentan, there was no statistical difference between groups in clinical trials. Thus, hepatic function monitoring is not required. Decreases to hemoglobin concentration and hematocrit can be associated with the use of ambrisentan, and, therefore, hemoglobin should be assessed prior to initiation of ambrisentan, at 1 month, and periodically thereafter [5].

Macitentan (Opsumit) is the most recent ERA to gain FDA approval in 2013. For all females, macitentan is available only through a restricted program called the Opsumit REMS Program because of the risk of embryo-fetal toxicity. The recommended dosage is 10 mg daily. For WCBP, providers must obtain and review pregnancy tests prior to starting therapy, monthly while on therapy and 1 month after discontinuation of therapy. It is recommended that liver function testing occur prior to starting macitentan and be repeated periodically at the discretion of the treating physician. Decreases in hemoglobin concentrations have occurred in patients taking macitentan. Hemoglobin should be assessed at baseline and repeated during treatment as clinically indicated [6]. Concomitant use of macitentan with strong CYP3A4 inducers, such as rifampin, should be avoided as they significantly reduce macitentan levels. Conversely, co-administration of strong CYP3A4 inhibitors like ketoconazole significantly increase macitentan exposure and should be avoided.

The most common side effects of the ERA class are edema and nasal congestion. Edema can often be managed with diuresis though the medication may ultimately need to be discontinued if it persists. Clinicians should pay close attention to educating patients about the potential to develop edema or experience worsening edema with the initiation of ERA therapy. Increased dyspnea and general sense of malaise may occur. These symptoms should trigger patients to contact their PH specialist office immediately. Tracking daily weights during ERA initiation is helpful to monitor for potential edema. Nasal congestion is also commonly associated with ERA treatment. Saline rinses can help to reduce tissue swelling in the nasal passages [7]. Nasal decongestants can potentially worsen the condition and must be avoided in this patient population. Steroid-based nasal sprays can help reduce swelling in some patients. For severe nasal congestion, consider referral to an otolaryngologist for other potential interventions. While some patients experience a degree of relief with these measures, intervention is typically temporary or ineffective. Dependent on the severity of the nasal congestion, therapy may need to be discontinued.

Phosphodiesterase-Type 5 Inhibitor (PDE-5i) Therapies

The PDE-5i drug class includes two different oral compounds, sildenafil (Revatio) and tadalafil (Adcirca). These medications are the least expensive PAH specific treatments. Sudden decrease or loss of hearing and vision has been reported in people taking PDE-5i. Patients are advised to seek a baseline eye examination prior to initiating therapy and periodically while on treatment. The most common side effects reported with the PDE5 inhibitors include headache, dyspepsia, epistaxis, diarrhea, and flushing. Epistaxis can be severe enough to require intervention such as nasal packing. Myalgia, which can be quite severe, is also reported, more often by patients on tadalafil versus sildenafil. Over the counter medications for headache, GI upset and myalgia may prove helpful. After initial exposure of this medication class, side effects generally subside within 1–2 weeks and can be managed successfully through this period. Importantly, patients are educated not to take PDE5 inhibitors in conjunction with nitrates of any form, or α-receptor antagonists due to the risk of systemic hypotension.

Sildenafil for pulmonary hypertension is supplied in a 20 mg tablet. The recommended dosage is 20 mg three times a day. There is clinical experience and data demonstrating dose related improvement with higher doses of sildenafil [8]. Because of the need for three times daily dosing, ongoing patient counseling should occur to assure continued medication compliance, particularly with the middle day dose.

Concomitant use of sildenafil with ritonavir and other potent CYP3A inhibitors is not recommended due to an increased potential for sildenafil-associated adverse events. Bosentan significantly decreases the plasma concentration of sildenafil when co-administered to patients with pulmonary hypertension [9]. Considerations for dose adjustment of sildenafil should be made if using these two medications in combination. When appropriate, clinicians should be certain patients understand not to use PDE5 inhibitors prescribed for erectile dysfunction in conjunction with those prescribed for PAH.

Tadalafil is supplied in a 20 mg tablet with recommended dosage of 40 mg once daily, which is helpful for improving medication compliance. To potentially improve tolerance throughout the day with tadalafil, consider dosing before bedtime for patients with significant headache. Dose adjustments may be required with co-administration of ritonavir. Clinicians should avoid use of CYP3A inhibitors and inducers, including ketoconazole, itraconazole, and rifampin.

Soluble Guanylate Cyclase Stimulator

Riociguat, a soluble guanylate cyclase (sGC) stimulator, was the first therapy approved to treat inoperable or persistent chronic thromboembolic pulmonary hypertension (CTEPH) (WHO Group 4). It is also approved to treat PAH WHO Group 1 patients. Due to teratogenicity effects, riociguat is only available through a restricted REMS program for female patients. WCBP must be taught about pregnancy avoidance and acceptable forms of birth control. A negative pregnancy test is required prior to starting therapy, monthly while on therapy and 1 month after discontinuation of therapy.

The recommended starting dose of riociguat is 1 mg three times daily, however for patients that may not tolerate the hypotensive effect of the drug, consider starting at 0.5 mg three times daily. Up titration of drug occurs by 0.5 mg dosages at intervals no sooner than 2 weeks as tolerated to a maximum dosage of 2.5 mg three times a day. Riociguat should not be taken in conjunction with nitrates in any form or PDE inhibitors due to risk of hypotension [10].

Precaution should be taken with concomitant use of ritonavir and ketoconazole, which can be associated with increased circulating levels of bioactive riociguat, resulting in systemic hypotension.

The most common reported side effects of riociguat are headache, GI upset, dizziness, nausea, hypotension, vomiting, and anemia. Though not mandated, some practices monitor for anemia at baseline and repeat during treatment as clinically indicated. Other less common side effects include hemoptysis, epistaxis, peripheral edema, and palpitations [10]. Patients should be counseled to report any sign of bleeding immediately. As hypotension is a more common

side effect of riociguat, home monitoring and periodic assessment by a SP nurse of vital signs and is advisable between clinic visits. There is no additional cost to the patient for this service.

Prostacyclin Analogues

The prostacyclin medications are more complex and historically have only been available in non-oral forms that include inhaled, subcutaneous and intravenous. Recently an oral formulation of treprostinil as monotherapy, marketed as Orenitram, was approved by the FDA.

PH program staff submits a referral and clinical documentation for all prostacyclin medications to an SP, who starts an insurance verification process. The PH coordinator initiates education, which is supplemented by SP cardiopulmonary nurse specialists. Patients placed on prostacyclin therapy require in-depth and extensive continuing education and close monitoring. Clinicians prescribing these medications must have adequate expert staff to support these therapies.

Inhaled and Oral Formulations

There are 2 inhaled prostacyclins, iloprost (Ventavis®), and treprostinil (Tyvaso®); each with a unique administration device [11, 12]. Patients are taught how to install medication into the device, operate the device and clean the components. Thorough education by health care providers trained to use the device is essential for maximum efficacy. Side effects of both inhaled prostacyclins are similar and are managed with the same regimens. Cough is the most common side effect and cause of discontinuation of therapy with inhaled prostacyclins. The PHC and SP nurse must take care to educate the patient on cough management, such as use of prescribed pretreatment bronchodilators [13].

Iloprost is delivered via the I-neb Adaptive Aerosol Delivery (AAD) System. The I-Neb incorporates AAD technology, which adjusts to the individual patient's breathing pattern to deliver iloprost, at a dose of either 2.5 mcg or 5.0 mcg six to nine times daily, using a single glass ampule of medication per treatment session. Patients are trained to perform treatments independently at home. Treatment times should take about 4–10 min. Improper technique or equipment issues can affect treatment times and efficacy. Patients are instructed to call their SP if this occurs.

Side effects of iloprost include flushing, coughing, and headache [11]. Technology exists to download information from the I-neb device to assess treatment compliance. Because patients must take a minimum of 6 treatments daily to provide benefit, it's important to assure adequate dosing adherence.

Inhaled treprostinil is delivered via an Optineb device, dosed four times daily. Patients are trained to deliver treatments independently at home. The medication, supplied as a liquid in plastic ampules, is inserted into the Optineb device once daily. The dosage of inhaled treprostinil is determined by the number of breaths patients take per treatment period. Typically patients get initiated on three breaths (18 mcg) four times daily. Depending on patient tolerance, the dosage is uptitrated by increasing the number of breaths at desired intervals. The recommended efficacious dose is 9 breaths (54 mcg) four times daily; treatment duration is 2–3 min. Most common reported side effects of inhaled treprostinil include coughing, headache, throat irritation and pain, and facial flushing [14]. Over the counter medication such as acetaminophen can be tried for headache complaints, and short acting β-agonists have been shown helpful in controlling cough associated with the treatments.

Oral treprostinil (Orenitram), approved as monotherapy in treatment-naive patients, is supplied as extended release tablets with the following four strengths: 0.125 mg, 0.25 mg, 1 mg, and 2.5 mg. A maximum dose is determined by tolerability and clinical response. Patients can be dosed either twice daily or three times daily. Abrupt discontinuation or sudden dose reductions may result in worsening PH symptoms. Most common adverse effects include headache, nausea, diarrhea, extremity pain, and flushing [15]. Oral treprostinil inhibits platelet aggregation thereby increasing the risk of bleeding. Its use is contraindicated in hepatically impaired patients, and patients should be counseled to take the medication with food and refrain from drinking alcohol.

Over the counter and prescriptive regimens should be used as needed to alleviate side effects. Downward dose adjustment of oral treprostinil is necessary if co-administered with the CYP2C8 enzyme inhibitor and lipid lowering therapy gemfibrozil.

Subcutaneous and Intravenous Formulations

Currently there are three IV and one SQ prostacyclin formulations available. Each has unique administration systems and pharmacologic action that will help guide clinician selection.

Infused prostacylin therapy requires extensive training by the PH coordinator and the SP nurse. Teaching includes mixing and storage of medication, pump operation, emergency procedures, aseptic technique, care of the central venous catheter (CVC) and central line dressing for IV formulations, signs of infection, up-titration schedule, side effect management and when to seek immediate medical assistance. Patients often experience significant side effects and may face various challenges with central line complications including infection or need for a replacement central line.

The most common side effects of infused prostacyclins therapy include flushing, headache, nausea, diarrhea, vomiting, hypotension, jaw pain, musculoskeletal pain (especially in feet and legs) and site pain with subcutaneous delivery.

Pharmacologic treatment with ondansetron and loperamide for the gastrointestinal effects may prove helpful. Gabapentin may be used to provide relief of commonly reported leg pain. Due to prostacyclin antiplatelet effects, patients should be monitored closely for thrombocytopenia and hypotension [16] and be counseled regarding the potential increase in bleeding risk.

In addition to patients receiving intensive training on managing the continuous infusion therapy at home, focus is also given to maintaining the CVC and subcutaneous site to avoid infection. Ongoing education on sterile technique and catheter and site care requires a team approach both from the PH specialist and SP nurses. Clinicians should have established protocols well understood by patients in the event a CVC site is infected or suspect. A plan is required in the event of interrupted drug therapy, as patients must seek immediate medical attention either via their PH Center or local emergency department. It is also reasonable to contact the patient's local emergency medical service (EMS) provider to notify them of the protocol for implementing prostacyclin therapy through a peripheral intravenous catheter under emergency conditions, particularly for patients living in rural areas. In the event of local site infection, oral antibiotics are often successful; however, in the event that an infection involves the CVC directly then line removal and parenteral antibiotics may be required.

Treprostinil administered subcutaneously is delivered via a small pump platform and is the only infused prostacyclin that does not require a central line. This form of prostacyclin delivery is initiated frequently in the outpatient setting, although patients often require extensive up-front training and education by both PHC and SP personnel. The possibility of side effects, including site pain, are communicated at the beginning of therapy and patients are taught strategies for managing these. In fact, infusion site pain is the most commonly reported adverse event with subcutaneous treprostinil and typically peaks in intensity 2–5 days after starting a new infusion site. Topical therapies like pluronic lecithin organogel (PLO gel) along with ice or heat packs, and acetaminophen, as needed, are often considered first line regimens. Step up regimens often include gabapentin, lidocaine patches, and tramadol if pain cannot be controlled otherwise. The use of medications such as histamine receptor antagonists and the use of a dry catheter pre-placement method has shown to be effective in improving site pain [17]. Patients are encouraged to maintain their SQ sites as long as possible to reduce site pain. Ongoing assessment should be performed to ensure the site is intact and drug is being absorbed, especially with those sites that have been in place for longer periods.

Epoprostenol, marketed as Flolan, or Veletri, is delivered intravenously. Both Flolan and Veletri are comprised of the same compound with different formulations and stability. Flolan is mixed daily and requires the use of ice packs changed twice a day to maintain stability. Veletri is stable at room temperature thus no ice packs are required and multiple cassettes can be mixed up to 7 days in advance of use when kept refrigerated. Patients initiated on epoprostenol require placement of a CVC, most commonly a *single*-lumen Hickman line. The half-life of epoprostenol is approximately 6 min [18]. This short half-life requires patients to be both vigilant and thoroughly educated on the infusion in order for it to be maintained safely at home. Abrupt withdrawal or reduction of dose may result in life threatening rebound pulmonary hypertension. Patients are typically initiated on a low dose and uptitrated as tolerated based on side effects and response to treatment. Generally a chronic stable dose is achieved and only small adjustments may be occasionally required.

Treprostinil, marketed as Remodulin, can be delivered subcutaneously or intravenously and has a half life of approximately 4 h [19]. This is a potential safety advantage for patients who do not live in close proximity of their PH center or in the case of an emergency. Starting dose and titration is similar to epoprostenol though chronic efficacious doses are generally two or more times that of epoprostenol [20, 21]. The IV formulation is mixed every other day. There is no mixing required for SQ Remodulin and the medication syringe is most often changed every 3 days. Dose adjustment may be necessary if inhibitors or inducers of CYP2C8 are co-administered with treprostinil.

The PHC will communicate with patients frequently between visits to monitor PH symptoms, medication side effects and determine how well the patient is tolerating dose increases. This information is communicated with the healthcare provider to determine any adjustments necessary to the titration schedule and the need for any medications to treat site pain or adverse medication effects.

Supportive Care

In addition to medication education, most patients will also require ongoing educational support regarding diet, exercise, pulmonary and cardiac rehabilitation, oxygen therapy, disability and palliative care or other end of life challenges, as indicated.

Anticogulation

In addition to education around specific PAH medical therapies, some patients will require anticoagulation, especially those patients with chronic thromboembolic pulmonary hypertension (CTEPH). In most cases, warfarin will be the anticoagulant of choice. However, newer factor Xa inhibitors are used more increasingly, although data remains lacking in regards to the efficacy of this drug class in the PAH popula-

tion. The PHC staff are well positioned to educate patients of importance of regular INR monitoring, and the potential for drug-drug and drug-food interactions.

Dietary Guidance

Most patients will be placed on a low sodium diet and often a fluid restriction if they have evidence of right ventricular failure and fluid retention. The PHC generally is responsible for this education, possibly in conjunction with a dietician, and includes instruction on measuring daily sodium intake and preparing low sodium meals. Patients are taught the importance of daily weights and immediately notifying the PH center of weight gain of >2 lbs. in 1 day or >5 lbs. in 1 week. Ongoing contact with patients regarding early awareness and management of fluid retention is critical in maintaining appropriate volume status.

Oxygen and Exercise Therapy

Some PAH patients will require oxygen therapy. The PHC works with the patient and oxygen supplier to obtain the most appropriate oxygen device for the patient, both at rest and with exertion. Extensive education will be required including the importance of preventing hypoxia and traveling with oxygen [22]. Pulmonary or cardiac rehabilitation may be ordered by the PH provider, but patients who cannot participate in medically monitored exercise programs need to be counseled about the benefit of exercise and their restrictions. The PHC often provides general guidelines for exercise including the need to stop or slow down if they experience chest pain, excessive dyspnea, or light-headedness [23].

Change in PAH Patient Status

The PH coordinator is also responsible for teaching patients about early recognition of changes in their status and when to seek emergency medical care. Some patients with significant activity intolerance and advanced disease may need to obtain temporary or permanent disability. If this is deemed appropriate by the treating physician and established guidelines, the PHC, preferably in conjunction with a social worker, will teach the patient how to begin the process and assist with completing disability forms.

Other Considerations

As a clinician, frustration can occur when the therapy that may be the most beneficial to a patient is not practical or available due to social or physical limitations. This typically comes into play when a prostanoid infusion is being considered, but can also be relevant with oral or inhaled treatments. Issues that may impede starting a therapy can include lack of support, age, drug dependency, history of non-compliance, or lack of dexterity from an underlying condition like systemic sclerosis. SP nurses can provide valuable insight into a patient's ability to handle a specific therapy through a home assessment and pre teaching on a therapy.

Caring for this patient population requires a tremendous amount of monitoring and follow up. Adopting a team approach inclusive of physicians, nurses, pharmacists, respiratory therapists, and other specialized providers such as social workers and SP professionals is necessary to make certain the patient's needs are being fully met. Establishing early in the care process a clear access route by which patients may contact their health care provider, PHC, and SP is critical to minimize the probability of avoidable problems. Finally, it is imperative that patients have a true understanding of their disease, are aware of all available options, and understand the implications associated with the various therapies.

Practical Issues for Inpatient and Outpatient Care of PAH Patients

In the United States, hospitalization rates for pulmonary hypertension (PH) have increased over the past decade [24]. This has occurred despite increased access to new PAH-specific medications and advances in medical therapy demonstrating improved survival in PAH patients [25]. Multiple studies have shown that even a single hospitalization is a predictor of mortality and readmission in this population [26, 27]. This section will discuss factors to consider to improve the safety of the inpatient environment for PAH patients and for a smooth transition to post-hospital care with the goal of reducing potentially avoidable hospitalizations.

Even highly experienced PH centers struggle to provide a safe inpatient environment for PAH patients and this is particularly true for patients receiving parenteral prostacyclins [28]. Furthermore, common occurrences such as systemic hypotension and atrial arrhythmias are managed very differently in PAH patients than in patients with other co-morbid conditions. PH physicians and team members should maintain close involvement in the care of their hospitalized patients regardless of where the patient is hospitalized. Programs should have a low threshold to transfer PAH patients that are hospitalized outside of their main institution. Patients and their caregivers must be educated and advised to be diligent in advocating for themselves to make sure they are receiving all the medications prescribed by the PAH provider and stay in contact with that provider during

any emergency room visit or hospitalization, even at their own center.

PH programs must employ a variety of strategies to maintain safety during hospitalizations. Strong consideration should be given to sequestering patients on a limited number of hospital units. The medical unit staff, both nursing and other allied health care professionals, should receive specific training in the disease state and administration of PAH medications with particular attention to the complexities characterizing infused prostacyclins. The program should have written policies and procedures for the administration of infused prostacyclins, and these policies should document the process for dose verification, schedule for cassette or syringe changes, type of infusion pumps utilized, management of drug interruption events and contact information for PH program staff and resources. Careful attention should also be given to training hospital transportation services and rapid response teams familiar with acute right ventricular heart failure and associated hemodynamic instability.

Initiating new PAH-specific medications in the hospital ahead of obtaining insurance approval can result in significant interruption to medical therapy after discharge. Excepting urgent cases, careful consideration should be given to delaying initiation of PAH specific therapy until insurance authorization is obtained. Equally important is confirmation of a long term, affordable co-pay with the pharmacy that will provide the therapy and the ability to obtain the medication immediately at discharge from either a mail order or local pharmacy. Even with insurance approval, the patient's co-pay cost may be prohibitive. Patients will then need to apply to outside programs for co-pay assistance, which involves a process that may require weeks to complete.

If a decision is made for the institution to dispense a medication through samples or institutional supply, this should be discussed with the patient's PH outpatient team to expedite authorization and co-pay assistance before the free supply is exhausted. In cases where insurance approval is denied, caution should be used for patients who express interest in paying out of pocket for medications, which occurs most commonly for PDE-5 inhibitor therapy. Patients need to be prepared to cover the cost indefinitely in the event that the medication is deemed beneficial despite insurance coverage denial. Providers should make every attempt to continue to appeal insurance denials at all levels until they have exhausted all options. Patients who have insurance through their employers but are denied approval for certain medications may advocate for coverage directly from within their local institutional Human Resources department.

Whatever the reason for hospitalization, thoughtful discharge assessment and planning can prevent re-admission. However, the scope and timing of follow-up will vary depending on the admitting diagnosis and condition of the patient upon discharge. For patients admitted with conditions other than sequela of PH or PAH treatment initiation, for example surgery, consideration should be given to transfer to the PH service prior to hospital discharge. Since patients frequently cannot be transferred to rehabilitation centers or skilled nursing facilities due to the expense and complexity of their PAH medications, they may require extended hospitalization.

The decision about discharge timing is made in conjunction with the PH team. Careful hand-off between the inpatient and outpatient teams is crucial to document timing of follow-up clinic appointments and designation of responsibility for monitoring the patient, laboratory tests and adverse events. When patients are admitted outside of the PH center, the discharge summary and testing should be reviewed and consideration should be given to having the patient return to PH clinic shortly after discharge.

In this population, the majority of hospital admissions are for worsening PH symptoms and management of right heart failure (RHF). While hospitalized, close attention should be given to recording accurate daily weights. The admission and discharge weights should be documented in the discharge summary for easy review and comparison in the outpatient setting. Patients should be advised to weigh themselves on their home scale immediately upon returning home and record daily weights thereafter.

On admission, careful assessment should be made of the patients adherence to both the prescribed outpatient diuretic and PAH regimen and sodium and fluid restriction recommendations. This can be done verbally with the patient and caregiver if present, but should be verified with pharmacy records. The goal is to determine if the patient is failing current medical therapy or failing to take it as directed. The answer to that question will guide the future treatment plan. If there is a perceived knowledge deficit about the importance of sodium in heart failure management, a nutrition consult may be helpful.

Managing Oxygen Therapy

The use of supplemental oxygen to maintain a $PaO_2 > 60$ mmHg remains part of the supportive care recommendations for treatment of PAH [29]. Resting, exertional and nocturnal hypoxemia should be assessed and documented as part of a comprehensive evaluation. Patients need to understand hypoxemia may be present even in the absence of dyspnea. Significant time should be devoted to selecting the appropriate oxygen delivery system, either stationary and/or portable to meet the patient's current medical needs and capacity, and maintain clinical status. There are numerous portable oxygen concentrators (POCs) now available

that vary in flowrate range, ability to deliver continuous vs. intermittent flow, size and weight. Generally, POC units capable of providing higher flowrates are heavier in weight. These devices may be insufficient to meet patient demand and other portable systems will need to be considered. Careful testing should be performed on the chosen system to ensure patients' needs are met prior to purchase or rental.

Access to Pulmonary and Cardiac Rehabilitation for the PAH Patient

Patients who have had prolonged hospitalizations with significant deconditioning may benefit from transfer to inpatient rehabilitation programs. However, inpatient rehabilitation programs may have limited experience caring for PH patients, inability to manage the complex medical regimen and may not be able to obtain PAH specific medications. The PH provider must determine if inpatient rehabilitation is a safe option for the patient, or they will be better cared for with home physical therapy and the eventual goal of enrolling in an outpatient rehabilitation program. SP nurses can be employed to assess and monitor the patient at home.

For patients who have not had an acute event requiring hospitalization, there is increasing evidence that formal exercise training is safe and improves symptoms and quality of life in patients with PH [29]. Generally, PH patients should be referred to a formal pulmonary or cardiac rehabilitation program to participate in safe medically monitored exercise. In practice, it can be challenging to find outpatient exercise programs for PH patients. One of the most important qualities of an exercise program is close proximity to the patient's home since they typically will need to attend the program 3 days a week for a minimum of 12 weeks, ideally followed by a long term maintenance program. This can present a challenge to the PH provider, since many patients live outside of their primary facilities catchment area. In these situations, the patient, PH team, and primary physician identifies a suitable local program. The American Association of Cardiovascular and Pulmonary Rehabilitation (AACVPR) provides a searchable online directory to assist in locating programs throughout the U.S.

While Medicare does not currently cover pulmonary or cardiac rehabilitation for a diagnosis of PAH or right heart failure, some private insurers may. Medicaid coverage varies from state to state. Pulmonary or cardiac rehabilitation may be covered by Medicare and private insurers for comorbidities other than PAH. Ordering pulmonary therapy or pulmonary physical therapy may provide the same rehabilitation program and be covered by Medicare. Careful attention should be given to ordering therapy and coding orders accurately to optimize insurance coverage. The diagnosis codes used to order treatment should include the medical diagnosis and more importantly, the functional abnormality that therapy will improve such as dyspnea, abnormal breathing pattern, generalized weakness or difficulty walking. The prescription should be written to indicate the functional abnormality. Ahead of sending a physician order for enrollment in rehabilitation, it is helpful to have a discussion with the program about the potential for insurance coverage. Programs less familiar with PAH will likely need assistance from the PH team to properly code the therapy. Denials for coverage should be reviewed to ensure that appropriate orders and codes were submitted originally.

Once insurance approval has been obtained, rehabilitation program-specific orders need to be carefully reviewed and adjusted. For example, many standard rehabilitation orders include administration of nitroglycerin for chest pain. This order may need to be deactivated for PAH patients and is contraindicated for patients actively received sildenafil, tadalafil or riociguat. Should standard rehabilitation include bending, lifting weights or working with high resistance bands, revisions may be required since these activities are generally avoided in PAH patients. It is also necessary to adjust the rehabilitation program standard vital sign parameters and provide specific instructions for oxygen requirements during exercise. The rehabilitation program should provide frequent updates to the PH program including attendance and progress data. Careful attention should be given to reviewing electrocardiogram tracings to ensure that the patient is not experiencing or has converted to a dysrhythmia. The PH program should document enrollment and completion dates of rehabilitation programs in the primary medical record. If available, patients should be encouraged to enroll in ongoing maintenance programs at the completion of the initial program. If this is not possible, the treating PH team should request a safe home exercise regimen be prescribed for the patient upon discharge.

Palliative and Hospice Care

There has been a significant increase in the number and use of palliative care programs in U.S. hospitals over the past 10 years [30]. The World Health Organization defines palliative care as "an approach that improves the quality of life of patients and their families facing the problems associated with life-threatening illness, through the prevention, identification and relief of suffering" [31]. The American College of Chest Physicians (AACP) Policy Statement on palliative care indicates that all patients with advanced lung disease should have access to palliative care services and they should be provided concurrently with life-prolonging care [32]. It is appropriate to use primary, secondary and tertiary palliative care services for symptomatic PAH patients.

When patients receiving maximum medical therapy continue to struggle with right heart failure and lung transplantation is not an option, it is appropriate to discuss referral for hospice care. The Johns Hopkins Hospital Palliative Care Service suggests that rather than try to predict a patients' survival, providers should ask themselves, "Would you be surprised if this patient died in the next 6 months?" If the answer is 'no', then discussion with the patient and referral to palliative care and or hospice services is appropriate.

Unfortunately, the ability of PAH patients to access inpatient and outpatient hospice services is variable in clinical practice. Admission to outpatient hospice is most often declined due to the exceedingly high cost and complexity of PH specific medications. Hospice programs are reimbursed at a daily rate that does not account for the administration of expensive medications. Regrettably, PH patients are often asked to choose between continuing PH medications and enrollment in hospice services. Nonetheless, the PH staff should aggressively investigate options for allowing PH patients to enroll in formal hospice programs near the end of life. The staff should work with the patient, caregivers, hospice program, SP and medication manufacturer to make every attempt to provide the patient with the support of hospice services. To guide these discussions, it is helpful to ask the following questions;

(i) Is the patient willing to discontinue PH medications now or ever?

(ii) Are there family or other close personal contact(s) that are willing and able to care for the patient at home?

(iii) Is the SP able to work with the health insurance company to provide financial coverage for PH medications? If the hospice program cannot provide coverage for PH medications, will the manufacturer consider that denial as uninsured or underinsured, and allow the patient to receive the medications through their patient assistance program?

(iv) Are creative ways available to provide the patient with PH medications?

(v) What will happen if the patient changes a decision about enrollment in hospice?

Unfortunately, sometimes patients may get the impression that they will no longer be able to visit or call their PH physician and coordinator once they enroll in hospice. It is helpful to have a proactive discussion about this with the hospice program and the patient. Patients are advised that while goals of care have changed, the close, long-term relationship with their PH team is unchanged.

Patients dying from refractory right heart failure develop significant ascites frequently despite high dose diuretic therapy. Abdominal ascites causes pain and can limit the patient's ability to eat, which, in turn, may exacerbate distress for the patient and their family. Palliative large volume paracentesis is an important option to maintain comfort. The PH program can assist with arranging routine, regular paracentesis at a facility close to the patient's home for comfort and convenience.

Access to PAH Medication

Ensuring access to PAH-specific medications is an essential aspect of supportive care for the PAH patient. These medications are expensive and generic forms are only starting to become available though still costly. Cost of and access to therapy are important determinants of adherence. In a survey conducted in Minnesota, Schomer et al. found that 26 % of adult consumers, compared to 5 % of physicians, reported that total drug costs were most important, compared to 63 % vs. 86 % for out-of-pocket costs. Financial hardship in purchasing prescription drugs was reported by 27 % of consumers [33]. Studies of the effects of the Medicare Part D coverage gap on medication use and adherence have been conducted in diabetes [34], hypertension and hyperlipidemia [35], and heart failure with diabetes [36]. All found a reduction in medication use and adherence for groups without support through the gap, compared to those with coverage through the gap. The high cost and lack of affordable generic alternatives makes PAH patients especially vulnerable to lapses in therapy.

Navigating Health Insurance

Private, commercial, and public (government) insurance usually includes prescription drug coverage. Health plans often contract with a pharmacy benefit manager (PBM) to manage their members' pharmacy claims. The PBM will contract with specific local and specialty pharmacies or may have their own dedicated specialty pharmacy. Using a different specialty pharmacy may result in higher co-pays, or may not be covered at all.

Public insurance includes Medicare (federally based) and Medicaid (state based). Original Medicare for persons over age 65 or disabled includes Part A for inpatient services and Part B for outpatient services and durable medical equipment. It covers 80 % of the cost of services with the remaining 20 % covered by the patient out of pocket, or by a supplemental plan, also known as a Medigap policy. Medicare Advantage Plans (otherwise known as Part C) are private managed care plans that replace Part A and B. In exchange for a limited provider network and managed care model, supplemental insurance is not needed,. A primary care provider (PCP) acts as a gatekeeper, and prior authorizations are required for specialty care, tests and procedures. Medicare Advantage Plans may also include Part D

(prescription drug coverage) (MA-PD). Medicaid is administered by the states (partially funded by the federal government) to provide health insurance to low income and/or disabled persons. It may act as the sole payor, or function as a secondary insurance to Medicare. Persons with both Medicare and Medicaid are termed "dual eligibles". Since Medicaid is administered by each state, coverage varies widely from state to state and even county by county within each state. A growing trend in Medicaid is to implement managed care, similar to the Medicare Advantage Plan model. Private health plans contract with Medicaid to provide health insurance coverage for their members. In some states, it's possible to file a managed care exemption so patients with complex health problems can remain with traditional Medicaid and not be limited to the restricted network of providers of a Health Maintenance Organization (HMO).

The Patient Protection and Affordable Care Act (ACA) resulted in significant changes that impact PAH patients. Components of the ACA that are especially relevant to PAH patients include making insurance more affordable through subsidies for low income persons, expanding Medicaid to those within 138 % of the federal poverty level (19 states have declined to expand Medicaid as of February 2014), eliminating pre-existing condition exclusions and higher rates, eliminating annual and life-time caps on benefits and the gradual closing of the Part D coverage gap or "donut hole" by 2020.

Prescription Drug Coverage

Medicare Part D covers prescription drugs, all administered through private insurance plans or PBMs. These plans can be purchased along with Original Medicare or a Medigap plan. A monthly premium is paid for the coverage. The annual deductible can vary from zero to a maximum of $310 for 2014 [37]. After the deductible is met, the plan pays a portion of the cost and the patient has co-insurance which is a percentage of the drug cost. In 2009, the median co-insurance was 30 % for specialty tier drugs [38]. A coverage gap, known as the donut hole begins when total drug spending (by the patient and the plan) reaches a set amount ($2850 in 2014, $2960 in 2015). In the coverage gap the patient is responsible for a higher percentage of the cost of their medications until they have reached the maximum out of pocket cost. In 2014, this cost is 47.5 % of the plan's cost of brandname drugs, decreasing to 45 % in 2015 due to the ACA. In addition to the percentage the patient pays, the manufacturer's discount payment of 50 % also counts toward the out-of-pocket costs, making it easier for the patient to get through the donut hole [39]. Once a set out-of-pocket maximum has been reached, catastrophic coverage automatically begins and the patient's contribution drops to 5 % of the drug cost. In 2014 the out-of-pocket maximum is $4550, in 2015 it will be $4700 [40]. Dual eligibles are automatically assigned a Medicare Part D plan and Medicaid covers the monthly premium for the Part D plan. Because they qualify for Medicaid, dual eligibles are not subject to deductibles or the coverage gap and co-pays are low for almost all prescriptions. Patients may be eligible for Extra Help with their prescription drug costs. Letters are sent out in May by the Social Security Administration (SSA) to alert patients that they may be eligible and should apply for Low Income Support (LIS) or the Medicare Savings Program (MSP), components of Extra Help. Patients can apply on-line (http://www.socialsecurity.gov) or at their local Medicaid office [41].

Disability

Most Americans have employer-based insurance or buy private individual plans if they are self-employed. Due to limitations from their disease, many PAH patients are unable to work and lose employer-based insurance coverage. They can continue this insurance through the Consolidated Omnibus Budget Reconciliation Act (COBRA); however, it is quite expensive. Patients must pay their premium in addition to the employer contribution. Due to reduced work hours or having to stop working altogether, this is generally unaffordable for most. Under the ACA, patients have the ability to buy insurance on state exchanges or the federal exchange and cannot be denied coverage due to a pre-existing condition.

When patients are no longer able to work due to their medical condition, they should apply for Social Security Disability (SSD) through the SSA [42]. Negotiating the disability process can be long and complicated for patients. There are several resources to assist patients, some specific to PAH (Table 21.1). Applicants must satisfy a work history requirement and a disability requirement. In order to collect SSD, one must have worked and paid Social Security payroll taxes (FICA). The benefit amount received is proportional to the amount paid into FICA. Social Security only pays for total disability, which is a complete inability to work, even with accommodations, and the disability is expected to last at least 1 year or to be fatal. At this point in time, the guidelines in the Blue Book (a manual that lists medical conditions that automatically qualify for disability) reference 3.09 Cor pulmonale secondary to chronic pulmonary vascular hypertension under the Respiratory Listing [43]. The qualifying evidence includes documentation of chronic and irreversible right ventricular overload or failure, electrocardiogram and imaging test results. In addition, mean PAP >40 mmHg or arterial hypoxemia (two arterial blood gas studies performed on room air, at rest and at least 3 weeks apart within 6 months) must be documented. For example, at less than 3000 ft above sea level, pCO_2 must be ≥ 40 mmHg and $pO_2 \leq 55$ mmHg. The Scientific Leadership Council of the Pulmonary Hypertension Association is advocating for policies that are more accurate and complete for PAH patients to meet the disability requirement. It may take 3–5 months to process disability claims and it is not unusual for the first disability claim to be denied. Patients should plan to appeal

Table 21.1 Disability and medicare resources

Agency or organization	Description	Contact information
Social Security Administration	SSD SSI	http://www.socialsecurity.gov 800 772-1213 Local social security office
Medicare	Official government site Information about Medicare, choosing plans and enrolling	http://www.Medicare.gov 800 633-4227
PSI-A.C.C.E.S.S. Advocating for chronic conditions, entitlements and social services	Direct representation and guidance for disability applications	http://www.patientservicesinc.org/For-Patients/ACCESS 888 700-7010 Legal support hotline 877 851-9065
Advocacy for patients with chronic conditions	Education, advice and advocacy relating to health insurance, disability and legal rights	http://www.AdvocacyforPatients.org 860 674-1370 Patient_Advocate@sbcglobal.net
Caring voice coalition	Insurance and disability counseling, patient support services, public advocacy and some legal assistance	http://www.CaringVoice.org 888 267-1440
Pulmonary hypertension association	Educational resources and patient advocacy	http://www.PHAssociation.org/Insurance Insurance Program 301 565-3005, x773 Insurance@PHAssociation.org
Medicare rights center	Free counseling and educational programs Assistance in English and Spanish	http://www.MedicareRights.org 800 333-4114

the initial denial. The specific PH resources for disability (Table 21.1) may be particularly helpful at this point.

Once permanent disability has been granted, Social Security Disability Income (SSDI) payments commence and the 2 year waiting period begins for Medicare benefits. Concurrently, patients are considered for Supplemental Security Income (SSI). This program provides low-income, disabled people with a very modest amount of money to meet basic needs. The program is funded by general tax revenue and not Social Security taxes. It is need-based and has no work history requirements. In most states, SSI automatically includes Medicaid and other government assistance programs, such as food stamps. In this case, Medicaid would act as the primary insurance during the 2 year waiting period for Medicare. Once the patient is eligible for Medicare, Medicaid becomes secondary and Medicare Part D takes over for prescription drug coverage.

PAH Medication Authorization and Referral Process

Parenteral prostanoids are covered under major medical plans; for example, Medicare Part B (at 80 %) and a secondary insurance (remaining 20 %). Coverage of inhaled prostanoids may vary depending on the plan. Oral medications are covered under the prescription drug plan. Some oral medications are available at local pharmacies (sildenafil and tadalafil) but the remainder are dispensed by SP's. Due to REMS requirements and the complexity of some therapies, the distribution may be restricted to a limited number of SP's. Patients on more than one PAH specific medication may need to interface with two or more pharmacies. For example, the PBM contracts with one SP for oral medications and the health plan contracts with a different SP for parenteral therapy. Not all local pharmacies stock expensive medications that are rarely dispensed; refills must be ordered well in advance to prevent interruption of therapy. To avoid potential lapses in therapy, it may be best to have all PAH medications dispensed by a SP. Required medication-specific referral forms are completed for most PAH medications and then submitted to the SP. Enrollment forms are mandated for medications with REMS requirements, and are sent to the specific program for each drug. These forms include both patient and prescriber information, insurance information, statement of medical necessity, diagnosis and the prescription. In addition, parenteral prostanoids require clinical documentation for evidence of medical necessity. Regardless of the current insurance, the standard of documentation must meet Medicare guidelines. If the patient becomes Medicare eligible in the future, this assures that all the needed clinical documentation is obtained before initiation of therapy. This documentation includes: (1) history and physical documenting signs and symptoms of PAH, progression of

disease and need for the requested therapy, (2) echocardiogram, (3) right heart catheterization, (4) calcium channel blocker statement (result of vasoreactivity testing during RHC or why this treatment is contraindicated), (5) ventilation/perfusion lung scan (preferred) or CT pulmonary angiogram to rule out CTEPH, (6) Antinuclear antibody test (ANA) for connective tissue disease screening. The SP will then submit the documentation to obtain insurance authorization for the therapy. However, in the case of managed care plans, the prescriber's office usually has to submit for authorization from the health plan or the medical group. In some cases, there is prolonged deliberation over who is "at-risk" to cover the therapy, the health plan or the medical group. Once the referral has "cleared", the SP notifies the patient and provides a benefits explanation, including responsibility for any co-pays or deductibles. Simultaneously, the prescriber office will be contacted so initiation of therapy can be scheduled. Close contact is needed with the SP at each step in the process. Submitting all required documentation with the referral will expedite clearance. Patients who have co-morbid lung or heart disease will require additional specific statements submitted outlining evidence that these conditions are not the primary cause of the PAH. Examples of such co-morbid conditions are obstructive sleep apnea, chronic obstructive lung disease, interstitial lung disease, sarcoidosis, left ventricular diastolic dysfunction and valvular heart disease.

PAH Patient Home Assessment and Therapy Demonstration

Oral PAH medications are covered under the prescription drug benefit, be it private, commercial, Medicaid or Medicare Part D and may be managed by a PBM. The prior authorization (PA) process allows the PBM to control cost and access to these expensive medications. The PBM contends that it ensures efficacy and patient safety. Most PAH medications require a PA, a very time consuming activity that places significant burden on staff. Annual or more frequent re-authorizations are often mandated and can result in medication interruption if not planned for ahead of time. A 2010 American Medical Association survey found that physicians spend an average of 20 h per week on prior authorizations [44]. Prior authorizations have become more common in Part D plans. In 2013, brand-name drugs required prior authorizations 21 % of time compared to 8 % in 2006 [44]. Given the complexity of the PA process, having a limited number of proficient staff will allow for a more efficient system. Mistakes can easily result in time consuming denials and appeals. Emerging sophisticated electronic medical record systems may be designed to alert involved parties to key components (such as WHO Group or Functional Class) that are necessary to satisfy PA requirements for a specific medication. Prescription drug plans and PBMs have set formularies that specify preferred medications in a class and may designate step therapy where one medication (often the least expensive) must be tried first before another medication can be used or added. Medications are placed in Tiers, which determine the amount of the co-pay (a set amount, such as $5–10) or co-insurance (a percentage, such as 25–50 %). Tier 1 is typically for generics with the lowest co-pay. Expensive, specialty medications (PAH therapies) mostly fall in the highest category, Tier 4, often with a co-insurance (20–50 %). In a literature review, Eaddy, et al. found that 18 out of 24 studies conducted between 1975 and 2008 found that increasing patient cost sharing had a statistically significant adverse effect on medication adherence [45]. In some cases, it is possible to request a Tier exception or adjustment if the patient's share of cost is unacceptable, especially for a life-sustaining medication for which there is no generic alternative. If the PA request is denied, the provider should appeal the denial. Some plans may be quick to deny an expensive medication on the initial request, but the denial may be overturned on appeal (also called redetermination) with little or no additional evidence. It is essential to obtain the complete denial letter and respond directly to the reason for denial. Table 21.2 lists the types of appeals that may be submitted. The denial letter must explain the appeal process and give directions about how to file the appeal. An expedited appeal must be adjudicated within 72 h and can be requested for urgent, life sustaining requests. A standard appeal must be adjudicated in 7 days. Successful appeals provide medical evidence to support the claim that the requested medication is preferred for a specific patient based on the patient's clinical condition, the properties of the medication (including potential side effects or drug-drug interactions) and evidence from the medical literature, including clinical trials.

If the appeal is denied, the next step may be to request an expedited independent (or outside) review. Maximus Federal Services is the Independent Review Entity (IRE) for all Medicare Part D appeals. If this fails, there are still mechanisms for further appeals that will be detailed in the denial letter. An alternate strategy after the denial of the first appeal is to request a peer-to-peer review with the medical director of the PBM or health plan and the prescriber. This may be difficult to arrange and coordinate, but it is often very effective since the PH specialist is speaking directly to a decision maker.

Even when successful with prior authorizations, patients' may face financial hardship in paying for their medications and medical care. Each PAH pharmaceutical company has patient assistance programs designed for uninsured and underinsured patients covered by private or commercial insurance. Table 21.3 lists the current pharmaceutical company patient assistance programs. If the patient is covered by government insurance, foundations can provide financial assistance based on need. In addition to co-pay assistance or coverage through the "donut hole", they may be able to provide assistance with premiums or refer patients to other assistance agencies. Caring Voice Coalition, in addition to providing insurance and disability counseling, provides co-pay and premium assistance as well as assistance with therapy appeals. Patient Services, Inc. (http://www.patientservices.org, 800 366-7741) provides financial assistance with premiums and co-pays for selected PAH medications. Chronic Disease Fund (http://www.cdfund.org; 877 968-7233) is another foundation that can assist underinsured patients with expensive therapies. Specialty pharmacies have patient assistance programs for parenteral therapy and should refer patients with financial needs related to other PAH therapies to the appropriate agencies (see Table 21.1).

Home assessment and therapy demonstration/pre-teaching visits by SP nursing are available to introduce the therapy, delivery system, and required daily routines. This visit can occur while the insurance clearance is in process.

Table 21.2 Medication appeal options

Type of appeal	Reason for denial	Response
Formulary exception	Requested medication is "non-formulary". Common for newly approved medications that have not yet been reviewed by the PBM for addition to their formulary	Present evidence why the requested medication is preferred either based on the characteristics of the medication, the patient's clinical condition or both
Plan exception	Requested medication is "not a covered benefit". This is an exclusion written into the plan	Review the Explanation of Benefits (EOB) Appeal is directed to the plan's administrators, for example, a Board of Trustees
Step edit	Plan has a requirement for step therapy. Another medication must be tried and failed before the requested medication can be authorized	Present evidence why the requested medication is preferred either based on the characteristics of the medication, the patient's clinical condition or both
Quantity override	The requested dose or quantity of pills exceeds the plan limit	Present evidence that the requested dose is safe and efficacious from the literature or has been effective for this particular patient
Medical necessity	The request does not meet the plan's criteria for medical necessity. For example, the diagnosis is contested (non-WHO Group I) or disease is not considered severe enough (Functional Class)	Present diagnostic testing that supports the diagnosis and descriptions of patient symptoms, especially activity intolerance

Table 21.3 Pharmaceutical company patient assistance programs

Pharmaceutical company	Medications	Name of program	Contact info
Actelion Pharmaceutics US, Inc.	Tracleer (bosentan) Opsumit (macitentan) Veletri (RTS epoprostenol) Ventavis (iloprost)	PAH Pathways	http://www.pahpathways.com 866 228-3546
Bayer HealthCare, LLC	Adempas (riociguat)	Aim Patient Support	http://www.Adempas-US.com 855 423-3672
Gilead Sciences, Inc.	Letairis (ambrisentan)	LEAP-Letairis Education and Access Program	http://www.letairis.com 866 664-5327
Pfizer, Inc.	Revatio (sildenafil)	RSVP Program-Reimbursement Solutions, Verification and Payment Program	888 327-RSVP
United Therapeutics Corporation	Orenitram (oral treprostinil) Remodulin (treprostinil) Tyvaso (inhaled treprostinil)	UT Assist	877 864-8437 87-UNITHER

The home assessment by the SP nurse can identify any concerns regarding the home environment or caregiver support system, which may influence the prescriber's determination of the most appropriate therapy. Depending on the needs of the PH provider and staff, the SP is available to augment patient education, specifically, teaching therapy administration to the patient and family in the hospital, clinic or home setting. The PH team should receive regular reports about the patient's progress, be notified of any problems or adverse events and informed when the patient/family is proficient and home visits are no longer required. Patients on chronic therapy have monthly phone contact with the SP to reorder medication and supplies and monitor dosing and adverse events. Any noted discrepancies from the prescribed plan will immediately be reported to the PH team. Additional home visits can be made as deemed necessary. The PH team can also develop specific patient protocols for the SP to implement and follow.

Pulmonary Hypertension Patient, Family and Caregiver Support Networks

A family caregiver is broadly defined as a friend or relative who provides unpaid assistance to a person with a chronic or disabling condition. In 2009, nearly 66 million Americans (three in 10 U.S. households) reported at least one person providing unpaid care as a family caregiver [46].

Chronic illness can affect relationships in a multitude of ways. Feelings of shock, anger, fear, and denial can be normal common responses to receiving a devastating medical diagnosis. The challenge lies in finding ways to address the illness as a team to limit resentment, frustration and isolation.

Discussing chronic illness is difficult and, at times, distressing. Ongoing honest dialogue is necessary for effective communication. Having a united front to approach and manage the acute and chronic life changes is paramount. It is important to direct feelings of frustration to the disease, not toward the patient or caregiver. Avoiding blame and guilt allows for interactions that lead to healthier relationships and lifestyles.

The unpredictability and uncertainty of chronic illness can lead to significant anxiety and fear for both the patient and their caregivers. Focusing on what is within their control can help strengthen, and even, improve the relationship. Living with a chronic condition may alter the relationship between partners in many ways:

- It may be difficult to share uncomfortable feelings and fears
- Changes can occur in the roles and responsibilities of the relationship
- Plans and expectations for the future are disrupted
- There may be changing sexual feelings and responses [47]

Chronic illness often places financial stress on the family ranging from bitterness to fear of the unknown. Caretakers may find themselves as the primary or sole financial earner if the patient has to reduce work hours or stop working altogether.

The balance of work and responsibilities can change dramatically when a person is no longer able to function at baseline. They may experience loss of identity, making it difficult to figure out where they fit into the current family structure. It's important for all family members, especially the patient, to feel they are in some way contributing to the household and relationships.

PAH is a progressive chronic disease that places a significant burden on patients and their caregivers. Distressing and debilitating symptoms for patients, including exertional dyspnea, fatigue, chest pain/discomfort, and feeling dizzy or lightheaded are common, causing physical and psychological harm [48]. The disabling nature of the disease can impact patients' relationships with family and friends, their ability to work and exercise, and their financial security [49]. Data from the multicenter US-based REVEAL Registry showed that clinical depression, defined as patients with the comorbid condition clinical depression and/or patients with the reported use of selective serotonin reuptake inhibitors as a concomitant medication, was present in 25.5 % of PAH patients [50].

Patient Support and Networks for PH

The PHA is a non-profit support, education, advocacy and awareness organization for patients and caregivers dealing with PAH. Their mission is to "find ways to prevent and cure pulmonary hypertension, and to provide hope for the pulmonary hypertension community through support, education, research, advocacy and awareness" [51]. It also serves as the accreditation body for the pulmonary hypertension comprehensive care (PHCC) initiative, a program established to credential centers with special expertise in pulmonary hypertension for achieving the overall goal of improving quality of care and outcomes for patients.

PHA provides comprehensive services and resources for patients, caregivers, families and friends. Some of these services include:

- Materials and e-courses for newly diagnosed patients
- The PAH Survival Guide
- Medical Education Programs (live and online)
- Connecting patients with in person, email and telephone support groups, chat rooms, message boards and a listserve.
- Patient and Caregiver mentoring programs created to connect via email.
- Age specific programs for children and young adults
- Advocacy Action Center [52]

Role of the Caregiver

PAH caregivers play a significant role in patients' medical care and self-management. They often serve as the ears, eyes and sometimes voice of the patient. First and foremost is the need to understand and be educated about the disease state. This can be accomplished in a variety of ways starting with the patient's health care providers, through patient organizations and associations, and attendance at local educational forums and support groups. It's important to understand and recognize the signs and symptoms of both the illness and its treatment in order to optimize patient care and compliance.

Family members and friends are best situated to monitor and understand how a patient's illness affects their daily life. Subtle changes in activities of daily living or symptoms are often noticed by caretakers before the patient recognizes them. Discussing these changes and, when appropriate, notifying the health care team in a timely fashion is critically important to the patient's health.

Helping track medication schedules, supplies, appointments and maintaining diaries will contribute to improved compliance with the prescribed medical regimen. Whenever possible, a family member or friend should accompany the patient to doctor visits to provide relevant information and partake in discussions with physicians and other health care providers. Often the patient alone will not be able to absorb the detailed information presented by the medical team, hence the need for a "second set of ears". Formulating questions in advance of appointments will allow for more efficient use of time with the medical team.

Effects of Living with Chronically Ill Patients on Caregivers

Serving as a caregiver can adversely affect emotional and physical health. Uninterrupted feelings of responsibility for a loved one's care and welfare may be burdensome. It may be difficult to share concerns with loved ones, leading to frustration and emotional isolation. Taking on more of the household and financial responsibilities may lead to a reduction in social and recreational activities. Ongoing levels of stress and a tendency to neglect self care leads to physical and mental exhaustion for caregivers.

A study commissioned by PHA Canada in late 2013 conducted online by pollster Harris, found 60 % of PAH patients reported they were either no longer able to work at all or partially stopped working due to their PAH. Close to 40 % of caregivers were forced to make employment changes to care for someone with PAH. Financial stability of those affected by PAH, many of whom were in their prime earning years, was of major concern to the surveyed participants [53]. Caregiver career advancement and plans may stagnate as a result of their changing lifestyle.

Studies consistently report higher levels of depressive symptoms and mental health problems among caregivers than among their non-caregiving peers [54–58]. Estimates show that between 40 and 70 % of caregivers have clinically significant symptoms of depression, with approximately one quarter to one half of these caregivers meeting the diagnostic criteria for major depression [59].

Of those surveyed by PHA Canada, more than 61 % of caregivers surveyed admitted that PAH led directly to social isolation and issues in relationships. Most respondents attributed these difficulties to the "invisibility" of PAH. Because there is a palpable lack of awareness about the disease, the ignorance lead to misunderstandings among friends, coworkers, and the overall public, all of which leads to a sense of social isolation [53]. These findings were supported further by Hwang and colleagues, who found that caregivers of PAH patients lack sufficient emotional support or information to meet the demands of caregiving [60]. Alternatively, caregiving can lead to positive outcomes. Existing relationships may be enriched and new ones developed. Providing care for a family member or loved one can offer personal fulfillment and a sense of accomplishment.

Caring for the Caregiver

In order to maintain and adequately manage the additional responsibilities of caring for a chronically ill family member, it is vitally important for caretakers to pay close attention to themselves. Without adequate sleep, good nutrition and regular exercise, caretakers are subject to physical and/or mental stress and illness. Leisure time, hobbies and interests and social support will better enable the caregiver to manage the stress in their lives.

Equally important is for caregivers to find and attend a support group that meets their individual needs. Research demonstrated that caregivers who actively participate in a support group are much better equipped to handle thoughts, feelings, and situations they encounter while caring for their loved ones. They are less likely to have negative feelings about their family member, such as anger and resentment, which can undermine the relationship between them, as well as affect the care they are able to offer [61].

Attending patient led support groups often provide fellowship for caregivers. There are more than 200 support groups alone listed on PHA's website. These meetings often host expert medical professionals and provide a forum for discussion on all PH related topics. Living with chronic illness presents many obstacles and challenges to both patients and caregivers. With adequate resources and coping strategies, families and support persons can lead fulfilling and gratifying lives.

References

1. Brown LM, Chen H, Halpern S, Taichman D, McGoon MD, Farber HW, Frost AE, Liou TG, Turner M, Feldkircher K, Miller DP, Elliott CG. Delay in recognition of pulmonary arterial hypertension: factors identified from the REVEAL Registry. Chest. 2011;140(1):19–26. doi:10.1378/chest.10-1166. Epub 2011 Mar 10.
2. Cordisco ME, Beniaminovitz A, Hammond K, Mancini D. Use of telemonitoring to decrease the rate of hospitalizations in patients with severe congestive heart failure. Am J Cardiol. 1999;84:860–2 [PubMed].
3. Tracleer [package insert]. South San Francisco: Actelion Pharmaceuticals US, Inc; 2012
4. Tracleer [package insert]. South San Francisco: Actelion Pharmaceuticals US, Inc; 2001.
5. Letairis [package insert]. Foster City: Gilead Sciences, Inc; 2007.
6. Opsumit [package insert].South San Francisco: Actelion Pharmaceuticals US, Inc; 2013.
7. Slavin R, Spector S, Bernstein L. The diagnosis and management of sinusitis: a practice parameter update. J Allergy ClinImmunol. 2005;116:S13–47.
8. Barnett C, Machado R. Sildenafil in the treatment of pulmonary hypertension. Vasc Health Risk Manag. 2006;2(4):411–22.
9. Gideon A Paul, J Simon R Gibbs, Alan R Boobis, Allifia Abbas, Martin R Wilkins,Br J Clin Pharmacol. 2005;60(1):107–112. doi:10.1111/j.1365-2125.2005.02383.xPMCID:PMC1884910
10. Adempas [package insert]. Whippany: Bayer Healthcare Pharmaceuticals Inc.; 2013.
11. Ventavis [package insert]. South San Francisco: Actelion Pharmaceuticals US, Inc.; 2013.
12. Tyvaso [package insert]. Research Triangle Park; United Therpeutics Corporation; 2013.
13. Poms A, Kingman M. Inhaled treprostinil for the treatment of pulmonary arterial hypertension. Crit Care Nurse. 2011;31(6):e1.
14. Tyvaso [package insert]. Research Triangle Park: United Therpeutics Corporation; 2013.
15. Orenitram [package insert]. Research Triangle Park: United Therapeutics Corporation; 2013.
16. Duarte J, Hanson R, Machado R. Pharmacologic treatments for pulmonary hypertension. Future Cardiology. 2013;9(3):335–49.
17. Mathier M, McDevitt S, Sagger R. Subcutaneous treprostinil in pulmonary arterial hypertension: practical considerations. J Heart Lung Transpl. 2010;29(11):1210–17.
18. Flolan [package insert]. Research Triangle Park: GlaxoSmithKline; 2011
19. Remodulin [package insert]. Research Triangle Park: United Therapeutics Corporation; 2011.
20. Tapson VF, Gomberg-Maitland M, McLaughlin VV, et al. Safety and efficacy of IV treprostinil for pulmonary arterial hypertension: a prospective, multicenter, open-label, 12-week trial. Chest. 2006;129:683–8.
21. Gomberg-Maitland M, Tapson VF, Benza RL, et al. Transition from intravenous epoprostenol to intravenous treprostinil in pulmonary hypertension. Am J Respir Crit Care Med. 2005;172:1586–9.
22. Mereles D, Ehlken N, Kreuscher S, et al. Exercise and respiratory training improve exercise capacity and quality of life in patients with severe chronic pulmonary hypertension. Circulation. 2006;114:1482–9.
23. Galiè N, Hoeper M, Humbert M, et al. Guidelines on diagnosis and treatment of pulmonary hypertension: the Task Force on Diagnosis and Treatment of Pulmonary Hypertension of the European Society of Cardiology and of the European Respiratory Society. Eur Heart J. 2009;30:2493–537.
24. George MG, Schieb LJ, Ayala C, Talwalkar A, Levant S. Pulmonary hypertension surveillance – United States, 2001–2010. Chest. 2014;146(2):476–95. doi:10.1378/chest.14-0527.
25. Benza RL, Miller DP, Barst RJ, Badesch DB, Frost AE, McGoon MD. An evaluation of long-term survival from time of diagnosis in pulmonary arterial hypertension from the REVEAL Registry. Chest. 2012;142(2):448–56.
26. Burger CD, Long PK, Shah MR, McGoon MD, Miller DP, Romero AJ, Benton WW, Safford RE. Characterization of first-time hospitalizations in patients with newly diagnosed. Pulmonary Arterial Hypertension in the REVEAL Registry. Chest. 2014. doi:10.1378/chest.14-0193.
27. Campo A, Mathai SC, Le Pavec J, Zaiman AL, Hummers LK, Boyce D, Housten T, Lechtzin N, Chami H, Girgis RE, Hassoun PM. Outcomes of hospitalisation for right heart failure in pulmonary arterial hypertension. Eur Respir J. 2011;38(2):359-6. Kingman MS, Tankersley MA, Lombardi S, Spence S, Torres F, Chin KS; Prostacyclin Safety Group. Prostacyclin administration errors in pulmonary arterial hypertension patients admitted to hospitals in the United States: a national survey. J Heart Lung

Transplant. 2010;29(8):841–6. doi:10.1016/j.healun.2010.03.008. Epub 2010 Apr 28.

28. Galiè N, Corris PA, Frost A, Girgis RE, Granton J, Jing ZC, Klepetko W, McGoon MD, McLaughlin VV, Preston IR, Rubin LJ, Sandoval J, Seeger W, Keogh A. Updated treatment algorithm of pulmonary arterial hypertension. J Am Coll Cardiol. 2013;62(25 Suppl):D60–72.

29. Grünig E, Lichtblau M, Ehlken N, Ghofrani HA, Reichenberger F, Staehler G, Halank M, Fischer C, Seyfarth HJ, Klose H, Meyer A, Sorichter S, Wilkens H, Rosenkranz S, Opitz C, Leuchte H, Karger G, Speich R, Nagel C. Safety and efficacy of exercise training in various forms of pulmonary hypertension. Eur Respir J. 2012;40(1):84–92.

30. Hughes MT, Smith TJ. The growth of palliative care in the United States. Annu Rev Public Health. 2014;35:459–75.

31. WHO Definition of Palliative Care. World Health Organization website. http://www.who.int/cancer/palliative/definition/en/. Accessed 2014.

32. Lanken PN, Terry PB, Delisser HM, Fahy BF, Hansen-Flaschen J, Heffner JE, Levy M, Mularski RA, Osborne ML, Prendergast TJ, Rocker G, Sibbald WJ, Wilfond B, Yankaskas JR, ATS End-of-Life Care Task Force. An official American Thoracic Society clinical policy statement: palliative care for patients with respiratory diseases and critical illnesses. Am J Respir Crit Care Med. 2008;177(8):912–27.

33. Schommer JC, Worley MM, Kjos AL. Decision-making during initiation of medication therapy. Research in Social and Adminsitrative Pharmacy. 2014;10:313–27.

34. Fung V, Mangione CM, Huang J, et al. Falling into the coverage gap: part D drug costs and adherence for medicare advantage prescription drug plan beneficiaries with diabetes. Health Services Research. 2010;45(2):355–75.

35. Li P, McElligott S, Bergquist H, et al. Effect of the medicare part D coverage gap on medication use among patients with hypertension and hyperlipidemia. Annals of Internal Medicine. 2012;156(11):776–84.

36. Zjang Y, Baik SH, Lave JR. Effects of the Medicare Part D coverage gap on medication adherence. American Journal of Managed Care. 2014;19(6):e214–24.

37. Medicare Part D Deductibles. Available at: http://www.medicare.gov/part-d/costs/deductible/drug-plan-deductibles.html. Accessed 8 Aug 2014.

38. Regnier SA. How does drug coverage vary by insurance type? Analysis of drug formularies in the United States. American Journal of Managed Care. 2014;20(4):322–31.

39. Medicare Part D Coverage Gap. Available at: http://www.medicare.gov/part-d/costs/coverage-gap/part-d-coverage-gap.html. Accessed 8 Aug 2014.

40. Medicare Part D Catastrophic Coverage. Available at: http://www.medicare.gov/part-d/costs/catastrophic-coverage/drug-plan-catastrophic-coverage.html. Accessed 8 Aug 2014.

41. Social Security Administration. Apply online for extra help with medicare prescription drug costs. United States Social Security Administration Disability Benefits Brochure, SSA Publication No. 05–10525. ICN 470142. Jan 2014.

42. Social Security Administration. Disability. SSA Publication No. 05–10029. ICN 456000. May 2014.

43. Disability Evaluation under Social Security. 3.00 Respiratory system – adult. Available at: http://www.ssa.gov/disability/professionals/bluebook/3.00-Respiratory-Adult.htm. Accessed 8 Aug 2014.

44. Bendix J. The prior authorization predicament. Med Econ. 8 July 2014. Available at: http://medicaleconomics.modernmedicine.com. Accessed 8 Aug 2014.

45. Eaddy MT, Cook CL, O'Day K, et al. How patient cost-sharing trends affect adherence and outcomes: a literature review. P&T. 2012.

46. American Family Physician. 2011. http://www.aafp.org/afp/2011/0601/p1309.

47. National Healthy Marriage Resource Center. 2008–2015. http://www.TwoOfUs.org/educational-content/articles/my-partner-was-just-diagnosed-with-a-chronic-illnessnow-what/index.aspx.

48. Studer SM, Migliore C. Quality of life in PAH: qualitative insights from patients and caregivers. Advances in Pulmonary Hypertension. 2012;10(4):222–6.

49. PHA Online University. http://www.phaonlineuniv.org/Journal/Article.cfm.

50. Badesch DB, Raskob GE, Elliott CG, et al. Pulmonary arterial hypertension: baseline characteristics from the REVEAL registry. Chest. 2010;137(2):376–87.

51. Pulmonary Hypertension Association. 2015. http://www.phassociation.org/homepage.

52. Pulmonary Hypertension Association. 2015. http://www.phassociation.org.

53. Pulmonary Hypertension Association. 2015. http://pulmonaryhypertensionnews.com/2014/05/08.

54. Schulz R, O'Brien AT, Bookwals J, Fleissner K. Psychiatric and physical morbidity effects of dementia caregiving: prevalence, correlates, and causes. The Gerontologist. 1995;35:771–91.

55. Marks N, Lambert JD, Choi H. Transitions to caregiving, gender, and psychological well-being: a prospective U.S. National study. Journal of Marriage and Family. 2002;64:657–67.

56. Pinquart M, Sorensen S. Differences between caregivers and non-caregivers in psychological health and physical health: a meta-analysis. Psychology and Aging. 2003;18(2):250–67.

57. Teri L, Logsdon R, Uomoto J, McCurry SM. Behavioral treatment of depression in dementia patients: a controlled clinical trial. Journal of Gerontology B: Psychological Science and Social Science. 1997;52:159–66.

58. Schulz R, Newsom J, Mittelmark M, Burton L, Hirsch C, Jackson S. Health effects of caregiving: the caregiver health effects study: an ancillary study of the Cardiovascular Health Study. Annals of Behavioral Medicine. 1997;19:110–6.

59. Zarit S. Assessment of family caregivers: a research perspective. In: Family Caregiver Alliance, editors. Caregiver assessment: voices and views from the field. Report from a National Consensus Development Conference (Vol. II). San Francisco: Family Caregiver Alliance; 2006. pp. 12–37.

60. Hwang B, Howie-Esquivel J, Fleischmann KE, Stotts NA, Dracup K. Family caregiving in pulmonary arterial hypertension. Heart Lung J Acute Crit Care. 2012;41(1):26–34.

61. Healthline. 2014. http://www.healthline.com/health/pulmonary-hypertension/guide-caregivers.

Kristina T. Kudelko, Roham T. Zamanian, and Vinicio A. De Jesus Perez

Exercise and Pulmonary Hypertension

Basics of Exercise Adaptation and Maladaptation

Normally, during exercise, cardiac output (CO) is expected to increase in order to augment oxygen delivery to peripheral muscles. The pulmonary vasculature accommodates this increase in pulmonary flow by recruiting more vascular units. Consequently, pulmonary arterial pressure (PAP) only mildly increases despite considerable increases in CO, and pulmonary vascular resistance (PVR) decreases during exercise. In patients with pulmonary hypertension (PH), the ability to recruit functional pulmonary vascular units is impaired. Hence, the mandatory increase in CO is less tolerated by the pulmonary vasculature, and PAP significantly increases, leading to an abrupt rise in PVR [1].

Furthermore, ventilation-perfusion mismatching is also thought to play a key role in exercise limitations in PH patients [2]. There is a relative hypoperfusion of well-ventilated lung units due to impaired pulmonary flow. "Dead space" ventilation is increased, leading to an increase in minute ventilation (VE) out of proportion to carbon dioxide output (VCO_2). This elevation in VE/VCO_2, a surrogate for ventilatory efficiency, as measured by cardiopulmonary exercise testing (CPET) has been well-described in the congestive heart failure literature [3, 4] and has been shown to have prognostic significance [5]. Reports have confirmed a similar elevation in chronic PH patients [2, 6]. Moreover, a reduced ventilatory efficiency (i.e. a high VE/VCO_2), alongside a depressed peak maximal oxygen consumption (VO_2), a surrogate for work capacity, depressed peak oxygen pulse (VO_2/heart rate [HR]), a surrogate for stroke volume, and early anaerobic threshold (AT) has been shown to correlate with severity of disease [2].

Exercise as Adjunct Therapy in PH

Exercise has been traditionally considered dangerous in PH patients for fear that these various impairments can lead to acute right ventricular compromise during exercise [1]. Importantly, PH patients can experience extreme dyspnea, dizziness, fatigue and even syncope during exercise, particularly during sudden, rigorous activity in an unsupervised setting. Walk distances as evaluated by the standardized 6 min walk test (SMWT), which have been shown to correlate with mortality [6], are significantly reduced. Quality of life (QOL) questionnaires address many aspects of physical capacity and perception. Scores on such questionnaires are substantially lower in PH patients and reliably track with mortality and time to clinical worsening [7]. Therefore, many experts have historically placed limitations on physical activity in PH patients. However, newer data have shed light on the potential benefits of low intensity, supervised, endurance-building exercise in a pulmonary rehabilitation setting in patients with PH [8–15].

Intensive Regimen

In a landmark study by Mereles et al. [11], 30 patients on stable pulmonary vascular-specific therapy for the treatment of pulmonary arterial hypertension (PAH) or chronic thromboembolic PH (CTEPH) were randomized to either an exercise and respiratory training program plus pulmonary

K.T. Kudelko, MD (✉)
Division of Pulmonary and Critical Care, Stanford University Medical Center, 300 Pasteur Road, Stanford, CA 94305, USA

Department of Medicine, Stanford University, Stanford, CA, USA
e-mail: kkudelko@stanford.edu

R.T. Zamanian, MD
Division of Pulmonary and Critical Care, Stanford University Medical Center, 300 Pasteur Road, Stanford, CA 94305, USA

V.A. De Jesus Perez, MD
Division of Pulmonary and Critical Care, Stanford University Medical Center, 300 Pasteur Road, Stanford, CA 94305, USA

Department of Medicine, Stanford University Medical Center, Stanford, CA, USA

© Springer International Publishing Switzerland 2016
B.A. Maron et al. (eds.), *Pulmonary Hypertension: Basic Science to Clinical Medicine*, DOI 10.1007/978-3-319-23594-3_22

education and non-intensive physical therapy (e.g. massage) versus pulmonary education and therapy alone. The first 3 weeks of the exercise program consisted of daily bike training, walking for 60 min 5 days/week, 30 min of isometric weight lifting (e.g., dumbbell use), and respiratory training sessions, which, collectively, required an inpatient hospital stay. A slightly less intensive exercise program was continued in the outpatient setting for another 12 weeks. Primary outcome measures were change in 6-min walk distance (SMWD) and QOL scores, which are a valid proxy marker of mortality [6, 7]. Patients were predominantly World Health Organization (WHO) functional class III (N = 22/30). At the end of 15 weeks, the intervention group demonstrated an increase from baseline in SMWD by +96 m compared to a decline of 15 m in the control group (p < 0.0001). Furthermore, many QOL dimensions improved significantly in the intervention group, particularly for physical functioning and vitality. Notably, patients tolerated the program well: although mild dizziness and reversible oxygen desaturation during exercise were noted, no major adverse events were reported.

Other studies have followed, implementing the Mereles et al. 15-week intervention protocol and finding similarly positive results [9, 10, 13]. One such study included WHO functional class IV patients in an effort to assess exercise safety in severe PH [10]. Notably, this study accepted WHO Group II (secondary to left heart disease) and III (secondary to lung disease) patients in addition to WHO Group I (PAH) and IV (CTEPH) patients. Twenty-five out of 183 patients (13.6 %) experienced adverse events. However, only one syncopal event and two self-limited episodes of supraventricular tachycardia seemed directly attributable to the inpatient exercise program. Furthermore, the 18 WHO functional class IV patients experienced a mean increase in SMWD of +63 m at the end of 15 weeks (p < 0.01) and 22 % were reclassified as WHO functional class III at the end of 3 weeks (p < 0.001). CPET parameters including peak VO_2, oxygen pulse, and maximal workload all significantly improved by the end of the study. These data support exercise training as efficacious in PH, even in severe disease, though not without risk. Hence, training should be closely monitored, preferably by a trained cardiopulmonary rehabilitation staff in a center equipped to handle emergencies, and tailored to each individual patient's abilities and limitations.

The effects of exercise training on survival was the focus of another similarly designed study [13] in which 58 PH patients of WHO Groups I-IV and WHO functional classes II-IV completed a 15-week training program and were then followed prospectively for 24 months. Overall, 2/58 patients in the training group died during the observation period, only one from right heart failure. The probability of survival by Kaplan-Meier analysis was 100 % at 1 year and 95 % at 2 years. This study was limited by the lack of a control group

but the authors concluded that low-dose, monitored exercise training is unlikely to worsen clinical outcome and may in fact serve as a powerful adjunct therapy. Secondary outcome measure results were similarly impressive: SMWD increased by +84 m (p < 0.001), mean WHO functional class improved from 2.9 to 2.6 (p < 0.01) and mean peak volume of oxygen consumption (VO_2) and workload capacity increased significantly by the end of 15 weeks.

In another investigation targeting connective tissue disease-associated PAH [16], a particularly progressive type of PAH with a 1-year mortality rate at least twice that of idiopathic PAH, structured exercise training for 15 weeks improved QOL scores, CPET parameters, and SMWD by +71 m (p = 0.003) at the end of 15 weeks [9]. Of specific interest, this study also examined the potential effects of exercise on survival. Overall and PAH-related survival rates were 100 % after 1 and 2 years and 73 % and 80 % after 3 years, respectively. These rates are substantially better than the quoted 1-year mortality rates of 12.5–17.0 % in CTD-APAH patients on PAH-specific therapy [16] and the 3-year mortality rate of 60 % of systemic sclerosis patients on therapy [17]. These authors acknowledged that their sample size was rather small and that they may have selected highly motivated and compliant patients. Nevertheless, given that parameters like resting heart rate and oxygen consumption significantly improved, they hypothesized that exercise therapy may have augmented right ventricular reserve.

Conventional Regime

An intensive 15-week protocol like the Mereles et al. protocol [11] may not be available to many PH patients. This lack of applicability drove other research groups to explore the potential benefits of a more conventional, strictly outpatient program [12, 14, 15]. A 12-week program consisting of 6 weeks interval training with treadmill walking, cycling and step climbing, followed by 6 weeks of additional aerobic exercise and resistance training in WHO Group I and IV PH patients did demonstrate a significant benefit [14]. Eleven PH patients randomized to the exercise arm increased their SMWD by +32 m compared to the 11 control PH patients whose SMWD decreased by 26 m (p < 0.003). Moreover, peak VO_2 increased in the rehabilitation group by 1.1 ml/kg*min versus a decline in the control group by −0.51 ml/kg*min (p = 0.02). No adverse events occurred during the exercise training sessions.

In another report, 23 women with WHO Group I pulmonary hypertension (i.e., pulmonary arterial hypertension) were randomized to a combined education/exercise combined (EXE) group or an education alone group (EDU) [15]. Patients in the EXE group participated in a 3x/week program for 10 weeks of intensive (70–80 % heart rate reserve) treadmill walking in addition to a weekly 60 min educational lecture series on various cardiopulmonary topics. Ninety percent of the EXE group demonstrated an increase in SMWD of at least 10 m, with 60 % achieving a ≥40 m increase. By contrast, no significant increase was found in the EDU group (p<0.008), while QOL scores and CPET parameters including peak work rate and time to exercise intolerance were also significantly improved only in the EXE group. A study using similar methods analyzed the effects of the EXE versus EDU regimen on fatigue severity indices [12]. After the 10-week intervention, the EXE group reported participation in higher levels of physical activity (p<0.05) and a substantial decline in fatigue severity (p=0.03). In that study, SMWD also improved in the EXE group by +53 m as compared to no significant change observed in the EDU group (p=0.003).

Muscle Dysfunction in PH

Deficits in muscle function are thought to significantly contribute to exercise limitations in PH patients. In the Mereles et al. study [11], hemodynamics by transthoracic echocardiogram (TTE) at rest did not change significantly within the groups while other exercise parameters including peak VO$_2$ and VO$_2$ at the anaerobic threshold (AT) improved significantly within the intervention group. This suggested that exercise training has positive effects on components other than cardiopulmonary hemodynamics per se, such as gas exchange efficiency, metabolism in skeletal muscle cells, and prevention of muscle atrophy [11].

Both respiratory and peripheral muscle weakness has been described in the PH literature [8, 18–22]. Mouth occlusion pressures (maximal inspiratory or [PImax] and expiratory pressures or [PEmax]) are surrogates for respiratory muscle strength, and are significantly impaired in idiopathic PAH patients independent of hemodynamics assessed by right heart catheterization (RHC) [18, 21]. Twitch mouth (TwPmo) and transdiaphragmatic pressures, measures of non-volitional respiratory strength, were also significantly depressed by up to 34 % in PAH and CTEPH patients compared with well-matched healthy controls [18]. The exact mechanisms of respiratory muscle weakness are unknown. Interestingly, hypocapnia is common at rest and with exertion in PH patients [18] in keeping with known higher VE and impaired ventilatory efficiency or VE/VCO$_2$ compared with controls [2]. This may lead to overuse and eventual fatigue of respiratory muscles as marked by reduced strength. Alternatively, tachypnea and concomitant hypocapnia may be the direct result of muscle weakness. Future studies are needed to legitimize these hypotheses.

Peripheral muscle abnormalities have been evaluated by both invasive and non-invasive measures [8, 19, 20, 22]. Ten idiopathic PAH patients and ten controls matched for age, sex, and activity level were subjected to lower leg imaging

by computed tomography (CT) and quadriceps muscle biopsy to assess for morphology as well as measures of volitional strength (maximal voluntary contraction [MVC]) and non-volitional strength (quadriceps twitch or TWq) in one report [20]. Leg biopsy served to examine fiber type and enzymatic activity, surrogates for aerobic versus anaerobic metabolism, as well as capillary density. Patients with IPAH displayed a lower proportion of Type I slow, oxidative and fatigue-resistant fibers (34 % in IPAH versus 50 % in controls, p=0.05), and a higher overall proportion of Type IIx fast, glycolytic, fatigable fibers (31 % in IPAH versus 21 % in controls), though the latter did not reach statistical significant (p=0.18). Enzymatic profiles were shifted toward more anaerobic metabolism although capillary density was similar to controls. MVC (p=0.05) and TWq (p=0.01) were diminished in IPAH patients. Interestingly, TWq correlated significantly with exercise capacity as measured by peak VO$_2$ (p=0.04) while no muscle characteristics correlated with hemodynamics, suggesting that peripheral muscle dysfunction rather than hemodynamics acts as a major limitation to exercise in PH patients.

Exercise Effects on Muscle Function

A few groups have explored the potential influence of exercise training on muscle function in PAH [8, 19, 22]. After a thrice-weekly program of cycling and quadriceps muscle training that lasted 12 weeks in 19 IPAH patients, exercise endurance time as assessed by a submaximal exercise test increased by 89 % (p<0.001) while no significant changes were recorded in CPET parameters or SMWD [8]. Quadriceps muscle endurance as measured in time increased markedly by 34 % after training (136±10 to 181±18 s, p=0.001) while strength as measured in torque increased only modestly by 13 % (94±7 to 106±8 Nm, p=0.005). On muscle biopsy, capillary number per myocyte notably increased by 30 % (p<0.001) (Fig. 22.1). The clinical implications of improvements in endurance in the absence of maximal exercise capacity have yet to be determined.

Conversely, in a smaller study [19], five IPAH patients participated in a thrice-weekly strength and endurance protocol for 12 weeks and displayed improvements on multiple measures of exercise capacity. Mean SMWD improved by 58 m (p=0.01), VE and VE/VCO$_2$ decreased by up to 20 % (p<0.05), and the proportion of Type IIx fibers decreased by 8 % (p=0.05). A decrease in the proportion of these glycolytic, fatiguable muscle fibers and an increase in the proportion of Type I oxidative, fatigue-resistant fibers at the end of this study may have contributed to a higher anaerobic threshold and hence improved exercise endurance and efficiency.

In a recent study, the Mereles et al. [11] 15-week exercise protocol was implemented in order to examine the specific

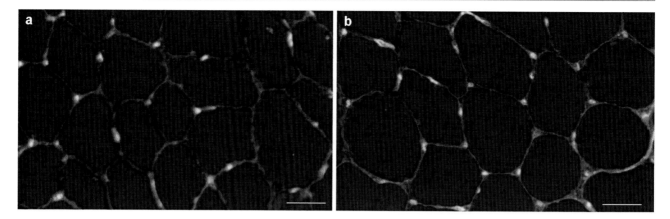

Fig. 22.1 Capillarization is increased in quadriceps muscle in one PH patient (**a**) before and (**b**) after exercise training (Adapted from de Man et al.[8]; Reproduced with permission of the European Respiratory Society)

effects of exercise on respiratory muscle function [22]. Seven PAH patients completed the 3-week inpatient, 12-week outpatient program with excellent compliance and no serious adverse events. Mean SMWD increased at the end of the study by 81 m (p<0.001). Measures of volitional respiratory strength including PEmax (p=0.02) were increased, alongside a trend towards an increase in PImax. Measures of nonvolitional respiratory strength including TwPmo and sniff nasal pressure also significantly increased, (p<0.04 and p<0.03, respectively). Increased proteolytic activity leading to atrophy of diaphragm muscle fibers as well as impaired fiber force-generating capacity of these fibers has been shown in both rats and humans [23]. Again, this may be in line with the hypothesis of increased ventilatory drive leading to muscle overuse and induction of muscle fiber loss of function [18].

Conclusions

Several barriers to efficient exercise in PH exist and are related to poor pulmonary vasculature reserve, impaired cardiac contractility, and peripheral and respiratory muscle dysfunction. As a result, prior consensus in the PH community has centered on exercise avoidance owing to concern that rigorous physical activity in the untrained patient may promote cardiopulmonary dysfunction and, possibly, sudden cardiac death. Intense, unsupervised exercise remains ill-advised in the contemporary era; however, more recent data supports beneficial effects of exercise in PH when patients are monitored, and when performed according to a disciplined and safe exercise regimen of both cardiac and strength training. Such benefits include improved cardiopulmonary fitness, quality of life, muscle strength, and even survival. An exercise prescription (Table 22.1) catered to each individual's PH severity and comorbidities is, thus, encouraged [24].

Management of Pregnancy in Pulmonary Hypertension

Hemodynamic Changes in Pregnancy

During the first 2 trimesters, there is an increase in blood volume up to 50 % that, together with a decrease in both pulmonary and systemic vascular resistance, results in an increased cardiac output [25, 26]. In the pregnant patient with PAH, the elevated pulmonary vascular resistance compounded with the increase in cardiac output results in substantially increased in pulmonary arterial pressure that may progressively overwhelm the right ventricle. The peri- and postpartum stages, in particular, are associated with right ventricular weakening due to increased cardiac preload from rapid increases in cardiac venous return mediated by uterine contractions during labor, shift of uteroplacental blood flow back to the systemic circulation, and withdrawal of vena cava compression by the gravid uterus [27, 28]. By contrast, blood *loss* associated with either vaginal (~500 ml) or cesarean (~1000 ml) delivery resulting in acutely decreased preload occurring in the setting of right ventricular failure may promote systemic hypotension and tissue hypoxia. Ultimately, the physician must be observant of these rapid and unpredictable shifts in cardiopulmonary hemodynamics and be prepared to rapidly intervene in order to prevent a catastrophic clinical outcome.

Incidence and Outcomes

Pregnancy remains one of the major triggers for the manifestation of PAH in previously asymptomatic patients with an estimated overall incidence of 1.1 in 100,000 women [27, 29–31]. Despite the availability of current PAH-specific therapies, PAH remains a major cause of mortality in pregnancy accounting for 30–56 % of all peripartum fatalities [32, 33].

Table 22.1 Example of exercise prescription for pulmonary rehabilitation in PH patients

Patients must be on optimized pharmacologic therapy and supplemental oxygen as needed before program enrollment
The exercise prescription should be based on symptom assessment and 6MWT or CPET
Exercise training should include low-intensity aerobic and strength training of the upper and lower extremities, as well as stretching, range of motion, and flexibility or respiratory muscle exercises
Low-intensity interval training can be used
The intensity of training can be advanced gradually to submaximal target levels, avoiding intensities leading to >70–80 % of HR reserve or peak HR higher than 120
Activities that lead to Valsalva-like maneuvers should be avoided to prevent sudden increases in intrathoracic pressure
Patients' SaO_2 (arterial oxygen saturation) should be kept higher than 90 % with exercise, and SaO_2 and HR monitoring should ideally be monitored continuously during exercise
Telemetry monitoring should be considered for persons with a history of arrhythmias
Caution must be undertaken to avoid falls for persons on anticoagulation therapy of disruption of intravenous vasodilator therapy
Exercise should be stopped immediately if the patient develops dizziness, presyncope, chest pain, hypertension or hypotension

Adapted and Reproduced from: Carolyn L. Rochester et al. [24], with permission from Elsevier

In addition, there is also a high risk for perinatal mortality of offspring born to PAH mothers given the stress on fetal growth and normal development due to reduced placental blood flow and oxygen delivery [34, 35]. Studies done prior to the availability of advanced PAH therapies have shown that elevated systemic pulmonary pressure (sPAP > 40 mmHg) and a higher NYHA functional class correlate positively with clinical deterioration and the need for an earlier delivery [36]. Premature delivery or termination of pregnancy may be necessary in some patients in the setting of clinical deterioration threatening their health and/or that of the unborn child. With the introduction of PAH-specific therapies to routine clinical practice, a reduction in PAH-related mortality during pregnancy has been observed, with one study reporting a mortality of rate of ~25 % vs. 50–70 % in the time period prior to availability of PAH-specific agents. In this study, use of advanced PAH therapies (e.g. prostanoids, ERAs) as well as calcium channel blockers in vasoreactive patients were associated with a better outcome [37]. Despite these encouraging observations, it is important to stress that PAH in pregnancy remains associated with an unacceptable rate of life-threatening complications and PAH patients should be counseled on use of available contraception methods to prevent pregnancy altogether or, if pregnant, strong consideration to early termination is often necessary.

Approach to Management of the Pregnant Patient with PAH

For the patients in whom pregnancy is pursued despite knowledge of the associated risks, it is imperative to establish an aggressive plan for frequent clinical monitoring by a multidisciplinary group that should include a PH expert, maternal-fetal medicine specialist, and cardiac anesthesiologist [38, 39]. The most frequent complications during pregnancy tend to occur during the second and early third trimester when the hemodynamic changes peak [33, 37]. In anticipation of this, visits during the first trimester should focus on assessing the need for either initiating or adjusting PAH-specific drugs as well as conventional therapies such as diuretics or anticoagulants. The latter is especially important given that pregnancy is a prothrombotic state with a fivefold risk of clotting events that could result in catastrophic outcomes in these clinically vulnerable patients [40, 41]. The choice of anticoagulant should be the result of a carefully-thought process and, when possible, in line with current consensus recommendations to minimize risks to the fetus, as some agents, such as warfarin, are associated with teratogenicity and should be avoided during early pregnancy. The most commonly used anticoagulants in pregnancy are either low or high molecular weight heparins since neither of these compound classes can cross the placental barrier [42, 43]. Despite lack of clear evidence, the general consensus is that anticoagulation should be initiated early in pregnancy, continued until the beginning to labor when it should be held to minimize blood loss during delivery period and restarted postpartum to prevent clot formation.

PAH Therapy in Pregnant Patients

Consensus guideline recommendations for determining optimal PAH-specific therapy for pregnant patients are lacking; however, currently available drugs offer a range of options of that can help the clinician optimize management of PAH during pregnancy. There are four FDA-approved available drug classes for the treatment of PAH: (1) phosphodiesterase 5 inhibitors (PDE5-I), (2) soluble guanylate cyclases (sGCs), (3) endothelin receptor antagonist (ERAs) and (4) prostanoids [44–46]. There are two currently available PDE5-I: sildenafil and tadalafil. Both agents are orally active and induce vasodilatation by increasing the availability of nitric oxide (NO) in the pulmonary circulation

[47]. Use of these agents during pregnancy appears to be safe based on several published clinical reports. Riociguat, the only available sGC in the market, is a vasodilator that synergizes with NO to increase vasodilation and reduce pulmonary vascular resistance [48, 49]. Studies in animals have shown that Riociguat is teratogenic and, therefore, its use is contraindicated in pregnancy. Similarly, all available ERAs (bosentan, ambrisentan and macitentan) are contraindicated in pregnancy since use of bosentan in mice is associated with birth defects such as craniofacial malformations, patent ductus arteriosus and other vascular malformations [46, 50–52]. The most potent of the available PAH specific drugs are the prostanoids, prostacyclin analogues that induce potent pulmonary and systemic vasodilatation. The available prostanoids can be found in various formulations: treprostinil is available as an oral (Orenitram) [53], inhaled, subcutaneous and intravenous agent whereas iloprost and epoprostenol are only available in inhaled and intravenous formulations, respectively [54–56]. While not all formulations have been tested in pregnancy, there have been multiple reports of prostanoids being safely used in pregnancy to treat PAH. At present, there are no well-controlled studies to evaluate teratogenic effects of prostanoids on pregnant women, a fact that has led the FDA to assign them a pregnancy risk category B (no documented evidence of harm in humans, teratogenic effects not seen in animals). Nevertheless, manufacturers of these drugs still advise caution when using any of these compounds in pregnant patients .

Pain Control and Method of Delivery

The most challenging stages of pregnancy for the clinical team managing PAH in pregnancy are labor and delivery, in which the goals of care should be to ensure the health of both mother and child by supporting cardiopulmonary hemodynamics [36, 38]. It is imperative that fetal monitoring is instituted throughout the course of labor for early detection of signs of fetal stress requiring immediate intervention. Pain control should also be instituted early as the sympathetic surge associated with pain can result in severe cardiac stress and ischemia. The choice of anesthesia to assist with pain control must also be weighted carefully as some agents can induce both profound systemic vasodilatation and myocardial suppression resulting in a substantial fall in cardiac output and tissue hypoxia [57]. When possible, regional anesthesia should be chosen over general anesthesia as the former can provide excellent pain control without the need for intubation that the latter entails [58–60]. However, one must be aware that common forms of regional anesthesia such as epidural spinal block carry the risk of inducing hypotension due to sympathetic blockade

and may adversely impact cardiopulmonary function. To avoid this complication, it is advised that the epidural anesthesia is administered slowly with while simultaneously monitoring the vitals signs of both the mother and fetus. Despite the ongoing debate concerning the optimal method of delivery, some physicians favor vaginal delivery as it presents the advantage of minimizing blood loss and preventing sudden changes in cardiac preload [61, 62]. On the other hand, cesarean delivery can be used to rapidly intervene in cases of severe fetal stress and to avoid severe hemodynamic swings induced by Valsalva maneuvers required to conduct vaginal delivery but it must be stressed that blood loss is higher with cesarean vs. vaginal delivery and this could result in hemodynamic complications ranging from hypotension to sudden cardiopulmonary collapse [39]. Finally, induction with oxytocin should be avoided as this can produce increases in pulmonary vascular resistance and tachycardia that could result in cardiopulmonary collapse and death [63, 64].

Contraception

Whether the patient is either considering or has already undergone successful pregnancy and delivery, it is imperative for the PH clinician to inform the patient of the risks associated with PAH in pregnancy and the rationale for contraception [65]. The current PAH guidelines recommend the simultaneous implementation of two different methods of contraception in female patients of reproductive age [44, 66]. Barrier methods such as condoms and spermicidal gels should not be used alone given their relatively high failure rate and should always be combined with other contraceptive methods such as the progesterone only pill, the etonogestrel-releasing subdermal implant or an intrauterine device (IUD).

Conclusion

A proposed algorithm for the management of the pregnant PH patient is shown in Fig. 22.2 [67]. It must be stressed that PAH is a strong predictor for mortality in pregnancy and should be avoided when at all possible by ensuring patient education and institution of dual contraceptive methods. In patients that choose to carry their pregnancy to term, it is imperative to assemble a multidisciplinary team that will closely monitor the patient's clinical course. Furthermore, timely institution of PAH specific therapies to achieve optimal control of cardiopulmonary hemodynamics should help mitigate the impact of volume gain and respiratory changes associated with pregnancy. Ultimately, the most important goal of care is to ensure that both mother

Fig. 22.2 Algorithm for the management of the pregnant patient with PH (Adapted from Zeenat Safdar et al. [67]; Reprinted by Permission of SAGE)

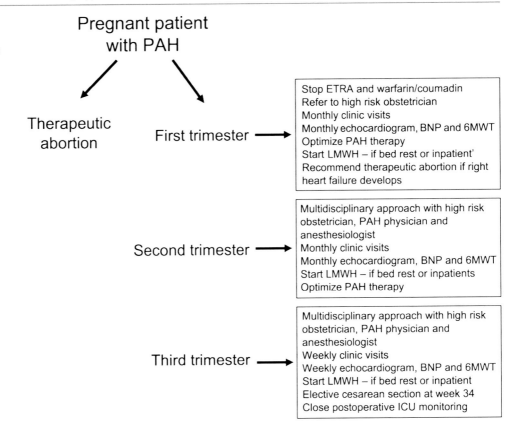

and fetus remain clinically stable throughout the pregnancy and delivery and that plans are in place to prevent future pregnancies.

Perioperative Management of the Patient with Pulmonary Hypertension

Background

It is well known that the presence of moderate PH increases the risk of morbidity and mortality in both cardiac and non-cardiac surgery. One study showed that, among 2,149 patients undergoing coronary artery bypass grafting (CABG), PH was a major predictor for perioperative mortality [68]. The EuroSCORE study has also shown that PH was an independent risk factor for perioperative mortality in patients undergoing cardiac surgery [69]. Perioperative mortality and complication rates for non-cardiac surgery have been estimated to range between 7 and 42 % in one study [70], and 14 and 18 % in another [71]. While the specific risk factors that influence the incidence of life-threatening complications for PH patient in the perioperative setting are not well established, it is critical for the PH specialist to initiate a thorough management protocol that will help prepare the anesthesia and surgical team for managing

acute complications related to pulmonary vascular and/or right ventricular disease.

Pre-operative Evaluation

A PH specialist should evaluate patients who require non-emergent surgery within a week of the planned surgery. This way, both patient and surgical characteristics can be thoroughly assessed and a multi-disciplinary team approach can be instituted.

Patient Characteristics

With regard to patient assessment, current functional status, comorbidities, and an evaluation of right heart function should be ascertained and updated immediately prior to surgery. New York Heart Association functional class and SWMD have been linked to PH outcomes in general [6, 72], and studies related to perioperative risk stratification have pointed to increased post-operative morbidity and mortality after surgery in NYHA class II or higher [70], and in patients with SMWD <399 m [73]. Often, the aim to improve functional class or SMWD after one office visit is an unrealistic expectation just prior to surgery, but a documented significant decline in either parameter suggests a decompensated state and is critical information that may result in the appropriate delay or cancellation of surgical intervention. Similarly, signs or symptoms of acute right heart failure such as peripheral edema, increased abdominal girth, new or worsening hypoxemia, and relative hypotension and tachycardia can be noted and treated with diuresis, supplemental oxygen and potentially augmentation of PH-specific therapy. Finally, identification of high-risk comorbidities like history of pulmonary embolism, chronic kidney disease and coronary artery disease [70, 71, 74] can assist in appropriate patient risk stratification.

A current transthoracic echocardiogram (TTE), basic laboratory tests including an N-terminal pro-basic natriuretic peptide (NT-pro BNP), an electrocardiogram (ECG) and an assessment of hemodynamics are also recommended preoperatively [75, 76], ideally within 6 to 12 months. On TTE, poorer surgical outcomes in PH patients have been linked to right ventricular hypertrophy (RVH) and a right ventricular myocardial performance index of >0.75 [70]. On ECG, right axis deviation is associated with increased morbidity [70], while a higher right atrial pressure (RAP) [73], pulmonary artery pressure (PAP) [71, 74] and right ventricular systolic pressure/systolic blood pressure ratio of >0.66 assessed by RHC is worrisome [70]. Laboratory tests can, of course, highlight new or progressive kidney or liver injury that may represent an exacerbation of right heart failure. Moreover, new or progressive anemia or alterations in acid–base status, both potentially adversely impactful on pulmonary vascular resistance (PVR), can also be identified.

Surgical Characteristics

Details of proposed anesthetic use, surgical approach, and duration of surgery are critical variables for planning and risk stratification of surgery in PAH patients. Not surprisingly, data have shown that prolonged time under anesthesia [70, 77] and intermediate (e.g. head and neck) and high (e.g. liver transplantation) versus low (e.g. cataract) risk operations (Table 22.2, [110]) are associated with worse surgical outcomes in PH patients [71, 74, 77]. Generally, the involvement of an anesthesiologist skilled in the management of PH is advised. This often warrants the transfer of the PH patient to a tertiary care center equipped to treat PH. Although there are no strict guidelines with respect to anesthesia type (e.g. general, neuraxial) or anesthetic agent delivery method per se, careful thought must be given to the potential effects on pulmonary versus systemic vascular resistance, sympathetic tone, right ventricular (RV) loading, and cardiac inotropy and chronotropy [78]. This is because the PH patient must be considered extremely sensitive to even minor alterations in vascular tone, heart rate, gas exchange, acid–base state and volume status. For example, patients with PH can decompensate acutely and irreversibly in response to an acute increase in vagal tone (e.g. nausea during intubation) or mismatch in ventilation-perfusion (V-Q) (e.g. prone positioning)

Table 22.2 Risk stratification in PH patients by type of surgery

| **Low-risk operations** |
| Dermatologic surgeries |
| Endoscopic procedures |
| Cataract surgery |
| Breast surgery |
| **Intermediate-risk operations** |
| Carotid endarterectomy |
| Head and neck surgery |
| Gynecologic surgery |
| Gastrointestinal/intraabdominal surgery |
| Orthopedic surgery |
| Prostate surgery |
| Thoracic surgery |
| **High-risk operations** |
| Emergent major surgery |
| Aortic or other major vascular surgery |
| Liver transplantation |
| Other major operations with anticipated large fluid shifts and/or blood loss |

Reproduced with permission from the Pulmonary Hypertension Association (PHA). Reprinted and Adapted from: McGlothlin et al. [110]

as these states can acutely decrease RV preload or induce hypoxia, respectively. Furthermore, the preoperative team need consider the appropriateness of PH-specific therapies, which is an assessment based, in part, on factors influencing effective drug delivery in the peri-operative period. A plan well in advance of surgery is ideal, one which takes into account severity of disease as well as patient comorbidities and current PH therapies.

Intraoperative Management

The primary objective during surgery is to preserve RV function. Most PH practitioners agree that four main tenets to intraoperative management of PH patients exist: maintenance of adequate RV preload, tolerable RV afterload, sufficient RV contractility and normal heart rate and rhythm [76, 78–80].

RV Preload

Ideal preload of the chronically stressed RV can be elusive as degree of RV remodeling varies greatly from patient to patient and amongst different types of PH. For instance, 5-year survival rates in the congenital heart disease population are thought to be considerably higher than in the idiopathic PH population [81] because of the benefit of years over months of RV adaptation to a high RV afterload or PVR. Hence, attentive tracking of central venous pressure (CVP) and fluid balance trends intra-operatively is advised. Large fluid shifts in either direction are not well-tolerated by the RV in PH. Hypotension can easily ensue because of an acute drop in preload (e.g. hemorrhage or induction) or a sudden large-volume bolus leading to acute RV strain and imminent ischemia and/or acute LV diastolic dysfunction related to interventricular dependence [82–84]. Adept anesthesiologists need to readily recognize and try to promptly offset such fluid shifts before the manifestation of acute RV failure.

RV Afterload

Most PH-specific therapies target RV afterload by way of pulmonary vascular vasodilatation and anti-proliferative effects [85]. Indeed, the central goal of any PH treatment plan is to actively reduce PVR. Peri-operatively, maintenance or reduction of PVR in PH patients is achieved in two ways: administration of PH-specific agents and avoidance of triggers of PVR elevation.

PH-Specific Agents: It is imperative that outpatient PH regimens are strictly adhered to in the operating room. Parenteral prostacyclins like epoprostenol and treprostinil are potent drugs that have been shown to improve multiple clinical parameters and survival in PH patients [86–91]. They are typically administered continuously and at a steady dose; any interruption in or accidental bolus of drug can lead to a PH crisis or acute hypotension, respectively. The correct management of parenteral prostacyclin pumps requires specialized training which should be addressed well in advance of surgery as, in the operating room, it is mandatory that physicians and nurses know how to quickly respond to an unexpected issue related to the infusion. Additionally, the peri-operative team should be familiar with the extensive side effect profile of the prostacyclins which includes, importantly, negative qualitative and quantitative platelet effects which can precipitate bleeding [92, 93]. These drugs are usually not started intra-operatively, as they can lead to hemodynamic instability when initiated and titrated up in dose. Similarly, the use of medications like endothelin receptor antagonists and phosphodiesterase (PDE)-5 inhibitors is typically saved for stable settings due to their longer half-lives and potential hemodynamic effects.

Inhalational agents, however, are routinely started peri-operatively in order to reduce RV afterload, salvage an acutely failing RV, and improve V-Q matching. Particularly in the cardiac surgery literature, inhaled nitric oxide, epoprostenol, iloprost and milrinone have been well-studied [94–99]. Cardiopulmonary bypass (CPB) is a unique circumstance that can significantly stress the pulmonary vasculature and increase PVR by way of atelectasis, ischemia-reperfusion injury, pulmonary embolism, and endothelial damage and capillary leak [83]. In addition, inotropy can be negatively impacted during CPB because of coronary artery bypass graft (CABG) failure and arrhythmia [83]. Thus, aggressive and anticipatory stabilization of the PVR during cardiac surgery is of utmost importance.

Inhaled nitric oxide (iNO) causes pulmonary vasodilatation by an augmentation of the cyclic GMP pathway. It is rapidly metabolized by oxyhemoglobin and deoxyhemoglobin and hence has no profound effects on systemic vascular resistance (SVR). Because of its short half-life, it can lead to rebound PH upon withdrawal [100], though this can be ameliorated with the overlap of another PH agent like the PDE-5 inhibitor sildenafil [101] once the patient is considered hemodynamically stable. Inhaled NO has demonstrated benefit in the heart transplant surgery [94] and CPB [96] settings. The main drawback of iNO is cost, and therefore more attention is being delivered to the inhaled prostacylins.

Inhalation versus intravenous administration of epoprostenol avoids the potentially harmful effects on SVR and platelets of the latter. It has been successfully used in RV failure and refractory hypoxia following cardiac surgery [95]. Disadvantages include requisite continuous administration given its short half-life and, in turn, rebound PH upon withdrawal. Inhaled iloprost, another synthetic prostacyclin, has the advantages of a half-life longer than epoprostenol and a cost less than iNO. One study demonstrated its benefit in mitral valve surgery [98] while another study directly compared iloprost to iNO in cardiac surgery and found it to be more effective [99].

Triggers of PVR Elevation: As aforementioned, the pulmonary vasculature is a highly dynamic environment, exquisitely sensitive to even the smallest perturbations in the environs. Because of this, avoidance of known triggers that adversely affect the PVR in the peri-operative period is paramount to RV health. Such triggers in include acidosis, hypercapnea, hypoxia, and anemia. Moreover, the act of intubation itself immediately places the PH patient at risk unless the operator is cognizant of the potential adverse effects on hemodynamics. To clarify, the contribution of peri-alveolar vessels accounts for the unique U-shaped distribution of PVR and lung volumes (Fig. 22.3, [78]). PVR is minimal at functional residual capacity (FRC) and increased at small and large lung volumes. At low lung volumes, including atelectasis, or at high or overdistended lung volumes, either distensibility or geometry of the small pulmonary vessels is impaired or altered, leading to turbulent flow, perhaps due to a neurohumoral signal [102]. Thus, bagging peri-intubation and subsequent ventilator manipulations must exclude extremes of tidal volumes and positive end-expiratory pressures. Finally, a sudden surge in sympathetic tone, as can occur with uncontrolled pain, is a distinct contributor to acute PVR elevation. An experienced anesthesiologist will engage in ardent pain and anxiety control in the PH patient [75]. The α-agonist dexmetomidine, an increasingly popular sedative in the ICU and operative settings due to its lack of effect on respiratory drive [103] has demonstrated hemodynamic benefits in patients with PH undergoing mitral valve surgery [104].

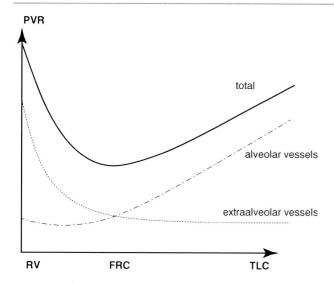

Fig. 22.3 Relationship is U-shaped between lung volumes and total PVR. *PVR* pulmonary vascular resistance, *RV* residual volume, *FRC* functional residual capacity, *TLC* total lung capacity (Adapted from Lars Fischer et al.[78]; Reprinted with permission of Wolters Kluwer Health)

RV Contractility

The majority of PH patients have impaired cardiac contractility at baseline. During surgery, the heart is further stressed by expected (e.g. intubation, CPB) and unexpected (e.g. pulmonary embolism, hemorrhage) events. Commonly, then, pharmacologic agents are utilized to preserve or augment RV function. Choice of such agents requires basic knowledge of potential effects on PVR.

Inotropes: Dobutamine is a synthetic β-1 and β-2 agonist that, at low doses, does not typically increase PVR [84, 105], however, may result in systemic hypotension due to systemic β-2 adrenoceptor activation and resultant vasodilatation of the systemic vasculature. Further, the β-1 effect can precipitate tachyarrhythmias. Therefore, vigilance is required upon initiation of dobutamine in the PH patient. Other adrenergic agonists like epinephrine and dopamine can often be substituted if hypotension is a concern as they have a less negative effect on SVR than dobutamine. However, at higher doses, dopamine can adversely affect PVR and also lead to tachyarrhythmia [84, 105], which is usually poorly tolerated by the acutely failing RV. Milrinone is a PDE-3 inhibitor that acts to increase intracellular cyclic-adenosine monophosphate (c-AMP) levels and hence intracellular calcium concentrations in the cardiomyocyte, leading to improved contractility. It is considered beneficial in PH patients because of its advantageous effects on inotropy and PVR. The main drawback to milrinone is that, unlike dobutamine and dopamine with half-lives of 2 min, its half-life is 2.5 h. Thus, sustained hypotension is a concern. Levosimendan is a calcium-sensitizing agent that binds to troponin C in cardiac myocytes, thereby increasing calcium effects in heart muscle. It

has been shown to improve hemodynamics in PH patients while mildly lowering PVR [75]. It, too, can cause hypotension. However, it has not yet been approved for use in the United States.

Vasopressors

Vasopressors are frequently employed alone or as adjunct therapy to inotropes if a sustained low SVR state ensues. Vasopressors like vasopressin, phenylephrine and norepinephrine are used to avoid or treat RV ischemia. Right ventricular blood flow, unlike that of the LV which is replenished in diastole, is equally replenished in diastole and systole. Thus, during systole, when the RVSP exceeds the SBP, right coronary perfusion is jeopardized and ischemia can set in [75, 105]. Given the chronically high PVR state in PH, the RV is particularly dependent on an adequate SVR for coronary perfusion. Vasopressin is commonly favored over phenylephrine and norepinephrine as it has been shown to lower or maintain PVR [83, 105]. However, there is no absolute contraindication to the use of any vasopressor in PH.

Rate and Rhythm

As is applicable to heart failure in general, the maintenance of an adequate heart rate in the PH patient is essential. Indeed, neither tachyarrhythmias, which prevent sufficient diastolic filling, nor bradyarrhythmias, which, alongside a low stroke volume, prevent sufficient cardiac output are well-tolerated by the RV in PH [75]. Even further, dysrhythmias are a poor prognosticator in PH [106]. In an unstable supraventricular tachycardia (SVT), Advanced Cardiac Life Support (ACLS) guidelines take precedence and cardioversion is recommended [107]. In a stable SVT, however, choice of pharmacologic intervention can be more complicated than usual. Beta-blockade, for instance, can profoundly inhibit RV inotropy and chronotropy to the point of hypotension and subsequent RV ischemia [76]. Centrally acting calcium channel blockade (e.g. verapamil) effects can be similar [75, 79, 80]. Amiodarone does have intrinsic beta-blockade activity but seems to be less negatively impactful on inotropy at least acutely. Digoxin conversely has reportedly positive inotropic effects, though its use in an emergency setting is usually limited by its longer time to onset of action. Data is limited with regard to dysrhythmia and heart rate management specifically in the peri-operative period, but the above principles should be considered.

Post-operative Management

The critical window of peri-operative morbidity and mortality in PH patients includes the hours to days following surgery [77, 108]. Volume shifts, bleeding, infection and sepsis, acute kidney injury and pulmonary embolism can devastate the already unstable RV. Hence, vigilance in the post-operative period is compulsory.

Monitoring

Patients with PH who are recovering from surgery should do so in an intensive care unit (ICU) setting to allow for close supervision. There are no strict guidelines with respect to type of monitoring (e.g. pulmonary arterial catheter (PAC)), though especially following high-risk surgeries, some form of RV surveillance is recommended [75, 76, 83, 109]. The goal is to follow trends of RV function. This can be achieved by central venous saturations off a central venous catheter or mixed venous saturations off a PAC coupled with the usual measures of perfusion including acid–base status, lactate levels, mean arterial pressures off an arterial line, and urine output. Alternatively, serial echocardiography is sometimes employed, via transesophageal or transthoracic probe. As aforementioned, strict observance and recording of fluid balance is also key to RV stability. Moreover, the ICU setting fosters the ideal preventative care bundles like thromboembolism prophylaxis, early extubation, pain management and sterile precautions, all of which are fundamental to good surgical outcomes.

Ambulatory PH Regimen

As soon as is possible post-operatively, the ambulatory PH medication regimen should be reinstituted to try to return the cardiopulmonary milieu to its usual state. Any interruptions or changes in chronic PH-specific therapy dosing can stress the RV and thus are avoided. However, some post-operative states and issues necessitate such changes. For example, when hypotension ensues, the longer-acting PDE-5 inhibitors that can drop SVR should be held and replaced by iNO. If a patient is being fed by nasogastric tube, endothelin receptor antagonists cannot be delivered because they are not easily crushed and hence withdrawal of this therapy must be accounted for. Finally, a patient who requires non-invasive positive-pressure ventilation cannot reliably use their inhaled prostacyclin device and therefore may need additional therapy. In sum, vigilant maintenance of the PH regimen serves to stave off post-operative cardiopulmonary complications.

Conclusions

Patients with PH are at increased risk for morbidity and mortality in the surgical setting and thus a detailed multidisciplinary approach to peri-operative management is warranted and should address both patient- and surgery-specific characteristics. Intra-operative care strategies should be centered on RV health. Triggers of acute PVR elevation must be minimized and therapeutics that preserve or increase cardiac contractility and decrease RV afterload should be readily and comfortably utilized. Post-surgical PH patients mandate close observation in the ICU, as complications are abundant in the post-operative setting. The theme of adherence to PH-specific therapy is relevant to the entire peri-operative course as acute withdrawal can prove to have devastating consequences.

References

1. Desai SA, Channick RN. Exercise in patients with pulmonary arterial hypertension. J Cardiopulm Rehabil Prev. 2008;28(1):12–6.
2. Sun XG, Hansen JE, Oudiz RJ, Wasserman K. Exercise pathophysiology in patients with primary pulmonary hypertension. Circulation. 2001;104(4):429–35.
3. Clark AL, Chua TP, Coats AJ. Anatomical dead space, ventilatory pattern, and exercise capacity in chronic heart failure. Br Heart J. 1995;74(4):377–80.
4. Metra M, Dei Cas L, Panina G, Visioli O. Exercise hyperventilation chronic congestive heart failure, and its relation to functional capacity and hemodynamics. Am J Cardiol. 1992;70(6):622–8.
5. Arena R, Myers J, Abella J, Peberdy MA, Bensimhon D, Chase P, et al. Development of a ventilatory classification system in patients with heart failure. Circulation. 2007;115(18):2410–7.
6. Miyamoto S, Nagaya N, Satoh T, Kyotani S, Sakamaki F, Fujita M, et al. Clinical correlates and prognostic significance of six-minute walk test in patients with primary pulmonary hypertension. Comparison with cardiopulmonary exercise testing. Am J Respir Crit Care Med. 2000;161(2 Pt 1):487–92.
7. Cenedese E, Speich R, Dorschner L, Ulrich S, Maggiorini M, Jenni R, et al. Measurement of quality of life in pulmonary hypertension and its significance. Eur Respir J. 2006;28(4):808–15.
8. de Man FS, Handoko ML, Groepenhoff H, Hul AJ V't, Abbink J, Koppers RJ, et al. Effects of exercise training in patients with idiopathic pulmonary arterial hypertension. Eur Respir J. 2009;34(3):669–75.
9. Grunig E, Maier F, Ehlken N, Fischer C, Lichtblau M, Blank N, et al. Exercise training in pulmonary arterial hypertension associated with connective tissue diseases. Arthritis Res Ther. 2012;14(3):R148.
10. Grunig E, Lichtblau M, Ehlken N, Ghofrani HA, Reichenberger F, Staehler G, et al. Safety and efficacy of exercise training in various forms of pulmonary hypertension. Eur Respir J. 2012;40(1):84–92.
11. Mereles D, Ehlken N, Kreuscher S, Ghofrani S, Hoeper MM, Halank M, et al. Exercise and respiratory training improve exercise capacity and quality of life in patients with severe chronic pulmonary hypertension. Circulation. 2006;114(14):1482–9.
12. Weinstein AA, Chin LM, Keyser RE, Kennedy M, Nathan SD, Woolstenhulme JG, et al. Effect of aerobic exercise training on fatigue and physical activity in patients with pulmonary arterial hypertension. Respir Med. 2013;107(5):778–84.
13. Grunig E, Ehlken N, Ghofrani A, Staehler G, Meyer FJ, Juenger J, et al. Effect of exercise and respiratory training on clinical progression and survival in patients with severe chronic pulmonary hypertension. Respiration; Int Rev Thoracic Dis. 2011;81(5):394–401.
14. Fox BD, Kassirer M, Weiss I, Raviv Y, Peled N, Shitrit D, et al. Ambulatory rehabilitation improves exercise capacity in patients with pulmonary hypertension. J Card Fail. 2011;17(3):196–200.
15. Chan L, Chin LM, Kennedy M, Woolstenhulme JG, Nathan SD, Weinstein AA, et al. Benefits of intensive treadmill exercise training on cardiorespiratory function and quality of life in patients with pulmonary hypertension. Chest. 2013;143(2):333–43.
16. Chung L, Liu J, Parsons L, Hassoun PM, McGoon M, Badesch DB, et al. Characterization of connective tissue disease-associated

pulmonary arterial hypertension from REVEAL: identifying systemic sclerosis as a unique phenotype. Chest. 2010;138(6): 1383–94.

17. Clements PJ, Tan M, McLaughlin VV, Oudiz RJ, Tapson VF, Channick RN, et al. The pulmonary arterial hypertension quality enhancement research initiative: comparison of patients with idiopathic PAH to patients with systemic sclerosis-associated PAH. Ann Rheum Dis. 2012;71(2):249–52.

18. Kabitz HJ, Schwoerer A, Bremer HC, Sonntag F, Walterspacher S, Walker D, et al. Impairment of respiratory muscle function in pulmonary hypertension. Clin Sci. 2008;114(2):165–71.

19. Mainguy V, Maltais F, Saey D, Gagnon P, Martel S, Simon M, et al. Effects of a rehabilitation program on skeletal muscle function in idiopathic pulmonary arterial hypertension. J Cardiopulm Rehabil Prev. 2010;30(5):319–23.

20. Mainguy V, Maltais F, Saey D, Gagnon P, Martel S, Simon M, et al. Peripheral muscle dysfunction in idiopathic pulmonary arterial hypertension. Thorax. 2010;65(2):113–7.

21. Meyer FJ, Lossnitzer D, Kristen AV, Schoene AM, Kubler W, Katus HA, et al. Respiratory muscle dysfunction in idiopathic pulmonary arterial hypertension. Eur Respir J. 2005;25(1):125–30.

22. Kabitz HJ, Bremer HC, Schwoerer A, Sonntag F, Walterspacher S, Walker DJ, et al. The combination of exercise and respiratory training improves respiratory muscle function in pulmonary hypertension. Lung. 2014;192(2):321–8.

23. de Man FS, van Hees HW, Handoko ML, Niessen HW, Schalij I, Humbert M, et al. Diaphragm muscle fiber weakness in pulmonary hypertension. Am J Respir Crit Care Med. 2011;183(10): 1411–8.

24. Rochester CL, Fairburn C, Crouch RH. Pulmonary rehabilitation for respiratory disorders other than chronic obstructive pulmonary disease. Clin Chest Med. 2014;35(2):369–89 [Review].

25. Robson S, Hunter S, Boys R, Dunlop W, Bryson M. Changes in cardiac output during epidural anaesthesia for caesarean section. Anaesthesia. 1989;44(6):475–9.

26. Robson SC, Hunter S, Boys RJ, Dunlop W. Serial study of factors influencing changes in cardiac output during human pregnancy. Am J Physiol. 1989;256(4 Pt 2):H1060–5.

27. Pritchard JA. Changes in the blood volume during pregnancy and delivery. Anesthesiology. 1965;26:393–9.

28. Clapp 3rd JF, Capeless E. Cardiovascular function before, during, and after the first and subsequent pregnancies. Am J Cardiol. 1997;80(11):1469–73.

29. Ueland K. Maternal cardiovascular dynamics. VII. Intrapartum blood volume changes. Am J Obstet Gynecol. 1976;126(6):671–7.

30. Pritchard JA. Blood volume changes in pregnancy and the puerperium. Iv. Anemia associated with hydatidiform mole. Am J Obstet Gynecol. 1965;91:621–9.

31. Lund CJ, Donovan JC. Blood volume during pregnancy. Significance of plasma and red cell volumes. Am J Obstet Gynecol. 1967;98(3):394–403.

32. McCaffrey RM, Dunn LJ. Primary pulmonary hypertension in pregnancy. Obstet Gynecol Surv. 1964;19:567–91.

33. Weiss BM, Zemp L, Seifert B, Hess OM. Outcome of pulmonary vascular disease in pregnancy: a systematic overview from 1978 through 1996. J Am Coll Cardiol. 1998;31(7):1650–7.

34. Gleicher N, Midwall J, Hochberger D, Jaffin H. Eisenmenger's syndrome and pregnancy. Obstet Gynecol Surv. 1979;34(10):721–41.

35. Lieber S, Dewilde P, Huyghens L, Traey E, Gepts E. Eisenmenger's syndrome and pregnancy. Acta Cardiol. 1985;40(4):421–4.

36. Jais X, Olsson KM, Barbera JA, Blanco I, Torbicki A, Peacock A, et al. Pregnancy outcomes in pulmonary arterial hypertension in the modern management era. Eur Respir J. 2012;40(4):881–5.

37. Bedard E, Dimopoulos K, Gatzoulis MA. Has there been any progress made on pregnancy outcomes among women with pulmonary arterial hypertension? Eur Heart J. 2009;30(3):256–65.

38. Warnes CA. Pregnancy and pulmonary hypertension. Int J Cardiol. 2004;97 Suppl 1:11–3.

39. Martinez MV, Rutherford JD. Pulmonary hypertension in pregnancy. Cardiol Rev. 2013;21(4):167–73.

40. Hellgren M, Blomback M. Studies on blood coagulation and fibrinolysis in pregnancy, during delivery and in the puerperium. I. Normal condition. Gynecol Obstet Invest. 1981;12(3):141–54.

41. Pechet L, Alexander B. Increased clotting factors in pregnancy. N Engl J Med. 1961;265:1093–7.

42. American College of O, Gynecologists. ACOG committee opinion: safety of lovenox in pregnancy. Obstet Gynecol. 2002; 100(4):845–6.

43. Bates SM, Greer IA, Hirsh J, Ginsberg JS. Use of antithrombotic agents during pregnancy: the seventh ACCP conference on antithrombotic and thrombolytic therapy. Chest. 2004;126(3 Suppl): 627S–44.

44. Montani D, Gunther S, Dorfmuller P, Perros F, Girerd B, Garcia G, et al. Pulmonary arterial hypertension. Orphanet J Rare Dis. 2013;8:97.

45. Zamanian RT, Kudelko KT, Sung YK, de Jesus PV, Liu J, Spiekerkoetter E. Current clinical management of pulmonary arterial hypertension. Circ Res. 2014;115(1):131–47.

46. Zijlstra WM, Ploegstra MJ, Berger RM. Current and advancing treatments for pulmonary arterial hypertension in childhood. Expert Rev Respir Med. 2014;22:1–14.

47. Archer SL, Michelakis ED. Phosphodiesterase type 5 inhibitors for pulmonary arterial hypertension. N Engl J Med. 2009;361(19): 1864–71.

48. Cannon JE, Pepke-Zaba J. Riociguat for pulmonary hypertension. Exp Rev Clin Pharmacol. 2014;7(3):259–70.

49. Conole D, Scott LJ. Riociguat: first global approval. Drugs. 2013;73(17):1967–75.

50. Casserly B, Klinger JR. Ambrisentan for the treatment of pulmonary arterial hypertension. Drug Des Devel Ther. 2009;2:265–80.

51. Liu C, Chen J. Endothelin receptor antagonists for pulmonary arterial hypertension. Cochrane Database Syst Rev. 2006;(3): CD004434.

52. Roberts KE, Preston IR. Safety and tolerability of bosentan in the management of pulmonary arterial hypertension. Drug Des Devel Ther. 2009;3:111–8.

53. de Jesus Perez VA. Understanding the pharmacokinetics of oral treprostinil in patients with pulmonary arterial hypertension. J Cardiovasc Pharmacol. 2013;61(6):471–3.

54. Baradia D, Khatri N, Trehan S, Misra A. Inhalation therapy to treat pulmonary arterial hypertension. Pharmaceut Patent Anal. 2012;1(5):577–88.

55. Galie N, Corris PA, Frost A, Girgis RE, Granton J, Jing ZC, et al. Updated treatment algorithm of pulmonary arterial hypertension. J Am Coll Cardiol. 2013;62(25 Suppl):D60–72.

56. Olschewski H. Prostacyclins. Handb Exp Pharmacol. 2013; 218:177–98.

57. Sorensen MB, Jacobsen E. Pulmonary hemodynamics during induction of anesthesia. Anesthesiology. 1977;46(4):246–51.

58. Krenz EI, Hart SR, Russo M, Alkadri M. Epidural anesthesia for cesarean delivery in a patient with severe pulmonary artery hypertension and a right-to-left shunt. Ochsner J. 2011;11(1):78–80.

59. Manohar MV, Vaidya A, Bakshi S. Revisiting epidural anaesthesia in a parturient with idiopathic pulmonary hypertension posted for caesarean section. Indian J Anaesth. 2014;58(2):235–6.

60. Maxwell BG, El-Sayed YY, Riley ET, Carvalho B. Peripartum outcomes and anaesthetic management of parturients with moderate to complex congenital heart disease or pulmonary hypertension*. Anaesthesia. 2013;68(1):52–9.

61. Smedstad KG, Cramb R, Morison DH. Pulmonary hypertension and pregnancy: a series of eight cases. Canadian J Anaesth = Journal canadien d'anesthesie. 1994;41(6):502–12.

62. Vongpatanasin W, Brickner ME, Hillis LD, Lange RA. The Eisenmenger syndrome in adults. Ann Intern Med. 1998;128(9): 745–55.

63. Roberts NV, Keast PJ, Brodeky V, Oates A, Ritchie BC. The effects of oxytocin on the pulmonary and systemic circulation in pregnant ewes. Anaesth Intensive Care. 1992;20(2):199–202.

64. Ross-Ascuitto N, Ascuitto RJ, Darnell J. A pregnant woman with moderate pulmonary hypertension. Pediatr Cardiol. 1995;16(1): 31–2.

65. Thorne S, Nelson-Piercy C, MacGregor A, Gibbs S, Crowhurst J, Panay N, et al. Pregnancy and contraception in heart disease and pulmonary arterial hypertension. J Family Plan Reprod Health Care/Facul Family Plan Reprod Health Care, Royal Coll Obstet Gynaecol. 2006;32(2):75–81.

66. Taichman DB, Ornelas J, Chung L, Klinger JR, Lewis S, Mandel J, et al. Pharmacologic therapy for pulmonary arterial hypertension in adults: CHEST guideline and expert panel report. Chest. 2014;146(2):449–75.

67. Safdar Z. Pulmonary arterial hypertension in pregnant women. Ther Adv Respir Dis. 2013;7(1):51–63 [Research Support, N.I.H., Extramural Review].

68. Reich DL, Wood Jr RK, Emre S, Bodian CA, Hossain S, Krol M, et al. Association of intraoperative hypotension and pulmonary hypertension with adverse outcomes after orthotopic liver transplantation. J Cardiothorac Vasc Anesth. 2003;17(6):699–702.

69. Roques F, Nashef SA, Michel P, Gauducheau E, de Vincentiis C, Baudet E, et al. Risk factors and outcome in European cardiac surgery: analysis of the EuroSCORE multinational database of 19030 patients. Eur J Cardio-thoracic Surgery : Off J Eur Assoc Cardio-thoracic Surg. 1999;15(6):816–22. [Multicenter Study Research Support, Non-U.S. Gov't]; discussion 22–3.

70. Ramakrishna G, Sprung J, Ravi BS, Chandrasekaran K, McGoon MD. Impact of pulmonary hypertension on the outcomes of non-cardiac surgery: predictors of perioperative morbidity and mortality. J Am Coll Cardiol. 2005;45(10):1691–9.

71. Lai HC, Lai HC, Wang KY, Lee WL, Ting CT, Liu TJ. Severe pulmonary hypertension complicates postoperative outcome of non-cardiac surgery. Br J Anaesth. 2007;99(2):184–90 [Research Support, Non-U.S. Gov't].

72. McLaughlin VV, Archer SL, Badesch DB, Barst RJ, Farber HW, Lindner JR, et al. ACCF/AHA 2009 expert consensus document on pulmonary hypertension a report of the American College of Cardiology Foundation Task Force on Expert Consensus Documents and the American Heart Association developed in collaboration with the American College of Chest Physicians; American Thoracic Society, Inc.; and the Pulmonary Hypertension Association. J Am Coll Cardiol. 2009;53(17):1573–619 [Consensus Development Conference Practice Guideline].

73. Meyer S, McLaughlin VV, Seyfarth HJ, Bull TM, Vizza CD, Gomberg-Maitland M, et al. Outcomes of noncardiac, nonobstetric surgery in patients with PAH: an international prospective survey. Eur Respir J. 2013;41(6):1302 [Multicenter Study].

74. Kaw R, Pasupuleti V, Deshpande A, Hamieh T, Walker E, Minai OA. Pulmonary hypertension: an important predictor of outcomes in patients undergoing non-cardiac surgery. Respir Med. 2011;105(4):619–24 [Comparative Study].

75. Hosseinian L. Pulmonary hypertension and noncardiac surgery: implications for the anesthesiologist. J Cardiothorac Vasc Anesth. 2014;28(4):1076–86 [Review].

76. McGlothlin D, Ivascu N, Heerdt PM. Anesthesia and pulmonary hypertension. Prog Cardiovasc Dis. 2012;55(2):199–217 [Review].

77. Price LC, Montani D, Jais X, Dick JR, Simonneau G, Sitbon O, et al. Noncardiothoracic nonobstetric surgery in mild-to-moderate pulmonary hypertension. Eur Respir J. 2010;35(6):1294–302 [Research Support, Non-U.S. Gov't].

78. Fischer LG, Van Aken H, Burkle H. Management of pulmonary hypertension: physiological and pharmacological considerations for anesthesiologists. Anesth Analg. 2003;96(6):1603–16 [Research Support, Non-U.S. Gov't Review].

79. Strumpher J, Jacobsohn E. Pulmonary hypertension and right ventricular dysfunction: physiology and perioperative management. J Cardiothorac Vasc Anesth. 2011;25(4):687–704 [Review].

80. Tonelli AR, Minai OA. Saudi guidelines on the diagnosis and treatment of pulmonary hypertension: perioperative management in patients with pulmonary hypertension. Ann Thorac Med. 2014;9 Suppl 1:S98–107.

81. McLaughlin VV, Presberg KW, Doyle RL, Abman SH, McCrory DC, Fortin T, et al. Prognosis of pulmonary arterial hypertension: ACCP evidence-based clinical practice guidelines. Chest. 2004;126(1 Suppl):78S–92 [Guideline Practice Guideline Review].

82. Lahm T, McCaslin CA, Wozniak TC, Ghumman W, Fadl YY, Obeidat OS, et al. Medical and surgical treatment of acute right ventricular failure. J Am Coll Cardiol. 2010;56(18):1435–46 [Research Support, N.I.H., Extramural Research Support, Non-U.S. Gov't Review].

83. Thunberg CA, Gaitan BD, Grewal A, Ramakrishna H, Stansbury LG, Grigore AM. Pulmonary hypertension in patients undergoing cardiac surgery: pathophysiology, perioperative management, and outcomes. J Cardiothorac Vasc Anesth. 2013;27(3):551–72 [Review].

84. Zamanian RT, Haddad F, Doyle RL, Weinacker AB. Management strategies for patients with pulmonary hypertension in the intensive care unit. Crit Care Med. 2007;35(9):2037–50 [Research Support, Non-U.S. Gov't Review].

85. Humbert M, Sitbon O, Simonneau G. Treatment of pulmonary arterial hypertension. N Engl J Med. 2004;351(14):1425–36 [Research Support, Non-U.S. Gov't Review].

86. Lang I, Gomez-Sanchez M, Kneussl M, Naeije R, Escribano P, Skoro-Sajer N, et al. Efficacy of long-term subcutaneous treprostinil sodium therapy in pulmonary hypertension. Chest. 2006;129(6):1636–43 [Clinical Trial Multicenter Study Research Support, Non-U.S. Gov't].

87. McLaughlin VV, Shillington A, Rich S. Survival in primary pulmonary hypertension: the impact of epoprostenol therapy. Circulation. 2002;106(12):1477–82 [Clinical Trial Research Support, Non-U.S. Gov't].

88. Sitbon O, Humbert M, Nunes H, Parent F, Garcia G, Herve P, et al. Long-term intravenous epoprostenol infusion in primary pulmonary hypertension: prognostic factors and survival. J Am Coll Cardiol. 2002;40(4):780–8 [Clinical Trial Research Support, Non-U.S. Gov't].

89. Barst RJ, Galie N, Naeije R, Simonneau G, Jeffs R, Arneson C, et al. Long-term outcome in pulmonary arterial hypertension patients treated with subcutaneous treprostinil. Eur Respir J. 2006;28(6):1195–203 [Comparative Study Randomized Controlled Trial].

90. Sadushi-Kolici R, Skoro-Sajer N, Zimmer D, Bonderman D, Schemper M, Klepetko W, et al. Long-term treatment, tolerability, and survival with sub-cutaneous treprostinil for severe pulmonary hypertension. J Heart Lung Transplant. 2012;31(7):735–43 [Research Support, Non-U.S. Gov't].

91. Barst RJ, Rubin LJ, McGoon MD, Caldwell EJ, Long WA, Levy PS. Survival in primary pulmonary hypertension with long-term continuous intravenous prostacyclin. Ann Intern Med. 1994;121(6):409–15 [Clinical Trial Multicenter Study Research Support, Non-U.S. Gov't Research Support , P.H.S.].

92. Chin KM, Channick RN, de Lemos JA, Kim NH, Torres F, Rubin LJ. Hemodynamics and epoprostenol use are associated with thrombocytopenia in pulmonary arterial hypertension. Chest. 2009;135(1):130–6.

93. Tamburrelli C, Crescente M, Izzi B, Barisciano M, Donati MB, de Gaetano G, et al. Epoprostenol inhibits human platelet-leukocyte mixed conjugate and platelet microparticle formation in whole blood. Thromb Res. 2011;128(5):446–51 [Research Support, Non-U.S. Gov't].

94. Ardehali A, Hughes K, Sadeghi A, Esmailian F, Marelli D, Moriguchi J, et al. Inhaled nitric oxide for pulmonary hypertension after heart transplantation. Transplantation. 2001;72(4):638–41.

95. De Wet CJ, Affleck DG, Jacobsohn E, Avidan MS, Tymkew H, Hill LL, et al. Inhaled prostacyclin is safe, effective, and affordable in patients with pulmonary hypertension, right heart dysfunction, and refractory hypoxemia after cardiothoracic surgery. J Thorac Cardiovasc Surg. 2004;127(4):1058–67 [Clinical Trial Comparative Study Research Support, Non-U.S. Gov't].

96. Fattouch K, Sbraga F, Sampognaro R, Bianco G, Gucciardo M, Lavalle C, et al. Treatment of pulmonary hypertension in patients undergoing cardiac surgery with cardiopulmonary bypass: a randomized, prospective, double-blind study. J Cardiovasc Med. 2006;7((2):119–23 [Comparative Study Randomized Controlled Trial].

97. Lamarche Y, Perrault LP, Maltais S, Tetreault K, Lambert J, Denault AY. Preliminary experience with inhaled milrinone in cardiac surgery. Eur J Cardiothorac Surg: Off J Eur Assoc Cardiothorac Surg. 2007;31(6):1081–7 [Research Support, Non-U.S. Gov't].

98. Rex S, Schaelte G, Metzelder S, Flier S, de Waal EE, Autschbach R, et al. Inhaled iloprost to control pulmonary artery hypertension in patients undergoing mitral valve surgery: a prospective, randomized-controlled trial. Acta Anaesthesiol Scand. 2008;52(1):65–72 [Comparative Study Randomized Controlled Trial].

99. Winterhalter M, Simon A, Fischer S, Rahe-Meyer N, Chamtzidou N, Hecker H, et al. Comparison of inhaled iloprost and nitric oxide in patients with pulmonary hypertension during weaning from cardiopulmonary bypass in cardiac surgery: a prospective randomized trial. J Cardiothorac Vasc Anesth. 2008;22(3):406–13 [Comparative Study Randomized Controlled Trial].

100. Miller OI, Tang SF, Keech A, Celermajer DS. Rebound pulmonary hypertension on withdrawal from inhaled nitric oxide. Lancet. 1995;346(8966):51–2 [Comparative Study Letter Research Support, Non-U.S. Gov't].

101. Namachivayam P, Theilen U, Butt WW, Cooper SM, Penny DJ, Shekerdemian LS. Sildenafil prevents rebound pulmonary hypertension after withdrawal of nitric oxide in children. Am J Respir Crit Care Med. 2006;174(9):1042–7 [Randomized Controlled Trial].

102. Linde LM, Simmons DH, Lewis N. Pulmonary hemodynamics in respiratory acidosis in dogs. Am J Physiol. 1963;205(5):1008–12.

103. Venn RM, Hell J, Grounds RM. Respiratory effects of dexmedetomidine in the surgical patient requiring intensive care. Crit Care. 2000;4(5):302–8 [Clinical Trial Controlled Clinical Trial Research Support, Non-U.S. Gov't].

104. But AK, Ozgul U, Erdil F, Gulhas N, Toprak HI, Durmus M, et al. The effects of pre-operative dexmedetomidine infusion on hemodynamics in patients with pulmonary hypertension undergoing mitral valve replacement surgery. Acta Anaesthesiol Scand. 2006;50(10):1207–12 [Randomized Controlled Trial].

105. Price LC, Wort SJ, Finney SJ, Marino PS, Brett SJ. Pulmonary vascular and right ventricular dysfunction in adult critical care: current and emerging options for management: a systematic literature review. Crit Care. 2010;14(5):R169 [Research Support, Non-U.S. Gov't Review].

106. Rajdev A, Garan H, Biviano A. Arrhythmias in pulmonary arterial hypertension. Prog Cardiovasc Dis. 2012;55(2):180–6 [Review].

107. Morrison LJ, Deakin CD, Morley PT, Callaway CW, Kerber RE, Kronick SL, et al. Part 8: advanced life support: 2010 international consensus on cardiopulmonary resuscitation and emergency cardiovascular care science with treatment recommendations. Circulation. 2010;122(16 Suppl 2):S345–421 [Consensus Development Conference Practice Guideline].

108. Minai OA, Venkateshiah SB, Arroliga AC. Surgical intervention in patients with moderate to severe pulmonary arterial hypertension. Conn Med. 2006;70(4):239–43.

109. Fox C, Kalarickal PL, Yarborough MJ, Jin JY. Perioperative management including new pharmacological vistas for patients with pulmonary hypertension for noncardiac surgery. Curr Opin Anaesthesiol. 2008;21(4):467–72 [Review].

110. McGlothlin D, De Marco T. Preoperative risk assessment of pulmonary arterial hypertension patients undergoing general surgery. Adv Pulm Hypertens. 2007;6(3):66–73.

Robert P. Frantz

Abbreviations

ASK   Apoptosis signal regulating kinase
NHLBI   National Heart Lung, and Blood Institute
NYHA   New York Heart Association
PA   Pulmonary artery
PAH   Pulmonary arterial hypertension
PH   Pulmonary hypertension
PVR   Pulmonary vascular resistance
RA   Right atrial
RV   Right ventricle
RVEDP   Right ventricular end diastolic pressure
RVEF   Right ventricular ejection fraction
VITA   Vascular Interventions/Innovations and Therapeutic
            Advances Program
WHO   World Health Organization

The field of pulmonary hypertension (PH) has progressed at an increasingly rapid pace in the days since intravenous epoprostenol made its astonishing 1995 debut. Despite the subsequent development of a range of alternative therapies, none has proven to be more effective. Recent explosive advances in the understanding of vascular biology have resulted in a seemingly bewildering tangle of pathways and putative therapeutic targets. This places the pulmonary hypertension community at the threshold of a new frontier that engenders both great excitement and a sense of obligation. For success to be achieved, this excitement must be paired with a bold spirit of innovation, cooperation, and a continued sense of urgency. In this chapter, important developments in the field will be discussed in the context of a proposed paradigm to

optimize the efficiency of the path ahead. Important directions in the field are summarized in Table 23.1.

Therapies thus far available for pulmonary hypertension have focused on vasodilation, despite the fact that the more severe forms of pulmonary hypertension are inevitably accompanied by vascular remodeling that results in reduction of the cross-sectional area of the pulmonary vascular bed. The subsequent development of right heart failure is usually ultimately responsible for pulmonary arterial hypertension (PAH)-related mortality. Non-vasodilator therapies could either target the pulmonary vascular remodeling process, the right ventricular response to the adverse pulmonary hypertension milieu, or both. Full restoration of normal pulmonary vascular resistance is not necessary; achieving a state in which the right ventricle (RV) is adequately coupled to the pulmonary vascular load, and preventing progression of RV dysfunction and the pulmonary vascular load would be adequate.

The Future of Clinical Trial Design

The move away from a vasodilator-centric view to approaches that target pulmonary vascular remodeling and/or the RV, combined with a wide array of possible therapeutic targets, creates several issues from a clinical trial perspective.

1. Trial organization and funding
2. Trial duration
3. Surrogate endpoints
4. Definitive endpoints
5. Patient selection
6. Patient recruitment strategies

Trial Organization and Funding

A July 2014 meeting in Bethesda, Maryland was inspired by the frustration of the pulmonary hypertension research

R.P. Frantz, MD
Division of Cardiovascular Diseases and Internal Medicine,
Mayo Pulmonary Hypertension Clinic,
Mayo Clinic College of Medicine, 200 First Street SW,
Rochester, MN, 55905, USA
e-mail: frantz.robert@mayo.edu

Table 23.1 Knowledge gaps, opportunities and strategies in pulmonary hypertension

Knowledge gap	Strategy	Example of present or future state
Unifying theory of PH across WHO groups	Cross-sectional deep phenotyping; consensus phenotypic definitions	NHLBI PVD phenomics; consensus documents [1]
Predicting PAH disease progression	Longitudinal deep phenotyping	Serial MRI as predictor of outcome [2]
	Serial biomarkers	Serial BNP or NTproBNP
Markers of progression of vascular remodeling and proliferation	PBMC and Serum OMIC signatures correlated with serial hemodynamics, outcome	Serial OMICS in clinical trials of therapeutic agents that include serial hemodynamics and outcome measures
	Lung vascular imaging	Lung FDG uptake [3]
Genetics of PH	GWAS; Exome sequencing	PAH susceptibility loci [4]
Pathobiology of PH	Network biology	MicroRNA-21 [5]
	Explanted lung tissue/serum analyses	Interleukin-33 [6]; CC Chemokine Ligand-2 [7]; PH breakthrough initiative [8]
Myocardial metabolism	PET	FDG uptake [9–12]
Peripheral muscle factors	MR spectroscopy; cardiopulmonary rehab	Skeletal muscle imaging [13–19]
Best RV function measures	RV imaging	Echo: TAPSE [20], RV strain [21], MRI: [22–25]
RV-PA coupling	Simplification of method	Hemodynamic predictors of outcome [26], and see Chap. 17
Exercise hemodynamics	Standardization, reporting of experience, relation to outcome	Invasive CPET in varied patient phenotypes [27–35]
Optimizing clinical trial recruitment in PAH	Understanding barriers, trial design, cultivating culture of participation	Patient interviews [36], Advocacy, Central repository for research options e.g., Clinicaltrials.gov, minimizing patient burden in trials

community at the slow pace of development of industry sponsored research in the non-vasodilator PH arena. This meeting brought together clinicians, clinical trialists, bench researchers, representatives of National Heart, Lung, and Blood Institute (NHLBI), and industry. The goal of this meeting was to showcase the range of most promising basic research and early translational data, learn from recent missteps, and set the framework for future innovative and collaborative approaches. Traditionally, most pulmonary hypertension drug trials have been industry initiated and funded. Future advances in pulmonary hypertension therapy may either result from repurposing of agents from other fields such as Oncology, or specific PH drug development within industry or academia. If already available compounds are either off patent or nearly so, then the interest of industry in developing them for PH is very limited and unlikely to occur if the PH community relies on industry alone to drive the funding. A classic and unfortunate recent example is that of imatinib for PAH indications. In the IMPRES study, imatinib was associated with a highly significant improvement in the primary endpoint of 6 min walk distance, despite most of the patients being on double or triple drug therapy that often included prostanoids [37]. The incidence of cerebral hemorrhage was higher in the treatment arm, with all such events occurring in patients also on warfarin. In addition, the time to clinical worsening endpoint trended in the wrong direction, reflecting an increased hazard of early hospitalization in the treatment arm. This was attributed to imatinib-related fluid retention,

although this could not be distinguished readily from PAH disease progression. In retrospect, a higher awareness of this issue could have allowed a contemporaneous diuretic approach analogous to that often employed during initiation of beta-blocker therapy in left heart failure. Future trials of repurposed agents must carefully consider known side effect profiles and be proactive about expected response to their development. In addition, the dropout rate in the imatinib treatment arm was high, and those patients were not subsequently followed for outcome. Future trials must make every effort to continue to collect data on patients that are withdrawn or who drop out, albeit recognizing that doing so can be logistically challenging. Discussing the importance of such follow up with patients a *priori* may enhance their willingness to continue to be followed for purposes of optimizing trial integrity, and should be a part of future trial design. Avoidance of clinical worsening endpoints that include components indistinguishable from disease progression must also be a key component of future trial design. Imatinib may have been further developed for PAH if it had not been close to going off patent, reducing interest of the pharmaceutical industry in further pursuing the concept.

In the future, academically driven consortiums will play an increasingly important role in drug development and clinical trial completion in pulmonary hypertension. Models for such consortiums are available, including the Eastern Cooperative Oncology Group and the Acute Respiratory Distress Syndrome Network. The National Heart, Lung, and

Blood Institute of the National Institutes of Medicine (NHLBI/NIH) models include the highly successful Heart Failure Research Network that, for example, completed the landmark RELAX trial studying sildenafil in the treatment of heart failure with preserved ejection fraction [38]. The successful NHLBI funded Pulmonary Arterial Hypertension Biorepository, spearheaded by Nichols at the University of Cincinnati Childrens Hospital, demonstrates the ability to pool biological and phenotypic resources that will help to speed the therapeutic discovery process. Although the REVEAL registry of PAH is industry funded, the steering committee is fully academic, and the extensive epidemiologic observations of that study demonstrate the value of a large number of PH centers contributing routinely obtained clinical phenotyping toward a common set of goals [39–58]. The recent NHLBI funded development of a consortium of pulmonary hypertension centers that will carefully phenotype a large cohort of patients with pulmonary hypertension across World Health Organization (WHO) Groups I, II, III and IV will include detailed genomic, proteomic and metabolomic characterization that promises to identify homologies that unite this seemingly disparate set of disorders. (RFA – HL-14-027: Redefining Pulmonary Hypertension Through Pulmonary Vascular Disease Phenomics [PVDOMICS]; nhlbi.nih.gov). The potential for a comprehensive "omics" approach is made possible by remarkable advances in high throughput technology, bioinformatics, and network biology. The discovery of microRNA-21 as a potentially important factor in pulmonary vascular disease represents an exciting example of such a novel approach [5, 59]. This effort promises to be complemented by the recent NHLBI decision to fund a network of centers to carry out multicenter trials in patients with pulmonary hypertension and also in patients with parenchymal lung disease. The visionary decision of the Pulmonary Hypertension Association to fund an additional center for the PVDOMICS network illustrates what it is hoped will be a burgeoning trend toward collaborative research approaches that may include academic, public non-profit/charitable organizations, private funding sources, and/or pharmaceutical industry collaboration. An additional example of this exciting trend is the NHLBI VITA initiative (Vascular Interventions/Innovations and Therapeutic Advances Program). (http://www.nhlbi.nih.gov/research/resources/vita.htm).

Trial Duration

The duration of therapy necessary to achieve a clinical endpoint depends upon the nature of that endpoint, the severity of illness of the population, their rate of disease progression, and whether they are already receiving reasonably effective therapy. It also depends upon the mode of action of the agent being studied, and the tolerability of that agent, which impacts the frequency of study drug discontinuation. The required therapy duration has increased steadily (e.g., 12 weeks to show a mortality benefit for epoprostenol or an improvement in 6 min walk with bosentan, vs. the 6 month placebo controlled phase for the imatinib study). Furthermore, the number of patients required to achieve adequate power, the length of time necessary to recruit them, and the number of centers that must be involved, have all increased and likely will continue to do so.

Surrogate Endpoints

"A surrogate does not an endpoint make" is the mantra of the clinical trialist when warning about the pitfalls of trial design [60]. Yet there is a tension between the need for properly conducted clinical trials with robust endpoints, and the difficulty of studying a rare disease that already has a host of (albeit ultimately inadequate) treatments available. This tension is exacerbated by the growing number of therapeutic targets and difficulty in establishing priorities. Surrogate endpoints are often useful in phase I and II studies in order to obtain early signals of biologic effect and efficacy. For vasodilator agents, acute changes in hemodynamics serve such a purpose. For pro-apoptotic and anti-proliferative agents, such straight forward surrogates are lacking. Accordingly, there is an unmet need for advances in the capacity to detect such effects prior to the point at which hemodynamic or clinical consequences are detectable. Systematic serial blood draws for biomarkers of response (known and to be discovered) should be a fundamental component of trials of anti-proliferatives in the future. Successful identification of changes in biomarkers that track with subsequent clinical response could help not only to sort which agents are most promising, but may also help to identify which patients are in fact responding to the agent. Baseline testing may also identify which patients are likely to respond, based upon genetic characteristics or other "omic" signatures. This "personalized medicine" approach has been particularly useful in cancer research and treatment. Tumor shrinkage is such a terrific surrogate for clinical response, that a study of a new cancer therapy can identify a subgroup of patients who respond, even if it is only 20 % of the studied population. If it were necessary as an early signal of efficacy to study every cancer therapy based upon survival of a whole treated cohort, many treatments that are useful only in a subset of patients would never have been identified as effective, since the power to detect clinical benefit in the entire cohort would be low. Consider the possibility that imatinib has a striking impact on outcome of 20 % of treated patients. Clear proof of that impact is difficult to achieve when there were many other patients who either did not tolerate the therapy or were non-responders. Hemodynamic effect is a tempting (albeit imperfect) surrogate in such a situation, but without a better methodology (e.g. biomarker of proliferative milieu) to identify *a priori* those probable responders, designing a trial that would recruit only likely responders, and then permit judicious application of the therapy, is difficult.

Definitive Endpoints

In the future, some clinical trials in PAH will utilize survival as the primary endpoint. Survival will be a primary endpoint because in the world of anti-proliferatives, a highly effective agent will have an impact on survival in an advanced PAH population within a feasible time frame and in a patient population of feasible size. Furthermore, one or more of such trials will be positive within the next decade. Is this a bold prediction? Perhaps, but it is not at all beyond the realm of possibility. At some point, a bold advancement will occur, revolutionizing the treatment of PAH. Consider the quandary of restenosis after coronary angioplasty. That recalcitrant problem was the Achilles heel of interventional cardiology for many years, and many compounds were tested without success. Then one day the sirolimus eluting stent was developed, and the world tilted.

The same will happen in PAH. How soon it will occur depends upon the success of the PAH community in fostering research, the degree of innovative thinking regarding trial design and drug discovery, the level of interest of scientists and clinicians in pushing the field, and the willingness of PAH patients to participate in clinical trials. Perhaps there is also an element of serendipity and luck. But as the old saying goes: "I am a great believer in luck. The harder I work, the more of it I seem to have."

In the future, the PAH community will continue to work hard, creating their own luck. Hospitalization as a critical component of a composite endpoint has recently thrice been a major driver of a positive outcome in PAH trials including the macitentan pivotal trial [61]. Two additional phase 3 studies achieving such an endpoint are not yet published as of this writing: AMBITION (AMBrIsentan and Tadalafil in patients with pulmonary arterial hypertensION) (up front combined ambrisentan and tadalafil) and GRIPHON (Prostacyclin (PGI2) Receptor agonist In Pulmonary arterial HypertensiON) study of the IP receptor agonist selexipag (phase 2 reference [62]). The expense and effort to successfully enroll and complete these studies represent landmark clinical trial efforts in PAH.

Patient Selection

Clinical trials will increasingly need to focus on those patients at significant risk of adverse outcome within a year.

The tendency in clinical trials has been to recruit patients that have long durations of disease and are therefore proven survivors. If that is combined with quite compensated clinical status, the trials are unlikely to meet efficacy endpoints within a set trial duration, and event driven trials will take too long to achieve an adequate number of events. Furthermore, patients who are fairly well compensated have little interest in trial participation.

Patient Recruitment Strategies

Trials will increasingly permit patients to be on a wide variety and number of PAH therapies, including parenteral prostanoids, since disease modifying agents will need to have demonstrable effects regardless of the background vasodilator therapy. This will make it easier to identify eligible patients in countries that have wide access to PAH therapies. If such patients are also at a point in their disease trajectory where they are seeking opportunity, then they will be more frequently willing to participate. This should facilitate trial launch, monitoring, and successful completion.

Assessment of Right Ventricular Function, Coupling, and Reserve

Quantitation of right ventricular function has historically been difficult, reflecting failure to perceive its importance in an LV-centric world, unusual geometry, and limitations in adequate visualization. As well discussed in earlier chapters, great strides have been made, including new echocardiographic tools such as strain, improve MRI techniques, sophisticated pressure volume loop analysis, and greater understanding of how changes in RV function over time correlate with clinical outcomes. The concept of coupling of the RV to the pulmonary circulation has also shed light. Measures of right ventricular function will increasingly play a role as exploratory endpoints of novel therapies and as secondary endpoints in phase III studies. From a clinical perspective, measurement of RV function will continue to gain acceptance as a critical component of longitudinal care. Recognition of the relationship between right ventricular function and outcome has become increasingly clear (Fig. 23.1). A desirable further development would be the creation of clear measures of right ventricular reserve. During exertion, cardiac output must increase in order to meet the needs of working muscle. Limitations in cardiac output response can manifest as dyspnea, lightheadedness, hypotension, and syncope. Noninvasive cardiopulmonary exercise testing can detect limitation in cardiac output response as manifested by a plateau in oxygen consumption, while invasive exercise testing can measure not only cardiac

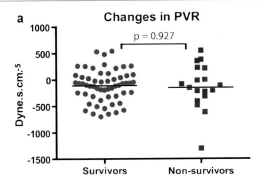

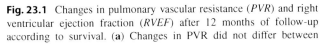

Fig. 23.1 Changes in pulmonary vascular resistance (*PVR*) and right ventricular ejection fraction (*RVEF*) after 12 months of follow-up according to survival. (**a**) Changes in PVR did not differ between survivors (*blue*) and nonsurvivors (*red*). (**b**) Survivors (*blue*) showed increased RVEF, whereas nonsurvivors (*red*) showed decreased RVEF during follow-up (Reproduced from [2] with permission from Elsevier)

output, but also right atrial and pulmonary artery pressures. If the right heart is unable to maintain compensation during exercise, the right atrial pressure may rise, PA pressure may rise and then start to fall, and cardiac output fails to augment appropriately. The relative merits of 6 min walk testing, non-invasive and invasive cardiopulmonary exercise testing in the assessment of adequacy of therapy remain under explored and should be studied further.

Implantable Hemodynamic Monitors

The CHRONICLE pilot study of an implantable pressure sensor in the RV shed light on the range and variability in right heart pressures at rest and with activity in PAH [63, 64]. This included the ability to measure right ventricular end – diastolic pressure, RV systolic pressure, and estimated pulmonary artery (PA) diastolic pressure. Beat to beat measurements during 6 min walks showed how right atrial pressure (as assessed by right ventricular end diastolic pressure) (RVEDP) can rise, associated with plateau in PA pressure and onset of dyspnea and lightheadedness, with recovery of these parameters with cessation of activity.

Cardiac output could be estimated by analysis of the RV pressure waveform [65]. Unfortunately this technology never made it to regulatory approval in this form.

However, the Cardiomems implantable pressure sensor (which can only measure PA pressure) has been approved for use in New York Heart Association (NYHA) class III left heart failure based upon results of the CardioMEMS Heart Sensor Allows Monitoring of Pressures to Improve Outcomes in NYHA Functional Class III Heart Failure Patients (CHAMPION) study [66, 67]. In this study, awareness of pulmonary artery pressures, with goal directed therapeutic modifications to lower pulmonary artery pressure, facilitated optimization of therapy. Whether frequent monitoring of PA pressure would have much utility in PAH is debatable, since PA pressure is much less important than right atrial (RA)

pressure and cardiac output. However, a project to examine the potential utility of remote PA pressure monitoring with the Cardiomems devices is currently under way as part of the NHLBI VITA initiative (Raymond L. Benza, PI). In theory the Cardiomems device could estimate cardiac output by pressure waveform analysis, but this has not been extensively studied. It is hoped that implantable hemodynamic monitors in PAH will continue to be explored.

Imaging of the RV during exercise is another approach to the idea of an "RV stress test". MRI compatible exercise testing is possible, and has provided interesting findings in performance athletes [68]. Whether RV imaging during exercise would provide added value in prognostication and assessment of adequacy of treatment in PAH is worthy of further investigation.

Disease Modifying Therapies

Beyond Vasodilation: Disease Modifying Therapies

Antiproliferative, pro-apoptotic, anti-inflammatory and metabolic approaches all hold promise in PAH, including pulmonary vascular, right ventricular and systemic perspectives. The explosion of understanding cellular pathways poses both tremendous promise and significant peril as the field evolves. Many of the pathways have complex, incompletely understood multisystem impact that raise the potential for off-target effects of novel therapeutic compounds that may not be fully predictable. The most promising compounds will have selective effects and/or activity that is manifest primarily under conditions of specific disease or pathologic stress. A detailed review of advances in myocardial and vascular pathophysiology is beyond the scope of this chapter. The most promising pathways and putative approaches are detailed in Chap. 21.

Apoptosis signal regulating kinase-1 (ASK-1) inhibition has a variety of effects on cardiovascular processes including

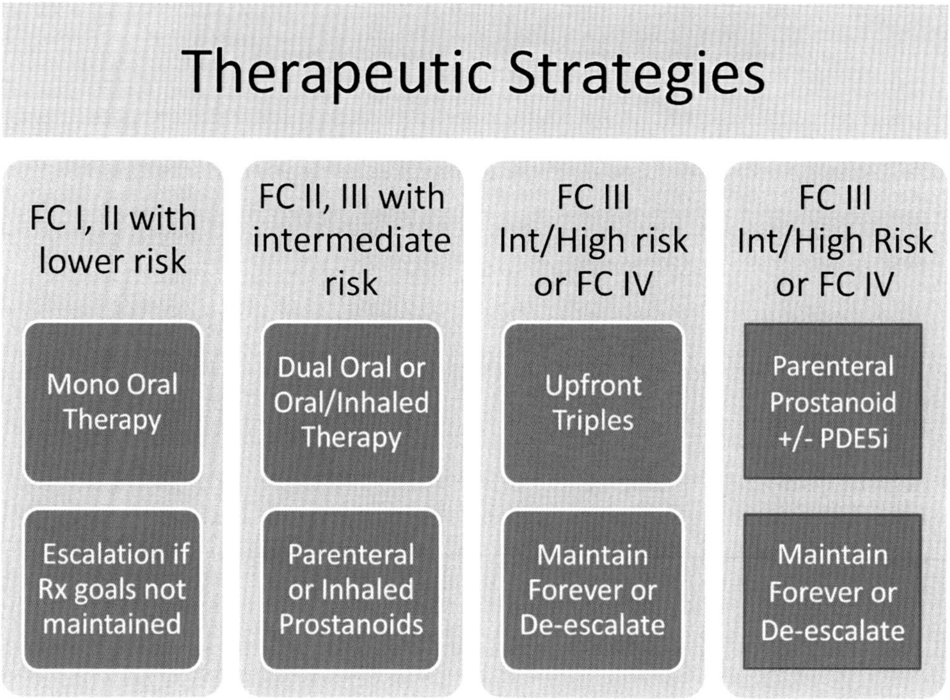

Fig. 23.2 Strategies in the treatment of pulmonary arterial hypertension. An emerging school of thought proposes earlier more aggressive therapy, e.g., initiating parenteral prostanoids plus two oral agents nearly simultaneously ("Upfront Triples"), and later de-escalating if feasible. If antiproliferatives achieve success, de-escalation could occur once the pulmonary vasculature has reverse remodeled

Therapeutic Strategies

FC I, II with lower risk	FC II, III with intermediate risk	FC III Int/High risk or FC IV	FC III Int/High Risk or FC IV
Mono Oral Therapy	Dual Oral or Oral/Inhaled Therapy	Upfront Triples	Parenteral Prostanoid +/- PDE5i
Escalation if Rx goals not maintained	Parenteral or Inhaled Prostanoids	Maintain Forever or De-escalate	Maintain Forever or De-escalate

cardiomyocyte hypertrophy [69]. ASK-1 is an important mediator of the adverse cellular effects of oxidative stress. In a variety of animal models of pulmonary hypertension, which are characterized by perturbations to the redox potential of pulmonary vascular cells and cardiomyocytes, small molecule ASK-1 inhibitors have had impressive effects on both the pulmonary vascular and right ventricular response. A phase II studies of an inhibitor of this pathway is currently underway, with results eagerly awaited (A Phase 2, Dose-Ranging, Randomized, Double-Blind, Placebo-Controlled Study of GS-4997 in Subjects With Pulmonary Arterial Hypertension; clinicaltrials.gov).

One significant limitation to systemic delivery of compounds with anti-proliferative and other pleiotropic effects is the potential for significant, and often unpredictable, off – target effects that may impede safety, tolerability, and adequate dosing. Inhalational delivery may obviate much of these concerns; inhaled iloprost and treprostinil are examples of this approach in the vasodilator arena. An example of developing efforts in the inhalational anti-proliferative space is the NHLBI VITA program-funded examination of PK10453, a nonselective platelet-derived growth factor receptor inhibitor that has shown promise in animal models of PAH [70].

The recognition of heart failure as a systemic disorder with abnormalities in peripheral skeletal muscle characteristics and derangements in metabolic pathways including insulin resistance, fatty acid and glycolytic pathways, mitochondrial function and iron metabolism has led to increasing awareness of possible therapeutic targets in left heart failure, many of which can likely be translated to right heart failure accompanying PAH [71].

The potential for pharmacologic approaches to peripheral muscle abnormalities is complemented by the developing evidence for physical rehabilitation strategies that indeed have demonstrated improvements in 6 min walk distance comparable or superior to that of pulmonary vasodilator therapies [13].

Therapeutic Strategies: Developing Paradigms

The surge in number of approved PAH therapies can be viewed as both a blessing and a curse. The blessing is the ability to tailor therapy to individual patient needs and tolerabilities. The curse is the difficulty in comparing therapies developed in silos without comparative trials, and the potential to undertreat or overtreat, creating competing perils of poor patient outcome, excessive side effects, and cost. A tension exists between proponents of an aggressive early versus stepwise therapeutic approach. This dilemma is further aggravated by inability to predict whether a patient currently well compensated on aggressive therapy would maintain that compensation long term if therapy were simplified. An example of these therapeutic options, and perhaps a reasonable compromise that includes the option of stepwise versus upfront aggressive triples [72] for higher risk patients, is illustrated in Fig. 23.2. However, the decision to de-escalate therapy in the clinically improved patient on aggressive therapy is always fraught, since there is no reliable way to predict long-term success with a less aggressive approach. In this regard, reliable markers of proliferative state and predictors of progression need further development.

Conclusions

Tremendous progress has been made with regard to vasodilator therapy in PAH, assessment of right ventricular function, development of network biology and 'omic' methodology, and discovery of pathways involved in pulmonary vasculopathy and right ventricular function. Expanding upon this knowledge and translating it into proven therapeutic strategies is the clear calling of the PH community as we move forward. Ultimately, and perhaps within the next decade, the approach to PAH will consist of four steps: (1) Aggressive upfront vasodilator therapy; (2) Remodeling of the pulmonary vascular bed via addition of anti-proliferative, pro-apoptotic, and anti-inflammatory therapies; (3) Therapeutic targeting of right ventricular adaptation; and (4) De-escalation of vasodilator therapy over the long-term in treatment responders. The future is bright; let us seize the opportunity and boldly push ahead.

References

1. Dweik RA, Rounds S, Erzurum SC, Archer S, Fagan K, Hassoun PM, et al. An official American Thoracic Society Statement: pulmonary hypertension phenotypes. Am J Respir Crit Care Med. 2014;189(3):345–55.
2. van de Veerdonk MC, Kind T, Marcus JT, Mauritz G-J, Heymans MW, Bogaard H-J, et al. Progressive right ventricular dysfunction in patients with pulmonary arterial hypertension responding to therapy. J Am Coll Cardiol. 2011;58(24):2511–9.
3. Zhao L, Ashek A, Wang L, Fang W, Dabral S, Dubois O, et al. Heterogeneity in lung (18)FDG uptake in pulmonary arterial hypertension: potential of dynamic (18)FDG positron emission tomography with kinetic analysis as a bridging biomarker for pulmonary vascular remodeling targeted treatments. Circulation. 2013;128(11):1214–24.
4. Germain M, Eyries M, Montani D, Poirier O, Girerd B, Dorfmuller P, et al. Genome-wide association analysis identifies a susceptibility locus for pulmonary arterial hypertension. Nat Genet. 2013; 45(5):518–21.
5. Parikh VN, Jin RC, Rabello S, Gulbahce N, White K, Hale A, et al. MicroRNA-21 integrates pathogenic signaling to control pulmonary hypertension: results of a network bioinformatics approach. Circulation. 2012;125(12):1520–32.
6. Shao D, Perros F, Caramori G, Meng C, Dormuller P, Chou P-C, et al. Nuclear IL-33 regulates soluble ST2 receptor and IL-6 expression in primary human arterial endothelial cells and is decreased in idiopathic pulmonary arterial hypertension. Biochem Biophys Res Commun. 2014;451(1):8–14.
7. Sanchez O, Marcos E, Perros F, Fadel E, Tu L, Humbert M, et al. Role of endothelium-derived CC chemokine ligand 2 in idiopathic pulmonary arterial hypertension. Am J Respir Crit Care Med. 2007;176(10):1041–7.
8. Austin ED, Rock MT, Mosse CA, Vnencak-Jones CL, Yoder SM, Robbins IM, et al. T lymphocyte subset abnormalities in the blood and lung in pulmonary arterial hypertension. Respir Med. 2010;104(3):454–62.
9. Lundgrin EL, Park MM, Sharp J, Tang WHW, Thomas JD, Asosingh K, et al. Fasting 2-deoxy-2-[18F]fluoro-D-glucose positron emission tomography to detect metabolic changes in pulmonary arterial hypertension hearts over 1 year. Ann Am Thorac Soc. 2013;10(1):1–9.
10. Bokhari S, Raina A, Rosenweig EB, Schulze PC, Bokhari J, Einstein AJ, et al. PET imaging may provide a novel biomarker and understanding of right ventricular dysfunction in patients with idiopathic pulmonary arterial hypertension. Circ Cardiovasc Imaging. 2011;4(6):641–7.
11. de Keizer B, Scholtens AM, van Kimmenade RRJ, de Jong PA. High FDG uptake in the right ventricular myocardium of a pulmonary hypertension patient. J Am Coll Cardiol. 2013;62(18):1724.
12. Wong YY, Raijmakers P, van Campen J, van der Laarse WJ, Knaapen P, Lubberink M, et al. 11C-Acetate clearance as an index of oxygen consumption of the right myocardium in idiopathic pulmonary arterial hypertension: a validation study using 15O-labeled tracers and PET. J Nucl Med. 2013;54(8):1258–62.
13. Fox BD, Kassirer M, Weiss I, Raviv Y, Peled N, Shitrit D, et al. Ambulatory rehabilitation improves exercise capacity in patients with pulmonary hypertension. J Card Fail. 2011;17(3):196–200.
14. Broskey NT, Greggio C, Boss A, Boutant M, Dwyer A, Schlueter L, et al. Skeletal muscle mitochondria in the elderly: effects of physical fitness and exercise training. J Clin Endocrinol Metab. 2014;99(5):1852–61.
15. Cannon DT, Howe FA, Whipp BJ, Ward SA, McIntyre DJ, Ladroue C, et al. Muscle metabolism and activation heterogeneity by combined 31P chemical shift and T2 imaging, and pulmonary O2 uptake during incremental knee-extensor exercise. J Appl Physiol. 2013;115(6):839–49.
16. Cordina R, O'Meagher S, Gould H, Rae C, Kemp G, Pasco JA, et al. Skeletal muscle abnormalities and exercise capacity in adults with a Fontan circulation. Heart. 2013;99(20):1530–4.
17. Parasoglou P, Xia D, Chang G, Regatte RR. 3D-mapping of phosphocreatine concentration in the human calf muscle at 7 T: comparison to 3 T. Magn Reson Med. 2013;70(6):1619–25.
18. Kemp GJ, Thompson CH, Stratton JR, Brunotte F, Conway M, Adamopoulos S, et al. Abnormalities in exercising skeletal muscle in congestive heart failure can be explained in terms of decreased mitochondrial ATP synthesis, reduced metabolic efficiency, and increased glycogenolysis. Heart. 1996;76(1):35–41.
19. van der Ent M, Jeneson JA, Remme WJ, Berger R, Ciampricotti R, Visser F. A non-invasive selective assessment of type I fibre mitochondrial function using 31P NMR spectroscopy. Evidence for impaired oxidative phosphorylation rate in skeletal muscle in patients with chronic heart failure. Eur Heart J. 1998;19(1):124–31.
20. Forfia PR, Vachiery J-L. Echocardiography in pulmonary arterial hypertension. Am J Cardiol. 2012;110(6 Suppl):16S–24.
21. Fine NM, Chen L, Bastiansen PM, Frantz RP, Pellikka PA, Oh JK, et al. Outcome prediction by quantitative right ventricular function assessment in 575 subjects evaluated for pulmonary hypertension. Circ Cardiovasc Imaging. 2013;6(5):711–21.
22. Peacock AJ, Crawley S, McLure L, Blyth K, Vizza CD, Poscia R, et al. Changes in right ventricular function measured by cardiac magnetic resonance imaging in patients receiving pulmonary arterial hypertension-targeted therapy: the EURO-MR study. Circ Cardiovasc Imaging. 2014;7(1):107–14.
23. Peacock AJ, Vonk Noordegraaf A. Cardiac magnetic resonance imaging in pulmonary arterial hypertension. Eur Respir Rev. 2013;22(130):526–34.
24. Rochitte CE, Hoette S, Souza R. Myocardial delayed enhancement by cardiac magnetic resonance imaging in pulmonary arterial hypertension: a marker of disease severity. Arq Bras Cardiol. 2013;101(5):377–8.
25. Surie S, Reesink HJ, Marcus JT, van der Plas MN, Kloek JJ, Vonk-Noordegraaf A, et al. Bosentan treatment is associated with

improvement of right ventricular function and remodeling in chronic thromboembolic pulmonary hypertension. Clin Cardiol. 2013;36(11):698–703.

26. Campo A, Mathai SC, Le Pavec J, Zaiman AL, Hummers LK, Boyce D, et al. Hemodynamic predictors of survival in scleroderma-related pulmonary arterial hypertension. Am J Respir Crit Care Med. 2010;182(2):252–60.

27. Lewis GD, Farrell L, Wood MJ, Martinovic M, Arany Z, Rowe GC, et al. Metabolic signatures of exercise in human plasma. Sci Transl Med. 2010;2(33):33ra7.

28. Lewis GD, Murphy RM, Shah RV, Pappagianopoulos PP, Malhotra R, Bloch KD, et al. Pulmonary vascular response patterns during exercise in left ventricular systolic dysfunction predict exercise capacity and outcomes. Circ Heart Fail. 2011;4(3):276–85.

29. Lewis GD, Shah RV, Pappagianopolas PP, Systrom DM, Semigran MJ. Determinants of ventilatory efficiency in heart failure: the role of right ventricular performance and pulmonary vascular tone. Circ Heart Fail. 2008;1(4):227–33.

30. Maron BA, Cockrill BA, Waxman AB, Systrom DM. The invasive cardiopulmonary exercise test. Circulation. 2013;127(10):1157–64.

31. Saggar R, Lewis GD, Systrom DM, Champion HC, Naeije R. Pulmonary vascular responses to exercise: a haemodynamic observation. Eur Respir J. 2012;39(2):231–4.

32. Tolle JJ, Waxman AB, Van Horn TL, Pappagianopoulos PP, Systrom DM. Exercise-induced pulmonary arterial hypertension. Circulation. 2008;118(21):2183–9.

33. Abudiab MM, Redfield MM, Melenovsky V, Olson TP, Kass DA, Johnson BD, et al. Cardiac output response to exercise in relation to metabolic demand in heart failure with preserved ejection fraction. Eur J Heart Fail. 2013;15(7):776–85.

34. Mohammed SF, Borlaug BA, McNulty S, Lewis GD, Lin G, Zakeri R, et al. Resting ventricular-vascular function and exercise capacity in heart failure with preserved ejection fraction: a RELAX trial ancillary study. Circ Heart Fail. 2014;7(4):580–9.

35. Schwartzenberg S, Redfield MM, From AM, Sorajja P, Nishimura RA, Borlaug BA. Effects of vasodilation in heart failure with preserved or reduced ejection fraction implications of distinct pathophysiologies on response to therapy. J Am Coll Cardiol. 2012;59(5):442–51.

36. Carroll R, Antigua J, Taichman D, Palevsky H, Forfia P, Kawut S, et al. Motivations of patients with pulmonary arterial hypertension to participate in randomized clinical trials. Clin Trials. 2012;9(3):348–57.

37. Hoeper MM, Barst RJ, Bourge RC, Feldman J, Frost AE, Galie N, et al. Imatinib mesylate as add-on therapy for pulmonary arterial hypertension: results of the randomized IMPRES study. Circulation. 2013;127(10):1128–38.

38. Redfield MM, Chen HH, Borlaug BA, Semigran MJ, Lee KL, Lewis G, et al. Effect of phosphodiesterase-5 inhibition on exercise capacity and clinical status in heart failure with preserved ejection fraction: a randomized clinical trial. JAMA. 2013;309(12):1268–77.

39. Badesch DB, Raskob GE, Elliott CG, Krichman AM, Farber HW, Frost AE, et al. Pulmonary arterial hypertension: baseline characteristics from the REVEAL Registry. Chest. 2010;137(2):376–87.

40. Barst RJ, Chung L, Zamanian RT, Turner M, McGoon MD. Functional class improvement and 3-year survival outcomes in patients with pulmonary arterial hypertension in the REVEAL Registry. Chest. 2013;144(1):160–8.

41. Barst RJ, Ivy DD, Foreman AJ, McGoon MD, Rosenzweig EB. Four- and seven-year outcomes of patients with congenital heart disease-associated pulmonary arterial hypertension (from the REVEAL Registry). Am J Cardiol. 2014;113(1):147–55.

42. Barst RJ, McGoon MD, Elliott CG, Foreman AJ, Miller DP, Ivy DD. Survival in childhood pulmonary arterial hypertension: insights from the registry to evaluate early and long-term pulmonary arterial hypertension disease management. Circulation. 2012;125(1):113–22.

43. Benza RL, Gomberg-Maitland M, Frost AE, Frantz RP, Humbert M, McGoon MD. Development of prognostic tools in pulmonary arterial hypertension: lessons from modern day registries. Thromb Haemost. 2012;108(6):1049–60.

44. Benza RL, Gomberg-Maitland M, Miller DP, Frost A, Frantz RP, Foreman AJ, et al. The REVEAL Registry risk score calculator in patients newly diagnosed with pulmonary arterial hypertension. Chest. 2012;141(2):354–62.

45. Benza RL, Miller DP, Barst RJ, Badesch DB, Frost AE, McGoon MD. An evaluation of long-term survival from time of diagnosis in pulmonary arterial hypertension from the REVEAL Registry. Chest. 2012;142(2):448–56.

46. Benza RL, Miller DP, Frost A, Barst RJ, Krichman AM, McGoon MD. Analysis of the lung allocation score estimation of risk of death in patients with pulmonary arterial hypertension using data from the REVEAL Registry. Transplantation. 2010;90(3):298–305.

47. Brown LM, Chen H, Halpern S, Taichman D, McGoon MD, Farber HW, et al. Delay in recognition of pulmonary arterial hypertension: factors identified from the REVEAL Registry. Chest. 2011;140(1):19–26.

48. Burger CD, Foreman AJ, Miller DP, Safford RE, McGoon MD, Badesch DB. Comparison of body habitus in patients with pulmonary arterial hypertension enrolled in the Registry to Evaluate Early and Long-term PAH Disease Management with normative values from the National Health and Nutrition Examination Survey. Mayo Clin Proc. 2011;86(2):105–12.

49. Burger CD, Long PK, Shah MR, McGoon MD, Miller DP, Romero AJ, et al. Characterization of first-time hospitalizations in patients with newly diagnosed pulmonary arterial hypertension in the REVEAL registry. Chest. 2014;146(5):1263–73.

50. Chung L, Liu J, Parsons L, Hassoun PM, McGoon M, Badesch DB, et al. Characterization of connective tissue disease-associated pulmonary arterial hypertension from REVEAL: identifying systemic sclerosis as a unique phenotype. Chest. 2010;138(6):1383–94.

51. Farber HW, Foreman AJ, Miller DP, McGoon MD. REVEAL Registry: correlation of right heart catheterization and echocardiography in patients with pulmonary arterial hypertension. Congest Heart Fail. 2011;17(2):56–64.

52. Farber HW, Miller DP, Meltzer LA, McGoon MD. Treatment of patients with pulmonary arterial hypertension at the time of death or deterioration to functional class IV: insights from the REVEAL Registry. J Heart Lung Transplant. 2013;32(11):1114–22.

53. Frost AE, Badesch DB, Barst RJ, Benza RL, Elliott CG, Farber HW, et al. The changing picture of patients with pulmonary arterial hypertension in the United States: how REVEAL differs from historic and non-US Contemporary Registries [Erratum appears in Chest. 2011 Oct;140(4):1106]. Chest. 2011;139(1):128–37.

54. Frost AE, Badesch DB, Miller DP, Benza RL, Meltzer LA, McGoon MD. Evaluation of the predictive value of a clinical worsening definition using 2-year outcomes in patients with pulmonary arterial hypertension: a REVEAL Registry analysis. Chest. 2013;144(5):1521–9.

55. Frost AE, Farber HW, Barst RJ, Miller DP, Elliott CG, McGoon MD. Demographics and outcomes of patients diagnosed with pulmonary hypertension with pulmonary capillary wedge pressures 16 to 18 mm Hg: insights from the REVEAL Registry. Chest. 2013;143(1):185–95.

56. Krowka MJ, Miller DP, Barst RJ, Taichman D, Dweik RA, Badesch DB, et al. Portopulmonary hypertension: a report from the US-based REVEAL Registry. Chest. 2012;141(4):906–15.

57. McGoon MD, Benza RL, Escribano-Subias P, Jiang X, Miller DP, Peacock AJ, et al. Pulmonary arterial hypertension: epidemiology and registries. J Am Coll Cardiol. 2013;62(25 Suppl):D51–9.

58. Poms AD, Turner M, Farber HW, Meltzer LA, McGoon MD. Comorbid conditions and outcomes in patients with pulmonary arterial hypertension: a REVEAL registry analysis. Chest. 2013;144(1):169–76.

59. Chan SY, White K, Loscalzo J. Deciphering the molecular basis of human cardiovascular disease through network biology. Curr Opin Cardiol. 2012;27(3):202–9.

60. Aronson JK. Biomarkers and surrogate endpoints. Br J Clin Pharmacol. 2005;59(5):491–4.

61. Pulido T, Adzerikho I, Channick RN, Delcroix M, Galie N, Ghofrani H-A, et al. Macitentan and morbidity and mortality in pulmonary arterial hypertension. N Engl J Med. 2013;369(9):809–18.

62. Simonneau G, Torbicki A, Hoeper MM, Delcroix M, Karlocai K, Galie N, et al. Selexipag: an oral, selective prostacyclin receptor agonist for the treatment of pulmonary arterial hypertension. Eur Respir J. 2012;40(4):874–80.

63. Frantz RP, Benza RL, Kjellstrom B, Bourge RC, Barst RJ, Bennett TD, et al. Continuous hemodynamic monitoring in patients with pulmonary arterial hypertension. J Heart Lung Transplant. 2008; 27(7):780–8.

64. Kjellstrom B, Frantz RP, Benza RL, Bennett T, Bourge RC, McGoon MD. Hemodynamic ranges during daily activities and exercise testing in patients with pulmonary arterial hypertension. J Card Fail. 2014;20(7):485–91.

65. Karamanoglu M, McGoon M, Frantz RP, Benza RL, Bourge RC, Barst RJ, et al. Right ventricular pressure waveform and wave reflection analysis in patients with pulmonary arterial hypertension. Chest. 2007;132(1):37–43.

66. Adamson PB, Abraham WT, Aaron M, Aranda Jr JM, Bourge RC, Smith A, et al. CHAMPION trial rationale and design: the long-term safety and clinical efficacy of a wireless pulmonary artery pressure monitoring system. J Card Fail. 2011;17(1):3–10.

67. Adamson PB, Gold MR, Bennett T, Bourge RC, Stevenson LW, Trupp R, et al. Continuous hemodynamic monitoring in patients with mild to moderate heart failure: results of The Reducing Decompensation Events Utilizing Intracardiac Pressures in Patients With Chronic Heart Failure (REDUCEhf) trial. Congest Heart Fail. 2011;17(5):248–54.

68. La Gerche A, Claessen G, Van de Bruaene A, Pattyn N, Van Cleemput J, Gewillig M, et al. Cardiac MRI: a new gold standard for ventricular volume quantification during high-intensity exercise. Circ Cardiovasc Imaging. 2013;6(2):329–38.

69. Taniike M, Yamaguchi O, Tsujimoto I, Hikoso S, Takeda T, Nakai A, et al. Apoptosis signal-regulating kinase 1/p38 signaling pathway negatively regulates physiological hypertrophy. Circulation. 2008;117(4):545–52.

70. Medarametla V, Festin S, Sugarragchaa C, Eng A, Naqwi A, Wiedmann T, et al. PK10453, a nonselective platelet-derived growth factor receptor inhibitor, prevents the progression of pulmonary arterial hypertension. Pulm Circ. 2014;4(1):82–102.

71. Doehner W, Frenneaux M, Anker SD. Metabolic impairment in heart failure: the myocardial and systemic perspective. J Am Coll Cardiol. 2014;64(13):1388–400.

72. Sitbon O, Jais X, Savale L, Cottin V, Bergot E, Macari EA, et al. Upfront triple combination therapy in pulmonary arterial hypertension: a pilot study. Eur Respir J. 2014;43(6):1691–7.

Index

© Springer International Publishing Switzerland 2016
B.A. Maron et al. (eds.), *Pulmonary Hypertension: Basic Science to Clinical Medicine*, DOI 10.1007/978-3-319-23594-3

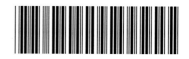